CLINICAL
NUTRITION

CLINICAL NUTRITION

Keith B. Taylor, D.M., F.R.C.P.
George DeForest Barnett Professor of Medicine
Stanford University

Luean E. Anthony, Ph.D.
Associate Professor of Nutrition and Assistant Professor of Surgery,
The University of Texas Health Science Center at Houston

McGraw-Hill Book Company
New York St. Louis San Francisco Auckland Bogotá Guatemala
Hamburg Johannesburg Lisbon London Madrid Mexico Montreal New Delhi
Panama Paris San Juan São Paulo Singapore Sydney Tokyo Toronto

Notice

Medicine is an ever-changing science. As new research and clinical experience broaden our knowledge, changes in treatment and drug therapy are required. The editors and the publisher of this work have made every effort to ensure that the drug dosage schedules herein are accurate and in accord with the standards accepted at the time of publication. Readers are advised, however, to check the product information sheet included in the package of each drug they plan to administer to be certain that changes have not been made in the recommended dose or in the contraindications for administration. This recommendation is of particular importance in regard to new or infrequently used drugs.

ISBN 0-07-063185-9

This book was set in Times Roman by Jay's Publishers Services, Inc.;
the editors were Anna R. Ferrera and Stuart D. Boynton;
the production supervisor was Jeanne Skahan.
R. R. Donnelley & Sons Company was printer and binder.

Library of Congress Cataloging in Publication Data

Taylor, Keith B.
  Clinical nutrition.

  Bibliography: p.
  Includes index.
  1. Nutrition disorders.   I. Anthony,
Luean E. II. Title. [DNLM: 1. Nutrition. 2. Diet
therapy. WB 400 T243c]
RC620.T38 1983   616.3′9   82–17109
ISBN 0–07–063185–9

CONTENTS

PREFACE

A recurrent theme in the past two decades has been the need for medical schools to provide education in the principles and clinical practice of human nutrition. This need has been expressed both by the general public and by concerned government and political leaders.

With some exceptions, such as pediatricians and gastroenterologists, practicing doctors have not acquired the knowledge or the motivation to apply nutritional principles to the treatment of their patients. This may in part be due to a persisting lack of easily accessible nutritional information which is relevant to clinical problems or which provides answers to the questions that patients ask. Surveys have shown, not unexpectedly, that the public regards physicians as the major source of nutritional information and complains that they do not provide such information. Many practitioners themselves have expressed a need for more easily available sources of nutritional information.

There are signs of change. Medical students are demanding courses in nutrition, and a few members of medical faculties throughout the country are now applying some of their time and effort to meeting these demands.

We have found that a major need has been a text which could be recommended to medical students and doctors, both to prepare them for an important professional function—namely, the provision of sound information about the biological aspects of nutrition to their patients—and to encourage awareness of nutritional matters in medical practice. These are the central goals of this book.

We have not attempted in this text to review the physiological and biochemical characteristics of nutrients, but appropriate references are provided. Nor do we emphasize the behavioral, cultural, and economic aspects of human nutrition with which a physician should be familiar in order fully to understand the needs of the population to whom he or she provides care. A list of suggested further reading is provided.

ACKNOWLEDGEMENTS

The authors are particularly grateful to the following colleagues who reviewed parts of the manuscript in its various stages, and offered valuable suggestions.

Drs. Rodney E. Kellems, Brian J. Rowlands, Eileen Brewer, Dennis Law, and Ms. Mary Schanler, Ms. Deborah Hunt, and Ms. Susan Warren.

They also wish to thank Kym Taylor who spent innumerable hours preparing the manuscript and Mary Carson, Becky Fullen and Margaret Warner for efficient secretarial support. The authors would like to thank the following for provision of the Color Figures indicated. (1) Dr. G. S. Gopalakrishna, (2) Dr. Bruce V. MacFadyen, Jr. and Dr. Stanley J. Dudrick, (3) Dr. David J. Atherton, (4) Dr. Harold H. Sanstead, (7) Dr. Samuel Dreizen, (10) Dr. Derek Jewell, (11, 12, 14, 15, 20) The Upjohn Company, Kalamazoo, Michigan, (12) Dr. Michael Latham, (13) Helen Keller International Incorporated, New York, New York, (16 to 18) Dr. John W. Farquhar, (20) Dr. Blair C. Rich.

Keith B. Taylor
Luean E. Anthony

CHAPTER 1

ASSESSMENT OF
NUTRITIONAL STATUS

CONTENTS

INTRODUCTION

Practicing physicians in the United States today generally assume that persons for whose medical care they are responsible are unlikely to be malnourished. As a consequence, time and thought are rarely devoted to taking a dietary history nor are even a few seconds of the physical examination set aside to consider how the person's physical state reflects a lifetime of exposure to numerous environmental variables, of which diet must be reckoned among the most important. A significant degree of obesity is usually described as "well-nourished," weight, if recorded at all, is not accompanied by a measurement of height, and assessment of skin-fold thickness is regarded as a research tool having no practical clinical value.

It should therefore occasion no surprise when it becomes evident that a substantial number of patients hospitalized for 2 weeks or more are allowed to develop protein-calorie malnutrition or that diagnostic procedures costing hundreds or even thousands of dollars are ordered to explore the possibility of intestinal malabsorption when a dietary history and caloric count would often provide an answer in far less time, at far less expense, and with far less discomfort to the patient.

This lack of interest in nutritional status extends to patients who develop often irreversible defects as a consequence of the long-term effects of gastrointestinal surgery. It applies particularly to patients who have had gastric resections. The nutritional evaluation of those subjected to intestinal bypass operations to treat obesity is frequently restricted to routine recording of subsequent weight loss, while gross nutrient deficiencies are allowed to develop in the meantime.

There are exceptions to this almost universal disregard of nutritional evaluation. Pediatricians and those who take care of newborn infants are concerned with nutritional status because the impact of malnutrition is evident, in general, much sooner in infants or young children than in adults. Medical and paramedical staff in intensive care units are also becoming increasingly familiar with the ways in which nutritional deficiencies express themselves and with how they must be treated or, better, prevented. The development of methods and materials which have made total parenteral feeding possible has been an important factor in raising the level of awareness of nutritional status, particularly in individuals receiving intensive care.

Recently there has been an encouraging proliferation of clinics devoted to problems related to nutrition, such as obesity, the hyperlipidemias, suspected food allergies, and anorexia, and to the long-term follow-up of patients who have undergone gastric or intestinal surgery and who have other gastrointestinal disorders associated with malnutrition, but the number of these clinics is still inadequate.

Nutritional status may be assessed for an individual, a group, or a population. Population studies, which are discussed at the end of this chapter, have the special advantage of being conducted by professional nutritionists who are trained in the appropriate methods and who are pursuing a defined goal with reasonable expectations of uncovering useful data. Individual assessments are usually made by medical and paramedical practitioners whose training, with the exception of clinical nutritionists, rarely emphasizes the importance of nutritional status. The majority of doctors have not been encouraged to develop the necessary skills or clinical judgment or to maintain a level of suspicion that malnutrition may be present.

The differences between the individual and the group approaches are listed in Table 1-1.

One insurance against overlooking the person on the threshold of developing significant nutritional deficiency is to be aware of those who are best described as being at high risk. Deficiencies of single nutrients are uncommon, with the exception of iron. However, deficiency of folacin or pyridoxine occurs in pregnancy, and deficiency of thiamine occurs in the alcoholic. Most states of deficiency comprise protein and calorie undernutrition, frequently accompanied by evidence of varying degrees of deficiencies of many essential nutrients. Some high-risk persons are listed in Table 1-2. Of course, this list is not exhaustive. Similar deficiencies may occur sporadically as a consequence of disease or dietary idiosyncrasy. The nutritional problems which occur in different age groups and as a consequence of pregnancy are discussed in more detail in Chapter 4.

DIETARY DATA AND EVALUATION

Dietary History

The practicing physician does not have the time and rarely has the expertise to take a detailed dietary history. When unexplained loss of weight, or clinical evidence of significant nutrient deficiency, is apparent or when patients with

TABLE 1-1
ASSESSMENT OF NUTRITIONAL STATUS

	Assessment of individuals	Assessment of groups

Food consumption	Dietary history:
	  Income
	  Home environment
	Presence of disease:
	  Infection
	  Locomotor
	  Depression
	  Gastrointestinal
	  Alcoholism
		Surveillance:
		  Food balance sheets
		  Food prices
		  Income scales
		  Household surveys

Physical assessment	Anthropometric
	  measurements (individuals):
		Anthropometric
		  measurements (groups):
		  Preschoolers
		  School-age children
		  Adults
		  Elderly people

	Clinical examination:
	  Evidence of:
	    Physical disease
	    Mental disease
	    Nutrient deficiency
		Vital statistics:
		  Mortality
		  Hospital admissions
		  Obvious disease
		    Goiter
		    Rickets

Supporting data	Laboratory and radiological
	  tests
		Laboratory and radiological
		  tests

Outcome	Assessment of:
	  Individual risk
	  Nutritional therapy
		Assessment of:
		  Community risk
		  Nutritional aid

diseases such as diabetes mellitus or chronic renal failure seek advice, it is usually necessary to enlist the help of the professional nutritionist or dietitian, who may use the techniques of 24-hour intake recall or the 3- to 5-day food intake record. But it is a simple matter, occupying only 1 to 2 minutes and often providing clinically useful information, to ask about the number of meals the patient eats each day, the times at which the meals are eaten, the size of the meals, and the consumption, in addition, of between-meal snacks. Questions about food preferences and dislikes and about suspected alimentary allergies should be posed. Cow's milk, eggs, fish, shellfish, chocolate, and various cereals, including corn, are the foods most commonly held culpable. The patient should be questioned about the amounts of green vegetables and salads that are consumed.

Alcohol consumption is generally best determined by inquiry about weekly purchases of beer, wine, and liquor rather than about daily consumption. There may be significant differences between the two, the latter being almost always underestimated.

TABLE 1-2
INDIVIDUALS AT HIGH RISK OF DEVELOPING NUTRITIONAL PROBLEMS

Age range	Disability	Consequences
Infants (0–1 yr)	Prematurity	Feeding difficulty; inadequate stores
	Birth defect	Feeding difficulty
Children (1–12 yr)	Chronic disease	Anorexia; failure to grow
	Malabsorption	Failure to grow; nutrient deficiencies
Adolescents* (13–20 yr)	Chronic disease	Anorexia; failure to grow; anemia
	Anorexia nervosa	Cachexia
	Pregnancy	Iron and folacin deficiency
Adults* (21–60 yr)	Obesity	Reduced physical activity; nutrient deficiencies in dieting or hospitalization
	Idiosyncrasy of diet	Nutrient deficiencies
	Real or imagined food allergy	Nutrient deficiencies
	Perimenopause	Calcium depletion; obesity
	Gastrointestinal disease	Nutrient deficiencies; anemia
	Gastrointestinal surgery	Nutrient deficiencies; anemia
	Renal dialysis	Prolonged nutrient losses
	Medication:	
	Catabolic steroids	Skeletal deficiencies
	Estrogens	Anorexia
	Aspirin	Gastrointestinal bleeding and iron deficiency
	Alcoholism	Nutrient deficiencies; impaired metabolism
	Pregnancy	Iron and folacin deficiency
Elderly (60+ yr)	Poor dentition	Reduced dietary intake and variety
	Depression	Anorexia
	Chronic disease	Anorexia
	Medication:	
	Cardiac	Anorexia
	Analgesics	
	Sedentary life	Reduced dietary intake
All ages	Serious trauma and surgery	Increased catabolism; protein-energy deficiency
	Inflammatory bowel disease	Anorexia; protein-losing enteropathy malabsorption; protein-energy deficiency, specific nutrient deficiencies
	Medication:	
	Cancer chemotherapy	Anorexia; protein-energy deficiency
	Anticonvulsants	Anemia; calcium deficiency

*Women of child-bearing age and pregnant women are also at high risk of developing anemia.

In addition, there is a growing practice of asking about salt consumption. This is clearly important in subjects with hypertension and cardiac, hepatic, or renal failure, but nutritionally aware doctors now ask about salt as a lead to recommending reduced sodium intake as prophylaxis against developing high blood pressure. This may be considered part of the recommended, prudent diet concept. Patients should be asked whether they like especially salty foods, use salt in cooking, or add salt at the table.

In the gastroenterology clinic we also ask routinely about the amounts of coffee and citrus juices consumed, since their use may frequently be associated with a tendency to complain of peptic esophagitis and variable diarrhea.

Answers to the foregoing questions provide a satisfactory dietary profile in the case of most white adult North Americans. It is usually a formidable task to obtain a satisfactory dietary history from an adolescent, however, because their eating habits are erratic and between-meal snacks (especially of milk and of foods and drinks of high carbohydrate, phosphate, and salt content) and raids on the refrigerator constitute a large part of their total intake but are difficult to recall. (For consideration of adolescents' nutritional problems, see Chapter 4.)

In the case of very sick patients, information relevant only to immediate diagnostic or therapeutic procedures is sought. This includes consumption of alcohol, both chronic and recent, and the size and nature of the most recent meals. If the patient is unable to respond, an accompanying relative, friend, or coworker may be able to give some information.

The diets of black and Latin American peoples differ significantly in content, in mode of preparation, and in proportions of individual constituents. Physicians working with populations of such persons become increasingly aware and attuned to this. Those who are not so familiar should seek help from a dietitian-nutritionist experienced in this matter. However, it is worthwhile having some working knowledge of the differences, and in the case of children good sources of reference are available [1,2]. This topic is addressed further in Chapter 4.

The eating habits of patients in general hospital wards have rarely been monitored or documented routinely in the past. Comments by the nursing staff are usually nonquantitative and are often not thoroughly scrutinized by the medical staff. Patients miss meals on account of diagnostic procedures, interruption by visits of medical or paramedical personnel, and inappropriate content or unappetizing presentation of meals. It is not surprising that there is good evidence that hospitalized patients become undernourished, sometimes to a degree which is life-threatening [3,4]. It is important to emphasize that increased energy and nutrient requirements, due to increased losses and often to very marked increases in metabolic demands, are likely to occur in the acute clinical setting. Fever, infections, burns, extensive wounds and other trauma, tumors, and catabolic drugs have all been implicated as responsible agents.

It is frequently possible to observe food trays at the bedside, to note what has been eaten and which foods have been rejected, and to ask why. A patient's dietary idiosyncrasies may thus be revealed. What people eat when they feel well may differ substantially from what they eat when they are sick. Some of these differences are determined by cultural factors, in which folklore, religious belief, taboo, and other prejudices may figure more prominently than we may like to believe. Examination of meal trays is also a valuable spot check of the quality of hospital food and of care taken in its preparation and presentation.

In intensive care units malnutrition was, until recently, even more prevalent than in general medical or surgical wards. The introduction of effective and relatively safe total parenteral feeding has overcome the difficulties of feeding seriously ill and semiconscious or stuporous patients by mouth. This subject and continuous feeding by nasogastric catheter are treated in detail in Chapter 3.

There are two final points to be made about taking a history. First, persons should be asked if they are consciously modifying their diets to lose or gain weight. Second, the effect of certain drugs on appetite in particular, and on intestinal absorption or metabolism to a lesser degree, is often forgotten. This topic receives detailed attention in Chapter 6 but is discussed briefly here, since it is frequently overlooked when taking a history.

Today it is particularly pertinent that many people are attempting to give up smoking cigarettes. Success is almost always accompanied by gain in weight, due mainly to increased consumption of calories, although metabolic changes may also result. Patients need counseling and encouragement and sometimes need to be given planned diets.

Other drugs that are significant because of their effect on nutrition fall into two categories. The first includes sex hormones now widely used by young and middle-aged women. If dosage is inadequately adjusted to the individual, estrogens may produce some of the gastrointestinal symptoms of pregnancy, such as loss of appetite and nausea. The second category comprises drugs used in the main by older subjects. The long-term treatment of heart failure with digoxin, an overdose of which produces profound gastrointestinal symptoms, and of arthritic diseases with analgesics and nonsteroidal anti-inflammatory drugs can result in significant depression of appetite in subjects in whom it may already be poor.

In taking a dietary history, therefore, specific questions should be asked about these drugs.

Twenty-Four-Hour Intake Recall

Dietitians and nutritionists use this technique extensively. Consumption in a single 24-hour period may not be representative of current weekly or monthly consumption, and, in addition, the data are subject to inaccuracies due to faulty memory and quantitative errors in assessing how much has been eaten. The use of models of various meals on serving plates to provide examples of sizes of helpings goes some way toward solving the latter problem. Retesting or testing over several days also improves the quality of data obtained from an individual. Obviously data obtained in this way are more reliable and, therefore, more useful in large group surveys than in assessing individual intake. Readers who wish to pursue the matter are referred to an excellent critical analysis by Marr [5].

Food Intake Record

This provides the best basis for proper evaluation of individual food consumption. It requires that the patient keep a record of everything eaten and drunk for 3 to 5 days, estimating the amounts in terms of small, medium, or large servings. After this period, studies have shown that compliance deteriorates. Ideally scales should be used to weigh each item, but this is not always feasible, and quantitative assessment in terms of helpings must be used. The limitations of this method are obvious. One important factor is the disruption of normal eating behavior which such record-keeping produces, especially if intake is weighed—a good example of the epigram "You can't get anything for nothing, not even an observation." The method is best applied to healthy subjects who are fairly well educated and competent or in special circumstances. The subject who lives alone is better able to meet the demands of this method than is a homemaker who cooks for an entire family, or someone who is involved in another kind of group living situation.

Analysis

Data obtained from patients in the different ways described must be analyzed to determine whether the subject is likely to be undernourished or overnourished. Until the use of tables of food composition and of recommended dietary allowances became accepted as the best means of establishing individual nutritional profiles, the usual method, which is still widely used, was based on the concept of the four major food groups: milk and milk products; meat, including fowl, fish, and eggs; vegetables and fruit; and grains, including bread, oatmeal and other cereals, potatoes, and rice. Sugar and extra fat were assessed separately, being regarded as sources only of calories and nowadays sometimes referred to derogatorily as "empty calories." This system of assessment is now regarded as outmoded for two important reasons: first, all meat products, formerly regarded as the main source of protein, may be partly or wholly replaced by mixtures of pulses or legumes and cereals; and, second, most milk products, such as whole milk and most cheeses, are seen in the light of current dietary concepts, including the "prudent diet," as being sources more of saturated animal fats than of protein. The food exchange system (see Chapter 2) goes a long way toward overriding these objections. However, a better procedure is to use food composition tables to calculate intake of calories and nutrients [6–9]. There are many sources of error, obviously. Error in estimate of sample size is a major one. Food analytical techniques are now very accurate, but seasonal differences in nutrient content of many foodstuffs occur and soil and species differences may cause variations in content. All foods of high water content are subject to significant variations, depending on their degree of hydration, and, finally, length of storage and cooking methods are sources of significant differences in nutritional value of food actually eaten.

If figures for the amounts of individual nutrients are obtained, a comparison can be made of tabulated Recommended Dietary Allowances (RDA) (Appendix 8) and recommended energy intake with mean height and weight (Appendix 2, Table 3).

It is important to stress that RDA figures have to be interpreted with the knowledge of how they are derived in mind. The estimations exceed the requirements of most individuals and meet the needs of nearly all the population. Intakes below the RDA are not necessarily inadequate, but the risk of inadequacy increases as intake falls below the level recommended as safe. The ability to predict a deficiency state from the value of the figure for any nutrient is low, therefore, unless the shortfall between the RDA and the amount consumed, estimated from dietary evaluation, is large.

In conclusion, it is clear that dietary assessment will rarely do more than help to explain observed anthropometric changes, including clinical evidence of malnutrition, or serve to emphasize the need to search for evidence of malnutrition by using clinical or laboratory techniques.

SYMPTOMS AND CLINICAL SIGNS OF MALNUTRITION

With some exceptions, clinical expressions of malnutrition are found mainly in patients who are grossly malnourished, but such gross malnourishment may occur in the hospital under the eyes of medical staff in the course of days or a few weeks and be overlooked. High-risk patients are those whose "weight for height" is less than 80 percent of standard or who have undergone serious recent weight loss of more than 10 to 15 percent of body weight or those who are acutely ill and obese and in whom subacute undernutrition may occur because the possibility is not entertained. The causes of increased metabolic demands, such as infections and burns, have already been addressed. When a change in medical or paramedical attendants occurs, the problem may be compounded or it may be resolved if the newcomer is alert and aware of potential nutritional problems, and if the patient's condition is still reversible.

Obesity or wasting may be assessed by nonquantitative clinical evaluation. However, available and simple anthropometric techniques (discussed under "Anthropometric Techniques," below) are preferable, since they provide a basis for longitudinal measurements which can be compared and, best of all, plotted on a flow sheet.

For convenience, physical examination is now considered by different structures.

Skin

The whole of the skin is accessible to the clinician. It cannot be overemphasized that the whole surface area of any patient should be inspected at the first examination, if possible. Such an inspection should be part of any thorough physical examination, but it is often overlooked.

Chronic wasting accompanied by loss of subcutaneous fat, the result of calorie or protein-calorie deficiency, results in fine wrinkling of the skin, especially in older subjects in whom the skin has lost its elasticity, and in the impression of hyperpigmentation (as the collapse of a colored balloon would make its color seem to deepen). If the skin seems unusually dark, the buccal mucosa should be scrutinized and the palmar creases examined for evidence of even greater pigmentation, which occurs in Addison's disease (hypoadrenalism). Buccal mucosal pigmentation tends to be patchy. In wasting in young people there may be much less redundant skin, but there is often excess hair growth, like fetal lanugo, most noticeable in girls with anorexia nervosa. This is commonly believed to be a heat-retaining mechanism compensating for loss of insulating fat. A tendency to excessive bruising may occur, in the absence of any other signs of deficiency of vitamin C or vitamin K, presumably as evidence of increased fragility of capillary walls or loss of strength of supporting connective tissue and, over bony protuberances, because of minor trauma and loss of protective fat. It should be emphasized that, in very wasted subjects, pressure and bony points should be well padded to avoid trauma-induced breaks in the skin, which may become infected and often heal very slowly. These lesions are very likely to occur when patients are moved during procedures such as radiological examinations, which are performed in partly darkened rooms with the patient lying on hard surfaces. An appearance identical with senile purpura may occur, especially on extensor aspects of the arms, on the backs of the hands, and at sites of venipuncture.

Dry, scaly skin may occur in subjects who are not malnourished, but if these changes appear for the first time in the appropriate setting or become markedly worse, they may indicate essential fatty acid deficiency. This is seen sometimes in subjects with severe chronic steatorrhea and sometimes in patients suffering from protein deficiency. "Flaky-paint skin" (Color Figure 1) is a change associated with more severe protein deficiency, both in children and adults. The cause is unknown.

In regions of the skin where sebaceous glands are dense, such as the nasolabial folds, the scalp, forehead, and eyebrows, the cheeks, the neck and the perianal region, deficiency of a number of essential nutrients may result in disturbances of secretory function which result in blocking of the ducts of sebaceous glands with plugs of dried sebum. There may be inflammation of the surrounding skin, and erythema, itching, and scaling may occur (Color Figure 2). Lack of essential fatty acids, which occurs in patients fed parenterally without adequate lipids and, rarely, in severe, untreated pancreatic or intestinal steatorrhea, is one cause. It occurs in experimental pyridoxine deficiency [10] and is seen occasionally in patients being treated with isoniazid or dialyzed for chronic renal disease, with pyridoxine deficiency believed to be the responsible factor. The condition does respond, although sometimes incompletely, to pyridoxine. In recent years zinc deficiency has also been implicated in the development of seborrheic dermatitis.

Acrodermatitis enteropathica is a rare condition of infancy and early childhood in which severe dermatitis with extensive ulceration of the extremities is associated with enterocolitis and diarrhea (Color Figure 3). It was usually fatal until the observation that large oral doses of zinc would induce remissions resulted in effective treatment of a disease now thought to be due to a defect in absorption of zinc. This led to recognition of the importance of zinc in the maintenance of biological functions [11].

Persisting mounds of keratin around hair follicles, which have the appearance of "goose pimples," are termed *follicular hyperkeratosis* (Color Figure 4). They occur in vitamin A deficiency and possibly in essential fatty acid deficiency and are therefore seen occasionally in an untreated patient with steatorrhea and occasionally in long-term hospitalized patients who become severely debilitated or are fed parenterally with carbohydrates and amino acids and no lipids.

Perifollicular hemorrhages and cutaneous petechiae (areas of extravasation of blood from capillaries, much smaller than a pin's head in size) are seen together almost exclusively in scurvy, due to deficiency of ascorbic acid. Petechiae alone may occur, of course, in thrombocytopenic purpura (due to a deficiency of blood platelets), but not perifollicular hemorrhages (Color Figure 5). Transient occlusion of the circulation to the forearm and hand, produced with an inflatable cuff, will sometimes reveal a latent tendency to petechial hemorrhage, as will the application of suction to the surface of the skin with a cup like a watchmaker's eyeglass, which has a sidearm through which negative pressure is applied. These tests may be positive in both thrombocytopenia and scurvy. A low activity of circulating prothrombin results not in petechiae but in bruising (ecchymosis) and extravasation of blood into tissues at any site (hematoma). This may occur as a consequence of deficient intake of vitamin K or, rarely, as a consequence of depressed synthesis of vitamin K by intestinal bacteria, of defective absorption of vitamin K, or of impaired hepatic synthesis of blood clotting factors.

The skin is shiny, thin, and often friable over areas of dependent edema. This may occur in protein-deficiency states, as a consequence of reduced plasma oncotic pressure due to low plasma albumin concentration, or in thiamine deficiency ("wet beriberi"), as a consequence of heart failure and, possibly, of increased capillary permeability (leakage).

Excessive skin pigmentation is seen in conditions other than wasting. In pellagra, due to deficiency of niacin (nicotinic acid and nicotinamide) or sometimes of its precursor, tryptophan, dermatitis is a major component. It is seen especially in areas of skin exposed to the actinic rays of the sun and around the orifices, such as the mouth and the anus. The extensor aspects of the arms, the backs of the hands, a V-shaped area below the front neckline (Casal's rosary), and a variable area around the back of the neck are the skin surfaces most affected. The skin becomes reddened (erythema), and there may be blistering, followed by peeling (desquamation). Reddened areas then become hyperpigmented in white-skinned people and depigmented in black-skinned people.

Another nutritional cause of pigmentation is the iron-storage disease hemochromatosis. The skin in this condition has a brown-gray color (café au lait), with brown hyperpigmentation of the flexures of the palms, similar to that seen in Addison's disease. Loss of axillary hair in males and changes of the pattern of the male pubic escutcheons to that of the female occur as a consequence of endocrine disturbance caused by male gonadal and possibly adrenocortical involvement.

An intriguing skin phenomenon is vitiligo, which is essentially depigmentation and is most apparent in the most pigmented areas, such as the forehead, the front of the neck, and the backs of the wrists and hands (Color Figure 6). Currently this phenomenon is unexplained. It occurs in pernicious anemia but is not responsive to cobalamin treatment; it also occurs in celiac-sprue but is not responsive to folacin. It is a useful signal, suggesting the need to further explore the nutritional status of a subject and particularly the need to check whether an underlying megaloblastic anemia is present.

Hair

Hair is an epidermal structure which sometimes reflects a state of nutritional deficiency. In kwashiorkor, reddening of normally black scalp hair occurs in black-skinned children. This may be of a transverse, linear distribution, an appearance which is termed the *flag sign*. It is seen occasionally in severely malnourished children in North America. In adults, excessive loss of scalp hair and body hair occur in protein-deficiency states. The scalp hair shows general thinning rather than patchy loss. The loss is due to failure of the hair follicle to hold its hair. There have been attempts to establish methods of quantifying hair pluckability as an index of protein deficiency. Some observations suggest that the ratio of actively growing hairs to those in a resting phase may decrease in protein-calorie malnutrition [12]. Restoration of a normal nutritional state is associated with recovery of hair color and of normal thickness and distribution.

Abnormalities of hair and hair distribution on the limbs and, less commonly, on the trunk occur in vitamin A–deficient states and in scurvy. As a consequence of follicular change due to disturbance of keratinization and, possibly, abnormal sebaceous gland activity, the hairs become coiled and corkscrew-like and may break short.

Nails

These are also epidermal structures which reflect nutritional state. Brittle nails are often thought to be an expression of some deficiency, but there is no valid evidence for this, nor does gelatin or any other so-called cure appear to be effective in correcting the problem. However, transverse ridging and an opaque, lackluster appearance of the nails may be associated with protein undernutrition. As isolated findings, they have no value as clinical signs, but they may sometimes serve as supportive evidence.

Spooning of the nails, so that they present a concave, dorsal surface, is sometimes found in the presence of a deficiency of iron, but it is a rare phenomenon in the United States. *Koilonychia,* as it is termed, seems to be more often seen in Britain.

Clubbing of the fingertips, so that the nails present a bulbous appearance, with the dorsal surface exaggeratedly convex, is found in chronic diseases of the respiratory system, the liver, and the intestines. It may be the first sign of cirrhosis or of celiac-sprue, but it is often congenital, in which case it has no known significance. Thus, observation of clubbing by itself has little clinical value.

Lips and Oral Structures

Cheilosis is a state of swelling and fissuring of the lips. It is usually painful, and bleeding may occur (Color Figure 7). It is claimed to be especially indicative of riboflavin deficiency. Proven, isolated riboflavin deficiency is exceedingly uncommon in North America or western Europe but since deficiency of all B-complex vitamins occurs in chronic alcoholics and in some patients with severe disease of the gastrointestinal tract, especially cancer, cheilosis is sometimes seen in such malnourished and sick patients. It often appears not to respond to treatment with vitamin B–complex preparations, but occasionally it may do so. There are many similar findings which have been observed in some human volunteers in whom specific nutrient deficiencies have been produced by special diets or by feeding them vitamin antagonists. Some of the better-known ones are listed in Table 1-3. Those listed are of importance because they may occur in other conditions or only very rarely in those conditions for which they have been claimed to be pathognomonic. Further, in many instances, they do not respond to treatment with repletion of the putative, deficient nutrient.

Angular stomatitis describes fissuring and ulceration of the angles of the mouth. Lack of riboflavin will produce these lesions, but it rarely occurs as an isolated deficiency. Loss of teeth (edentulousness) or dentures which are too

TABLE 1-3
DIAGNOSTIC MANIFESTATIONS WHICH HAVE LIMITED OR NO CLINICAL VALUE IN NORTH AMERICA

Finding	Deficiency
Angular stomatitis	Riboflavin
Cheilosis	Riboflavin
Koilonychia	Iron
Magenta tongue	Riboflavin
Seborrheic dermatitis	Pyridoxine Riboflavin Other B vitamins Zinc Essential fatty acid
Bitot's spot	Vitamin A

shallow, both of which allow the opposing surfaces of the lips to become chronically boggy with saliva, may result in similar changes (Color Figure 7). Some patients with chronic iron-deficiency anemia also develop such changes, which respond to treatment.

Noma is a condition in which gangrenous breakdown of soft tissues between the oral mucosa and skin occurs, usually in the region of the lips or cheeks, with the formation of fistulas. It is seen in grossly undernourished, very sick infants and children.

Tongue

The tongue is large in subjects with hypothyroid goiter, which may be a consequence of iodine deficiency. In untreated pellagra the tongue may also be swollen and edematous and is frequently deeply fissured, with superadded infection. These changes respond to treatment with niacin. The surface of the tongue may lose its normal papillae and become smooth, sore, and sometimes raw, presumably as a consequence of inadequate repair of the specialized epithelial surface (Color Figure 8). In the North American clinical setting this glossitis is usually due to isolated or combined deficiencies of iron, cobalamin, and folacin and is common in untreated celiac-sprue. In most patients there is restoration of the normal surface following treatment, though it may take some months. The soreness disappears within days of starting appropriate treatment. Some believe that the excessive ice eating (pagophagia) of iron-deficient women is an attempt to relieve minor soreness of the tongue and mouth.

The cause of color changes in the tongue is a controversial matter. In severe iron-deficiency anemia and untreated pernicious anemia the tongue is pale (Color Figure 8), but if anemia is not pronounced, the color of the tongue may be a fiery red in folacin deficiency and sometimes in untreated pernicious anemia (Color Figure 9).

In some chronic, undernourished alcoholics and occasionally in other patients in whom nutritional status is very poor and in whom there may be a deficiency of vitamin B complex, such as those who have had extensive gastrointestinal surgery, who have esophageal carcinoma, or who have had large-dose cancer chemotherapy, there may be cheilosis and, in addition, the tongue may be violet-red (magenta) in color and show some depapillation (Color Figure 10). No convincing trials of individual nutrient therapy for this condition have been reported. Improvement does not seem to occur when large doses of the B-group vitamins are given together, but it may follow restoration of general nutritional status toward normal.

Recurrent, painful small lesions, called *aphthous ulcers,* may be found on the tips or lateral margins of the tongue, the palate, and other parts of the oral mucosa. They occur most frequently in association with celiac-sprue and inflammatory bowel disease and may be a sign of nutritional deficiency.

Examination of the gums as part of the clinical examination for nutritional deficiency is valuable only in checking for overt deficiency of ascorbic acid. In established scurvy the gums are usually swollen, ulcerated, and bleeding (Color Figure 11). If the teeth are well looked after, gingivitis is minimal, and in the absence of teeth no changes occur at all.

Teeth

The state of the teeth provides no useful information about nutritional status other than that they display brown mottling in fluorosis (Color Figure 20), which is the result of excessive intake of fluoride as a consequence of diet or high fluoride content of supplies of drinking water. The presence of dental caries suggests too low a fluoride intake but may, of course, occur because of poor dental care and possibly frequently repeated exposure to sugar during the day.

The dental finding of most nutritional significance is lack of adequate teeth or of poorly fitting dentures, both of which may result in a subject's inability to chew food. Sometimes, especially in older people, such a finding may adequately explain loss of weight.

Thyroid

Thyroid enlargement, or goiter (Color Figure 12), occurs in inland areas where the effects of deficiency of iodine in soil and water have not been corrected by some program of iodination of table salt. Areas of endemic goiter are now virtually nonexistent in North America and Great Britain. Occasionally, a patient is seen who has been exposed to a goitrogenic agent, which blocks uptake of iodine by the thyroid. Such agents are present in green vegetables of the genus *Brassica* (e.g., cabbage and brussels sprouts).

Salivary Glands

In chronic protein-deficient states in adults, the parotid glands may be enlarged. This is seen in some undernourished alcoholic patients, but is otherwise rare.

Eyes

A common cause of blindness in some parts of the world, particularly in Central America and southeast Asia, is a deficiency of vitamin A, which leads to xerophthalmia, in which the conjunctival surfaces of the eyes become dull and dry. Subsequently, infection and poor integrity of the cornea (keratomalacia) progress to perforation into the anterior chamber of the eye, which leads to dislocation and even extrusion of the lens and irremediable blindness. The earliest ocular evidence of vitamin A deficiency is small, whitish foamy plaques called *Bitot's spots,* which form bilaterally in the conjunctiva lateral to the iris, outside the limbus, in the horizontal midline of each eye (Color Figure 13). They are not pathognomonic of vitamin A deficiency, occurring also as a result of conjunctival irritation or infection [13].

Bones and Joints

In the infant and child, rickets, due to lack of vitamin D and underabsorption of calcium, expresses itself as exaggerated convexity of the frontal bones of the skull (craniotabes or bossing) and enlargement of the costochondral junctions to form the so-called rachitic rosary (Color Figure 14). The ribs at the attachments of the diaphragm may be permanently bowed inward to form a bilateral groove of the chest wall called *Harrison's sulcus*. In severe cases, pelvic narrowing occurs, which in the female may later complicate pregnancy and delivery because of a narrowed birth canal. In toddlers the shafts of the femurs and the tibias become bowed (Color Figure 15). An early, frightening manifestation of craniotabes is the ease with which the frontal bones can be depressed by firm pressure with thumb or finger. Fortunately, the depressed area does revert to its former conformation on releasing the pressure. Treatment with a source of vitamin D and exposure to sunlight should be begun when this sign is elicited.

In adults with osteomalacia, due usually to intestinal malabsorption resulting from pancreatic or small intestinal disease, the long bones or vertebrae may be tender to pressure and sometimes spontaneous pain may be intractable, though it usually responds to intravenous calcium infusions.

In scurvy, hemorrhages into skin and gums may be accompanied by bleeding below the periosteum, producing tenderness and spontaneous pain. Infants having scurvy may be fractious, are often febrile, and respond violently to chance pressure on an affected area. Persistent swelling around large joints may sometimes occur following repeated subperiosteal bleeding. Significant sub-periosteal hemorrhages do not seem to occur in scorbutic adults, but hemor-rhages into muscles may occur and produce tenderness. The cardiac pain and sometimes sudden death occurring in scurvy have been ascribed to small hemorrhages in the myocardium.

Abdomen

Wasting due to caloric deficiency (marasmus) may be evident on examining the anterior abdominal wall. Palpation and percussion are used to assess the size of the liver and spleen. A large liver may be due to fatty infiltration as a consequence of alcohol abuse or may be found, in infants and children, in association with protein deficiency. A large and tender liver may be associated with heart failure. A palpable and, by inference, enlarged spleen is found in 15 to 25 percent of subjects with a significant degree of iron-deficiency anemia.

Rectal Examination

Proctoscopy may reveal the appearance of inflammation of the rectal mucosa in untreated pellagra, indistinguishable from "nonspecific" ulcerative colitis or even amebiasis by inspection. This responds rapidly to treatment with niacin.

Central and Peripheral Nervous System

Deficiency of a number of nutrients may be associated with mild or severe organic psychoses.

Korsakoff's syndrome, or psychosis, which occurs in chronic alcoholics and consists of confabulation and loss of memory, especially for recent events, may respond in part to treatment with massive doses of thiamine. Complete recovery is rare. Instances of cobalamin deficiency may, rather uncommonly, be seen in which mental derangement is the predominant symptom. Screening of psychotic patients, especially in institutions, may reveal a small but significant number of patients with untreated cobalamin deficiency due to the lesion of pernicious anemia. The early signs may be loss of recent memory, irritability, other personality changes, and mild confusion, but they may progress to severe psychosis and paranoid delusions.

An important part of the clinical picture in pellagra is dementia, sometimes of a violent and paranoid kind, which responds rapidly to treatment with niacin. Folacin deficiency may also be associated with mental disturbance; depression and irritability have been noted in experimental folacin deficiency.

Depression and lethargy are also a major component of scurvy and respond to ascorbic acid. It has been suggested that this may be due to an induced defect in the synthesis of norepinephrine from dopamine by hydroxylation, since the responsible enzyme, dopamine β-hydroxylase, requires ascorbic acid [14].

Widespread application of total parenteral nutrition has resulted in the emergence of two conditions, in both of which changes of consciousness predominate: hypophosphatemia and nonketotic hyperosmolar syndrome. Both have a serious prognosis, and early recognition is lifesaving.

Hypophosphatemia may occur as a consequence of inadequate phosphate in fluids used for infusion, if there has been too enthusiastic infusion of amino acids or glucose to previously starving patients. The consequent fall in serum phosphate is accompanied by a major disturbance of glycolytic phosphorylation, concentrations of 2,3-diphosphoglycerate in red blood cells fall, and the oxygen saturation curve is shifted to the left, so that tissue anoxemia results. Patients so affected may have convulsions and become comatose [15]. Precipitating factors are previous severe undernutrition and massive infusions of amino acids and glucose. This phenomenon is also discussed in Chapter 3.

A second cause of occasional stupor or coma is nonketotic hyperosmolar syndrome. This occurs in older subjects receiving total parenteral nutrition. The kidneys may retain glucose until high plasma concentrations are attained. An osmotic diuresis then results in loss of sodium, leading to hypotension. The double onslaught of hyperosmolarity and hypotension results in obtundation and sometimes in irreversible coma and death.

Prevention consists of avoiding sudden, massive intravenous infusions of glucose. Excess amounts of calcium or magnesium in the plasma may also cause stupor or coma.

Wilson's disease (hepatolenticular degeneration), discussed in Chapters 16 and 18 is due to deposition of excessive amounts of copper in the liver parenchyma and the basal ganglia of the brain. The neurological consequences are incoordination of all movements, sometimes tremors similar to those seen in Parkinson's disease, and, rarely, impaired mentation.

Convulsions and Migraine

We include these disturbances of central nervous function under clinical signs of malnutrition, although there may be no abnormal signs associated with them at the time of physical examination.

Convulsions due to pyridoxine deficiency in infants were correctly attributed to a defectively formulated milk substitute [16]. Available infant feeding formulas now contain adequate amounts of pyridoxine.

Alcohol excess or withdrawal are other causes of convulsions (see Chapter 17), and convulsions may also occur in hypophosphatemia, a complication of total parenteral nutrition.

Some subjects develop migraine following ingestion of certain foods. This observation, together with the increase in migrainous attacks noted with allergies of the respiratory tract, suggests that gastrointestinal allergy may be responsible. Cow's milk and chocolate are common offenders. The evidence is incomplete.

Special Senses and Cranial Nerves

Impairment of smell and taste may occur as a result of zinc deficiency. This may occur in total parenteral nutrition, unless infusions of trace elements are provided, and also in some patients with intestinal malabsorption. Deficiency of vitamin A is associated with similar disturbances but is very rarely seen in the United States. In untreated pernicious anemia loss of taste, responding to treatment with cobalamin, sometimes occurs. Rarely function of the optic nerve is disturbed by cobalamin deficiency; this may occur in untreated pernicious anemia, with resulting loss of vision.

Disturbances of Spinal Cord Function

Demyelination of long neural fibers in the spinal cord may occur in cobalamin deficiency. The pyramidal tracts (motor) and posterior columns (sensory tracts carrying information about position, vibration, and light touch) are selectively affected. The condition is described as subacute combined degeneration and, in pernicious anemia, when anemia is also present, as combined systems disease. Punctate hemorrhages may also occur in the region of areas of demyelination. The result is weakness, especially of the lower limbs, and loss of position sense, making walking unsteady and even impossible in poor light. The deep tendon reflexes are brisk, and the plantar reflexes upgoing (positive Babinski sign).

Cobalamin therapy may produce minimal, partial, or complete recovery. It has been claimed that similar changes may occur with folacin deficiency alone [17]. This remains unconvincing, but there are undoubtedly similar cases on record in which progressive long-tract nervous degeneration has occurred in spite of massive replacement of all known nutrients [18]. It has been suggested that deficiencies of hitherto unidentified nutrients may be responsible, possibly involving substances possessing a pteridine group other than folacin [19].

Peripheral Nervous System

Disturbances of peripheral nerve function (peripheral neuropathy) occur in a number of nutrient deficiency states, pure or mixed. Some are of predominantly sensory type, so that reduced sensation (hypesthesia), absent sensation (anesthesia), abnormal or inappropriate sensation (paresthesia), or inappropriate unpleasant sensation (hyperpathia) occur. Others are of predominantly motor type, so that failure to stand up may be a first sign. Patients complain of numbness, persistent tingling, difficulty in handling small objects, and weakness. Sometimes they complain of intermittent sharp pains or nagging, chronic pain. Motor nerve disorders with true weakness are common in thiamine deficiency ("dry beriberi"), in which the leg muscles, especially the quadriceps, are most affected. In general, repletion with appropriate nutrients leads to better recovery of peripheral nerve lesions than those of the spinal long tracts. Deficiencies of cobalamin, pyridoxine, and thiamine may all be associated with peripheral sensory neuropathy of the "glove-and-stocking" type, which well describes the peripheral distribution, starting in the extremities. Sensory testing of response to touch, pinprick, and hot and cold allows mapping of the affected areas and a semiobjective means of measuring response to treatment.

Deficiency of pantothenic acid (rare in North America) may produce paresthesia, described as the "burning feet syndrome" [20].

ANTHROPOMETRIC TECHNIQUES

The value of these techniques is that they provide quantitative data. They should permit (1) comparisons of the data for one individual with norms derived from populations of various sizes (these may have both diagnostic and prognostic value and may provide a valid base for recommendations for change), and (2) longitudinal records of an individual from which rates of growth and other parameters of maturation and gains or losses of weight may be derived.

Much ingenuity has been expended in constructing formulas which derive values, within defined limits of variation, from measurements such as height and weight, mid-upper arm circumference, skin-fold thickness at various sites, and so on, and also from certain biochemical tests. Genetically determined factors increase the variance of the mean of all these derived values, and this is particularly evident when data are compared for different ethnic groups. For example, studies have shown that the adipose–lean muscle mass ratios for black and white males in the United States are significantly different [21]. In spite of these differences there is a high probability, on the basis of the data given in weight-height reference charts, that an adult whose weight is 20 percent above standard is significantly overweight and, therefore, obese and is endowed with the health risks of obesity, and if the weight of an adult is the same percentage below standard, the probability is high that the individual is significantly underweight, emaciated, and at nutritional risk.

These data are recorded routinely in obstetric and pediatric offices, clinics, and wards. They are best plotted on standard charts such as those designed by the National Center for Health Statistics, samples of which are shown in Figures 1-1 through 1-6. These charts provide a good means of following rates of growth. They are especially valuable in (1) the care of infants who are not thriving because of food intolerance or disorders of intestinal malabsorption and (2) the management of children with metabolic diseases, such as diabetes mellitus, or chronic diseases, such as juvenile rheumatoid arthritis, chronic renal disease, or inflammatory bowel disease; in the latter group fluctuations of appetite occur which may pass unnoticed unless an objective record is kept.

In the case of adults, there is growing recognition that a more meaningful and accessible display of recorded weight is needed than a figure on a clinic visit sheet or a chart of vital signs.

Weight is measured on balance-beam scales, the calibration of which should be frequently checked. There is merit in repeated weighing of any individual on the same scales. The subject should be unclothed or in underclothes and stockinged feet. In clinical practice it is still necessary sometimes to remind medical and nursing staff that loss of weight may be masked by the development of edema, which may in the very sick patient be misinterpreted as a gain in weight. Evidence of edema must be sought for, and it should not be forgotten that in the recumbent individual the area over the sacrum is the best place to look.

Height is measured in the case of infants and toddlers with the subject supine, looking straight up. Older children and adults are measured erect, using a horizontal arm that moves vertically on a calibrated scale; the heels should be on the ground, the buttocks, shoulders, and back of the head should touch the vertical scale, and the horizontal arm should rest lightly on the crown of the head, displacing any scalp hair. An elegant and valuable addition is a standardized photograph of the subject being measured, since it provides an unequaled record for subsequent comparisons. The expense has prevented wide application to clinical practice.

Skin-fold Thickness and Measurements of Upper Arm Circumference

There are elaborate methods of assessing the relative amounts of fat and lean muscle in the body. One is to weigh the subject in air and then totally immersed in water and to use the weight difference and reference tables to derive estimates of body fat [22,23]. Lean body mass has been assessed by measuring amounts of

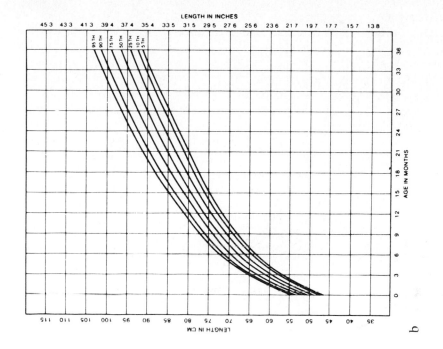

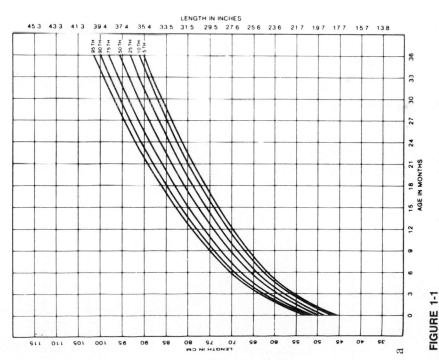

FIGURE 1-1

Length percentiles by age (a) for girls from birth to the age of 36 months and (b) for boys from birth to the age of 36 months.

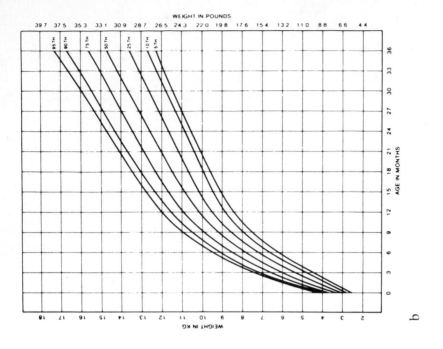

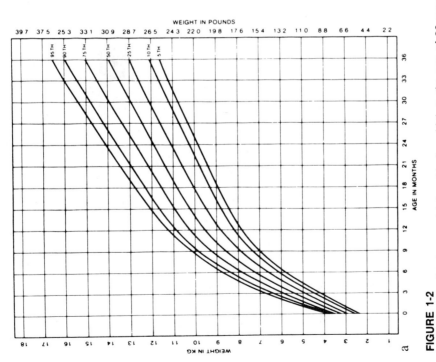

FIGURE 1-2
Weight percentiles by age (a) for girls from birth to the age of 36 months and (b) for boys from birth to the age of 36 months.

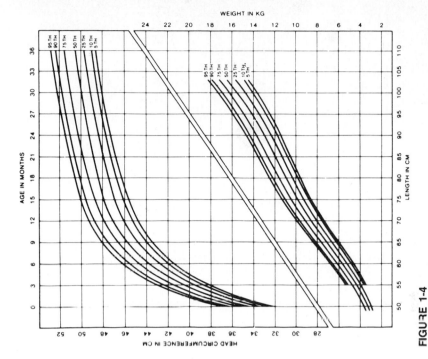

FIGURE 1-4

(Top) Head circumference percentiles by age for boys from birth to 36 months. (Bottom) Weight percentiles by length for boys from birth to 36 months.

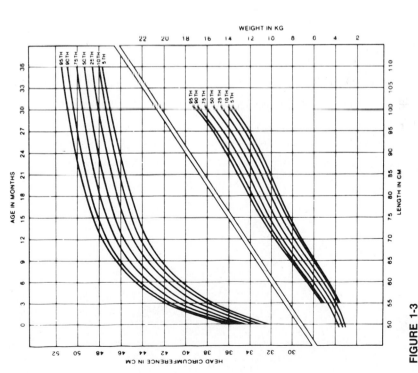

FIGURE 1-3

(Top) Head circumference percentiles by age for girls from birth to 36 months. (Bottom) Weight percentiles by length for girls from birth to 36 months.

23

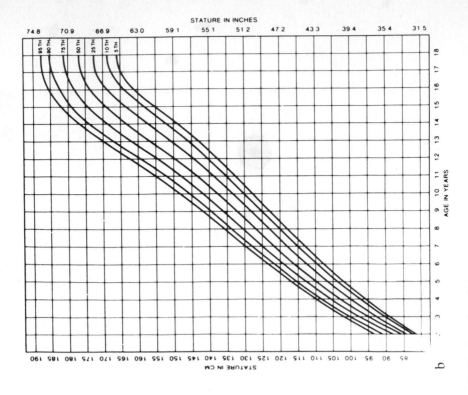

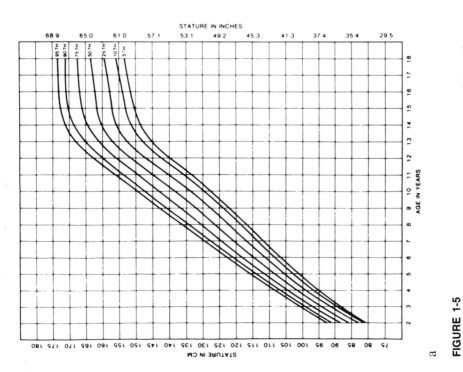

FIGURE 1-5
Stature percentiles by age (a) for girls from the age of 2 to 18 years and (b) for boys from the age of 2 to 18 years.

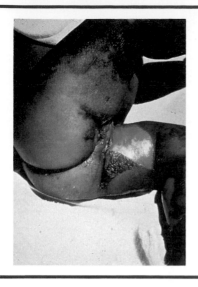

1

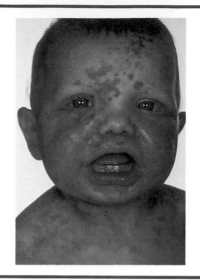

3

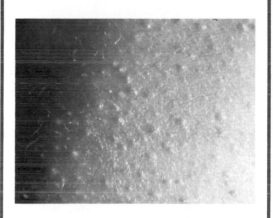

2

4

1 Flaky paint dermatosis

2 Seborrheic dermatitis

3 Acrodermatitis
  enteropathica

4 Follicular
  hyperkeratosis

5 Perifollicular
  hemorrhages

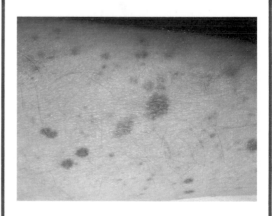

5

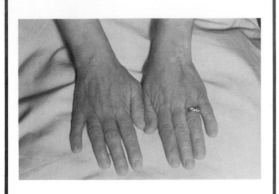

6

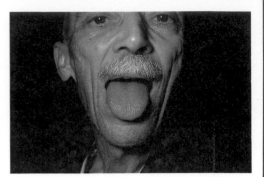

9

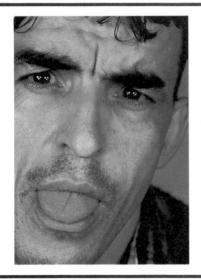

7

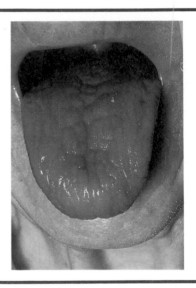

10

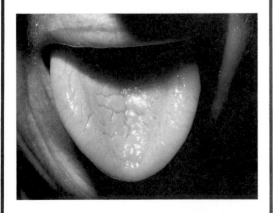

8

6 Vitiligo
7 Cheilosis and angular
   stomatitis
8 Pale glossitis
9 Fiery red glossitis
10 Magenta tongue

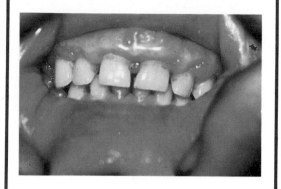

11

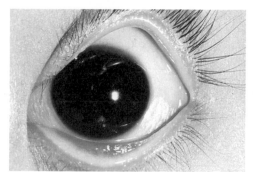

13

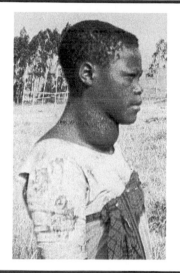

12

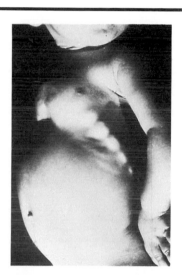

14

11 Scorbutic gums

12 Goiter

13 Bitot's spot

14 Rachitic rosary

15 Rachitic bowlegs,
note angle of feet

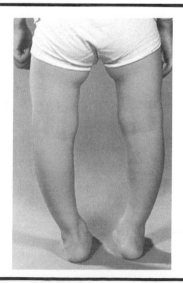

15

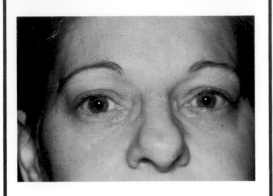

16

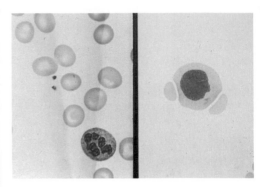

19

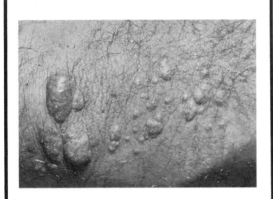

17

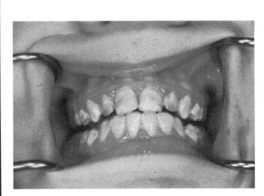

20

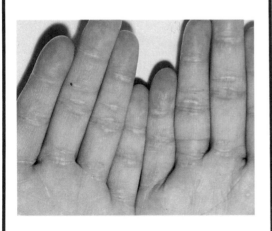

18

16 Xanthelasma

17 Eruptive xanthoma

18 Palmar xanthoma

19 Hypersegmentation of polymorphonuclear leukocyte and megaloblast in folate or cobalamin deficiency

20 Mild fluorosis - mottling of teeth

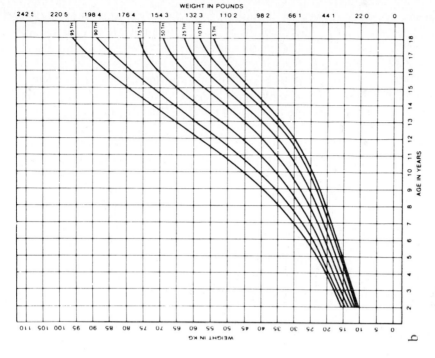

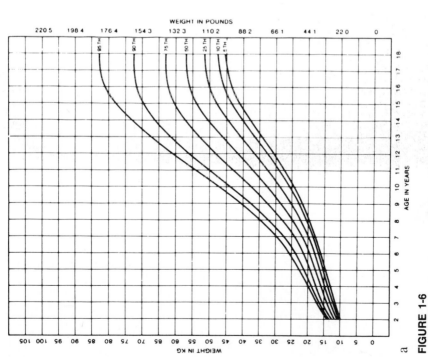

FIGURE 1-6
Weight percentiles by age (a) for girls from the age of 2 to 18 years and (b) for boys from the age of 2 to 18 years.

25

the naturally occurring potassium radioisotope ^{40}K with a total-body gamma scintillation counter [24]. These methods have no application currently to clinical practice. However, measurements of skin-fold thickness at defined sites provide a satisfactory index of body fat, which closely relates to energy reserves.

Skin calipers (Figure 1-7) are used to measure skin-fold thickness. The skin is pinched and pulled away from underlying muscle, and then the calipers are applied 1 cm from the ridge of skin thus formed. A reading is made 3 seconds after application of the calipers to standardize any effects produced by deformation of tissue. The most-used site, because it does not require that the subject be undressed, is over the triceps muscle, midway between the tip of the acromion of the scapula and the ulnar olecranon (Figure 1-7). Arm circumference is measured at the same site with an inelastic tape measure. Care must be taken to keep the tape in a horizontal plane (the arm hangs relaxed at the

FIGURE 1-7
Skin calipers and site of triceps skin-fold measurement.

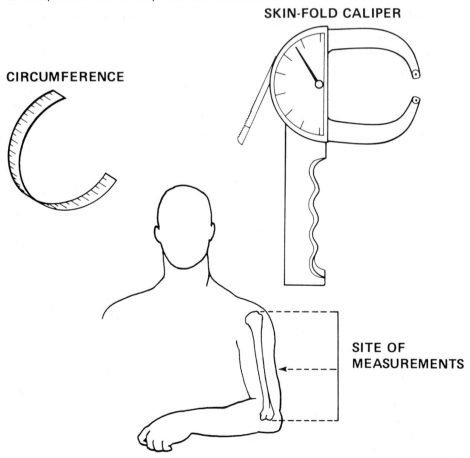

SKIN-FOLD CALIPER

CIRCUMFERENCE

SITE OF
MEASUREMENTS

subject's side) and not indent the skin. The measurement is recorded to the nearest millimeter. The average of three readings is recorded. The value is read off a standardized skin-fold thickness table which allows for sexual dimorphism (Table 1-4). For clinical purposes the result is classified as obese or as normal, or as depleted fat reserves. The sexual dimorphism of the triceps skin-fold is established by the age of 3 years.

If skin-fold calipers are unavailable, a rough index of subcutaneous fat may be obtained by picking up in the fingers a skin fold over the iliac crest of the pelvic bones. It should be no thicker than the little finger of the subject.

The circumference of the upper arm at the midpoint expresses muscle mass

TABLE 1-4

STANDARDS FOR TRICEPS FAT FOLD

(All Values Expressed in Millimeters)

Age, yr (or mo)	Triceps skin-fold percentile*									
	Male					Female				
	5th	15th	50th	85th	95th	5th	15th	50th	85th	95th
0–5 mo	4	5	8	12	15	4	5	8	12	13
6–17 mo	5	7	9	13	15	6	7	9	12	15
$1\frac{1}{2}$–$2\frac{1}{2}$	5	7	10	13	14	6	7	10	13	15
$2\frac{1}{2}$–$3\frac{1}{2}$	6	7	9	12	14	6	7	10	12	14
$3\frac{1}{2}$–$4\frac{1}{2}$	5	6	9	12	14	5	7	10	12	14
$4\frac{1}{2}$–$5\frac{1}{2}$	5	6	8	12	16	6	7	10	13	16
$5\frac{1}{2}$–$6\frac{1}{2}$	5	6	8	11	15	6	7	10	12	15
$6\frac{1}{2}$–$7\frac{1}{2}$	4	6	8	11	14	6	7	10	13	17
$7\frac{1}{2}$–$8\frac{1}{2}$	5	6	8	12	17	6	7	10	15	19
$8\frac{1}{2}$–$9\frac{1}{2}$	5	6	9	14	19	6	7	11	17	24
$9\frac{1}{2}$–$10\frac{1}{2}$	5	6	10	16	22	6	8	12	19	24
$10\frac{1}{2}$–$11\frac{1}{2}$	6	7	10	17	25	7	8	12	20	29
$11\frac{1}{2}$–$12\frac{1}{2}$	5	7	11	19	26	6	9	13	20	25
$12\frac{1}{2}$–$13\frac{1}{2}$	5	6	10	18	25	7	9	14	23	30
$13\frac{1}{2}$–$14\frac{1}{2}$	5	6	10	17	22	8	10	15	22	28
$14\frac{1}{2}$–$15\frac{1}{2}$	4	6	9	19	26	8	11	16	24	30
$15\frac{1}{2}$–$16\frac{1}{2}$	4	5	9	20	27	8	10	15	23	27
$16\frac{1}{2}$–$17\frac{1}{2}$	4	5	8	14	20	9	12	16	26	31
$17\frac{1}{2}$–$24\frac{1}{2}$	4	5	10	18	25	9	12	17	25	31
$24\frac{1}{2}$–$34\frac{1}{2}$	4	6	11	21	28	9	12	19	29	36
$34\frac{1}{2}$–$44\frac{1}{2}$	4	6	12	22	28	10	14	22	32	39

*These percentiles were derived from data obtained for white subjects in the United States Ten-State Nutritional Survey of 1968 to 1970. In this survey, obesity in adults was defined as a fat fold greater than the 85th percentile.

Source: Adapted from A. Frisancho, Triceps skin fold and upper arm muscle size norms for assessment of nutritional status, Am. J. Clin. Nutr., 27:1052, 1974.

TABLE 1-5

STANDARDS FOR UPPER ARM CIRCUMFERENCE

(All Values Expressed in Millimeters)

Age midpoint, yr	Arm muscle circumference percentiles*				
	5th	15th	50th	85th	95th
Males					
0.3	81	94	106	125	133
1	100	108	123	137	146
2	111	117	127	138	146
3	114	121	132	145	152
4	118	124	135	151	157
5	121	130	141	156	166
6	127	134	146	159	167
7	130	137	151	164	173
8	138	144	158	174	185
9	138	143	161	182	200
10	142	152	168	186	202
11	150	158	174	194	211
12	153	163	181	207	221
13	159	169	195	224	242
14	167	182	211	234	265
15	173	185	220	252	271
16	186	205	229	260	281
17	206	217	245	271	290
21	217	232	258	286	305
30	220	241	270	295	315
40	222	239	270	300	318
Females					
0.3	86	92	104	115	126
1	97	102	117	128	135
2	105	112	125	140	146
3	108	116	128	138	143
4	114	120	132	146	152
5	119	124	138	151	160
6	121	129	140	155	165
7	123	132	146	162	175
8	129	138	151	168	186
9	136	143	157	176	193
10	139	147	163	182	196
11	140	152	171	195	209
12	150	161	179	200	212
13	155	165	185	206	225
14	166	175	193	221	234
15	163	173	195	220	232
16	171	178	200	227	260
17	171	177	196	223	241
21	170	183	205	229	253
30	177	189	213	245	272
40	180	192	216	250	279

*These percentiles were derived from data obtained for white subjects in the United States Ten-State Nutritional Survey of 1968 to 1970.

Source: A. Frisancho, Triceps skin fold and upper arm muscle size norms for assessment of nutritional status, Am. J. Clin. Nutr., 27:1052, 1974.

and subcutaneous fat. The formula for deriving that part of the cross-sectional area of the upper arm at that level which is fat is obviously the total area minus the muscle area:

$$\text{Arm muscle area} = \frac{[\text{circumference (cm)}]^2}{4\pi}$$

$$\text{Mid-upper-arm muscle circumference} = \text{arm circumference (cm)}$$
$$- \pi \, [\text{skin-fold thickness (cm)}]$$

The significance of this value is classified as normal or as reduced muscle reserve. Alternatively, the mid-upper-arm muscle circumference is obtained: Charts and tables of mid-arm muscle circumferences in adults have been derived from data obtained in the United States Ten-State National Nutrition Survey (1968–1970) by Frisancho [25] (Table 1-5). Sexual dimorphism of mid-arm muscle circumference appears by about the age of 13 years.

LABORATORY AND SPECIAL TESTS

Routine

Useful information about nutritional status may be obtained from many laboratory tests which are performed routinely in standard clinical laboratories. The advantages of these tests are that clinical staff are familiar with the techniques for obtaining samples, the proper storage of samples in order to keep errors due to deterioration to a minimum, and the interpretation of the laboratory data. An added advantage is that laboratories perform a sufficiently large number of estimations to maintain a high degree of quality control, so that reliable data are obtained. Tests which fall into this category are listed in Table 1-6.

Routine hematological data include red and white blood cell counts, platelet counts, hemoglobin levels, packed red cell volume (hematocrit), and examination of a stained film of the peripheral blood to determine the morphology of both red and white cells and the distribution of different types of white cells. Small red cells, low in hemoglobin content, are associated with deficiency of iron; abnormally large, variably shaped red cells, high in hemoglobin content, are associated with deficiencies of cobalamin or folacin. Examination of bone marrow cells taken from the iliac crest, vertebra, or sternum may provide corroborative evidence and also an index of iron status, since absence of iron demonstrated by a negative result on staining with ferrocyanide is a good indicator of depleted body stores of iron.

Direct measurement of iron, cobalamin, and folacin contents of serum is now widely available. Body stores of folacin are better reflected by red cell folacin than serum folacin content.

Tests of hepatobiliary function, which are routinely available, include serum bilirubin, alkaline phosphatase, and various transaminases.

TABLE 1-6

ROUTINE LABORATORY TESTS WHICH PROVIDE INFORMATION
ABOUT NUTRITIONAL STATUS

Serum electrolytes:	Hematological indexes:
Sodium	Hemoglobin
Potassium	Hematocrit
Calcium	Red cell count
Phosphorus	White cell count and
Magnesium	differential
Serum proteins:	Thrombocytes
Albumin	Serum iron
Transferrin	Serum vitamins:
C3 component of complement	Cobalamin
Coagulation proteins	Folacin (erythrocyte folacin)
Prothrombin	
Factors VII, IX, X	
Serum lipids:	
Cholesterol	
Triglycerides	

Nitrogen Balance

In patients without complications of renal injury or failure or of severe bowel
disease associated with protein-losing enteropathy, it is possible to derive an
approximate estimate of nitrogen balance from protein intake and the output of
urea in the urine (see Appendix 3). This is best done over a 3-day period and
requires complete collections of urine.

$$\text{Nitrogen balance} = \frac{\text{protein intake (g)}}{6.25}$$
$$- [\text{24-hour urinary urea N (g)} + 4] \quad \text{(from Ref. 26)}$$

There are other formulas. One, with which it is claimed very close
approximation to daily nitrogen requirements can be made, derives nitrogen loss
from blood urea, urinary urea, and proteinuria [27]. It has been applied only
when intravenous amino acids are being used and varies according to the
preparation being used.

In practice, these methods only have value in the management of patients if
the patients remain in a hypercatabolic state for several days or longer; these
methods apply especially to those patients with continuing severe infections or
burns.

In patients with renal disease it is best to use the patient's own appraisal and
complaints, blood pressure readings, levels of serum albumin, and, less
importantly, values of blood urea, creatinine, potassium, and bicarbonate as
indexes of nutritional status.

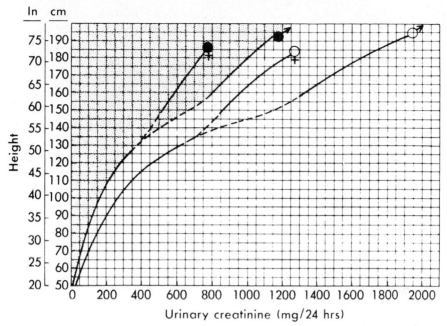

FIGURE 1-8
Creatinine-height index reference standard (all ages). Broken line represents extrapolated data. Stippled areas represent severe muscle mass deficit (60 percent standard). ♂ = average (standard). *From R. L. Weinsier, and C. E. Butterworth, Handbook of Clinical Nutrition, Mosby, St. Louis, 1981; data adapted from F. E. Viteri and J. Alvardo: Pediatrics 46:696, 1970, and B. R. Bistrian, et al.: Surg. Gynecol. Obstet. 141:512, 1975.)*

In patients with protein-losing gastroenteropathy due to inflammatory disease or malignancy, the levels of serum albumin and of rapid turnover proteins such as transferrin and the C3 component of the complement system are the most useful indicators of inadequate nitrogen retention.

The creatinine-height index provides a means of estimating muscle or lean body mass and is based on the observed direct relation between the amount of creatinine excreted in the urine in 24 hours and the total muscle mass [28]. The estimated urinary creatinine in relation to height is compared with a plot of standard values in Figure 1-8.

Tests of Intestinal Absorption

These are also discussed in Chapter 15. The most useful, as indexes of possible nutrient deficiency, are the following:

1 *Measurement of total fat in a 72-hour collection of feces from the patient, who must be eating 100 g fat daily:* Values above 18 g indicate steatorrhea and raise the possibility of malabsorption of nutrients. The defect may be in pancreatic secretion, biliary secretion, the intestinal mucosa, or lymphatic drainage, or it may be due to bacterial overgrowth in the upper small bowel.

2 *Oral D-xylose test:* This is performed by giving the fasting subject 25 g D-xylose in 100 ml water and collecting urine for 5 hours. Twenty percent or more of the dose should appear in the urine in this time. A lower figure indicates intestinal mucosal disease. In pancreatic and biliary disease the results should be within the normal range.

3 *Serum carotene concentration:* This is a relatively simple measurement. Figures above 50 mg/dl tend to exclude intestinal malabsorption, but lower figures may be due to malabsorption or recent absence of carotene from the diet.

4 *Urinary excretion test of cobalamin:* This test is often called the *Schilling test* after its originator [29]. The fasting subject is given a 0.5-μg oral dose of radiocobalt-labeled cobalamin, followed by an intramuscular "flushing" dose of unlabeled cobalamin (usually 1 mg) 2 hours later. The proportion of the administered radioactivity excreted in the urine during the next 24 hours provides an accurate measure of cobalamin absorption. Urine is collected for 24 hours, and the amount of radioactivity excreted is expressed as a percentage of the total amount in the oral dose. A result above 10 percent indicates normal absorption. Most subjects with pernicious anemia, in which there is a deficiency of intrinsic factor (IF), excrete less than 2 percent in the urine.

When biologically active IF is given with the oral dose of radiocobalt-labeled cobalamin to IF-deficient individuals, absorption of the labeled cobalamin is enhanced and the percentage of urinary excretion is increased toward or into the normal range. By using two 0.5-μg oral doses of cobalamin labeled with a different radioisotope of cobalt, such as ^{57}Co and ^{58}Co, to one of which has been added a preparation of biologically active (usually hog) exogenous IF, it is possible to perform the two tests at the same time. The absorption of cobalamin alone and complexed with IF is thus estimated by measuring the difference in the amounts of the two radioactive isotopes appearing in the urine in 24 hours. This technique can to some extent obviate the problem of any tests requiring complete collections of urine for 24 hours—namely, the lost urine specimen—since the ratio of the two isotopes indicates whether the subject lacks IF. For instance, if the ratio is near unity, there is no lack of IF, regardless of the total amount of radioactivity excreted, whereas if there is a significant excess of the isotope labelling the cobalamin complexed with IF, the patient has a deficiency of IF.

Special Laboratory Tests

Immunological Tests There is evidence that depression of the normal immune response may occur in protein-energy malnutrition (PEM) and in some specific nutrient deficiencies. Cell-mediated immunity is more depressed than humoral immunity. In infants and children the thymus gland and other lymphatic tissue, such as the tonsil, may be much reduced in size in PEM [30], and there is a reduction in number of circulating thymus-derived lymphocytes (T cells) and in their response to stimulation [31,32]. A deficiency of zinc, which is sometimes associated with PEM, may be associated with similar changes, which are reversed by zinc supplementation [33,34].

By contrast, humoral immunity is impaired little, or not at all, and the number of circulating bone-marrow-derived lymphocytes (B cells) is barely affected, if at all. The antibody response to most ingested antigens is apparently normal [35], although some components of the complement system, which is involved in antigen-antibody interactions, may be depleted in PEM [36]. The concentrations of circulating immunoglobulins either are within the normal range or are elevated if there has been continuing exposure to infection and infestation [35]. However, this is a currently complex though very interesting topic, particularly in relation to the secretion of the immunoglobulin IgA, which is secreted in a special form (SIgA) by gastrointestinal, bronchial, and other internal mucosal surfaces and which appears to exert a protective action against invasion by microorganisms and to control their numbers. The comprehensive review by Gross and Newberne [35], already cited, should be consulted.

The depression of T-cell function (cellular immunity) in PEM has been used as an index of malnutrition in hospitalized patients. The delayed-type, cutaneous hypersensitivity reaction has been used as a measure of T-cell function. A battery of antigens, to one or more of which almost all adult Americans have become sensitized by previous exposure, comprises purified tuberculoprotein (PPD), mumps, *Candida,* and streptokinase-streptodornase. Standard amounts are injected intradermally at standard sites on the flexor surfaces of the forearms, and results are read 24 and 48 hours after the time of injection. Readings taken only at 48 hours may sometimes give false-negative results, since some reactions subside rapidly after a peak at 24 hours. A positive result is one in which there is a thickening of the skin (induration) at the center and usually a peripheral zone of reddening, or erythema. The diameter of the induration is measured by using a millimeter scale and the ball-point technique, i.e., drawing a ball-point pen toward the center (site of injection) from two separate peripheral starting points until resistance is encountered [37]. The diameter is recorded each time the test is done with the same antigen in the same concentration. Many regard any induration at 48 hours as a positive test, while others set arbitrary standards of 5- or 10-mm diameter. However, in the case of mumps antigen, erythema alone is considered a positive result. Recording the dimensions at each test permits comparison and obviates the need for arbitrary evaluation. A negative test is one in which there is no induration or, in the case of mumps antigen, no erythema. When all such skin tests are negative, the subject is described as being *anergic* (i.e., as having no reaction).

In addition, tests have been done using a powerful artificial contact sensitizing agent, dinitrochlorobenzene (DNCB). An alcoholic solution of known strength is applied to the skin; after two weeks and, if appropriate, at intervals thereafter, test solutions of DNCB are applied to a standardized area on the forearm. This technique assesses the functions of the T-cell-mediated sensitization mechanism and of the recognition or efferent limb of the immune response. The depression of response to all skin tests observed in children with PEM has thus been successfully applied to hospitalized children and adults in the United States as a measure of nutritional status [38], and it has been noted, for instance, in malnourished patients with cancer that parenteral feeding is associated with conversion of negative to positive tests in a significant number of patients [39]. The results of these tests must be interpreted as one indication of possible malnutrition. The underlying cause for the immune depression may be partly or wholly the elevated concentrations of cortisol which have been demonstrated in PEM and which occur following trauma. It has been shown that whereas major surgery depresses the skin response, severe caloric restriction does not [40]. This suggests that skin tests should not be performed any sooner than several days after significant physical trauma. Clearly, further evaluation of the importance of these tests is needed.

Measurement of Specific Nutrients Measurement of specific nutrients is currently not widely available, and, in consequence, a profile of the nutrient status of an individual is impossible to obtain, except in a few centers. These measurements comprise three categories:

1 Measurements of the nutrient in tissue samples, usually blood, urine, or blood cells.

2 Measurements of the nutrient or one of its metabolic products in the urine after giving an oral or parenteral loading dose of the nutrient.

3 Measurement of the efficiency of an enzyme reaction in which the nutrient or product of the nutrient is a cofactor. This may be done in vivo or in vitro. When it is done in vivo, a loading dose of the appropriate substrate is given in an attempt to overload the impaired kinetics of the reaction and amplify the defect. Blood or urinary concentrations of a metabolite that are quantitatively or qualitatively abnormal may thus be estimated. In vitro comparison of the rates of reaction with and without addition of the deficient nutrient in a biologically active form may provide evidence of deficiency.

Few of the methods currently available are free from important criticism.

In the case of trace elements, such as zinc or chromium, interpretation of the data obtained by such techniques as atomic absorption spectrophotometry is also open to criticism, since matters of compartmental distribution and biological half-lives for all of them have yet to be established with confidence.

POPULATION STUDIES AND SURVEYS

A full description and evaluation of nutrition surveys applicable to groups would be out of context in this book. However, the value of surveys of populations from which patients are referred is to increase awareness of what sort of nutritional background may be anticipated, so that an appropriate history can be taken and potentially informative laboratory tests can be performed.

Techniques

Sources of information which are useful for assessment of nutritional status are shown in Table 1-7. It is apparent that what health professionals in clinical medicine need to know is derived from dietary surveys, food habits, anthropometric data, and clinical and laboratory nutrition surveys, but they should be familiar with local beliefs and prejudices and with fads about food, especially as they affect individuals at special risk of developing nutritional deficiencies, such as pregnant or lactating women, infants and preschool children, and, especially nowadays, adolescents.

In North America evidence of overt nutritional disease other than dental caries and obesity is uncommon, if we exclude chronic alcoholics. Depending on the ranges of normal values which are used, there is, however, a variable amount of subclinical nutritional deficiency which constitutes an iceberg phenomenon, and this, in terms of the impact of superimposed diseases, surgical interventions, or other traumas which are associated with reduction in intake of nutrients, or the impact of old age, may have great clinical importance.

Recent Findings in the United States

The Ten-State Nutrition Survey of 1968 to 1970 was conducted by a specially constituted nutrition program of the Department of Health, Education, and Welfare in response to direction by the U.S. Congress. The survey focused on low-income groups in the population of 10 states, but some higher-income groups were also included. The clinical evaluation of some 40,000 individuals of different age and sex was achieved. The greatest population was white, the next black, and the smallest Latin American.[41]

Evidence of nutritional deficiency correlated with low income, but despite low income levels, black children were found, in general, to be taller than white children and to have more advanced skeletal and dental development. This finding emphasizes the need to develop specific standards for black children, and possibly for other ethnic groups.

Evidence of iron-deficiency anemia was found in adolescent and adult males, and of low vitamin A nutriture in Mexican-Americans, especially in Texas. Low vitamin C levels were found in old people. Dietary histories of old people suggested the possibility of nutritional deficiencies, which did not express themselves clinically or biochemically, however. These results have been criticized on the grounds that little evidence of signs of clinical deficiency was revealed by the survey and that laboratory criteria of deficiency may need to be revised downward.

Subsequently, the first Health and Nutrition Examination Survey in the United States was conducted, starting in 1971, with the objective of assessing and monitoring the nutritional status of the U.S. population longitudinally. The nutrition survey is made up of four parts: (1) dietary intake based on a 24-hour recall and food-frequency questionnaire, (2) biochemical levels of various

TABLE 1-7
SOURCE OF INFORMATION FOR ASSESSMENT OF NUTRITIONAL STATUS

Source	Information	Nutritional implications	Population
Food balance sheets Agricultural data	Food production Cash crops Production of staples Food imports-exports	Food supplies available	National
Socioeconomic data Marketing Distribution Storage	Availability and distribution of foods	Unequal consumption by groups	Groups in the community
Cultural data and patterns of food consumption	Beliefs and prejudices Ignorance	Improper and underutilization	Groups Families Individuals
Dietary surveys Household surveys	Food consumption Distribution within the family Nutrient value Food preparation	Variations in consumption Distribution within the family	Groups Families Individuals
Vital statistics	Morbidity Mortality	Risks to community Identification of high-risk groups	National Regional
Clinical nutrition surveys	Signs of deficiency	Deficiency disease	Groups Individuals
Anthropometric studies	Physical development	Impaired development due to malnutrition	Groups Individuals
Laboratory tests	Levels of nutrients; nutrient-dependent metabolism in tissues	Nutrient supplies and metabolic function	Groups Individuals
Medical information	Epidemiological	Nutrition-disease interrelationships	National Regional Groups

Source: Derived from WHO Tech. Rep. Ser. no. 258, 1963.

nutrients based on assays of blood and urine samples, (3) clinical signs of possible nutritional deficiency disease (as observed by an examining physician), and (4) anthropometric measurements. A so-called national probability sample of 28,943 persons from the age of 1 to the age of 74 years was selected from 65 different locations in the 48 contiguous states. Results obtained, including information on methods, tables, a descriptive summary of the tables, and an index, were published in a series, *Advancedata from Vital and Health Statistics of the National Center for Health Statistics,* in order to make some of the data easily accessible in tabular and partly processed forms. Full data are available for further analysis to those with support staff and computer capability. To date, dietary intake, clinical and biochemical findings, anthropometric data, hemoglobin, serum iron and transferrin-saturation data, and serum cholesterol levels, all evaluated in relation to socioeconomic characteristics, are among the data that have been published in partly processed form. In addition, many medically related socioeconomic studies have been derived from the raw data, such as the use of medical and family planning services.

A system of risk categories is being developed in an attempt to estimate the sensitivity of clinical signs in detecting possible deficiencies and to determine how specific a sign is in indicating a specific nutrient deficiency [42]. Preliminary results suggest that high-risk signs of nutrient deficiency are rare, with the exception of papillary atrophy of the tongue and goiter. These were present to a significant degree in older black people. Moderate-risk signs suggesting, but not establishing, the presence of degrees of deficiencies of B-complex vitamins, ascorbic acid, vitamin A, vitamin D, and iodine were also more common in blacks than whites. An important result of the Survey was the identification of black women as a group at high risk of obesity.

Anyone interested in any aspects of these ongoing surveys should follow the publications of the National Center for Health Statistics.

REFERENCES

1 Fomon, S. J., and T. A. Anderson: *Practices of Low-Income Families in Feeding Infants and Small Children with Particular Attention to Cultural Subgroups,* Department of Health, Education, and Welfare, Public Health Service, Maternal and Child Health Services, Rockville, Md., 1972.

2 Queen, G. S.: Culture, economics and food habits, J. Am. Diet. Assoc., 33:1044, 1957.

3 Leevy, C. M., L. Cardi, O. Frank, R. Gellene, and H. Baker: Incidence and significance of hypovitaminemia in a randomly selected municipal hospital population, Am. J. Clin. Nutr., 17:259, 1965.

4 Weinsier, R. L., E. M. Hunker, C. L. Krumdieck, and C. E. Butterworth, Jr.: Hospital malnutrition: A prospective evaluation of general medical patients during the course of hospitalization, Am. J. Clin. Nutr., 32:418, 1979.

5 Marr, J. W.: Individual dietary surveys: Purposes and methods, World Rev. Nutr. Diet., 13:105, 1971.

6 Watt, B. K., and A. L. Merrill: *Composition of Foods, raw, processed, prepared,* U.S. Department of Agriculture Handbook no. 8, U.S. Government Printing Office, Washington, 1963.

7 Posati, L. P. and M. L. Orr: *Composition of Foods—raw, processed, prepared—Dairy and Egg Products,* U.S. Department of Agriculture Handbook no. 8-1, U.S. Government Printing Office, Washington, 1976.

8 Marsh, A. C., A. K. Moss, and E. W. Murphy: *Composition of Foods—raw, processed, prepared—Spices and Herbs,* U.S. Department of Agriculture Handbook no. 8-2, U.S. Government Printing Office, Washington, 1977.

9 Paul, A. A., and D. A. T. Southgate: *McCance and Widdowson's Composition of Foods,* 4th ed., 1978 and supplements.

10 Vilter, R. W., J. F. Mueller, H. S. Glazer, T. Jarrold, J. Abraham, C. Thompson, and V. R. Hankins: The effect of vitamin B_6 deficiency induced by desoxypyridoxine in human beings, J. Lab. Clin. Med., 42:335, 1953.

11 Moynahan, E. J.: Acrodermatitis enteropathica. A lethal inherited human zinc-deficiency disorder, Lancet, 2:399, 1974.

12 Crounse, R. G., A. J. Bollet, and S. Owens: Quantitative tissue of human malnutrition using scalp hair roots, Nature, 228:465, 1970.

13 Rodger, F. C., H. Scriduzzafao, A. D. Graves, and A. A. Fazal: A reappraisal of the ocular lesion known as Bitot's spot, Br. J. Nutr., 17:4, 1963.

14 Dixit, V. M.: Cause of depression in chronic scurvy, Lancet, 2:1077, 1979.

15 Silvis, S. E., and P. V. Paragas, Jr.: Paresthesia, weakness, seizures and hypophosphatemia in patients receiving hypoalimentation, Gastroenterology, 62:513, 1972.

16 Coursin, D. B.: Convulsive seizures in infants with pyridoxine deficient diet, J. Am. Med. Assoc., 154:406, 1954.

17 Manzoor, M., and J. Runcie: Folate responsive neuropathy, Br. Med. J., 1:11, 1976.

18 Badenoch, J.: Steatorrhea in the adult, Br. Med. J., 2:879, 1960.

19 Cooke, W. T.: The neurological manifestations of malabsorption, Postgrad. Med. J., 54:760, 1978.

20 Hodges, R. E., W. B. Bean, M. A. Ohlson, and R. Bleiler: Human pantothenic acid deficiency produced by omega-methyl pantothenic acid, J. Clin. Invest., 38:1421, 1959.

21 Garn, S.: Human biology and research in body composition, Ann. N.Y. Acad. Sci., 110:429, 1963.

22 Keys, A., and J. Brozek: Body fat in adult men, Physiol. Rev., 33:245, 1953.

23 Siri, W. E.: *Advances in Biological and Medical Physics,* Academic, New York, 1956, p. 239.

24 Anderson, E. C., and W. H. Langham: Estimation of total body fat from potassium-40 content, Science, 133:1917, 1961.

25 Frisancho, A. R.: Triceps skinfold and upper arm muscle size norms for assessment of nutritional status, Am. J. Clin. Nutr., 27:1052, 1974.

26 Mackenzie, T., G. Blackburn, and J. P. Flatt: Clinical assessment of nutritional status using nitrogen balance, Fed. Proc., 33:683, 1974.

27 Lee, H. A., and T. F. Hartley: A method of determining daily nitrogen requirements, Postgrad. Med. J., 51:441, 1975.

28 Viteri, F. E., and J. Alborado: The creatinine height index: Its use in the estimation of the degree of protein depletion and repletion in protein calorie malnourished children, Pediatrics, 46:696, 1970.

29 Schilling, R. F.: Intrinsic factor studies. II. The effect of gastric juice on the urinary excretion of radioactivity after the oral administration of radioactive vitamin B_{12}, J. Lab. Clin. Med., 42:860, 1953.

30 Smythe, P. M., G. G. Brereton-Styles, H. J. Grace, A. Mafoyane, M. Schonland, H. M. Coovadia, W. E. R. Loening, M. A. Parenb, and G. H. Vos: Thymolymphatic deficiency and depression of cell-mediated immunity in protein-calorie malnutrition, Lancet, 2:941, 1971.

31 Sellmeyer, E., E. Bhettay, A. S. Truswell, D. L. Meyers, and J. D. L. Hansen: Lymphocyte transformation in malnourished children, Arch. Dis. Child. 47:429, 1972.

32 Das, M., E. R. Stiehm, T. Borut, and S. A. Feig: Metabolic correlates of immune dysfunction in malnourished children, Am. J. Clin. Nutr. 30:1949, 1977.

33 Golden, M. H. N., A. A. Jackson, and B. E. Golden: Effect of zinc on thymus of recently malnourished children, Lancet, 2:1057, 1977.

34 Golden, M. H. N., B. E. Golden, P. S. E. G. Harland, and A. A. Jackson: Zinc and immunocompetence in protein-energy malnutrition, Lancet, 1:1226, 1978.

35 Gross, R. L., and P. M. Newberne: Role of nutrition in immunologic function, Physiol. Rev., 60:198, 1980.

36 Sirisinha, S., R. Suskinel, R. Edelman, C. Charupatana, and R. E. Olson: Complement and C3 proactivation levels in protein-calorie malnutrition, Lancet, 1:1016, 1973.

37 Sokal, J. E.: Measurement of delayed skin-test responses, N. Engl. J. Med., 293:501, 1975.

38 Bistrian, B. R., G. L. Blackburn, N. S. Scrimshaw, and J. P. Flatt: Cellular immunity in semi-starved states in hospitalized adults, Am. J. Clin. Nutr., 28:1148, 1975.

39 Souchon, E. A., E. M. Copeland, and P. Watson: Intravenous hyperalimentation as an adjunct to cancer chemotherapy with 5-fluorouracil, J. Surg. Res., 18:451, 1975.

40 Nair, K. S., and J. S. Garrow: Depression of cellular immunity as an index of malnutrition in surgical patients, Br. Med. J., 282:698, 1981.

41 *Highlights. Ten-State Nutrition Survey 1968–1970,* Department of Health, Education, and Welfare, Health Services and Mental Health Administration, Center for Disease Control, Atlanta, 1972.

42 Lowenstein, F. W.: Preliminary clinical and anthropometric findings from the first Health and Nutrition Survey, USA, 1971–1972, Am. J. Clin. Nutr., 29:918, 1976.

CHAPTER 2

TOOLS FOR NUTRITION COUNSELING

CONTENTS

INTRODUCTION

The amount of time the physician can spend with patients who require dietary counseling is limited. Fortunately, the patient can be referred to a registered dietitian (R.D.) for dietary assessment and information. The registered dietitian is well-prepared, from an educational and professional standpoint, to provide individualized, professional guidance to people in adjusting their daily food consumption to meet their health needs. A registered dietitian may be found in several settings: in a hospital or clinic, in a public health agency, or in private practice, relating to the medical community through referrals.

In dietetics, "tools of the trade" include a working knowledge of food composition, exchange lists, and food group guides. Recommended Dietary Allowances (RDAs) [1] and U.S. Recommended Daily Allowances (U.S. RDAs) are additional aids in the delivery of nutritional care. Some basic tools for planning an adequate diet and/or evaluating a diet are discussed in this chapter.

TABLES OF FOOD COMPOSITION

It is now over 100 years since the first food composition tables were published in 1878, by König in Germany. These were followed by the classic American tables compiled by Atwater and Woods in 1896. Food composition tables provide average nutrient values, based on quantitative analysis of many samples of each food item. Most include data for a minimum of five vitamins (ascorbic acid, vitamin A, thiamine, riboflavin, and niacin) and two or more minerals (calcium and iron) as well as for food energy, protein, carbohydrate, and lipid content (see Appendix 9).

The U.S. Department of Agriculture periodically issues food composition tables; the most recent major publication is Handbook No. 8, *Composition of Foods—Raw, Processed, Prepared* [2]. Handbook No. 8 is being updated, and sections are released as they are ready; "Cholesterol Content of Foods" [3] and "Vitamin E Content of Foods" [4] have already been released. USDA Handbook No. 456 [5] is based on Handbook No. 8 and presents values for foods in household measures (cups, tablespoons, etc.) rather than 100-g portions, thus making the information more accessible to the consumer.

EXCHANGE LISTS

Using tables of food composition to calculate nutrient intake from dietary histories or individual dietary patterns is very time-consuming unless a computer is used. A more convenient tool for the rapid estimation of calories, protein, fat, and carbohydrate in records of dietary intake is the system of exchange lists. The exchange lists were originally designed for use in the calculation of diabetic diets [6], but they have found widespread use in the calculation of other therapeutic diets, especially fat-restricted and weight-reduction diets. The exchange lists were recently updated and revised by committees from the American Diabetes Association, the American Dietetic Association, the National Institute of Arthritis, Metabolism, and Digestive Diseases, and the National Heart and Lung Institute of the U.S. Department of Health and Human Services [7]. These revised exchange lists stress foods of low-cholesterol and low-fat content with lower energy values.

The term *exchange* is used in the sense of "substitute." Each exchange list includes a number of measured foods of similar energy and nutritive value which can be substituted interchangeably in meal plans.

TABLE 2-1
NUTRIENT COMPOSITION OF EXCHANGE LISTS

Exchange list	Protein, g	Fat, g	Carbohydrate, g	Energy, kcal
List 1: Milk exchanges	8	Trace	12	80
List 2: Vegetable exchanges	2	—	5	25
List 3: Fruit exchanges	—	—	10	40
List 4: Bread exchanges	2	—	15	70
List 5: Meat exchanges	7	3	—	55
Medium-fat meat	—	Omit $\frac{1}{2}$ fat exchange		
High-fat meat	—	Omit 1 fat exchange		
List 6: Fat exchanges	—	5	—	45

The following six major exchange lists have been designated:

List 1: Milk exchanges (nonfat, low-fat, and whole milk)
List 2: Vegetable exchanges (all nonstarchy vegetables)
List 3: Fruit exchanges (all fruits and fruit juices)
List 4: Bread exchanges (bread, cereal, pasta, starchy vegetables, and prepared foods)
List 5: Meat exchanges (lean meat, medium-fat meat, high-fat meat, and other protein-rich foods)
List 6: Fat exchanges (polyunsaturated, saturated, and monounsaturated fats)

Table 2-1 summarizes the calorie, protein, fat, and carbohydrate values assigned to each exchange list. These figures are weighted averages for the various foods included in each list. The use of the exchange list on a national basis has simplified patient education and communication among health professionals. However, exchange lists are intended for use by the patients in consultation with a registered dietitian or other health professional. Unless patients receive guidance as to how to adjust for individual needs, exchange lists are not particularly useful.

Table 2-2 presents the foods included in each exchange list. The amount of each exchange for vegetables is ½ cup, and for meat is 1 oz. For each of the exchange lists, the specified amount varies with the food. The usual serving size for meat for menu planning is 3 or 4 oz; thus, three or four meat exchanges may be included in one serving. Starchy vegetables are included in the bread list. Sugar-rich foods (soft drinks, candies, cake, etc.) are not included in any of the exchange groups, since they should not be included in diets for people with diabetes. Table 2-3 gives exchange substitutions for high-sugar-content foods, and Table 2-4 gives additional diet exchanges for desserts.

One drawback to exchange lists is that many foods that are popular with particular ethnic groups, food "combinations," and commercially available foods cannot be correctly assigned to a single exchange list. Some food

(Text continues on p. 49.)

TABLE 2-2
EXCHANGE LISTS

List 1: Milk exchanges (includes nonfat, low-fat, and whole milk)

One exchange of milk contains 12 g carbohydrate, 8 g protein, a trace of fat, and 80 kcal. Those items in *italics* are nonfat.

Nonfat fortified milk
Skim or nonfat milk	1 cup
Powdered (nonfat dry, before adding liquid)	⅓ cup
Canned, evaporated skim milk	½ cup
Buttermilk made from skim milk	1 cup
Yogurt made from skim milk (plain, unflavored)	1 cup

Low-fat fortified milk
1% fat fortified milk (omit ½ fat exchange)	1 cup
2% fat fortified milk (omit 1 fat exchange)	1 cup
Yogurt made from 2% fortified milk (plain, unflavored) (omit 1 fat exchange)	1 cup

Whole milk (omit 2 fat exchanges)
Whole milk	1 cup
Canned, evaporated whole milk	½ cup
Buttermilk made from whole milk	1 cup
Yogurt made from whole milk (plain, unflavored)	1 cup

List 2: Vegetable exchanges

One exchange of vegetables contains about 5 g carbohydrate, 2 g protein, and 25 kcal. This list shows the kinds of vegetables to use for one vegetable exchange. 1 exchange = ½ cup. (Starchy vegetables are included in the bread exchange list.)

Asparagus	Greens:	Rhubarb
Bean sprouts	Beet	Rutabaga
Beets	Chards	Sauerkraut
Broccoli	Collards	String beans, green or yellow
Brussels sprouts	Dandelion	Summer squash
Cabbage	Kale	Tomatoes
Carrots	Mustard	Tomato juice
Cauliflower	Spinach	Turnips
Celery	Turnip	Vegetable juice cocktail
Cucumbers	Mushrooms	Zucchini
Eggplant	Okra	
Green pepper	Onions	

The following raw vegetables may be used as desired:

Chicory	Escarole	Radishes
Chinese cabbage	Lettuce	Watercress
Endive	Parsley	

List 3: Fruit exchanges

One exchange of fruit contains 10 g carbohydrate and 40 kcal.

Apple	1 small	Mango	½ small
Apple juice	⅓ cup	Melon	
Applesauce (unsweetened)	½ cup	Cantaloupe	¼ small
Apricots, fresh	2 medium	Honeydew	⅛ medium

TABLE 2-2 (Continued)

List 3: Fruit exchanges

Apricots, dried	4 halves	Watermelon	1 cup
Banana	½ small	Nectarine	1 small
Berries		Orange	1 small
Blackberries	½ cup	Orange juice	½ cup
Blueberries	½ cup	Papaya	¾ cup
Cranberries	*	Peach	1 medium
Raspberries	½ cup	Persimmon, native	1 medium
Strawberries	¾ cup	Pineapple	½ cup
Cherries	10 large	Pineapple juice	⅓ cup
Cider	⅓ cup	Plums	2 medium
Dates	2	Prunes	2 medium
Figs, fresh	1	Prune juice	¼ cup
Figs, dried	1	Raisins	2 tbsp
Grapefruit	½	Tangerine	1 medium
Grapefruit juice	½ cup		
Grapes	12		
Grape juice	¼ cup		

*May be used as desired if no sugar is added.

List 4: Bread exchanges (includes bread, cereal and starchy vegetables)

One exchange of bread contains 15 g carbohydrate, 2 g protein, and 70 kcal. Those items in *italics* are *low-fat*.

Bread
White (including French and Italian)	1 slice
Whole wheat	1 slice
Rye or pumpernickel	1 slice
Raisin	1 slice
Bagel, small	½
English muffin, small	½
Plain roll, bread	1
Frankfurter roll	½
Hamburger bun	½
Dried bread crumbs	3 tbsp
Tortilla, 6 in	1

Cereal
Bran flakes	½ cup
Other ready-to-eat unsweetened cereal	¾ cup
Puffed cereal (unfrosted)	1 cup
Cereal (cooked)	½ cup
Grits (cooked)	½ cup
Rice or barley (cooked)	½ cup
Pasta (cooked): spaghetti, noodles, macaroni	½ cup
Popcorn (popped, no fat added)	3 cups
Cornmeal (dry)	2 tbsp
Flour	2½ tbsp
Wheat germ	¼ cup

Crackers
Arrowroot	3
Graham, 2½ in square	2
Matzo, 4 × 6 in	½

TABLE 2-2 (Continued)

List 4: Bread exchanges (includes bread, cereal and starchy vegetables)

Oyster	20
Pretzels, 3⅛ in long × ⅛ in diameter	25
Rye wafers, 2 × 3½ in	3
Saltines	6
Soda, 2½ in square	4
Dried beans, peas, and lentils	
Beans, peas, lentils (dried and cooked)	½ cup
Baked beans (canned), no pork	¼ cup
Starchy vegetables	
Corn	⅓ cup
Corn on cob	1 small
Lima beans	½ cup
Parsnips	⅔ cup
Peas, green (canned or frozen)	½ cup
Potato, white	1 small
Potato (mashed)	½ cup
Pumpkin	¾ cup
Squash, winter, acorn, or butternut	½ cup
Yam or sweet potato	¼ cup
Prepared foods	
Biscuit, 2 in diameter (omit 1 fat exchange)	1
Corn bread, 2 × 2 × 1 in (omit 1 fat exchange)	1
Corn muffin, 2 in diameter (omit 1 fat exchange)	1
Crackers, round butter type (omit 1 fat exchange)	5
Muffin, plain small (omit 1 fat exchange)	1
Potatoes, french fried, length 2 to 3½ in (omit 1 fat exchange)	8
Potato or corn chips (omit 2 fat exchanges)	15
Pancake, 5 × ½ in (omit 1 fat exchange)	1
Waffle, 5 × ½ in (omit 1 fat exchange)	1

List 5: Meat exchanges

Lean meat: One exchange of lean meat (1 oz) contains 7 g protein, 3 g fat, and 55 kcal. Items in *italics* are *low-fat*.

Beef: Baby beef (very lean), chipped beef, chuck, flank steak, tenderloin plate ribs, plate skirt steak, round (bottom, top), all cuts rump, spare ribs, tripe	1 oz
Lamb: Leg, rib, sirloin, loin (roast and chops), shank, shoulder	1 oz
Pork: Leg (whole rump, center shank), ham, smoked (center slices)	1 oz
Veal: Leg, loin, rib, shank, shoulder, cutlets	1 oz
Poultry: Meat without skin of chicken, turkey, Cornish hen, guinea hen, pheasant	1 oz
Fish:	
Any fresh or frozen	1 oz
Canned salmon, tuna, mackerel, crab, and lobster	¼ cup
Clams, oysters, scallops, shrimp	5 or 1 oz
Sardines, drained	3
Cheeses containing less than 5% butterfat	1 oz
Cottage cheese, dry and 2% butterfat	¼ cup
Dried beans and peas (omit 1 bread exchange)	½ cup

Medium-fat meat: For each exchange of medium-fat meat omit ½ fat exchange.

Beef: Ground (15% fat), corned beef (canned), rib eye, round (ground commercial)	1 oz

TABLE 2-2 (Continued)

List 5: Meat exchanges	
Pork: Loin (all cuts tenderloin), shoulder arm (picnic), shoulder blade, Boston butt, Canadian bacon, boiled ham	1 oz
Liver, heart, kidney, and sweetbreads (these are high in cholesterol)	1 oz
Cottage cheese, creamed	¼ cup
Cheese: Mozzarella, ricotta, farmer's cheese, Neufchâtel	1 oz
Parmesan	3 tbsp
Egg (high in cholesterol)	1
Peanut butter (omit 2 additional fat exchanges)	2 tbsp
High-fat meat: For each exchange of high-fat meat omit 1 fat exchange.	
Beef: Brisket, corned beef (brisket), ground beef (more than 20% fat), hamburger (commercial), roasts (rib), steaks (club and rib)	1 oz
Lamb: Breast	1 oz
Pork: Spare ribs, loin (back ribs), pork (ground), country-style ham, deviled ham	1 oz
Veal: Breast	1 oz
Poultry: Capon, duck (domestic), goose	1 oz
Cheese: Cheddar types	1 oz
Cold cuts	4½ × ⅛ in slice
Frankfurter	1 small

List 6: Fat exchanges			

One exchange of fat contains 5 g fat and 45 kcal. To plan a diet low in saturated fat, select only those exchanges that appear in *italics* because they are *polyunsaturated*.

Margarine, soft, tube, or stick†	1 tsp	Butter	1 tsp
Avocado (4 in diameter)‡	⅛	Bacon fat	1 tsp
Oil: corn, cottonseed, safflower,		Bacon crisp	1 strip
soy, sunflower	1 tsp	Cream, light	2 tbsp
Oil, olive‡	1 tsp	Cream, sour	2 tbsp
Oil, peanut‡	1 tsp	Cream, heavy	1 tbsp
Olives‡	5 small	Cream cheese	1 tbsp
Almonds‡	10 whole	French dressing§	1 tbsp
Pecans‡	2 large whole	Italian dressing§	1 tbsp
Peanuts‡		Lard	1 tbsp
Spanish	20 whole	Mayonnaise§	1 tsp
Virginia	10 whole	Salad dressing,	2 tsp
Walnuts	6 small	mayonnaise type	2 tsp
Nuts, other‡	6 small	Salt pork	¾-in cube
Margarine, regular stick	1 tsp		

†Made with corn, cottonseed, safflower, soy, or sunflower oil only.
‡Fat content is primarily monounsaturated.
§If made with corn, cottonseed, safflower, soy, or sunflower oil, can be used on fat-modified diet.
Source: Adapted from Exchange Lists for Meal Planning, American Diabetes Association and American Dietetic Association, 1976.

TABLE 2-3
SUGARS AND SWEETS

	Amount	kcal	Equivalent fruit exchanges
Carbonated soft drink	8 oz	90	2
Chocolate, sweet	1 oz	147	3½
Honey	1 tbsp	64	1½
Jams, jellies, preserves	1 tbsp	55	1½
Syrup	1 tbsp	58	1½
Sugar	1 tbsp	46	1

TABLE 2-4
ADDITIONAL DIET EXCHANGES
Desserts

Food	Serving size	Exchanges per serving
Cookies		
Animal crackers	10	1 bread
Oreo, Hydrox	2	1 bread
Lorna Doone	3	1 bread + 1 fat
Ginger Snaps	3	1 bread
Fig Newton	1½	1 bread
Toll House (Nestlé 12-oz package)	2	1 bread
Ice cream (vanilla, chocolate, strawberry)	½ cup	1 bread + 2 fat
Ice milk	½ cup	1 bread + 1 fat
Ice cream cone (unfilled)	1	1 bread
Popsicle (twin)	3 oz	1 bread
Jelly beans	10	1 bread
Keebler tart shell	3 in	1 bread + 1 fat
Jello	¼ cup	1½ bread
Pie	⅙ pie	3 bread + 2 fat
Cake (average, iced)	⅛ cake	4 bread + 3 fat
Cake doughnut	1	1 bread + 1 fat
Glaced sweet roll	3 in	2½ bread + 1 fat
Sherbet	3 oz	2 fruit
Sugar	2 tsp	1 fruit
Syrup	1½ oz	3 fruit
Jelly	½ oz	1 fruit

TABLE 2-5
ADDITIONAL DIET EXCHANGES FOR MAIN DISHES AND MEAL ACCOMPANIMENTS

	Serving size	Exchanges per serving
Aunt Jemima		
French toast	2	1 meat + 1½ bread
Original waffles	2	1 bread + 1 fat
Betty Crocker		
Lasagna hamburger helper mix	⅕ package	2 bread
Creamy noodles 'n tuna		
hamburger helper mix	⅕ package	2 bread + 2 fat
Birdseye frozen vegetables		
French-style green beans with		
mushrooms	3 oz	1 vegetable
Mixed vegetables with onion sauce	2.6 oz	2 vegetable + 1 fat
Chinese-style vegetables	3.3 oz	1 vegetable
Mexican-style vegetables	3.3 oz	1 bread
French-fried potatoes	17 pieces	1½ bread + 1 fat
General Mills		
Bisquick	1 cup	4 bread + 2 fruit + 3 fat
Green Giant		
Frozen broccoli in cheese sauce	3½ oz	½ low-fat meat
Frozen creamed peas	3½ oz	1 bread + 1 fat
Heinz		
Beans, Boston style	¼ cup	½ meat + 1 bread
Beans and franks	¼ cup	1 meat + 1 bread + 1 fat
Beef stew	1 cup	1½ meat + 2 bread + ½ fat
Chicken stew with dumplings	1 cup	1 meat + 1 bread
Chili con carne with beans	1 cup	2 meat + 2½ bread + 1½ fat
Spaghetti in tomato sauce and		
cheese	1 cup	2 bread + 1 fat
Kraft		
Macaroni and cheese mix		
(prepared)	¾ cup	2 bread + ½ high-fat meat + 2 fat
American-style spaghetti		
dinner mix (prepared)	1 cup	3 bread + 1 fat
Blue-cheese dressing	1 tbsp	2 fat
Catalina French dressing	1 tbsp	1½ fat
Italian-style dressing	1 tbsp	2 fat
La Choy		
Beef chow mein	1 cup	1 meat + 1 vegetable
Fried rice	½ cup	2 bread
Shrimp chow mein	1 cup	½ meat + 1 bread
Minute		
Precooked rice mixes (beef-		
flavored, spanish, chicken-flavored)	½ cup	2 meat + 1 fat
Morton		
Beef dinner	1	4 meat + 1½ bread
Chicken pot pie	1	2 meat + 2½ bread + 3 fat
Fish dinner	1	3 meat + 2 bread

TABLE 2-5 (Continued)

	Serving size	Exchanges per serving
Fried chicken dinner	1	4 meat + $1\frac{1}{2}$ bread + $\frac{1}{2}$ fat
Turkey dinner	1	2 meat + $2\frac{1}{2}$ bread + 3 fat
Mrs. Paul's		
Frozen fish sticks	4 sticks	1 medium-fat meat + 1 bread
Ore-Ida		
Frozen onion rings	$2\frac{1}{2}$ oz	1 bread + 2 fat
Pepperidge Farm		
Butter crescent rolls	1 roll	1 bread + $1\frac{1}{2}$ fat
Club rolls	1 roll	2 bread
Twin french rolls	$\frac{1}{5}$ roll	1 bread
Stouffer's		
Chicken pie	1 pie (10 oz)	$2\frac{1}{2}$ meat + 3 bread + 4 fat
Escalloped chicken and noodles	$\frac{3}{4}$ cup	2 meat + 1 bread + 2 fat
Lasagna	$\frac{1}{4}$ package (8 oz)	3 meat + 2 bread

companies, however, publish information about the "exchange list" value of their products. Tables 2-5 and 2-6 provide additional exchange information for commercially available and "fast-food" products.

Individuals who consume alcohol may wish to substitute alcoholic beverages for other exchanges (see Table 2-7).

Since the exchanges focus on energy in the form of fat, protein, and carbohydrate, meals based on these lists may not provide adequate amounts of other essential nutrients. In nutrition education programs using the exchange system, the vitamin A and vitamin C content of fruits and vegetables must be stressed and food sources of other vitamins and minerals emphasized as well. The importance of making diversified choices within each group must also be explained. Generally, the exchange system has been very useful for planning diets for individuals with special needs, and it is usually easier to live with on a long-term basis than other diet plans.

FOOD GROUP GUIDES

Food-grouping systems are used to translate nutritional needs or nutritional standards like the Recommended Dietary Allowances into practical guidelines for food intake. Since people think of nutrition in terms of foods, instead of a list of amounts of required nutrients, food groups are designed so that individuals fulfilling the guidelines will consume adequate quantities of essential nutrients.

Both the United States and Canada until recently used the "basic-four" food group system. This system classified foods into the following four groupings: milk, meat, fruits and vegetables, and breads and cereals. It also established the

TABLE 2-6
ADDITIONAL DIET EXCHANGES FOR FAST-ORDER MEALS

Food	Exchanges per serving
Burger King	
Hamburger	$1\frac{1}{2}$ meat + $1\frac{1}{2}$ bread + $\frac{1}{2}$ fat
Whopper	3 bread + 3 meat + 4 fat
French fries	2 bread + $2\frac{1}{2}$ fat
Chocolate milk shake	$4\frac{1}{2}$ bread + $1\frac{1}{2}$ fat
Dairy Queen	
Small burger	1 meat + 2 bread + 1 fat
Double burger	2 meat + 2 bread + 1 fat
Kentucky Fried Chicken	
Original 3-piece dinner	4 bread + 6 meat + $2\frac{1}{2}$ fat
McDonald's	
Egg McMuffin	2 meat + $2\frac{1}{2}$ bread
Hamburger	1 meat + 2 bread + 1 fat
Quarter pounder	3 meat + 2 bread + 1 fat
Big Mac	3 meat + 3 bread + 3 fat
Filet O' Fish	2 meat + $2\frac{1}{2}$ bread + 2 fat
Pizza Hut	
Cheese pizza	
Individual	
Thick crust	$9\frac{1}{2}$ bread + $7\frac{1}{2}$ meat
Thin crust	$8\frac{1}{2}$ bread + 6 meat
$\frac{1}{2}$ of 13 in	
Thick crust	$7\frac{1}{2}$ bread + 7 meat
Thin crust	7 bread + 5 meat

TABLE 2-7
ALCOHOLIC BEVERAGES

Beverage	Amount, oz	Exchange
Beer	8	1 bread
Champagne	4	1 bread
Gin, dry	$1\frac{1}{2}$	1 bread + 1 fruit
Manhattan	$3\frac{1}{2}$	2 breads + $\frac{1}{2}$ fruit
Martini	$3\frac{1}{2}$	2 breads
Scotch	$1\frac{1}{2}$	$2\frac{1}{2}$ fruit
Vermouth, dry	$3\frac{1}{2}$	1 bread + 1 fruit
Wine, dry	$3\frac{1}{2}$	2 fruit

requirements for portion size and number of servings (see Table 2-8). Although there was only one group of fruits and vegetables in this food guide, the need to select dark-green leafy and deep-yellow vegetables for vitamin A and fruits or vegetables that are good sources of ascorbic acid was emphasized. The combination of the minimum number of servings from each food group was thought to provide a nutritionally balanced diet that approached the RDAs for protein, calcium, vitamin A, thiamine, riboflavin, niacin, and ascorbic acid. Adjustments in serving sizes could be made to meet the differing nutritional

TABLE 2-8
BASIC-FOUR FOOD GROUPS WITH NUTRIENT PATTERN AND RECOMMENDED QUANTITY

Nutrients	Quantity	Comments
Milk group		

Calcium
Protein
Phosphorus
Riboflavin
	Servings: Three or more for children, four or more for teenagers and pregnant or lactating women, two or more for adults
	Serving size:
	  Milk or yogurt, 8 oz
	  Cheese, 1 oz
	  Cottage cheese, ice cream, or
	  custard, 1½ cups
		Butter is not included in this group, as it is a fat and does not contain other essential nutrients.

Meat group		

Protein
B vitamins
Iron
	Servings: Two or more
	Serving size:
	  Meat, poultry, or fish, 3 oz
	  Eggs, 2
	  Peanut butter, 2 tbsp
	  Lentils or beans, ½ cup
		Legumes, nuts, and soy extenders can be substituted for meat, although the protein has a lower biological value than meat has. These foods can be combined with animal or grain products to increase protein quality.

Vegetable and fruit group		

Vitamin A
Vitamin C
Carbohydrate
(fiber)
Iron
	Servings: Four or more
	Serving size:
	  Vegetable or fruit, ½ cup
	  Citrus juice, 4 oz
	  Medium-size fruit, 1
	  Dark-green or yellow vegetables,
	  ½ cup
		One serving daily should be vitamin C–rich (e.g., citrus fruits). Vitamin A–rich foods (e.g., leafy green and yellow vegetables) should be consumed three to four times per week.

Grain group		

Carbohydrate
(fiber)
B vitamins
Iron
	Servings: Four or more
	Serving size:
	  Bread, 1 slice
	  Cereal, ½ cup
		Whole-grain and enriched products are recommended grain foods.

needs of nearly all individuals. Additional energy could be obtained by choosing more than the minimum number of servings from the four food groups. The requirement of premenopausal women for iron was not met by following the recommended amounts, since it is difficult to meet this requirement by eating only ordinary foods.

The basic-four food group guide was a nutrition education tool which provided both a plan for teaching consumers how to choose an adequate diet and an easy way to evaluate a day's meal pattern for healthy individuals. It was not designed to be an absolute measure of dietary quality. It was adapted to the usual dietary pattern in the United States and Canada and was recognized as not being applicable to subgroups who did not follow the usual pattern. A more serious criticism, which has made the basic-four food group system outmoded, is that changes in dietary concepts have occurred in response to current knowledge of the potential hazards of high consumption of animal fats. Further, the idea of the "prudent-diet," as well as economic pressures, has encouraged partial replacement of meat by vegetable protein. Milk should still be regarded as a valuable source of calcium and protein, but its use as whole milk rather than low-fat or non-fat milk should be discouraged.

In terms of practicality, a modified basic-four system has much to commend it, and it is to be hoped that similar ones which emphasize the prudent-diet concept will gain recognition.

RECOMMENDED DIETARY ALLOWANCES (RDAs)

The Recommended Dietary Allowances (RDAs) represent levels of nutrients and energy intake thought to be adequate for the nutritional needs of practically all healthy Americans. The levels are set by the Food and Nutrition Board of the National Research Council and are continually updated in accordance with the most current scientific research (see Appendix 8). RDAs are *not requirements;* requirements are actual physiological needs which differ for each individual. RDAs are best thought of as guidelines which have been set high enough to provide a margin of safety so that the actual needs of most healthy individuals are met. Furthermore, RDAs are best used to evaluate diets of groups of people and not diets of individuals. Assessment of the nutritional status of a particular person (as opposed to a population group) must be made on an individual basis using additional clinical and biochemical evidence (see Chapter 1). Some investigators have used *two-thirds* of the RDA as the breaking point between adequate and inadequate intake. This criterion is arbitrary and must be used cautiously to express dietary adequacy.

RDAs have been established for healthy persons, and they do not consider the needs of persons suffering from chronic disease or recovering from illness. Routine hospital menus are usually planned to meet the RDAs for adults, but they do not ensure adequate intake for all patients.

Moreover, the RDAs do not establish the proportion in which carbohydrate, fat, and protein should be consumed as sources of energy. RDAs are not established for all nutrients known to be essential to humans and it is even possible that some vital nutrients remain to be discovered. In the final analysis, however, it is helpful for health professionals to be familiar with the RDAs, as well as their uses and limitations, so that they can be used as tools in working with patients.

NUTRITION LABELING AND U.S. RECOMMENDED DAILY ALLOWANCES (U.S. RDAs)

Nutrition labeling of most foods is voluntary but is required by the Food and Drug Administration (FDA) for (1) products for which a nutritional claim is made (low-calorie, low in cholesterol), (2) products that have been fortified (when a nutrient not normally present in a food is added, such as vitamin D to milk), and (3) products that have been enriched (nutrients are added to replace those lost during processing, such as thiamine, riboflavin, niacin, and iron to wheat flour). Over 200 foods have an FDA *standard of identity,* which is a standard "recipe" specifying mandatory limits and ingredients in a food. The standards also allow for optional ingredients. The mandatory ingredients of a food with a standard of identity need not be listed on the label; however, optional ingredients must be listed. Margarine, ice cream, peanut butter, jelly, soda water, macaroni and noodle products, and mayonnaise are examples of foods with standards of identity.

Nutrition labeling must include the following information specified per serving size (Figure 2-1): the amount of protein, carbohydrate, and fat in grams;

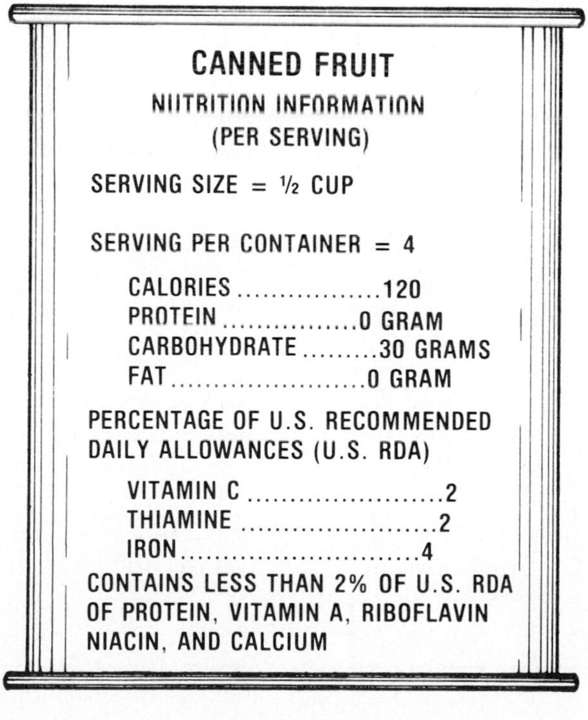

FIGURE 2-1
A nutrition label containing the minimum information allowed.

CANNED FRUIT

NUTRITION INFORMATION
(PER SERVING)

SERVING SIZE = ½ CUP

SERVING PER CONTAINER = 4

CALORIES 120
PROTEIN ....0 GRAM
CARBOHYDRATE ....30 GRAMS
FAT......................0 GRAM

PERCENTAGE OF U.S. RECOMMENDED
DAILY ALLOWANCES (U.S. RDA)

VITAMIN C 2
THIAMINE 2
IRON..........................4

CONTAINS LESS THAN 2% OF U.S. RDA
OF PROTEIN, VITAMIN A, RIBOFLAVIN
NIACIN, AND CALCIUM

the number of calories; and the percentage of the Recommended Daily Allowances (U.S. RDA) of 7 vitamins and minerals. Information for 12 other vitamins and minerals and for cholesterol, fatty acids, and sodium content is optional (Figure 2-2).

U.S. RDAs are the FDA's simplified version of the Recommended Dietary Allowances (RDAs) set by the Food and Nutrition Board in 1968. They replace the Minimum Daily Requirements (MDRs) previously used by the FDA in labeling. Actually, there are three sets of U.S. RDAs: (1) for adults and children over the age of 4 years, (2) for infants and children under the age of 4 years, and (3) for pregnant and lactating women. Those for infants and children are used on baby foods and special vitamin-mineral supplements for infants and small children. The most familiar are those used for adults and children over 4 years of age (Table 2-9). The U.S. RDA for a given nutrient is the highest RDA of that nutrient for children and adults, excluding pregnant and lactating women; thus, with a few exceptions, the RDA for 18-year-old males became the U.S. RDA.

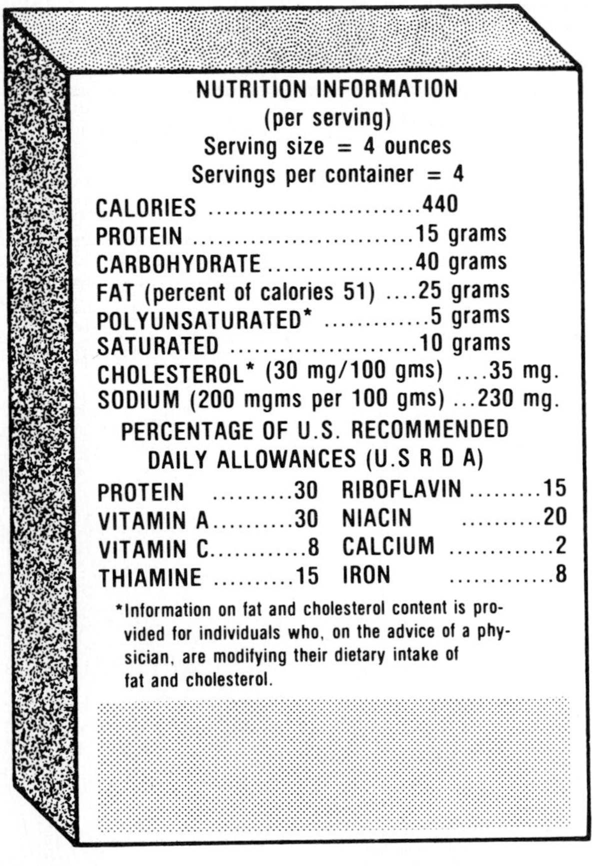

FIGURE 2-2
Label showing fatty acid and cholesterol declaration by standard format.

NUTRITION INFORMATION
(per serving)
Serving size = 4 ounces
Servings per container = 4

CALORIES 440
PROTEIN ....15 grams
CARBOHYDRATE ....40 grams
FAT (percent of calories 51) ....25 grams
POLYUNSATURATED* ....5 grams
SATURATED ....10 grams
CHOLESTEROL* (30 mg/100 gms) ....35 mg.
SODIUM (200 mgms per 100 gms) ...230 mg.

PERCENTAGE OF U.S. RECOMMENDED
DAILY ALLOWANCES (U.S R D A)

PROTEIN	30	RIBOFLAVIN	15
VITAMIN A	30	NIACIN	20
VITAMIN C	8	CALCIUM	2
THIAMINE	15	IRON	8

*Information on fat and cholesterol content is provided for individuals who, on the advice of a physician, are modifying their dietary intake of fat and cholesterol.

TABLE 2-9
U.S. RECOMMENDED DAILY ALLOWANCES
FOR ADULTS AND CHILDREN OVER 4 YEARS
OF AGE

Nutrients	U.S. RDA
Must be listed on label	
Protein	65 g*
Vitamin A	5000 IU
Vitamin C (ascorbic acid)	60.0 mg
Thiamine (vitamin B_1)	1.5 mg
Riboflavin (vitamin B_2)	1.7 mg
Niacin	20.0 mg
Calcium	1.0 g
Iron	18.0 mg
May be listed on label	
Vitamin D	400 IU
Vitamin E	30 IU
Vitamin B_6	2.0 mg
Folacin (folic acid)	0.4 mg
Vitamin B_{12}	6.0 μg
Phosphorus	1.0 g
Iodine	150 μg
Magnesium	400 mg
Zinc	15 mg
Copper	2.0 mg
Biotin	3.0 mg
Pantothenic acid	10.0 mg

*For proteins with a protein efficiency ratio (PER) less than that of casein (<2.5), the U.S. RDA is 65 g. For foods providing high-quality protein such as meat, fish, poultry, eggs, and milk (PER ⩾2.5), the U.S. RDA is 45 g. Proteins with a PER less than 20% that of casein may not be expressed on the label as a percent of U.S. RDA.
Source: Federal Register, 38(13), Jan. 19, 1973.

Examination of these standards reveals that for some age and sex groups, U.S. RDAs are even higher than the RDAs.

Eating 100 percent of the U.S. RDA for the 7 listed vitamins and minerals does not ensure an adequate diet, since these 7 are just a few of the more than 40 essential nutrients. In addition, the consumer must be conscious of the serving size for which the percent of U.S. RDAs is listed. The serving size may be much smaller or larger than that which is normally eaten.

Nutrition labeling is a relatively easy way for consumers to learn which foods are good sources of a particular nutrient, which foods provide the most nutrients for the money spent, and which foods provide the most nutrients in proportion to the energy content. Such labels can serve as guidelines for selection of a nutritionally balanced diet.

INDEX OF NUTRITIONAL QUALITY

Nutritionists at Utah State University have developed the Index of Nutritional Quality (INQ) to help quantify a "nutritious food" [8]. The INQ was developed to identify foods that have a beneficial nutrient:energy ratio, or nutrient:calorie ratio, relative to a standard. The INQ expresses nutrient density as a numerical ratio or a "bar" graph. The standard reference is an energy level of 1000 kcal. The reference values for adults for specific nutrients are the RDAs converted into an allowance per 1000 kcal (Table 2-10).

For example, a 1000-kcal portion of fluid whole milk contains 54 g protein, while 25 g is the suggested allowance for protein per 1000 kcal. The resultant INQ for milk protein, 2.2 (54/25) is independent of serving size.

By exploiting the INQ, an assessment of the ability of a food to meet dietary

TABLE 2-10
SINGLE-VALUE NUTRIENT ALLOWANCES PER
1000 kcal

Nutrient	Amount
Vitamin A	400 μg R.E.
Vitamin D	4 μg
Vitamin E	4 mg αT.E.
Vitamin C	30 mg
Thiamine	0.5 mg
Riboflavin	0.6 mg
Niacin	7 mg N.E.
Vitamin B_6	1.0 mg
Folacin	200 μg
Vitamin B_{12}	1.5 μg
Calcium	450 mg
Phosphorus	450 mg
Magnesium	150 mg
Iron	8 mg
Zinc	8 mg
Iodine	75 μg
Protein	25 g
Carbohydrate	137.5 g
Fat	39.0 g
Oleic acid	12.25 g
Linoleic acid	10.0 g
Saturated fatty acids	14.25 g

Source: R. G. Hansen and B. W. Wyse, J. Am. Diet.
Assoc., 76:223, 1980.

needs is possible. Indeed, an INQ equal to 1.0 or more for any nutrient indicates that the food has a beneficial nutrient-energy ratio for that particular nutrient. Moreover, this concept is particularly applicable to the formulation of weight-reduction diets.

"NORMAL" VERSUS "USUAL" DIETS

Dietary intake patterns and food habits vary widely from one nation to another as well as from individual to individual. There is no single diet pattern which must be followed to ensure adequate intake of nutrients. The essential nutrients are usually widely dispersed in nature and can be obtained from many combinations of foods.

In the United States, diet has changed markedly in this century (Figure 2-3). According to estimates made by the U.S. Department of Agriculture two major changes have occurred: (1) consumption of meat, poultry, fish, dairy products, sugar and other sweeteners, fats and oils, and processed fruits and vegetables has increased, and (2) consumption of grain products, potatoes and sweet potatoes, fresh fruit and vegetables, and eggs has decreased [9]. The current American diet is estimated to provide about 40 percent of the calories as fat, about 20 percent as sugar, 500 to 700 mg of cholesterol per day, and 8 to 10 g of salt [10].

FIGURE 2-3
Calories from energy-yielding nutrients (per capita civilian consumption). (*From L. Page and B. Friend, BioScience, 28; p. 196, 1978.*)

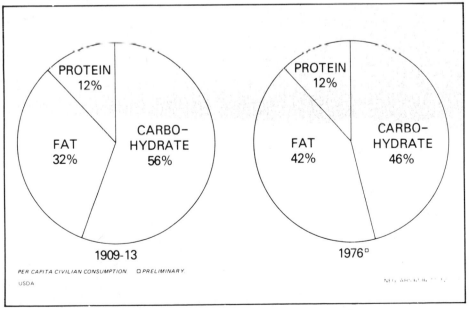

TABLE 2-11
DIETARY GOALS FOR THE UNITED STATES

1. To avoid overweight, consume only as much energy (calories) as is expended; if overweight, decrease energy intake and increase energy expenditure.

2. Increase the consumption of complex carbohydrates and "naturally occurring" sugars from about 28 percent to about 48 percent of energy intake.

3. Reduce the consumption of refined and other processed sugars by about 45 percent to account for about 10 percent of total energy intake.

4. Reduce overall fat consumption from approximately 40 percent to about 30 percent of energy intake.

5. Reduce saturated-fat consumption to account for about 10 percent of total energy intake and balance that with polyunsaturated and monounsaturated fats, which should account for about 10 percent of energy intake each.

6. Reduce cholesterol consumption to about 300 mg per day.

7. Limit the intake of sodium by reducing the intake of salt (sodium chloride) to about 5 g per day (2 g sodium).

Source: Select Committee on Nutrition and Human Needs, U.S. Senate, Dietary Goals for the United States, 2d ed., December 1977.

In 1977, responding to the concerns that these changes were not necessarily for the better and that overnutrition played a role in the etiology of coronary heart disease, obesity, cancer, and stroke, the Senate Select Committee on Nutrition and Human Needs [11,12] issued dietary goals for the United States. The goals stipulated that Americans should eat less food; they specifically stipulated that Americans should eat less fat, particularly saturated fat, less cholesterol, less sugar, and less salt and that they should increase their consumption of fruits, vegetables, grain products, and unsaturated oils (Table 2-11).

Implementation of the goals would require the following changes in food selection and preparation:

1 Increased consumption of fruits and vegetables and whole grains

2 Decreased consumption of meats and increased consumption of poultry and fish

3 Decreased consumption of foods high in fat and partial substitution of polyunsaturated fat for saturated fat

4 Substitution of nonfat milk for whole milk

5 Decreased consumption of butterfat, eggs, and other high-cholesterol sources

6 Decreased consumption of sugar and foods high in sugar

7 Decreased consumption of salt and of foods high in salt content

The dietary goals cannot be used to plan diets; they must be used in conjunction with dietary guidelines, such as the RDAs, in a planning scheme, such as the basic-four food groups (Table 2-8).

It is difficult to devise actual meal plans to take all goals into account and to maintain, at least initially, consumers' satisfaction with their meals. However, diets based on the dietary goals and RDAs have been published [13,14]. A day's food for an adult male (20 to 54 years old), as served, which complies with the goals and meets the RDAs for energy, vitamin A, thiamine, riboflavin, niacin, ascorbic acid, calcium, and iron is shown in Table 2-12.

Clearly, few people in the United States presently consume diets that are as high in carbohydrate content and as low in fat and sugar content as specified in the dietary goals. Between 1965 and 1975 changes in food consumption, as indicated by annual food disappearance data, of eggs, butter, lard, margarine, vegetable oils, vegetables, and fruit were in the direction set by the goals. Whether these trends will continue remains to be seen.

TABLE 2-12
SAMPLE MEALS FOR A DAY FOR A MAN AGED 20-64
MEETING THE DIETARY GOALS

Breakfast
   Cereal, 2 cups (with sugar*)
   Skim milk, 1 cup
   Toast, 3 slices
   Margarine*
   Juice, ½ cup
   Coffee or tea, if desired

Lunch
   Macaroni salad, 1 cup
    (contains macaroni, ⅓ egg, 2 tbsp kidney beans, salad oil)
   Vegetable, ½ cup
   Bread, 3 slices
   Margarine
   Milk, ½ cup

Dinner
   Lean meat, poultry, or fish,† 5 oz
   Potato, ½ cup
   Other vegetable or salad, ½ cup
   Bread, 3 slices
   Margarine
   Cake
   Coffee or tea, if desired

Snack
   Biscuits, 3
   Juice, ½ cup

   *About 2 tbsp of sugar or other sweets such as syrup, jams, and jellies and 3½ tbsp of fats and oils per day may be added to foods during preparation or at the table.
   †Meat and poultry (or fish) are served on alternate days.
   Source: B. Peterkin, The dietary goals and food on the table, Food Technol. 32:34, 1978.

VEGETARIAN DIETS

Health professionals are encountering increasing numbers of vegetarians, particularly young adults, who adopt this eating pattern out of philosophical and/or religious conviction. Most vegetarians believe that their dietary practices are more healthful, and there is some support in the scientific literature for this view. Vegetarians have been shown to have lower blood cholesterol levels than nonvegetarians [15], and the incidence of heart disease among vegetarian Seventh-Day Adventist males has been reported to be substantially less than that of the average male population in California [16].

Part of the cholesterol-lowering effect of a vegetarian regimen may be due to the tendency to consume less total fat, less saturated fat, more polyunsaturated fat, and less cholesterol than nonvegetarians [17]. Vegetarians usually consume more dietary fiber, and diets high in fiber content have been associated with reductions in blood cholesterol levels in controlled studies [18]. Vegetarians also have a decreased incidence of many cancers [19].

The types of vegetarianism are as diverse as the motivations of their adherents. Some individuals abstain only from red meat, or from red meat and poultry, while continuing to eat fish. Lacto-ovo-vegetarians will avoid flesh foods but consume milk, cheese, and eggs. Lacto-vegetarians eat milk and cheese but not eggs, and ovo-vegetarians eat eggs but no dairy products. Strict or pure vegetarians, or vegans, avoid all foods of animal origin.

Vegetarianism is a reason for clinical and nutritional concern when it is practiced in an extreme form and when it is implemented at an early age. Planning a nutritionally adequate diet is more difficult as food choices become more restrictive. The greatest risk results from undue reliance on a single plant food source. Infants and children on restrictive vegetarian diets are of particular concern because they are more likely to develop clinical deficiencies with symptoms and signs and may show slower rates of growth and development. For example, children with vitamin D and calcium deficiencies are especially prone to rickets [20].

A major nutritional concern has focused on the protein content of vegetarian diets. Vegan diets require careful planning to provide adequate supplies of lysine, tryptophan, and sulfur-containing amino acids, the amino acids generally lacking in plant foods. Wheat tends to be low in lysine and high in methionine, relative to the body's needs, while beans tend to be high in lysine and low in methionine. Combining wheat and beans in one dish or one meal is referred to as mutual supplementation of dietary proteins, or as utilizing the *complementary* value of proteins. Frances Lappe offers a guide to complementing proteins in *Diet for a Small Planet* [21]. Vegetarian diets rely heavily on four groups of plant foods: legumes (including beans and peas), grains and cereals, fruits and vegetables, and nuts and seeds. Legumes are a good source of tryptophan and the sulfur-containing amino acids. Nuts and seeds and, generally speaking, cereal grains are good sources of tryptophan and sulfur-containing amino acids, but they are low in lysine. The food patterns of many cultures combine these effectively: the lentils and rice of India, the corn, beans, and rice of Mexico, and the soybean products and rice of Asian countries are examples that have been emulated by many American vegetarians. The North American practices of eating cereal with milk, macaroni with cheese, and a peanut butter sandwich with milk combine plant and animal sources of protein. These practices provide all the essential amino acids in one meal. Meat, therefore, is not essential as a source of dietary protein.

Other nutrients likely to be of marginal content in all-plant diets are vitamin B_{12}, vitamin D for children not exposed to sunlight, riboflavin, calcium (especially for children and women), and iron for women of childbearing age. Vitamin B_{12} is of special concern for the vegetarian, since it is found only in foods of animal origin. Milk and eggs are satisfactory sources, but the vegan should consume vitamin B_{12}–fortified soybean milk or a vitamin B_{12} supplement. Recently, some packaged cereals have been fortified with this vitamin.

Enough vitamin B_{12} will have been stored in the liver of an adult who has eaten animal products from birth to last many years should he or she become a strict vegetarian; it would be years before signs of deficiency appeared. However, since vitamin B_{12} deficiency can severely damage the nervous system, a strict vegetarian is well advised to consume a source of vitamin B_{12}.

Adequate riboflavin and calcium can be provided by generous servings of most green leafy vegetables. A lacto-vegetarian would obtain most of the adult RDA for calcium from two servings of milk and cheese, but a vegan would need regular servings of dried beans, certain seeds such as sesame seeds, and certain nuts such as almonds to obtain the same amount of calcium. Soybean milk also contributes calcium and vitamin D (see Table 2-13).

Although iron in meats is better absorbed than iron in plant foods, studies of vegetarians have shown no greater incidence of iron-deficiency anemia among strict vegetarians than among nonvegetarians [22] Many beans, seeds, nuts, green leafy vegetables, dried fruits, and grain products supply iron. Foods that might be included in vegetarian diets as sources of iron are listed in Table 2-13.

Williams has compared the percentage of total calories from protein, fat, and carbohydrate in a sample lacto-ovo-vegetarian menu as compared to a typical nonvegetarian menu (Table 2-14). The total calories and calories per meal are essentially the same in both of the menus, but the percentage of the calories from carbohydrate is higher (55 percent versus 45 percent) and from fat lower (32 percent versus 43 percent) in the vegetarian menu. In planning the nonvegetarian menu, Williams made no attempt to plan an "adequate diet"; instead the menu is patterned after the choices that many Americans make every day. It is high in fat, sugar, and salt and low in several nutrients, including calcium and iron.

Vegetarian diets can be nutritionally adequate and appealing to the palate. Health professionals must be ready and willing to help vegetarians obtain the necessary information to plan adequate diets.

TABLE 2-13
SOME VEGETARIAN SOURCES OF CALCIUM AND IRON

	Calcium, mg	Iron, mg
Beans		
Navy beans (cooked), ½ cup	48	2.5
Seeds		
Mature soybeans (cooked), ½ cup	37	1.3
Nuts		
Sesame seeds (whole), ½ cup	1160	10.5
Sesame seeds (hulled), ½ cup	110	2.4
Almonds, ½ cup	166	3.3
Soybean milk, 1 cup	60	1.5
Vegetables		
Spinach (cooked), ½ cup	*	2.0
Beet greens (cooked), ½ cup	*	1.4
Dandelion greens (cooked), ½ cup	126	1.6
Kale (cooked), ½ cup	74	0.6
Mustard greens (cooked), ½ cup	97	1.3
Collards (cooked), ½ cup	126	0.8
Broccoli (cooked), ½ cup	144	0.6
Dried fruits		
Dried apricots (cooked), ½ cup	25	2.0
Dried figs (uncooked), 1 large	26	0.6
Prunes (uncooked), 4	14	1.1
Raisins, ½ oz	9	0.5
Cereals and breads		
Rice, brown (cooked), ⅔ cup	7	0.3
Oatmeal (cooked), 1 cup	22	1.4
Wheat germ, ¼ cup	18	2.4
Whole wheat bread, 1 slice	25	0.8

*Calcium in spinach and beet greens is present as insoluble calcium oxalate and cannot be absorbed.

Source: Adapted from E. R. Williams, Making vegetarian diets nutritious, Am. J. Nursing, 75: 2168, 1975.

TABLE 2-14
SAMPLE MENUS: LACTO-OVO-VEGETARIAN AND TYPICAL AMERICAN

	Calories	Protein, g	Fat, g	Carbohydrate, g
Lacto-ovo-vegetarian				
Breakfast*				
Orange juice, ½ cup	60	1	tr†	15
Oatmeal (cooked), 1 cup	130	5	2	23
Honey, 1 tsp	22	tr	0	6
Skim milk, 1 cup	90	9	tr	12
Whole wheat toast, 1 slice	60	3	1	12
Peanut butter, 1 tbsp	95	4	8	3
Hot cereal beverage	0	0	0	0
Total	457	22	11	71
Lunch				
Meatless split-pea soup, 1 cup	145	9	3	21
Sandwich				
Whole wheat bread, 2 slices	120	6	2	24
Cheddar cheese, 1 oz	115	7	9	1
Mayonnaise, ½ tbsp	33	tr	3	1
Lettuce leaves, 2	10	1	tr	2
Raw green pepper, ½ pod	7	tr	tr	2
Raw apple	70	tr	tr	18
Fig bars, 2	100	2	2	22
Whole milk, 1 cup	160	9	9	12
Total	760	34	28	103
Dinner				
Spanish soybeans over rice and bulgur‡	461	18	17	61
Spinach and mushroom salad				
Raw spinach, 1 cup	13	1	tr	2
Oil in dressing, 1 tbsp	125	0	14	0
Skim milk yogurt, 1 cup	125	8	4	13
Raw peach, 1	35	1	tr	10
Apple juice, 1 cup	120	tr	tr	30
Mushrooms, ⅓ cup	9	1	tr	1
Total	878	29	35	117
Grand total	2095	85	74	291
% of total calories §		16%	32%	55%
Typical American				
Breakfast				
Orange juice, ½ cup	60	1	tr	15
Egg (scrambled), 1	110	7	8	1
Bacon, 2 slices	90	5	8	1
Toast, 1 slice	60	3	1	12
Butter, 1 pat	35	tr	4	tr
Jelly, 1 tbsp	50	tr	tr	13

TABLE 2-14   (Continued)

	Calories	Protein, g	Fat, g	Carbohydrate, g
Typical American				
Coffee, 1 cup				
(Cream, 1 tbsp)	30	1	3	1
(Sugar, 1 tsp)	13	0	0	4
Total	448	17	24	47
Lunch				
Chicken noodle soup, 1 cup	220	8	6	33
Sandwich				
White bread, 2 slices	120	6	2	24
Bologna, 2 slices	80	3	7	tr
Mayonnaise, ½ tbsp	33	tr	3	1
Lettuce leaves, 2	10	1	tr	2
Potato chips, 10	115	1	8	10
Chocolate chip cookie, 1	50	1	2	7
Soft drink, 12 oz	145	0	0	37
Total	773	20	28	114
Dinner				
Ground beef, 3 oz	245	21	17	0
Mashed potatoes, ½ cup	93	2	4	12
Green peas, ½ cup	58	5	1	10
Iceberg lettuce wedge	15	1	tr	3
Blue-cheese dressing, 1 tbsp	75	1	8	1
Apple pie, 1 slice	350	3	15	51
Coffee, 1 cup				
(Cream, 1 tbsp)	30	1	3	1
(Sugar, 1 tsp)	13	0	0	4
Total	879	34	48	82
Grand total	2100	71	100	243
% of total calories §		13%	43%	45%

*Vegetarian breakfast from U. D. Register and L. M. Sonnenberg, The vegetarian diet: Scientific and practical considerations, J. Am. Diet. Assoc., 62:253, 1973.

†tr = trace.

‡Recipe (1/8) from F. M. Lappe, Diet for a Small Planet, rev. ed., Ballantine, New York, 1975.

§Values total over 100% because figures are rounded.

Source: E. R. Williams, Making vegetarian diets nutritious, Am. J. Nursing, 75:2168, 1975.

REFERENCES

1 *Recommended Dietary Allowances,* 9th ed., National Academy of Sciences, Food and Nutrition Board, Washington, 1980.

2 Watt, B. K., and A. L. Merrill: Handbook no. 8, Composition of Foods—raw, processed, prepared, U.S. Government Printing Office, Washington, 1963.

3 Feeley, R. M., P. E. Criner, and B. K. Watt: Cholesterol content of foods, J. Am. Diet. Assoc., 61:134, 1972.

4 McLaughlin, P. J., and J. L. Weihrauch: Vitamin E content of foods, J. Am. Diet. Assoc., 75:647, 1979.

5 Adams, C. F.: *Nutritive Value of American Foods in Common Units,* Department of Agriculture Handbook 456, U.S. Government Printing Office, Washington, 1975.

6 American Diabetes Association and American Dietetic Association: *Meal Planning with Exchange Lists,* American Dietetic Association, Chicago, 1950.

7 American Diabetes Association and American Dietetic Association: *Exchange Lists for Meal Planning,* American Diabetes Association, Chicago, 1976.

8 Hansen, R. G., and B. W. Wyse: Expression of nutrient allowances per 1,000 kilocalories, J. Am. Diet. Assoc., 76:223, 1980.

9 Page, L., and B. Friend: The changing United States diet, Bioscience, 28:192, 1978.

10 Hegstead, D. M.: Dietary goals—a progressive view, Am. J. Clin. Nutr., 31:1504, 1978.

11 Select Committee on Nutrition and Human Needs, U.S. Senate: *Dietary Goals for the United States,* U.S. Government Printing Office, Washington, February, 1977.

12 Select Committee on Nutrition and Human Needs, U.S. Senate: *Dietary Goals for the United States,* 2d ed., U.S. Government Printing Office, Washington, December, 1977.

13 Peterkin, B.: The dietary goals and food on the table, Food Technol., 32:34, 1978.

14 Dwyer, J: Diets for children and adolescents that meet dietary goals, Am. J. Dis. Child, 134:1073, 1980.

15 Hardinge, M. G., and F. J. Stare: Nutritional studies of vegetarians 2. Dietary and serum levels of cholesterol, Am. J. Clin. Nutr., 2:83, 1954.

16 Phillips, R. L., F. R. Lemon, W. L. Beeson, and J. W. Kuzma: Coronary heart disease mortality among Seventh-Day Adventists with differing dietary habits: Preliminary report, Am. J. Clin. Nutr., 31:S191, 1978.

17 Hardinge, M. G., H. Crooks, and F. J. Stare: Nutritional studies of vegetarians 4. Dietary fatty acids and serum cholesterol levels, Am. J. Clin. Nutr., 10:516, 1962.

18 Grande, F., J. T. Anderson, and A. Keys: Effect of carbohydrates of leguminous seeds, wheat, and potatoes on serum cholesterol concentrations in man, J. Nutr., 86:313, 1965.

19 Phillips, R. L.: Role of life-style and dietary habits in risk of cancer among Seventh-Day Adventists, Cancer Res., 35:3513, 1975.

20 Erhard, D.: The new vegetarians part one—vegetarianism and its medical consequences, Nutr. Today, 8:4, Nov.–Dec., 1973.

21 Lappe, F. M.: *Diet for a Small Planet,* rev. ed., Ballantine Books, New York, 1975.

22 Hardinge, M. G., and F. J. Stare: Nutritional studies of vegetarians 1. Nutritional physical and laboratory studies, Am. J. Clin. Nutr., 2:73, 1954.

CHAPTER 3

NUTRITIONAL SUPPORT: SUPPLEMENTAL, ENTERAL, AND PARENTERAL

CONTENTS

INTRODUCTION

When the conventional foods and beverages consumed do not meet an individual's nutrient requirements, a nutritional supplement may be necessary to augment nutrient intake. For some patients who are unable to eat a normal diet, a conventional diet can be modified so that it can be fed through a small-bore feeding tube, or commercially available defined formula diets can be administered in that way. Other patients with disorders of the gastrointestinal tract who are unable to absorb an oral diet efficiently need partial or complete nourishment via the parenteral route. The indications, principles, and techniques that are necessary for rational and adequate nutritional support by other than conventional means are discussed below.

ORAL NUTRITIONAL SUPPLEMENTS

A supplement is usually a commercially formulated liquid or powder containing one or more nutrients in a concentrated form. Most supplements are nutritionally incomplete and should be used in conjunction with the regular diet of patients who cannot eat enough to meet nutrient needs. The patient's requirements may be normal, as in the case of poor appetite or problems of mastication, or increased, as in sepsis or with severe burns or other excessive tissue damage. Some supplements may be ingested between meals, or with meals, in place of low-caloric beverages. Others may be added to food or beverages to increase nutrient density. Modular supplements provide a single nutrient (carbohydrate, fat, or protein) and may be mixed with food, beverages, or other liquid formulas to increase the intake of that nutrient and/or the caloric density.

Supplemental feedings should not be used as a replacement for food. The objective is to encourage the patient to return to a normal diet as quickly as possible. Snacks (milk shakes, sandwiches, etc.) should be used instead of supplemental feedings when possible. Many of these products are excessively sweet, so that many patients object to their use over an extended period. Some products supply only certain nutrients; others meet the National Research Council's Recommended Dietary Allowances (RDAs) for vitamins and minerals if used in specified amounts. See Tables 3-1 and 3-2 for specific nutritional information about these products.

Examples of nutritional supplements include the following:

Sustacal Liquid: A palatable, lactose-free, high-protein, nutritionally complete formula that can be drunk or given by tube.

Sustacal Powder: A milk-based, high-protein powder which can be mixed with milk.

Meritene: A palatable, milk-based, high-density, nutritionally complete formula sometimes used as a between-meal supplement but which may be used as a complete diet for tube feeding.

Carnation Instant Breakfast: A low-cost, palatable, oral supplement which provides one-third of the National Research Council's RDAs when mixed with 8 oz of whole milk at recommended dilutions.

Delmark Eggnog: A high-calorie, high-protein, palatable supplement when mixed with whole milk.

Hepatic Aid: A low-protein soluble powder that must be mixed with water. It contains controlled amounts of branched-chain and aromatic amino acids for use in patients with liver disease. Each packet contains 560 kcal, 14.5 g protein, and no vitamins, electrolytes, or indigestible fiber.

Amin-Aid: A low-protein water-soluble powder specifically formulated for use in patients with renal failure. Each package contains the minimum daily requirement for the eight essential amino acids plus 0.25 g of histidine and provides 0.8 g of nitrogen and 680 kcal. Amin-Aid contains no vitamins and no indigestible fiber. This product is very hypertonic and should be administered cautiously. It is expensive.

Examples of modular calorie supplements include the following:

MCT oil: A high-calorie (115 kcal/tbsp) supplement consisting of triglycerides of medium-chain (8 to 10 carbons in length) fatty acids. It does not contain essential fatty acids. Medium-chain triglycerides require less enzymatic and bile salt action for digestion than conventional long-chain fatty acids and are transported directly to the liver by the portal circulation. Absorption of conventional fats in foods requires intestinal micellar formation and a chylomicron transport mechanism via the lymphatics. MCT facilitates the nutritional management of a variety of disorders characterized by impaired hydrolysis and absorption of dietary fat. The recommended dosage is 3 or 4 tbsp daily. A dietitian should be consulted, since MCT oil is usually mixed with foods and beverages.

Microlipid: A safflower oil emulsion which is a concentrated fat source of calories, containing 135 kcal per 2 tbsp. Microlipid contains essential fatty acids and may be used to meet the fatty acid requirements of patients receiving intravenous parenteral nutrition who can absorb ingested fat.

Polycose: A carbohydrate supplement which consists of glucose polymers from hydrolyzed corn starch. It contains 2 kcal/ml. Polycose is low in electrolytes and can be easily mixed with many foods and beverages to increase the caloric density of the diet without significantly increasing the volume of the diet.

TUBE FEEDING

Patients who will not or cannot eat but have a functioning gastrointestinal tract are candidates for tube feeding. The diet fed can be a conventional diet which has been processed in a food blender or a liquid diet designed to provide essential nutrients in a form that will easily pass through a tube.

Indications and Patient Selection

Initial steps in identifying patients in need of total or supplemental nutritional support are an appropriate medical history, a dietary review, and a physical examination. Those with anorexia due to chronic illnesses or neoplastic disease, those who have just experienced trauma or major burns, and those who are about to undergo or who have just undergone surgery to the head and neck for

(*Text continues on p. 72.*)

TABLE 3-1
NUTRITIONAL SUPPLEMENTS
(Nutritional Analysis per 100 ml)

	Instant breakfast* (Carnation)	Eggnog* (Delmark)	Sustacal powder* (Mead Johnson)	Amin-Aid† (McGaw)	Hepatic Aid† (McGaw)
Protein					
g	5.66	6.25	8.1	1.94	4.26
% of calories	21.0	21.0	24.0	4.0	10.4
Sources	Nonfat dry milk Whole milk	Nonfat dry milk Whole milk Egg white and yolk solids	Nonfat milk Whole milk	Essential amino acids includes 0.074 g of histidine	Essential and non-essential amino acids
Carbohydrate					
g	13.2	15.42	18.2	32.4	28.7
% of calories	50.0	51.0	54.0	64.0	69.8
Sources	Sucrose Corn syrup solids Lactose	Whole milk Nonfat dry milk Maltodextrin Sugar	Sucrose Corn syrup solids Lactose	Maltodextrin Sucrose	Maltodextrin Sucrose
Lactose, g	9.0	NA	11.6	0	0
Fat					
g	3.0	3.75	3.3	7.03	3.6
% of calories	26.0	28.0	22.0	32.0	19.8
Sources	Whole milk	Whole milk Egg yolk solids Soybean oil Cottonseed oil	Milk fat	Soybean oil	Soybean oil
Calories	106	121	133	200	164
Nitrogen-total calorie ratio, g:kcal	1:117	1:121	1:103	1:802	1:254
Nitrogen-nonprotein calorie ratio, g:kcal	1:92	1:95	1:78	1:254	1:226

TABLE 3-1 (Continued)

	Instant breakfast* (Carnation)	Eggnog* (Delmark)	Sustacal powder* (Mead Johnson)	Amin-Aid† (McGaw)	Hepatic Aid† (McGaw)
Osmolality, mOsm/kg H_2O	677	NA	756	900	900
Minerals					
-Sodium, mg (meq)	91.0 (4.0)	91.7 (3.98)	122.2 (5.3)	< 0.6 meq	Trace
-Potassium, mg (meq)	276.0 (7.1)	262.5 (6.73)	340.0 (8.7)	< 0.6 meq	Trace
Comments	Milk-based powder Three envelopes provide: 100% RDAs for vitamins and minerals Flavors: Vanilla Strawberry Chocolate malt Coffee Eggnog	Milk-based powder Flavors: Orange	High-protein powder 803 ml provides: 100% RDAs for vitamins and minerals Flavors: Vanilla Chocolate	High-calorie essential amino acid powder Low in protein and electrolytes Recommended for use in renal failure Flavors: Berry Strawberry Orange	High-calorie amino acid powder (high in branch-chain and low in aromatic amino acids) Recommended for use in liver failure Flavors: Chocolate Eggnog Custard

*Mixed with whole milk as directed.
†Mixed with water as directed.
Note: NA, data not available.

TABLE 3-2

MODULAR SUPPLEMENTS

(Nutritional Analysis per 100 ml or tbsp)

	Carbohydrate modules				Fat modules		Protein module
	Polycose liquid (Ross)	Polycose powder (Ross)	Hy Cal (Beechum)	Cal Powder (General Mills)	MCT oil (Mead Johnson)	Microlipid (Organon)	Casec (Mead Johnson)
Amount	100 ml	1 tbsp (8 g)	100 ml	100 ml	100 ml	100 ml	1 tbsp (4.7 g)
Protein							
g	0	0	Trace	0	0	0	4.1
Source			NA				Calcium caseinate
Carbohydrate							
g	50	7.5	60.2	62.5	0	0	0
Source	Glucose polymers	Glucose polymers	Glucose	Glucose			
Fat							
g	0	0	Trace	0	93.3	50.0	Trace
Source			NA		Fractionated coconut oil	Safflower oil Monoglycerides and diglycerides Soy lecithin	Milk fat
Calories, kcal	200	32	295	228	774 (2 kcal/ml)	450	17
Osmolality, mOsm/kg H_2O	847	NA	2781	NA, varies with flavor	598	32	NA
Minerals							
Sodium, mg (meq)	62.0 (2.7)	8.8 (0.38)	8.3 (0.36)	26.0 (1.1)	0	0	7.1 (0.3)
Potassium, mg (meq)	5.39 (0.13)	3.1 (0.08)	0.6 (0.02)	13.0 (0.33)	0	0	NA

Note: NA, data not available.

TABLE 3-3

INDICATIONS FOR TUBE FEEDING

Neurological or psychiatric
Central nervous system disorders
Cerebrovascular accidents
Neoplasms
Severe depression
Anorexia

Oropharyngeal or esophageal
Neoplasms
Trauma or fractures
Head and neck irradiation
Palliative chemotherapy

Gastrointestinal
Chronic pancreatitis
Inflammatory bowel disease
Short-bowel syndrome
Neonatal intestinal diseases
Malabsorption
Preoperative bowel preparation
Fistulas

Burns

Chemotherapy or radiotherapy

Renal failure

Hepatic failure

malignant disease are obvious candidates for tube feedings; however, many apparently well-nourished individuals undergo subtle changes in nutritional status following an acute illness. Nutritional assessment that includes measurement of both anthropometric and biochemical parameters should be used to identify patients who need nutritional intervention (see Chapter 1).

Next, the appropriate route of delivery must be determined. Ideally, the oral route is preferred, but in many instances, the patient is unable to swallow or is unable to meet his or her increased metabolic requirements orally. Table 3-3 lists clinical situations in which administration of nutrients by tube is indicated. Even the unconscious patient, in whom the protective gag reflex is absent, may be safely nourished via a nasogastric tube if carefully monitored [1]. Tube feedings are generally contraindicated in patients who can be fed by mouth or in patients with adynamic ileus, intestinal obstruction, intractable vomiting, and proximal high-output enterocutaneous fistulas.

Tube Feeding Routes

The feeding tube can be inserted through the nares, and food administered by the nasogastric, nasoduodenal, or nasojejunal routes, or after an esophagostomy, gastrostomy, or jejunostomy the tube can be inserted through the respective surgically created opening into the stomach or jejunum and food administered through these routes.

Intubation by the nasogastric route is the simplest and most widely used approach to enteral feeding. The technique imposes negligible trauma, requires a minimum of equipment, and is rapid and relatively safe. The disadvantage is that the tube can be readily removed by the disoriented or uncooperative patient. Small-bore (5 through 9 French) flexible tubes made from silicone or polyurethane are readily inserted, and placement can be confirmed without much difficulty. Confirmation of the position of the tube in the stomach is achieved by (1) aspirating the gastric contents, (2) listening with a stethoscope over the epigastrium while injecting air through the tube, and (3) in doubtful cases, in which the gag reflex is absent, taking a chest x-ray which includes the diaphragm.

Nasoenteric tube placement generally requires the use of a longer mercury-weighted feeding tube which is initially placed in the stomach and passes into the intestine by peristalsis. This passage requires time but usually occurs within 24 hours in most patients [2]. Confirmation of tube placement can be made by x-ray examination.

Feeding ostomies are done by surgical insertion. They are indicated when an obstruction in the mouth, pharynx, or esophagus makes insertion through the nares impossible or when long-term feeding is anticipated. Ostomies are also invisible between feeds when the patient is dressed.

A cervical esophagostomy is a surgically created, skin-lined canal at the lower border of the neck which extends to just below the cervical esophagus. The feeding tube is passed through this opening into the stomach for each feed and is removed after the feed. Since the tube does not remain in place permanently, erosions of the esophagus are minimal and there are no problems of drainage of gastrointestinal secretions, which can cause skin excoriation [3].

Gastrostomy tube placement bypasses the intrathoracic part of the gastrointestinal tract. Foodstuffs are fed via a French catheter (no. 20 through no. 26 in caliber) inserted through the anterior abdominal wall directly into the stomach, which allows the foodstuffs full access to the digestive and absorptive processes. The major complications are reflux aspiration and peritonitis. Dumping (see Chapter 15) may occur if the gastrostomy tube is passed in error through the pylorus and the patient is fed as if it were in the stomach [4].

Some patients have problems which preclude access to the stomach, such as gastric cancer, peptic ulcer, or chronic nausea and vomiting. Jejunostomies must be handled carefully because volume, rate of feeding, and osmolality must be considered. An important advantage of jejunostomy feeding is decreased risk of esophageal reflux, which reduces the risk of aspiration. Depending on the location of the tip of the tube, a partially digested formula may be recommended for jejunostomy feeding. It is advisable to start with a diluted formula at a diminished flow rate. Continuous drip feeding is often recommended because the function of the stomach as a reservoir is lost. Since the small intestine can adapt to changes in volume better than to changes in concentration, it is recommended that the volume of the formula be increased before caloric concentration [5].

Mode of Administration

The volume and concentration of formulas delivered by tube feeding should be individually tailored to the patient and should be based on the patient's prior feeding intake, the feeding site and formula selected, and the patient's current medical status. A patient who has not been fed orally for several weeks or who has consumed minimal amounts of food requires a period of adaptation to refeeding before full volume and strength can be tolerated. In addition, a patient's current medical status influences his or her response to volume and concentration.

Isotonic formulas are more easily tolerated and do not require the degree of dilution necessary with hypertonic solutions. Furthermore, since the duodenum and jejunum are more sensitive than the stomach to both volume and osmolality, enteric feeds should have low osmolality and should be delivered by continuous drip.

Generally, tube feeds should be initially one-quarter to one-half strength (25 to 50 ml per hour) for a minimum of 8 hours. If the patient tolerates this regimen (no nausea, diarrhea, or glucosuria), the rate can be increased by 25 ml per hour every 8 to 12 hours. When the desired rate is reached, the strength can be increased to tolerance. Concentration and rate of flow should not be increased at the same time [6].

Intermittent feeding allows the patient greater freedom of movement between feeding times. When this method is used, the prescribed volume of formula is infused over a period of 20 to 30 minutes and is delivered by a slow gravity drip. The initial volume and frequency are usually 200 ml of formula containing 0.5 kcal/ml, administered every 4 to 6 hours, and the concentration, volume, and frequency are advanced as tolerated. Gravity feeds can also be delivered by continuous drip over a 16- to 24-hour period. However, rates of flow may be inconstant and should be checked frequently [7]. Use of an infusion pump is desirable because a constant drip rate can be maintained and accidental delivery of a bolus is less likely. Drip rates should be checked frequently (every hour) for accuracy. Continuous feeding can be started with an initial 24-hour volume of 1200 ml at a concentration of 0.5 kcal/ml. Feedings delivered directly into the distal duodenum or proximal jejunum should always be given by continuous pump infusion to reduce the risk of dumping.

The most important precaution in tube feeding is to ensure that the patient is in a proper position. Elevating the upper torso or head at a 45° angle or greater is wise in order to avoid aspiration. If it is not possible to raise the patient, the head of the bed should be elevated with blocks or mechanically [8].

Patients receiving enteral feeds should be monitored carefully; it is necessary to check the intake daily. Observations should be made regarding glucosuria, hematological values, electrolyte status, and the overall state of hydration. If a patient has bloating, nausea, or diarrhea, the tube feeding should be stopped and the symptoms investigated. Tube feeding must be stopped if the patient vomits.

Details of techniques for delivery of formula diets can be found in articles by Sandler [9] and Rombeau and Barot [10].

Formula Selection

The multitude of formula diets commercially available makes it difficult to be familiar with all of them. Since almost all clinical problems can be handled with a small number of mixtures, it is better to be familiar with the generic features of the formulas. A clinical dietitian should be consulted for assistance in choosing the optimal diet that meets the patient's complete nutritional requirements.

The clinically important variants in diet formulations are their lactose content, their osmolality, and the molecular form of their substrates. The intestinal brush border of many adults, especially blacks, Chinese, and those of Mediterranean origin, may be deficient in the enzyme lactase, which causes intolerance to lactose-containing diets.

The osmolality of the infused solution is an important consideration in patients being fed at sites distal to the pylorus. It has been emphasized that hyperosmolar solutions delivered directly into the small bowel may cause rapid fluid and electrolyte shifts which result in severe diarrhea and systemic effects similar to those of the dumping syndrome [10]. This problem can be minimized by starting with dilute solutions and increasing the concentration over a period of 2 to 3 days.

Finally, the molecular composition of the substrates in available formula diets varies widely. A diet that is fed intragastrically and is based on intact protein, starches, and long-chain fatty acids is usually well tolerated if the patient's proteolytic and lipolytic functions are intact. These high-molecular-weight forms tend to be low in osmolality and inexpensive, and provide about 1 kcal/ml. Hospital diets that have been processed in a food blender can also be used if bulk is needed and if the caliber of the feeding tube (> 12 French) will accommodate the high viscosity of the solution. An important hazard of diets prepared in a food blender is bacterial contamination.

Diets composed of protein isolates from casein, soybean, or egg white, together with oligosaccharides and long-chain fatty acids, are lactose-free. These diets are also minimally hyperosmolar, are well tolerated, and provide 1 kcal/ml. These formulas require normal proteolytic and lipolytic function for proper utilization.

Patients with impaired digestive or absorptive capacity, such as those with pancreatic-biliary dysfunction or short-bowel syndrome, need predigested or elemental nutrient sources. Protein hydrolysates containing added amino acids or a synthetic crystalline amino acid solution are absorbed readily. Nonprotein calorie sources are supplied as glucose oligosaccharides, medium-chain triglycerides, and soy or safflower oil. For optimal delivery, chemically defined hyperosmolar diets require gradual increases in concentration, and they provide 1 kcal/ml at full strength.

Nutritionally Complete Formulas for Oral or Tube Feeding Containing Intact Nutrients Nutritionally complete formulas, which are designed to provide adequate nutrients for maintenance, are available for oral or tube feeding. These formulas generally have low residue levels and provide approximately 30 percent of their calories from fat and 12 to 16 percent from protein. Products vary widely in lactose content, osmolality, and palatability, but in adequate volumes, these formulas meet or exceed the National Research Council's RDAs. Osmolality may range from 300 to 450 mOsm. These products require intact digestive and absorptive capacity, since nutrient sources are whole proteins, complex carbohydrates, and triglyceride fats. See Table 3-4 for a listing of products that contain lactose and Table 3-5 for a listing of those that are lactose-free.

Nutritionally Complete Formulas for Oral or Tube Feeding Containing Hydrolyzed Protein or Amino Acids Nutritionally complete formulas containing hydrolyzed protein or amino acids are sometimes called *elemental diets*. A better designation is *defined formula diet* [11]. These formulas are nutritionally complete powders that provide an easily digested liquid diet when mixed with water. Most are clear liquids, have minimal residue levels, and are lactose-free. Ingredients may include amino acids, hydrolyzed protein, polysaccharides, essential fatty acids, vitamins, and minerals. These nutrients require minimal digestion and are readily absorbed.

Most products are unpalatable and are best administered as tube feedings rather than as liquids to be taken by the patient orally. High-nitrogen varieties are available for patients with increased nitrogen requirements. These formulas provide the National Research Council's RDAs when consumed in calorically adequate volumes. However, the RDAs are designed to provide guidelines for maintenance of healthy individuals, and stress, disease, or injury may significantly alter an individual's nutrient requirements. Since exact requirements in hypercatabolic states are unknown, initial and follow-up nutritional assessment is essential for monitoring the adequacy of dietary management. Table 3-6 provides a listing of products containing hydrolyzed nutrients.

Cost of Enteral Feeding Products A major factor in the use of enteral feeding products is their cost. It is possible to feed a patient a nutritionally complete enteral diet for a few dollars a day. For a daily intake of 3000 kcal, an elemental diet costs from $12 to $25 daily, as compared with $5 for meal-replacement formulas and more than $100 for total parenteral nutrition [12]. If enteral feeding is compared to the cost of parenteral nutrition, enteral feeding is a relatively inexpensive form of nutritional support for both critically and chronically ill patients. However, it is important to use an appropriate formula that meets the physiological and metabolic needs of the patient. The use of an expensive predigested formula in a patient with a normally functioning gastrointestinal tract is wasteful!

Problems and Complications

The complications associated with tube feeding can be divided into three categories: mechanical, gastrointestinal, and metabolic (Table 3-7). Mechanical problems associated with the tube itself can cause nasopharyngeal discomfort, along with sinusitis or otitis [13]. Luminal obstruction can occur from residual feeding or from any particulate matter, such as a drug being administered. Because of the small caliber of many of these tubes, it is difficult to flush them once they become obstructed; in order to prevent obstruction, the tube should be flushed whenever feeding is interrupted. Cranberry juice has been found to be more effective than water as a flushing agent.

Tube displacement is another common problem. It is unusual for a mercury-weighted nasoduodenal tube to reflux spontaneously into the stomach. However, if it is positioned in the first section of the duodenum or if the mercury tip has been removed for fluoroscopic placement, the tube can reflux into the stomach during coughing or vomiting.

Gastrointestinal side effects, including distention, cramping, vomiting, and diarrhea, are the most frequent complications of tube feeding [14]. The most common diet-related causes of these symptoms are unrecognized lactose intolerance or rapid infusion of a hyperosmolar formula. Other causes are bacterial contamination, excessive lactose in the formula, and too rapid introduction of feedings.

Metabolic and fluid-electrolyte imbalances, such as hypernatremia, hyperchloremia, azotemia, and dehydration, have also been described as complications of tube feeding. Therapy consists of addition of free water to the dietary regimen, usually through dilution of the formula. Tube-fed patients must be given enough fluids so that they maintain an acceptable urinary output and excretion of nitrogen waste products. Monitoring of blood urea nitrogen, creatinine, electrolytes, hematocrit, urine specific gravity, and body weight should be done, particularly in tube-fed patients who are unconscious or who, for other reasons, cannot experience thirst [15].

Diets in which carbohydrate is the primary calorie source may cause glucose intolerance. Diabetic patients may need increased insulin dosage. Hyperglycemic hyperosmolar nonketotic coma may occur in patients being tube fed. Patients with conditions such as cardiac failure and hepatic or renal disease will require appropriate modification of their tube feeding regimen in order to avoid fluid overload, azotemia, or hyperphosphatemia. Special amino acid mixtures are available for use in patients with renal disease or with poorly functioning livers (see Table 3-1).

PARENTERAL FEEDING

Parenteral feeding is the most effective method of providing nutrients when abnormalities of the gastrointestinal tract do not allow feeding by the enteral route or when dysfunction of the alimentary tract occurs following abdominal surgery or trauma. Strictly speaking, parenteral feeding describes any route

(*Text continues on p. 86.*)

TABLE 3-4
NUTRITIONALLY COMPLETE FORMULAS FOR ORAL OR TUBE FEEDING CONTAINING INTACT NUTRIENTS AND LACTOSE
(Nutritional Analysis per 100 ml)

	Sustagen* (Mead Johnson)	Formula II (Cutter)	Nutri-1000* (Cutter)	Compleat-B (Doyle)	Meritene liquid (Doyle)	Meritene powder* (Doyle)
Protein						
g	11.1	3.8	3.8	4.0	6.0	6.9
% of calories	24.0	15.0	15.0	16.0	26.0	26.0
Sources	Nonfat milk Whole milk Calcium caseinate	Nonfat dry milk Beef Egg yolks	Skim milk Sodium caseinate	Beef Nonfat milk	Concentrated skim milk Sodium caseinate	Nonfat milk Whole milk
Carbohydrate						
g	31.7	12.3	10.6	12.0	11.5	11.9
% of calories	68.0	49.0	38.0	48.0	46.0	45.0
Sources	Corn syrup solids Glucose Lactose	Sucrose Carrots Orange juice concentrate Green beans Wheat flour	Skim milk Sucrose Corn syrup solids	Sucrose Maltodextrin Vegetables Fruit Orange juice Lactose	Corn syrup solids Sucrose Lactose	Corn syrup solids Lactose
Lactose, g	11.1	3.8	5.3	2.4	5.7	10.4
Fat						
g	1.6	4.0	5.2	4.0	3.3	3.5
% of calories	8.0	36.0	47.0	36.0	30.0	29.0
Sources	Milk fat	Corn oil Egg yolks	Corn oil Hydrogenated coconut oil Monoglycerides and diglycerides Soy lecithin	Corn oil	Vegetable oil Monoglycerides and diglycerides	Milk fat
Calories	186	100	110	100	100	107
Nitrogen-total calorie ratio, g:kcal	1:104	1:165	1:174	1:156	1:104	1:96
Nitrogen-nonprotein calorie ratio, g:kcal	1:80	1:140	1:149	1:131	1:79	1:71
Osmolality, mOsm/kg H_2O	1334	435–510	500	490	550–610	690

Volume required to provide 100% RDAs, ml	946	2000	1920	1600	1200	1107
Minerals						
Sodium, mg (meq)	127.0 (5.5)	63.0 (2.7)	53.0 (2.2)	156.3 (6.79)	91.7 (3.98)	96.1 (4.2)
Potassium, mg (meq)	370.0 (9.5)	191.0 (4.9)	147.8 (3.6)	130.0 (3.37)	166.7 (4.27)	296.1 (7.6)
Chloride, mg (meq)	250.0 (7.0)	190.0 (E.4)	120.0 (3.1)	81.0 (22.9)	166.7 (4.7)	219.0 (6.2)
Calcium, mg	338.0	110.0	115.0	62.5	125.0	230.0
Phosphorus, mg	254.0	95.0	90.0	168.8	125.0	192.0
Magnesium, mg	42.0	20.0	20.0	25.0	33.0	38.5
Iodine, μg	16.0	7.5	7.5	9.38	12.5	14.5
Manganese, mg	0.5	0.02	0.13	0.25	0.3	0.38
Copper, mg	0.2	0.1	0.1	0.13	0.2	0.19
Zinc, mg	2.1	0.75	0.8	0.94	1.2	1.4
Iron, mg	1.9	1.3	0.9	1.13	1.5	1.7
Vitamins						
Vitamin A, IU	528.0	250.0	264.3	313.0	415.0	481.0
Vitamin D, IU	42.0	24.0	21.1	25.0	33.0	38.0
Vitamin E, IU	5.0	2.1	1.6	1.9	2.5	2.9
Vitamin K, μg	26.0	NA	NA	NA	NA	NA
Ascorbic acid, mg	32.0	3.9	4.8	5.6	7.5	8.7
Folic acid, μg	40.0	20.0	21.1	25.0	33.3	38.4
Thiamine, mg	0.40	0.08	0.11	0.14	0.19	0.22
Riboflavin, mg	0.45	0.08	0.11	0.16	0.2	0.24
Vitamin B_6, mg	0.53	0.14	0.11	0.19	0.24	0.29
Vitamin B_{12}, μg	1.6	0.3	0.32	0.38	0.5	0.8
Niacin, mg	5.3	1.0	1.1	1.25	1.6	1.9
Choline, mg	53.0	NA	19.0	18.8	8.3	20.5
Biotin, mg	0.03	NA	0.02	0.02	0.03	0.03
Pantothenic acid, mg	2.6	0.48	0.5	0.62	0.8	1.0
Comments	Low residue Requires mixing Flavors: Chocolate Vanilla	Moderate residue Ready to feed Flavors: Orange	Low residue Ready to feed Flavors: Chocolate Vanilla	Moderate residue Ready to feed Unflavored	Low residue Ready to feed Flavors: Chocolate Vanilla Eggnog	Low residue Requires mixing Flavors: Chocolate Vanilla Eggnog Plain

*Vanilla-flavored.
Note: NA, data not available.

TABLE 3-5
NUTRITIONALLY COMPLETE FORMULAS FOR ORAL OR TUBE FEEDING CONTAINING INTACT NUTRIENTS—LACTOSE-FREE
(Nutritional Analysis per 100 ml)

	Sustacal liquid (Mead Johnson)	Isocal (Mead Johnson)	Osmolite (Ross)	Ensure* (Ross)	Ensure Plus* (Ross)
Protein					
g	6.0	3.4	3.7	3.7	5.5
% of calories	24.0	12.9	14.0	14.0	14.7
Sources	Ca and Na caseinate Soy protein isolate	Ca and Na caseinate Soy protein isolate	Ca and Na caseinate Soy protein isolate	Ca and Na caseinate Soy protein isolate	Ca and Na caseinate Soy protein isolate
Carbohydrate					
g	13.8	13.0	14.3	14.0	20.0
% of calories	55.0	50.0	54.6	54.5	53.3
Sources	Sucrose Corn syrup solids	Corn syrup solids	Hydrolyzed corn syrup	Corn syrup solids Sucrose	Corn syrup solids Sucrose
Lactose, g	1.5				
Fat					
g	2.3	4.4	3.8	3.7	5.3
% of calories	21.0	37.0	31.4	31.5	32.0
Sources	Soy oil	Soy oil MCT oil	MCT oil Corn oil Soy oil	Corn oil	Corn oil
Calories	100	106	106	106	150
Nitrogen-total calorie ratio, g:kcal	1:104	1:195	1:178	1:178	1:171
Nitrogen-nonprotein calorie ratio, g:kcal	1:79	1:170	1:154	1:154	1:145
Osmolality, mOsm/kg H_2O	625	300	300	450	600
Volume required to provide 100% RDAs, ml	1080	1890	2000	2000	2000
Minerals					
Sodium, mg (meq)	92.5 (4.0)	52.1 (2.2)	53.9 (2.3)	74.0 (2.9)	106.0 (3.1)
Potassium, mg (meq)	205.6 (5.27)	130.0 (3.2)	104.9 (2.7)	127.0 (3.25)	190.0 (4.9)

Chloride, mg (meq)	156.0 (4.38)	124.2 (2.8)	80.3 (2.1)	106.0 (2.99)	159.0 (4.48)
Calcium, mg	100.0	62.0	52.8	53.0	63.0
Phosphorus, mg	91.67	52.0	52.8	53.0	63.0
Magnesium, mg	37.5	21.0	21.1	21.0	31.7
Iodine, μg	13.89	7.5	7.93	7.9	10.6
Manganese, mg	0.28	0.25	0.21	0.21	0.21
Copper, mg	0.19	0.10	0.11	0.11	0.16
Zinc, mg	1.39	1.0	1.59	1.59	2.38
Iron, mg	1.67	0.94	0.95	0.95	1.43
Vitamins					
Vitamin A, IU	463.9	260.0	264.2	264.2	264.3
Vitamin D, IU	36.9	21.0	21.1	21.1	21.2
Vitamin E, IU	2.8	4.0	3.2	3.2	4.8
Vitamin K, μg	4.0	12.0	10.0	10.0	16.0
Ascorbic acid, mg	5.6	15.6	15.9	16.0	15.9
Folic acid, μg	36.9	20.8	21.1	21.1	21.1
Thiamine, mg	0.14	0.2	0.16	0.16	0.26
Riboflavin, mg	0.17	0.23	0.18	0.18	0.28
Vitamin B_6, mg	0.19	0.26	0.21	0.21	0.32
Vitamin B_{12}, μg	0.56	0.79	0.63	0.63	0.95
Niacin, mg	1.94	2.58	2.11	2.11	3.17
Choline, mg	16.0	26.0	50.0	50.0	50.0
Biotin, mg	0.028	0.02	0.02	0.02	0.03
Pantothenic acid, mg	0.97	1.29	0.53	0.53	0.85
Comments	Low residue	Low residue	Low residue	Low residue	Low residue
	Ready to feed	Ready to feed	Ready to feed	Ready to feed	High caloric density
	Flavors:	Unflavored	Unflavored	Flavors:	Ready to feed
	Chocolate			Vanilla	Flavors:
	Vanilla			Black walnut	Vanilla
	Eggnog			Chocolate	Chocolate
				Flavor packets	Flavor packets
				available	available

*Vanilla flavored.
†Mixed with water as directed.
Note: NA, data not available.

TABLE 3-5 (Continued)

	Nutri-1000* (Cutter)	Renu (Organon)	Precision HN† (Doyle)	Precision Isotonic† (Doyle)	Precision LR† (Doyle)
Protein					
g	3.9	3.3	4.4	2.9	2.63
% of calories	15.0	14.0	16.7	12.0	9.5
Sources	Ca and Na caseinate Soy protein isolate	Ca and Na caseinate Soy protein isolate	Egg white solids	Egg white solids	Egg white solids
Carbohydrate					
g	10.5	13.0	21.6	14.4	24.9
% of calories	38.0	50.0	82.2	60.0	89.2
Sources	Corn syrup solids Sugar	Maltodextrin Corn syrup solids Corn and malt syrup	Maltodextrin Sucrose	Glucose oligosaccharides Sucrose	Maltodextrin Sucrose
Lactose, g					
Fat					
g	4.7	4.0	0.13	3.0	0.16
% of calories	47.0	36.0	1.1	28.0	1.3
Sources	Corn oil Soybean oil Monoglycerides and diglycerides	Soy oil Monoglycerides and diglycerides	Partially hydrogenated soybean oil Monoglycerides and diglycerides	Partially hydrogenated soybean oil Monoglycerides and diglycerides	Partially hydrogenated soybean oil Monoglycerides and diglycerides
Calories	106	100	105	96	111
Nitrogen-total calorie ratio, g:kcal	1:170	1:189	1:150	1:208	1:264
Nitrogen-nonprotein calorie ratio, g:kcal	1:145	1:164	1:125	1:183	1:239
Osmolality, mOsm/kg H$_2$O	380	330	557	300	525 (orange)
Volume required to provide 100% RDAs, ml	3000	2000	2850	1560	1710
Minerals					
Sodium, mg (meq)	68.0 (2.9)	50.0 (2.17)	100.0 (4.1)	76.9 (3.5)	70.0 (3.0)
Potassium, mg (meq)	140.0 (3.6)	125.0 (3.21)	91.0 (2.2)	96.2 (2.5)	87.0 (2.3)

Chloride, mg (meq)	NA	65.0 (1.86)	120.0 (3.2)	103.0 (3.0)	112.0 (3.2)
Calcium, mg	50.0	50.0	35.0	64.0	58.4
Phosphorus, mg	50.0	50.0	35.0	64.0	58.4
Magnesium, mg	20.0	20.0	14.0	25.6	23.4
Iodine, µg	7.5	7.5	5.3	9.6	8.8
Manganese, mg	0.13	NA	0.14	0.26	0.24
Copper, mg	0.1	0.2	0.07	0.13	0.12
Zinc, mg	0.75	1.0	0.53	0.96	0.88
Iron, mg	0.9	1.0	0.63	1.2	1.05
Vitamins					
Vitamin A, IU	265.0	300.0	176.0	321.0	292.0
Vitamin D, IU	21.2	25.0	14.0	26.0	23.5
Vitamin E, IU	1.6	2.0	1.1	1.9	1.8
Vitamin K, µg	15.7	VA	3.5	6.4	5.9
Ascorbic acid, mg	4.8	60.0	3.2	5.8	5.3
Folic acid, µg	20.0	40.0	14.0	26.0	23.0
Thiamine, mg	0.1	0.13	0.08	0.14	0.13
Riboflavin, mg	0.1	0.14	0.09	0.17	0.15
Vitamin B_6, mg	0.1	0.15	0.11	0.19	0.18
Vitamin B_{12}, µg	0.3	0.4	0.21	0.38	0.35
Niacin, mg	1.0	1.5	0.7	1.3	1.17
Choline, mg	19.0	NA	3.5	6.4	5.8
Biotin, mg	0.02	0.03	0.01	0.02	0.02
Pantothenic acid, mg	0.5	0.8	0.35	0.64	0.58
Comments	Low residue Ready to feed Flavors: Vanilla Chocolate	Low residue Ready to feed Flavors: Imitation vanilla	Low residue High protein Requires mixing Flavor: Citrus fruit	Low residue Requires mixing Flavors: Vanilla Orange	Low residue Requires mixing Flavors: Cherry Lemon Lime Orange

*Vanilla flavored.
†Mixed with water as directed.
Note: NA, data not available.

TABLE 3-6
NUTRITIONALLY COMPLETE FORMULAS FOR ORAL OR TUBE FEEDING CONTAINING HYDROLYZED PROTEIN OR AMINO ACIDS
(Nutritional Analysis per 100 ml)

	Vital* (Ross)	Vivonex HN* (Eaton)	Vivonex STD* (Eaton)	Flexical* (Mead Johnson)	Vipep* (Cutter)
Protein					
g	4.2	4.3	2.1	2.2	2.5
% of calories	16.7	17.7	8.2	9.0	10.0
Sources	Hydrolyzed soy, whey and beef	Crystalline amino acids	Crystalline amino acids	Hydrolyzed casein Amino acids	Peptides Amino acids
Carbohydrate					
g	18.5	21.1	23.0	15.4	17.6
% of calories	74.0	81.5	90.5	61.0	68.0
Sources	Oligosaccharides Polysaccharides Sucrose	Glucose oligo-saccharides	Glucose oligo-saccharides	Corn syrup solids Modified tapioca starches	Corn syrup solids Sucrose Potassium gluconate Cornstarch Tapioca flour
Lactose, g	0.05	0	0	0	0
Fat					
g	1.0	0.1	0.1	3.4	2.5
% of calories	9.3	0.78	1.3	30.0	22.0
Sources	Sunflower oil	Safflower oil	Safflower oil	MCT oil Soy oil	MCT oil Corn oil
Calories	100	100	100	100	100
Nitrogen-total calorie ratio, g:kcal	1:150	1:150	1:300	1:279	1:250
Nitrogen-nonprotein calorie ratio, g:kcal	1:124	1:123	1:275	1:260	1:225
Osmolality, mOsm/kg H$_2$O	450	810 (unflavored) 850–910 (flavored)	550 (unflavored) 580–610 (flavored)	550	520
Volume required to provide 100% RDAs, ml	1500	3000	1800	2000	2000

Minerals

Sodium, mg (meq)	38.3 (1.7)	77.1 (3.4)	86.0 (3.7)	35.0 (1.6)	75.0 (3.2)
Potassium, mg (meq)	116.7 (3.0)	70.2 (1.8)	117.0 (3.0)	125.0 (3.2)	85.0 (2.1)
Chloride, mg (meq)	66.7 (1.9)	185.8 (5.2)	133.6 (5.2)	100.0 (2.8)	170.0 (4.8)
Calcium, mg	66.7	33.3	55.5	60.0	60.0
Phosphorus, mg	66.7	33.3	55.5	50.0	50.0
Magnesium, mg	26.7	13.3	22.2	20.0	20.0
Iodine, µg	10.0	5.0	8.3	7.5	7.5
Manganese, mg	0.13	0.09	0.16	0.25	0.13
Copper, mg	0.13	0.07	0.11	0.1	0.1
Zinc, mg	1.0	0.5	0.83	1.0	0.75
Iron, mg	1.2	0.6	1.0	0.9	0.9

Vitamins

Vitamin A, IU	333.3	166.7	277.8	250.0	250.0
Vitamin D, IU	26.7	13.3	22.2	20.0	20.0
Vitamin E, IU	2.0	1.0	1.7	2.3	1.5
Vitamin K, µg	130.0	2.2	3.7	12.5	7.5
Ascorbic acid, mg	6.0	2.0	3.3	15.0	4.5
Folic acid, µg	26.7	13.3	22.0	20.0	0.2
Thiamine, mg	0.1	0.5	0.08	0.19	0.8
Riboflavin, mg	0.11	0.6	0.09	0.22	0.9
Vitamin B_6, mg	0.13	0.7	0.11	0.25	0.1
Vitamin B_{12}, µg	0.4	0.2	0.33	0.75	0.3
Niacin, mg	1.33	0.67	1.11	2.5	1.0
Choline, mg	10.8	2.5	4.1	25.0	14.25
Biotin, mg	0.02	0.01	0.02	0.02	0.02
Pantothenic acid, mg	0.07	0.33	0.56	1.25	0.5

Comments	High protein	High protein	Low fat	Low residue	Peptide formula diet
	Low residue	Low fat	Low residue	Requires mixing	Low residue
	Requires mixing	Low residue	Requires mixing	Unflavored	Requires mixing
	Flavor:	Unflavored	Unflavored		Flavors:
	Banana	Flavor packets	Flavor packets		Orange
	Flavor packets	available	available		Strawberry
	available				Custard

*Mixed with water as directed.

TABLE 3-7
COMPLICATIONS OF TUBE FEEDING

Complication	Therapy
Mechanical	
Nasopharyngeal irritation	Give ice chips, topical anesthetics, decongestants
Luminal obstruction	Flush, replace tube
Mucosal erosions	Reposition tube, give ice water lavage, remove tube
Tube displacement	Replace tube
Aspiration	Discontinue tube feeding
Gastrointestinal	
Cramping or distention	Change formula if patient is lactose-intolerant, reduce infusion rate
Vomiting or diarrhea	Reduce infusion rate, dilute formula, add antidiarrheal agents
Metabolic	
Hypertonic dehydration	Increase free water
Glucose intolerance	Give insulin, reduce infusion rate
Hyperosomolar nonketotic coma	Discontinue tube feeding
Hepatic encephalopathy	Decrease amount of protein
Renal failure	Decrease phosphate, magnesium, potassium; restrict protein
	Give essential amino acid solution
Cardiac failure	Reduce sodium content, restrict fluid

other than the gastrointestinal tract, such as, for example, subcutaneous and intramuscular injections, which have been used for administering electrolytes, vitamins, or iron. However, intravenous feeding is the most satisfactory parenteral feeding method and is essentially synonymous with parenteral feeding. Although it is not possible to supply all nutritional needs via peripheral vein, total parenteral feedings through a central vein can provide complete nourishment for individuals.

Indications

Meng [16] suggested that parenteral nutrition should be considered if the patient:

1 Has an abnormality of the gastrointestinal tract such as the following:
   a Inability to ingest food or an abnormality which makes it unwise to ingest food, e.g., as the result of an obstruction or peritonitis
   b Inability to retain ingested food, e.g., vomiting, diarrhea, or a fistula
   c Impaired digestion and absorption, e.g., malabsorption syndromes
   d Edema due to malnutrition

2 Is being prepared for surgery and is nutritionally depleted and emaciated

3 Has undergone surgery or trauma, especially burns or multiple fractures

4 Is a neonate with congenital anomalies who is about to undergo or who has just undergone surgery

5 Is in a coma, has anorexia nervosa, or refuses to eat

6 Requires supplementation because of inadequate oral feeding, as occurs in patients with cancer, especially those receiving chemotherapy or radiation therapy, and in those with renal or hepatic failure.

To this list should be added patients with acute and severe inflammatory bowel diseases, particularly ulcerative colitis. In general one should consider total parenteral nutrition (TPN) for patients in the high-risk categories mentioned. Any patient who has been, or might be, deprived of adequate oral intake for 7 days or more or who has had a recent (acute) loss of 10 percent or more of body weight as a result of inadequate nutrition or who weighs 80 percent or less than his or her ideal body weight should also be considered.

Administration

Standardized methodology has maximized the effectiveness and minimized the morbidity associated with TPN. These methods include strict adherence to aseptic techniques for catheter insertion and care; precise monitoring of the patient's response to carbohydrate, fat, protein, fluid, and electrolyte infusion; and utilization of a "team approach".

Route of Administration The safest and most effective technique for long-term infusion of hypertonic nutrient solutions (1800 to 2400 mOsm per liter) in adults and in infants weighing more than 4.5 kg (10 lb) has been infraclavicular, percutaneous, subclavian, venous catheterization. In patients being treated at the University of Texas, a 2-inch-long no.14 gauge needle is inserted under the middle third of the clavicle into the subclavian vein. An 8- to 10-inch-long no.16 gauge polyethylene catheter is advanced through the needle in the subclavian vein into the midportion of the superior vena cava. Detailed descriptions of the subclavian catheterization technique are beyond the scope of this discussion. However, the basic principles of catheter insertion and care are as follows:

1 Catheters should always be placed and subsequently handled using completely aseptic techniques.

2 Infraclavicular percutaneous puncture is best accomplished with the patient positioned head-down at a 15° angle (Trendelenburg position) to allow hydrostatic dilatation of the subclavian vein.

3 The catheter should be demonstrated radiologically to be positioned in the superior vena cava prior to commencing total parenteral nutrition with hypertonic fluids.

4 The catheter used for TPN should not be used to withdraw blood, to measure central venous pressure, or to administer any medication as a bolus.

5 Meticulous care and maintenance of the catheter should include removal of the dressing over the entrance site every 2 to 3 days and changing the administration tubing. The skin around the entrance site should be cleaned with ether or acetone, and the skin should be prepared with povidone-iodine. Antimicrobial ointment should be reapplied around the catheter, and the sterile occlusive dressing should be replaced.

If this procedure is used, catheters can remain in place safely for periods in excess of 60 days with an infection rate of less than 2.2 percent [17]. In patients who require central venous catheterization for periods of less than 60 days, a percutaneously placed polethylene catheter can be used. When patients require TPN for periods longer than 60 days, the line should be changed electively to minimize risks of infection. Patients requiring long-term TPN (home hyperalimentation) usually have a surgically implanted Broviac-Scribner silicone catheter or Hickman catheter.

Excellent accounts of catheter insertion techniques can be found in articles by Daly and Long [18], Duke and Dudrick [19], and Grant [20].

Infusion Apparatus   The nutrient solutions can be delivered from bottles or plastic bags by gravity flow, by a propulsion pump, or by air pressure. The current practice is to use a controlled infusion pump. The equipment is provided with monitoring features and warning alarms to give visual and auditory cues to both the patient and clinical personnel in order to prevent or to minimize complications. A 0.22-μm disposable millipore filter is generally utilized in the infusion line as close to the catheter as possible to prevent infusion of contaminants.

Infusion Rate   The optimal infusion rate for glucose is 0.5 to 0.75 g/kg per hour, although 0.35 g/kg per hour has been proposed to avoid hyperglycemia and urinary spillage [21]. The rate depends on the individual patient's condition. Insulin must be administered to patients who are insulin-resistant as a consequence of trauma or infection. The dose of insulin is based on urinary glucose loss. Insulin may be added to the infusion solution.

Less is known about optimal infusion rates for amino acids. It has been suggested that 0.02 to 0.03 g of nitrogen per kilogram per hour may be given continuously during a 24-hour period. In most patients, except those with renal and cardiac disease, 3 liters of solution are given in a 24-hour period. On the first day, 1 liter is administered, on the second day, 2 liters, and on the third and succeeding days 3 liters. Additional fluid is given when needed during the first 2 days. A continuous infusion rate of 125 ml per hour provides 3 liters in 24 hours.

The rate of infusion of fat emulsions may be maintained at 0.1 to 0.5 g/kg per hour. The initial amount of fat should be 0.5 g/kg per day; it is increased stepwise to 1, 1.5, 2, and 2.5 g/kg per day over 4 or 5 days. Plasma triglycerides should be measured before each incremental change is made. The increase in amount should be postponed when hypertriglyceridemia is observed.

Guidelines for Clinical Management   Monitoring and careful record keeping are essential for the success of a program of TPN. At the initiation of TPN, basic guidelines include accurate measurements of the patient's temperature, pulse rate, respiratory rate, and blood pressure at least every 4 hours; of the patient's fractional urinary sugar and acetone concentrations at least every 6 hours; of the patient's fluid balance at least every 8 hours; and of the patient's body weight at the same time and under the same conditions each day. Serum electrolyte concentrations, blood urea nitrogen, and blood glucose levels should be determined at least daily until they are stable and thereafter every 2 or 3 days. It is also advisable to evaluate hepatic function (bilirubin, serum aspartate aminotransferase, serum alanine aminotransferase, and alkaline phosphatase) and serum calcium, phosphorus, magnesium, albumin, and globulin concentrations initially and weekly thereafter. Measurements of hemoglobin concentration and hematocrit together with the red blood cell indexes, white blood cell count, differential leukocyte count, and peripheral blood smear examination and a prothrombin determination should be done initially and at least weekly thereafter. Measurements of serum osmolality, electrolytes, protein, and nitrogen may be helpful in the progressive monitoring and therapy of patients in whom complicated metabolic derangements have developed. Periodic measurements of arterial and central venous pressures, arterial blood gases, pH, and ammonia may be necessary or desirable in the management of critically ill patients with cardiovascular, respiratory, or metabolic derangements. If lipid is infused, the patient's ability to clear lipids should be assessed by checking the serum triglyceride level. It should be within the normal range within 12 hours of infusing the emulsion. The patient's platelet count should be checked weekly if lipid is being infused regularly.

The TPN Team   Experience has indicated that the optimum care of the patient requiring TPN is best assured by a nutrition support team consisting of a physician, a pharmacist, a nurse, and a dietitian [22].

The physician is responsible for evaluating each patient's nutritional status and assessing the need for TPN. The team physician either inserts the catheter or is responsible for ensuring that only those trained in catheter insertion are permitted to do so. Orders relevant to this therapy are written by the physician, including the prescribing of solutions and the clinical and laboratory parameters that are to be monitored.

The pharmacist is responsible for interpreting the order, formulating the solutions, and ensuring delivery to the clinical area. The pharmacist's ability to maintain quality control in the preparation of the solutions and to keep accurate records of administration, and the pharmacist's knowledge of the incompatibilities of the solutions with pharmacological agents are essential to successful therapy.

The nurse must have an adequate knowledge and understanding of the clinical application of TPN and must be skilled in the procedural aspects of TPN. The nurse is responsible for supervising the administration of the solutions to the patient and for assisting in educating the floor nurses about TPN therapy. The nurse is also responsible for monitoring specific nursing parameters, for recognizing and reporting signs and symptoms of potential complications, and for providing psychological support to the patient and the family.

The dietitian who functions as a member of the nutrition support team must have skills in assessing the nutritional status of patients, must possess a working knowledge of nutrient metabolism, should be familiar with the various laboratory tests that have significance for nutritional therapy, should have the ability to function as a consultant, and should be very knowledgeable about the composition, value, and limitations of the various dietary supplements, defined formula diets, and tube feedings.

Nutritional Considerations

Specific nutrient requirements must be borne in mind if one is to formulate an appropriate TPN solution. The caloric requirement for the resting adult patient whose weight is in an acceptable range, whose activity is restricted, and who has little or no fever or conditions that might lead to a hypermetabolic state is 25 to 30 kcal/kg per day [23]. Infants and young children require approximately 100 to 150 kcal/kg per day to maintain their body weight. Many centers use the Harris-Benedict equations to calculate basal energy expenditure (BEE) (see Appendix 2).

$$\text{Men's BEE} = 66 + (13.7 \times W) + (5 \times H) - (6.8 \times A)$$
$$\text{Women's BEE} = 655 + (9.6 \times W) - (1.7 \times H) - (4.7 \times A)$$

where W = actual weight, kg
H = height, cm
A = age, years

However, these values approximate the requirement for a nonstressed hospital patient who remains in bed. Ambulation increases metabolic expenditures by about 20 percent. Fever increases metabolic requirements by 11 to 13 percent for each degree centigrade that body temperature is elevated. Major stress increases requirements by up to 20 percent, peritonitis by 50 percent, and significant burns by 100 percent [24]. Blackburn and associates have recommended $1.75 \times \text{BEE}$ as the energy requirements needed to achieve an anabolic state in patients on TPN [25].

Consideration must also be given to the ratio of nitrogen (in grams) to nonprotein calories (in kilocalories). A ratio of 1:250 to 1:300 is found in the normal diet. However, in individuals who are significantly underweight or who are stressed by trauma, burns, or infection, the nitrogen-calorie ratio may have to be decreased to 1:150 to allow nitrogen equilibrium or positive nitrogen balance [23].

Both the amount of protein infused and its composition are important for determining the protein requirement of a patient receiving TPN. Customarily, patients requiring TPN are given 12 to 15 g of nitrogen (75 to 95 g protein), and most patients will achieve a positive nitrogen balance. Because the means for measuring nitrogen balance are available to the clinician (see Appendix 3), adjustments to achieve a positive nitrogen balance can be made. Amino acid solutions containing both essential and sufficient nonessential amino acids to balance the mixture (the solutions approximate an "ideal" protein) are used as a protein source.

Absolute fat requirements are important with respect to adequate delivery of essential fatty acids. Seven and one-half grams of linoleic acid per day or approximately 4 percent of the total daily energy has been recommended [26].

Requirements for vitamins in TPN have not been established. Furthermore, patients who require TPN are under stress, are nutritionally depleted, are critically ill, are septic, or are subject to any combination of these conditions, which may further alter vitamin requirements. Generally, the type and dose of vitamins given to patients receiving TPN are based on assumptions made from oral requirements previously established. Generally, 1 to 2 ml of several commercially available water-soluble B-complex vitamin preparations will fulfill the daily requirements for this important group. Vitamin B_{12} may be administered intramuscularly in doses of 100 to 200 μg monthly or added (usually with folacin) in a dosage of 100 μg weekly to bottles of nutrients containing no other vitamins. The usual weekly dosage of folacin is 2.5 mg. Vitamin C requirements are 60 mg daily. This water-soluble vitamin is available as a mixture with B-complex vitamins. A commercially available emulsion of the fat-soluble vitamins A, D, and E (Multi-Vitamin Infusion, USV Laboratories) can be administered twice weekly for fat-soluble vitamin maintenance. Vitamin K preparations are often administered intramuscularly. Weekly doses should be adjusted to the patient's prothrombin time and are usually in the range of 10 to 15 mg weekly. A new product—M.V.I.-12 (USV Laboratories)—containing 12 vitamins, including biotin, folic acid, and vitamin B_{12}, is available and can be used daily by diluting it in 500 to 1000 ml of intravenous dextrose, saline, or similar infusion solutions.

Electrolyte requirements for TPN vary widely in individual patients and depend on the volume and type of fluid loss, preexisting deficits, cardiovascular, renal, and endocrine status, and the type and amount of nutrients given. It is essential to monitor plasma electrolyte levels at frequent intervals in order to afford a rational basis for adjusting dosages. The usual adult phosphorus requirement is 10 to 12 mmol (20 to 24 meq of dibasic phosphorus) per liter of TPN solution. The amount infused should be 1.5 times the calcium infusion. The usual calcium requirement is 15 to 20 meq per day. Therefore, about 30 meq per day of phosphate will be required because of reciprocal relationships between serum calcium and phosphate levels. The recommended daily requirement for magnesium is approximately 24 meq for adults. In patients without excessive loss, 60 to 100 meq of sodium per day are adequate. Less sodium should be given to patients with renal insufficiency or cardiovascular diseases. For potassium a dosage of 120 meq per day is adequate for most patients [21].

Attention must also be given to the addition of minerals and other micronutrients to the solutions given patients on prolonged TPN. Currently, no standard recommendation or preparation including these minerals is available. Iron is required at levels of 1 to 2 mg per day and may be administered intramuscularly or intravenously as iron salts or as an iron-dextran complex. Zinc may be required at levels of 2 to 4 mg or more per day. Other trace elements for which requirements have been suggested include iodine, copper, manganese, chromium, and selenium.

Finally, in administration of nutrients, fluid requirements must be considered. The quantity of water that corrects for losses by excretion (urine and feces) and insensible water loss and achieves proper tissue hydration of a normal adult is about 100 ml per 100 kcal per day or about 2600 ml. The fluid volume usually given to an adult TPN patient is about 3 liters per day or 30 to 45 ml/kg per day. Attention to urinary output and observation of fluid retention will provide information about appropriate daily fluid loads.

Formulation of Nutrient Solutions

The hypertonic nutrient solution most commonly used for parenteral feeding consists of approximately 20 to 25 percent dextrose (the caloric source), 4 to 5 percent crystalline amino acids or protein hydrolysates (the nitrogen source), and 1 to 3 percent minerals and multiple vitamins (Table 3-8). Each unit of base solution provides approximately 5.25 to 6.0 g of nitrogen and 900 to 1000 kcal in 1100 ml of water. Aminosyn, FreAmine, Travasol, and Veinamine are commercially available crystalline amino acid mixtures (see Table 3-9). In addition, there are specific amino acid mixtures available for treatment of patients with renal and liver failure.

The nutrient solutions are usually prepared from commercially available stock products under the auspices of the pharmacy, where meticulous, aseptic mixing technique can be monitored. The standard additions to each unit of base solution are listed in Table 3-8. While it is possible to illustrate such a "standard" TPN solution, the specific water, electrolyte, calorie, and nitrogen requirements of each patient must be individualized so that avoidable metabolic derangements do not occur during the course of therapy [19].

When the TPN mixture for a typical adult patient who has no significant cardiovascular, hepatic, or renal dysfunction or metabolic abnormality is formulated, 40 to 50 meq of sodium and 30 to 40 meq of potassium are usually added to each unit of the base solution. Sodium administration, however, is reduced or temporarily omitted in patients with congestive heart failure, liver failure, or severe edema. Potassium, phosphorus, and magnesium administration is often reduced or omitted in patients with compromised renal function. Some crystalline amino acid solutions are prepared as the chloride and hydrochloride salts, and there exists a significant risk of hyperchloremic

TABLE 3-8
TYPICAL BASIC TPN FORMULA FOR AN ADULT

Component	Amount
Base solution, 1 unit	
Amino acid solution (crystalline), 8.5%	500 ml
Dextrose solution, 50%	500 ml
Additions to each unit of base solution	
Sodium (chloride and/or acetate, lactate, bicarbonate salt)	50 meq
Potassium (acetate, lactate, chloride, acid phosphate salt)	30–40 meq
Magnesium (sulfate)	10–20 meq
Phosphate (potassium acid salt)	10–20 mMol
Additions to one unit of base solution daily	
M.V.I.-12 (concentrate) containing:	10 ml
Vitamin A	3300 IU
Vitamin D	200 IU
Vitamin E	10 IU
Vitamin C	100 mg
Thiamine	3.0 mg
Riboflavin	3.6 mg
Pyridoxine	4.0 mg
Niacinamide	40.0 mg
Pantothenic acid	15.0 mg
Biotin	60 μg
Folacin	400 μg
Vitamin B_{12}	5 μg
Calcium gluconate	1 g
Zinc sulfate	5 mg
Copper sulfate	2 mg
Optional additions to daily nutrient regimen	
Vitamin K	10 mg
Iron (iron-dextran)	1–2 mg
Supplements during week	
Intralipid, 10%	500 ml (2–3 times/week)

metabolic acidosis when additional sodium requirements are satisfied solely by adding sodium chloride to these solutions. There are other crystalline amino acid solutions available that contain most or all of the amino acids as acetate salts, which has greatly reduced the incidence of hyperchloremic metabolic acidosis. The importance of the precise composition of the formulated nutrient solution and the exact nutritional and electrolyte requirements of each individual patient

TABLE 3-9
COMPOSITIONS OF CRYSTALLINE AMINO ACID INFUSIONS

	Aminosyn 7% (Abbott)	Aminosyn 10% (Abbott)	FreAmine II 8.5% (McGaw)	Travasol 5.5% (Travenol)	Travasol 8.5% (Travenol)	Veinamine 8% (Cutter)	Nephramine 5.1% (McGaw)
Protein, g	7	10	8	5.5	8.5	8	5
Nitrogen, g	1.1	1.6	1.2	0.9	1.4	1.3	0.6
Potassium, meq	0.5	0.5	—	—	—	3.0	—
Sodium, meq	—	—	1.0	—	—	4.0	0.6
Phosphate, mmol	—	—	2.0	—	—	—	—
Magnesium, meq	—	—	—	—	—	0.6	—
Chloride, meq	—	—	—	2.2	3.4	5.0	—
Acetate, meq	—	—	—	3.5	5.2	5.0	—
Osmolarity, mOsm/liter	700	1,100	850	—	—	950	420
pH	5.3	5.3	6.6	6.0	6.0	6.2–6.6	6.0
Amino acids, mg							
Essential							
Isoleucine	510	720	590	263	406	493	560
Leucine	660	940	770	340	526	347	880
Lysine	510	720	870	318	492	667	640
Methionine	280	400	450	318	492	427	880
Phenylalanine	310	440	480	340	526	400	886
Threonine	370	520	340	230	356	160	400
Tryptophan	120	160	130	99	152	80	200
Valine	560	800	560	252	390	253	650
Nonessential							
Tyrosine	44	44	—	22	34	—	—
Alanine	900	1,280	600	1,140	1,760	—	—
Arginine*	690	980	310	570	880	749	—
Histidine*	210	300	240	241	372	237	—
Proline	610	860	950	230	356	107	—
Serine	300	420	500	—	—	—	—
Glycine	900	1,280	1,700	1,140	1,760	3,387	—
Cysteine*	—	—	20	—	—	—	—
Aspartic acid	—	—	—	—	—	460	—
Glutamic acid	—	—	—	—	—	426	—
Trace elements, μg							
Zinc	12–14	3–6	82–404	NA	14	13–15	NA
Copper	—	—	0.9–8.5	NA	—	1.3–1.5	NA
Chromium	NA	—	0.2	NA	NA	0.8–2.4	NA
Manganese	NA	NA	0.3	NA	NA	NA	NA

*Considered nonessential for adults but essential for infants.
Note: NA, data not available; —, not detectable or negligible.

must be thoroughly appreciated in order to prevent iatrogenic metabolic complications.

TPN, in contrast to isotonic dextrose therapy, can result in hypophosphatemia when solutions devoid of phosphate are used. Phosphorus is an intracellular anion that is essential in promoting protein synthesis in patients receiving TPN. Hypophosphatemia does not occur as a result of increased urinary losses of phosphorus, but develops secondary to "trapping" of the phosphorus in newly synthesized protein. Thus, severely malnourished patients given TPN are at the highest risk of developing this complication. Under ordinary circumstances, phosphorus should be added to each unit of base solution as potassium acid phosphate or sodium acid phosphate in doses of 15 to 30 meq per liter, but in severely malnourished patients 30 to 50 meq should be added to each liter of solution. In adults 4 to 5 meq of calcium (as the gluconate) is added to one unit (e.g., 1000 ml) of nutrient solution per day. Calcium should always be added to parenteral feeding regimens of infants and children in order to provide 3 to 4 meq per kilogram of body weight daily.

One vial of a mixture containing fat-soluble and water-soluble vitamins suitable for parenteral administration is added to only one unit of the nutrient solution daily. Since each vial contains vitamins in therapeutic dosages [27], it is not necessary or advisable to administer more than one ampule to a patient per day.

Trace-element deficiency may become manifest clinically late in the course of parenteral nutrition or early if significant deficits preexist. Zinc sulfate and copper sulfate are added to one unit of nutrient solution daily to assure adequate intake of these elements [28]. Trace elements such as iodine and manganese are present as contaminants in most parenteral solutions and may or may not be added routinely to the nutritional regimen. Not all of the trace-element stock solutions are available commercially, and if they are needed in a nutrient solution, the pharmacist must prepare them with aseptic techniques.

Appropriately computed doses of iron can be added to the TPN solution or can be given in depot as iron-dextran by deep intramuscular injection. In patients with hemoglobin concentrations less than 10 g/dl, it is advisable to restore normal red cell mass by transfusing whole blood or packed erythrocytes prior to initiating TPN. In some patients it may be necessary to give occasional transfusions of packed erythrocytes or whole blood during the course of prolonged TPN therapy. This should be done through a separate transfusion line.

In the United States, intravenous fat emulsions (Intralipid and more recently Liposyn) have been approved by the Food and Drug Administration only in recent years. Ten percent and twenty percent Intralipid (soybean oil) and Liposyn (safflower oil) solutions provide 1.1 kcal/ml and 2.2 kcal/ml, respectively. The standard unit for both Intralipid (Cutter Laboratories) and Liposyn (Abbott Laboratories) is a 500-ml container, and typically 2 to 3 units are administered per week. Lipid emulsions are used for the prevention of essential fatty acid deficiency and can be an alternative calorie source. Intravenous fat is usually infused as a separate solution through a Y connector into the tubing of a central or peripheral line containing other solutions. Since these emulsions have an osmolality of 280 mOsm, they can be infused through a peripheral vein. Very few patients who receive fat are intolerant of the preparation. The contraindications to its use are limited to those with acute liver disease and/or acute and chronic pulmonary insufficiency.

Complications

Potential complications fall into three categories: technical, septic, and metabolic. If an experienced TPN team carefully monitors patients, adheres strictly to aseptic techniques, and has a sound knowledge of nutrient requirements, most complications can be prevented.

Technical Complications   Subclavian catheterization is associated with a variety of complications, the most common of which is pneumothorax. Pneumothorax may be visible on the chest x-ray which must be done following insertion of the catheter, but it is possible to have a slow leak into the pleural space, in which case symptoms are not apparent until hours later. Other technical complications include hydrothorax, carotid or subclavian artery laceration, mediastinal hematoma, phrenic or brachial plexus nerve damage, or thoracic duct injury. The patient must be monitored closely for signs of respiratory distress, hypotension, a slow-growing hematoma, or neurological complaints.

Air embolism is a potentially fatal complication which can occur during the insertion of catheters into the central venous system or during the time the line is open for changing tubing. Prevention is accomplished by positioning patients flat in bed or in the Trendelenburg position and by having them perform a Valsalva maneuver whenever the line is open.

Septic Complications   Septic complications are the most frequent and most potentially dangerous complications in patients receiving TPN. Numerous studies have now demonstrated that most sepsis originates in the skin and that the organisms grow down the catheter and infect the blood or the fibrin sleeve around the tip of the catheter [29]. Additional sources of sepsis include ongoing septic foci in the patient, such as intraabdominal abscesses or urinary tract infections, and contaminated nutrient solutions. However, the TPN system should be considered first in the differential diagnosis of fever. A complete assessment includes physical assessment by the physician; removal and culture of the TPN solution (a new bottle and new tubing may be established); a chest x-ray; cultures of urine, sputum, and drainage from wounds; and blood cultures from the peripheral vein and from the catheter.

In general there are two types of catheter sepsis; the first is bacterial and involves skin organisms such as *Staphylococcus epidermidis, Aerobacter, Klebsiella,* and other nosocomial organisms. In the presence of a fever spike, removal of the catheter without antibiotic therapy is generally sufficient, provided there is no septic thrombophlebitis. If catheter sepsis is neglected and a septic endovasculitis has been established, this should be treated as any other endovasculitis, with intravenous antibiotics for between 2 and 6 weeks. Fungal septicemia is a more difficult problem and requires the abandonment of the central venous administration of nutrients. If an obvious source of infection other than the catheter is identified, it may be appropriate to continue TPN therapy and treat the infection with antibiotics.

Metabolic Complications The most common metabolic complications usually involve glucose. Significant hyperglycemia (blood glucose > 300 mg percent) or hypoglycemia (blood glucose < 60 mg percent) occurs in 15 percent and 9 percent of cases, respectively [30]. Patients with decreased insulin secretion or increased insulin resistance, as in pancreatitis, liver disease, or sepsis, are predominantly at risk for hyperglycemia. An extreme but rare complication of hyperglycemia is osmotic diuresis and dehydration that result in hyperosmotic coma.

Hypoglycemia may occur when the infusion is interrupted for as little as 15 to 30 minutes [20] as a result of technical or mechanical complications (kinking or clotting of the line). In order to avoid hypoglycemia, patients should be "weaned" by gradually decreasing the infusion rate prior to discontinuation of therapy.

Most of the other metabolic complications are deficiency states that result from inadequate administration of fat, vitamins, or minerals. Essential fatty acid deficiency can be prevented by providing linoleic acid in the form of a lipid emulsion. Water-soluble and fat-soluble vitamins, as well as trace elements such as zinc, copper, iodine, iron, manganese, and chromium, should be an integral part of the TPN regimen.

In conclusion, it must be emphasized that TPN is a lifesaving measure which carries potentially life-threatening risks. It should not be initiated unless the indications for it are strong; once the decision is made, it should be implemented without delay, and finally, and very importantly, it should be discontinued as soon as the indications for it have ceased.

REFERENCES

1 Day, S., and M. Bucknell: Feeding the unconscious patient, Proc. Nutr. Soc., 30:184, 1971.
2 Dobbie, R. P., and J. A. Hoffmeister: Continuous pump-tube enteric hyperalimentation, Surg. Gynecol. Obstet., 143:273, 1976.
3 Bush, J.: Cervical esophagostomy to provide nutrition, Am. J. Nurs., 79:109, 1979.
4 Torosian M. H., and J. L. Rombeau: Feeding by tube enterostomy: a collective review, Surg. Gynecol. Obstet., 150:918, 1980.
5 Chernoff, R.: Nutritional support: formulas and delivery of enteral feedings. II. Delivery systems, J. Am. Diet. Assoc., 79:430, 1981.
6 Chernoff, R.: Enteral feeding, Am. J. Hosp. Pharm., 37:65, 1980.
7 Griggs, B. A., and M. C. Hoppe: Update: nasogastric tube feeding, Am. J. Nurs. 79:481, 1979.
8 Chernoff, R.: Nutrition and the cancer patient, J. Can. Diet. Assoc., 40:139, 1979.

9 Sander, J. T.: Specific techniques for delivery of liquid diets, in *Nutrition in Clinical Surgery*, M. Deitel (ed.), Williams & Wilkins, Baltimore, 1980.

10 Rombeau, J. L., and L. R. Barot: Enteral nutrition therapy, Surg. Clin. North Am., 61:605, 1981.

11 Hill, G. L., I. Pickford, G. A. Young, C. J. Schorah, R. L. Blackett, L. Burkinshaw, J. V. Warren, and D. B. Morgan: Malnutrition in surgical patients, Lancet, 1:689, 1977.

12 Michel, L., A. Serrano, and R. A. Malt: Nutritional support of hospitalized patients, N. Engl. J. Med., 304:1147, 1981.

13 Padilla, G. V., M. Grant, H. Wong, B. W. Hansen, R. L. Hanson, N. Bergstrom, and W. R. Kubo: Subjective distresses of nasogastric tube feeding, J. Parenteral Enteral Nutr., 3:53, 1979.

14 Heymsfield, S. B., R. A. Bethel, J. D. Ansley, D. W. Nixon, and D. Rudman: Enteral hyperalimentation: an alternative to central venous hyperalimentation, Ann. Intern. Med., 90:63, 1979.

15 Gault, M. H., M. E. Dixon, M. Doyle, and W. M. Cohen: Hypernatremia, azotemia and dehydration due to high-protein tube feeding, Ann. Intern. Med., 68:778, 1973.

16 Meng, H. C.: Parenteral nutrition: principles, nutrient requirements, and techniques, Geriatrics, 30:97, 1975.

17 Copeland, E. M., B. V. MacFadyen, Jr., and S. J. Dudrick: The use of hyperalimentation in patients with potential sepsis, Surg. Gynecol. Obstet., 138:377, 1974.

18 Daly, J. M., and J. M. Long, III: Intravenous hyperalimentation: techniques and potential complications, Surg. Clin. North Am. 61:583, 1981.

19 Duke, J. H., Jr., and S. J. Dudrick: Parenteral feeding, in *Manual of Surgical Nutrition*, W. F. Ballinger et al. (eds.), Saunders, Philadelphia, 1975.

20 Grant, J. P.: *Handbook of Total Parenteral Nutrition*, Saunders, Philadelphia, 1980.

21 Meng, H. C.: Parenteral nutrition: principles, nutrient requirements, techniques and clinical applications, in *Nutritional Support of Medical Practice*, H. A. Schneider, C. E. Anderson, and D. B. Coursin (eds.), Harper & Row, Hagerstown, Md. 1977.

22 Dudrick, S. J., B. V. MacFadyen, Jr., E. A. Souchon, D. Englert, and E. M. Copeland: Parenteral nutrition techniques in cancer patients, Cancer Res., 37:2440, 1977.

23 Kinney, J. M.: Energy requirements for parenteral nutrition, in *Total Parenteral Nutrition*, J. E. Fischer (ed.), Little, Brown, Boston, 1976.

24 Guild, R. T., and J. J. Cerda: Total parenteral nutrition in *Nutrition and Medical Practice*, L. A. Barness (ed.), Avi Publishing, Westport, Conn. 1981.

25 Blackburn, G. L., R. R. Bistrian, B. S. Maini, H. T. Schlamm, and M. F. Smith: Nutritional and metabolic assessment of the hospitalized patient, J. Parenteral Enteral Nutr., 1:11, 1977.

26 Bowles, M: Hyperalimentation, J. Arkansas Med. Soc., 77:61, 1980.

27 American Medical Association: Multivitamin preparations for parenteral use. A statement by the Nutrition Advisory Group, J. Parenteral Enteral Nutr., 3:258, 1979.

28 American Medical Association: Guidelines for essential trace element preparations for parenteral use. A statement by the Nutrition Advisory Group, J. Parenteral Enteral Nutr., 3:263, 1979.

29 Fischer, J. E.: Hyperalimentation, Med. Clin. North Am., 63:973, 1979.

30 Law, D. H.: Current concepts in nutrition (TPN), N. Engl. J. Med., 297:1104, 1977.

CHAPTER **4**

NUTRITIONAL ASPECTS OF PREGNANCY, LACTATION, INFANCY AND CHILDHOOD, ADOLESCENCE, MIDDLE AGE, AND OLD AGE

CONTENTS

PREGNANCY

Concern about eating habits in pregnancy is probably as old as history. Many of the taboos and proscriptions do not seem, by contemporary criteria, to have been in the best interests of the pregnant woman. In primitive societies there have always been food taboos. In the western world, throughout most of the last three centuries, pregnancy was regarded as a plethoric state, best treated by bloodletting, when this was in fashion, and more recently by restricted diets [1]. More rational reasons to restrict the diet included reducing fetal growth in order to make labor easier, especially in women with contraction of the bony pelvis as a result of rickets, and reducing the risk of preeclamptic toxemia. Subsequently, the obstetrician's interest in nutrition appears to have waned as the use of caesarean section to avoid difficult labor gained favor.

The realization that a woman's nutritional status during pregnancy profoundly influences her own health as well as that of her infant is of recent origin [2]. Since a pregnant woman is ideally under the continuing care of a physician for a prolonged period of time and since she is highly motivated to understand and accept advice, the prenatal patient presents the physician with a unique opportunity to teach sound nutritional principles, which can offer benefits extending far beyond the duration of pregnancy and can have a lasting influence on her and on her family.

Assessment of Maternal Nutritional Status

Since there is much accumulated evidence that poor nutrition, at the inception of pregnancy and during gestation, influences the outcome of pregnancy, good prenatal care includes evaluation of maternal nutritional status.

Gross nutritional deficiency is rarely found in the United States, but subclinical malnutrition is not rare. When evaluating the nutritional status of a pregnant woman it is important to recognize the factors which can put the patient into the category of increased nutritional risk and to determine which patients may need special evaluation and/or nutritional care.

Recently, the American College of Obstetricians and Gynecologists (A.C.O.G.) in cooperation with the American Dietetic Association (A.D.A) prepared a booklet, *Assessment of Maternal Nutrition* [3], which contains as one of its more important features a listing of nutritional risk factors during pregnancy. In taking a medical history, it is helpful to keep in mind that an obstetrical patient is at nutritional risk if:

1 She is an adolescent (15 years old or less).
2 She has been pregnant three or more times during the past two years.
3 She has a history of poor obstetrical or fetal performance.
4 She is economically disadvantaged (an income below the poverty level or a recipient of local, state, or federal assistance, such as Medicaid or a U.S. Department of Agriculture food program, e.g., WIC).
5 She is a food faddist who ingests a bizarre or nutritionally restrictive diet.

6 She is a heavy smoker, drug addict, or alcoholic.

7 She follows a therapeutic diet for a chronic systemic disease.

8 She has a prepartum weight at the first prenatal visit that is below 85 percent or above 120 percent of the ideal weight for her height and body build.

She is *very likely* to be at nutritional risk if:

1 She has a low or deficient hemoglobin or hematocrit. (A low value is a hemoglobin below 11.0 g/dl and a hematocrit below 33 percent; a deficient value is a hemoglobin below 10.0 g/dl and a hematocrit below 30 percent.)

2 She has experienced inadequate weight gain during pregnancy, i.e., any weight loss or a gain of less than 1 kg (2 lb) per month.

3 She has experienced excessive weight gain during pregnancy, i.e. above 1 kg per week.

4 She is planning to breast-feed her infant.

Fundamental to nutritional assessment is an evaluation of dietary intake. Detailed information can be obtained by using a 24-hour intake recall (see Chapter 1). From a clinical perspective, *qualitative* information based on her intake of major food groups and of essential nutrients, her consumption of unusual foods, or an unconventional dietary pattern can suggest whether nutritional handicaps may affect the patient's health.

Physical evidence of poor nutrition tends to appear late and is often subtle and nonspecific. Physical signs of deficiency may be masked by changes peculiar to a normal pregnancy (see Chapter 1, under "Physical Examination and Clinical Signs of Malnutrition").

During the course of pregnancy many biochemical and physiological changes take place which cause values obtained from standard hematological and biochemical tests to appear abnormal when compared to the values obtained in healthy nonpregnant women. In addition, lack of established standards for healthy pregnant women limits the value of many laboratory tests. Both maternal plasma volume and red cell volume begin to increase shortly after conception. Plasma volume rises to a peak of 39 to 50 percent above the nonpregnant level early in the third trimester, after which there is little or no increase [4]. In contrast, red cell volume increases in a linear pattern throughout pregnancy and by term is 17 to 40 percent above its initial level [5]. As a consequence of the differential rates of increase of these two blood components, the concentration of many substances in the blood decreases. For example, hemoglobin concentration (expressed as grams per deciliter of blood) decreases, as does the concentration of blood proteins. In addition, maternal renal function is altered; excretion of some blood components falls and excretion of others rises. Serum cholesterol levels rise during pregnancy but fasting levels of blood glucose decrease. Cardiac output increases because of an accelerated heart rate and a larger stroke volume [6]. If no physical symptoms of deficiency, or consequences to the course or outcome of pregnancy, are observed when serum nutrient levels differ from the norm, their clinical significance is difficult to determine. Further information on this topic is available in *Laboratory Indices of Nutritional Status in Pregnancy* [4].

Nutritional Requirements

It has been accurately pointed out by Beal [7] that adequate information is not available for defining nutritional requirements of the pregnant woman. The present recommendations are calculations based largely on the interpretation and judgment of individuals or "expert committees." Variations in recommendations from one country or expert committee to another testify to the paucity of firm data. Differentiation between mean levels and optimal levels is ultimately essential but is at the present time difficult.

Energy Requirement and Weight Gain   One of the most important topics to be discussed at the first prenatal visit with a physician is the patient's expected weight gain during the pregnancy. On the basis of her prepregnancy weight she should be advised to aim for a definite range. If the patient has any high-risk nutritional problems which are discovered at this initial visit, it is advisable to refer her to a registered dietitian for in-depth nutrition counseling.

Essentially all major human studies have documented a positive correlation between total maternal weight gain and birth weight of the fetus; prepregnant weight is also related to birth weight. Evidence in humans comes partly from "natural experiments" such as war and famine, which are accompanied by maternal malnutrition. Infants born in those circumstances have had correspondingly significantly lower birth weights. Several current nutritional intervention trials conducted in various areas of the world indicate that protein-calorie supplementation during pregnancy to populations of women whose nutritional status is known or presumed to be deficient significantly increases the mean birth weight.

Weight gain is at best a crude index of nutritional status, providing little information regarding nutrients other than energy. Birth weight is also an imprecise index of fetal development. Regardless of these facts, birth weight still remains the most significant indicator of maternal nutrition.

Optimal weight gain in pregnancy has been the subject of considerable speculation. The fewest obstetrical complications occur in association with an "average" weight gain, so that it is likely that "average" and "optimal" are similar. Data regarding average weight gain in single pregnancies show remarkable degrees of consistency. Chesley [8] found the average weight gain to be 11 kg. This value is similar to that reported by the Committee on Maternal Nutrition of the Food and Nutrition Board of the National Research Council [9]. Hytten and Leitch [6] suggested 12.5 kg for healthy primigravidas who are eating without restriction.

The temporal *pattern* of weight accumulation is more important than total weight gain. The optimum is a minimum gain of 1 to 2 kg during the first trimester, then a steady linear gain averaging 400 g per week until term (Figure 4-1). Women who are obese before becoming pregnant are not advised to

PRENATAL WEIGHT GAIN GRID

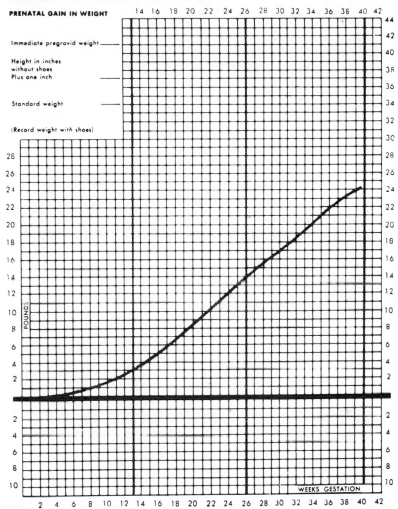

FIGURE 4-1
Pattern of normal prenatal weight gain. (*From Committee on Maternal Nutrition, Food and Nutrition Board, National Research Council, National Academy of Sciences, Maternal Nutrition and the Course of Pregnancy, U.S. Government Printing Office, Washington, D.C., 1970.*)

restrict energy intake. The incidence of infants with a low birth weight is higher among women whose weight gain is low. Furthermore, energy intakes below 36 kcal per kilogram of body weight impair protein utilization in pregnancy [10].

During pregnancy, the increase in body weight is derived from both the products of conception and the mother's body tissue. At term (40 weeks) the average gain in maternal body weight is 12.5 kg, of which the fetus, placenta, and amniotic fluid as well as the maternal tissue fluid account for 7.3 kg. The rest

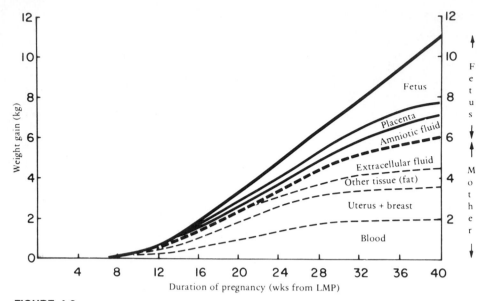

FIGURE 4-2
Pattern and components of average maternal weight gain during pregnancy. LMP = last menstrual
period. (*From R. M. Pitkin, Clin. Obstet. Gynecol., 19:489, 1976.*)

of the gain in body weight, which is not accounted for by these increments,
represents maternal stores, including about 4 kg of fat [11] (see Figure 4-2).

The Recommended Dietary Allowance (RDA) for energy intake for pregnant and nonpregnant women is summarized in Table 4-1 and the RDA for
pregnant women provides 300 kcal above the age-specified recommendation for
nonpregnant women.

Protein   The need for additional protein during pregnancy is clear, but
estimates of the quantity needed vary with the methods used. The "factorial"
approach (see Appendix 4), in which total protein accumulation during
pregnancy is calculated from the nitrogen contents in the maternal and fetal
compartments, estimates the total protein accumulation during pregnancy to
term to be about 1 kg. Dividing the total known protein accumulation by the
duration of pregnancy yields a value of approximately 4 g per day (that is, about
0.5 g of nitrogen per day). Adjusting this figure for individual variation,
efficiency of conversion of dietary protein to tissue protein, and varying
biological quality of protein, leads to an estimate of about 10 g per day as the
additional quantity of protein needed during pregnancy. If balance studies are
used (see Appendix 4), the estimations of protein requirements are two or three
times those calculated by the factorial method. If these balance studies are valid,
they suggest that pregnancy involves nitrogen storage in unknown sites. In view
of the uncertainty regarding protein storage, the current RDA presumes the
higher values and suggests 30 g per day in addition to the basic protein allowance
(Table 4-1).

TABLE 4-1
RECOMMENDED DIETARY ALLOWANCES

	Nonpregnant females					
	11–14 yr*	15–18 yr†	19–22 yr†	23–50 yr†	Pregnancy	Lactation
Energy, kcal	2200	2100	2100	2000	+300	+500
Protein, g	46	46	44	44	+30	+20
Vitamin A, RE	800	800	800	800	+200	+400
Vitamin D, μg	10	10	7.5	5	+5	+5
Vitamin E, mg α-TE	8	8	8	8	+2	+3
Ascorbic acid, mg	50	60	60	60	+20	+40
Folacin, μg	400	400	400	400	+400	+100
Niacin, mg NE	15	14	14	13	+2	+5
Riboflavin, mg	1.3	1.3	1.2	1.2	+0.3	+0.5
Thiamine, mg	1.1	1.1	1.1	1.0	+0.4	+0.5
Vitamin B_6, mg	1.8	2.0	2.0	2.0	+0.6	+0.5
Vitamin B_{12}, μg	3	3	3	3	+1	+1
Calcium, mg	1200	800	800	800	+400	+400
Phosphorus, mg	1200	800	800	800	+400	+400
Iodine, μg	150	150	150	150	+25	+50
Iron, mg	18	18	18	18	‡	‡
Magnesium, mg	300	300	300	300	+150	+150
Zinc, mg	15	15	15	15	+5	+10

*Weight, 46 kg (101 lb); height, 162 cm (62 in).
†Weight, 55 kg (120 lb), height 163 cm (65 in).
‡30–60 mg of supplemental iron per day is recommended.

Source: Food and Nutrition Board, Recommended Dietary Allowances, 9th ed., National Academy of Sciences, Washington, 1980.

Vitamins The B vitamins thiamine, riboflavin, and niacin are important components of the diet during pregnancy because of their role in energy production. Pyridoxine (vitamin B_6) and folacin are needed for protein synthesis and, thus, for fetal development and growth; folacin and cobalamin are involved in synthesis of red blood cells, and vitamin C is essential for the formation of collagen. The biochemical roles and other functions of these water-soluble vitamins are described in Appendix 6. The RDAs for all of these are increased during pregnancy (see Table 4-1).

Folacin (folic acid) is the only nutrient for which the RDA during pregnancy is *twice* the nonpregnant allowance. The role that folic acid plays in DNA synthesis and in erythrocyte maturation is particularly important during pregnancy. Dietary survey data suggest that the usual American diet has a marginal folic acid content; hence, many experts recommend supplements of 200 to 400 μg per day. The Committee on Nutrition of the American College of Obstetricians and Gynecologists [12] has suggested that folic acid supplementation, particularly high-risk patients, such as those of low socioeconomic status, those with a multiple pregnancy, and those with chronic hemolytic anemia, is a reasonable prophylactic measure.

Megaloblastic anemia in pregnancy is most often due to a deficiency of folacin, but cobalamin must be considered in making the diagnosis. Concern about meeting the recommendation for cobalamin is probably unnecessary in women whose diets contain animal products, but supplementation should be considered by strictly vegetarian women who become pregnant.

For nonmilk drinkers, vitamin D is the only other vitamin for which supplementation should be considered. However, since excess prenatal intakes of vitamin D have been related to hypercalcemia in infants [13], caution must be used.

Minerals   Table 4-1 indicates increases in the RDAs for the minerals calcium, phosphorus, iodine, iron, magnesium, and zinc. Needs for other minerals are also increased but specific estimates have not been established.

Calcium and Phosphorus   The recommended increase in dietary calcium and phosphorus during pregnancy is 400 mg per day for each, which represents an increase of 50 percent. As with protein, attempts to estimate requirements by balance studies indicate a higher need than if the calcium content of the fetus, tissue, and fluids is measured. The measured total is about 30 g [14]. Most of the accumulation of calcium occurs in the fetus during the latter part of pregnancy, with an estimated average accumulation of 300 mg daily during the last trimester.

Some argue that the calcium allowance is set too high, since apparently successful pregnancies occur in many other cultures with calcium intakes substantially below those recommended. A likely explanation probably relates to the large calcium reservoir in the maternal skeleton, of which the 30 g needed for pregnancy represents about 2.5 percent [15]. However, in many other cultures the diets consumed also contain less phosphorus and protein, which would serve to reduce calcium loss in the urine. Clinical manifestations of osteomalacia in multiparous women have been reported [16], and neonatal bone density may be related to the adequacy of maternal calcium consumption during pregnancy [17].

The current RDA of 1200 mg calcium can be provided by 1 qt of milk or equivalent dairy products. However, women who do not or cannot consume milk or milk products must rely on other sources. Since calcium present in plant sources may not be totally available for absorption, individuals such as strict vegetarians require calcium supplementation.

Little concern has been expressed about the phosphorus requirement because of its widespread availability from foods such as animal protein, dairy products, and snack items. The RDA is set to provide a calcium-phosphorus ratio of 1.

Iron   The growing fetus and placenta and expanded maternal red cell mass increase the requirement for iron during pregnancy (see Table 4-2). Thus, despite the fact that iron is no longer lost by menstruation, the pregnant woman needs to absorb 540 mg of extra iron during her pregnancy.

As pointed out in Chapter 10, it is not easy to satisfy the usual dietary iron requirements of women. The amount of iron consumed in the usual American diet is 6 mg per 1000 kcal, and in order to meet the RDA for nonpregnant women (18 mg), 3000 kcal would have to be consumed—an unrealistic figure! Since the RDA during pregnancy is greater than 18 mg, iron supplementation in amounts of 30 to 60 mg of elemental iron daily is routinely prescribed throughout pregnancy and for 2 to 3 months postpartum. The elemental iron content of several commonly used preparations is ferrous fumarate, 33 percent; ferrous sulfate (nonexsiccated), 20 percent; and ferrous gluconate, 12 percent (see Table 10-7). In addition, increased vitamin C intake has been shown to improve iron absorption. Therefore, the pregnant woman should be encouraged to include in her diet a generous intake of foods with a high vitamin C content (see Appendix 6).

However, the universal need for supplemental iron in pregnancy is questioned both in the United States and in Europe. The red cell mass increases by 20 to 30 percent in pregnancy and the plasma volume by 40 to 45 percent, so that some hemodilution is inevitable [18]. The observed temporary fall in serum ferritin concentration may be, at least in part, due to this hemodilution. Administration of iron during pregnancy has been shown to reduce the incidence of anemia [19], though falls in serum ferritin levels are not thereby prevented [20]. However, it has not been shown that maternal supplementation with iron results in a more favorable outcome of the pregnancy [21].

Those who now insist that there is no need for iron supplementation in pregnancy usually qualify this by emphasizing that women who commence pregnancy in an iron-depleted state should be given iron. The difficulty is recognition of those at risk. Some recent studies of adolescents [22] have shown good evidence for iron depletion, possibly as a consequence of faulty diet, and in such individuals, supplementation with iron (and folacin) is very important. Although direct evidence in older females is not currently available, on the

TABLE 4-2
IRON BALANCE DURING PREGNANCY

Extra iron in:	Iron, mg
Product of conception	370
Maternal blood	290
Total	660
Less iron "saved" by cessation of menstruation	120
Total	540

Source: Committee on Maternal Nutrition, Food and Nutrition Board, Maternal Nutrition and the Course of Pregnancy, National Academy of Sciences, National Research Council, Washington, 1970.

theoretical grounds already presented, there seems to be a good case to be made for iron supplementation.

Sodium   Sodium metabolism in pregnancy is complicated and often misunderstood. The older and more traditional view holds that pregnancy is characterized by insidious sodium retention, which increases vascular reactivity and may lead to blood vessel constriction, with resultant preeclampsia and toxemia. The more current theory, based on evidence that pregnancy is a salt-wasting state, holds that inadequate sodium intake in the face of excessive losses leads to hypovolemia (abnormal decreased volume of blood fluids) and to compensatory vascular contraction. Hence, this theory holds that sodium intake should be increased somewhat in pregnancy.

Although there is no RDA for sodium, pregnant women are now advised to salt their food "to taste." As total food intake increases, so too will sodium intake increase. The edema seen in a large proportion of pregnant women, usually late in pregnancy, should be treated with support stockings or bedrest but *not* with salt restriction or diuretics.

Special Nutritional Concerns during Pregnancy

Preconceptional Underweight   Women with a low prepregnancy weight (10 percent or more under ideal weight for her height) have an increased risk of having low-birth-weight infants and other complications [23,24]. As Pitkin pointed out [25], the hazards presented by the underweight obstetrical patient have been underemphasized and frequently the underweight patient goes unnoticed by health professionals. A recent study of 654 women by Brown et al. [24] indicates that women who began pregnancy at less than 80 percent of standard weight or at 80 to 90 percent of standard weight delivered infants of a younger gestational age and of lower birth weight than did women of normal weight who gained the same amount of weight. The incidence of low birth weight was approximately twice as high among infants born to underweight women as to women of normal weight gaining the same amount of weight (see Table 4-3).

Data gathered to date indicate that the effects of prepregnancy weight and pregnancy weight gain are independent and additive [26,27]. These findings suggest that underweight women should be urged to replenish their own stores as well as to gain the recommended amount for pregnancy. If an underweight woman has not gained 10 lb by the twentieth week of gestation, she should be regarded as a high-risk case. The patient should be referred to a nutritionist for appropriate measures to augment weight gain.

Preconceptional Obesity   The obese woman entering pregnancy faces increased risks of several complications, especially hypertensive disorders and diabetes mellitus [28]. The Committee on Maternal Nutrition [9], however, concluded that there is no advantage in prescribing weight-reduction regimens for obese patients during pregnancy and that such regimens should be

TABLE 4-3
INFLUENCE OF PREPREGNANCY WEIGHT STATUS ON WEIGHT GAIN DURING
PREGNANCY AND ON GESTATIONAL AGE AND BIRTH WEIGHT OF INFANTS

Prepregnancy weight status	Total no.	Weight gain, kg	Gestation, weeks	Birth weight, g	Percentage of low birth weight (< 2501 g)
Very underweight	155	12.6 ± 0.27	38.9 ± 0.3	2976 ± 48	12.9 (N = 20)
Moderately underweight	243	12.9 ± 0.32	38.9 ± 0.2	3020 ± 41	16.5 (N = 40)
Normal weight	247	12.6 ± 0.5	39.5 ± 0.1	3234 ± 32	6.9 (N = 17)
Significance level*		NS	$p < 0.032$	$p < 0.0001$	$p < 0.0005$

*Statistical significance of differences between mean vlaues obtained for normal weight and underweight women.
Note: Results are reported as mean ± SE.
Source: J. E. Brown, H. N. Jacobson, L. H. Askue, and M. G. Peick, Influence of pregnancy weight gain on the size of infants born to underweight women, J. Obstet. Gynecol., 57:13, 1981.

undertaken only *after* termination of pregnancy. If most women were to follow the RDAs for energy and nutrients, they should achieve a desirable pattern of weight gain. One hazard of "dieting" for obese women during pregnancy is ketonemia resulting from catabolism of fat stores [29]. Ketosis is poorly tolerated by the fetus, and women with acetonuria during pregnancy have children who do not score as well on IQ tests at the age of 4 as children of nonacetonuric women [14].

Weight Gain During Pregnancy   Although the length of gestation is the most important factor determining birth weight, the weight gain of the mother during pregnancy is the second most significant. In the Collaborative Perinatal Study of over 53,000 women and their infants [30], when maternal weight gain was 15 lb or less, 16 percent of the infants weighed less than 2500 g. The proportion dropped to 8 percent when the maternal gain was 16-25 lb, to 4 percent with a maternal gain of 26-35 lb, and to 3 percent when the maternal gain during pregnancy was 36 lb or higher. Naeye [31] further examined 44,565 of those cases and found that optimal weight gain, taken as the rate associated with the lowest perinatal mortality, was 30 lb for very thin mothers (prepregnancy weight <90 percent of the Metropolitan Life Insurance Company's desirable values), 20 lb for normally proportioned mothers, and 16 lb for overweight mothers (>135 percent of desirable values). The perinatal mortality rates increased when mothers gained more than 32 lb at term, regardless of their "weight for height" prior to pregnancy. Naeye concluded that a woman's optimal weight gain in pregnancy depends upon her body build and that optimal weight gain of an overweight woman is about half that of a very thin woman. There are some problems, however, in interpreting the data from this report. The study did not take into consideration the health of the women studied, their age, their parity, or their nutritional histories. The study did not distinguish between overweight due to obesity and overweight related to a large, lean body as would be seen in some very muscular women. It is necessary to consider these factors because the optimal weight gains suggested for women are different from those recently recommended in the United Kingdom (27 lb) [6] and by others in the United States (20 to 25 lb) [9]. It would appear that further studies are needed in this difficult and complex field before present recommendations regarding optimum weight gain in pregnancy can be modified with confidence.

Even more serious than the risks associated with excessive weight gain during pregnancy are the risks imposed on the fetus when energy intake is limited and weight gain is severely restricted. A restriction in energy intake often means that the supply of other essential nutrients will be inadequate. *At least* 2000 kcal of *well-chosen* foods is necessary to supply the recommended intake of protein, vitamins, and minerals [32].

Anemia   Anemia occurs frequently in pregnancy [33], and the majority of these cases are nutritional in origin, with a deficiency of iron being the most common cause. A second related cause is acute blood loss from hemorrhage and a third less common cause of anemia is a deficiency of folacin.

A characteristic microcytic, hypochromic anemia is produced by a deficiency of iron. A diagnosis of iron-deficiency anemia is made on the basis of a hemoglobin concentration value of 11 g or less per deciliter of blood, a hematocrit value of 33 percent or less, and the appearance of characteristic red blood cells on a stained peripheral blood smear. A serum iron level of below 50 to 60 μg/dl and less than 15 percent saturation of transferrin are usually indicative of iron-deficiency anemia if other causes of decreased serum iron are ruled out [34]. Iron-deficiency anemia is treated with 200 mg iron per day, as three 0.2-g tablets of either ferrous sulfate or ferrous fumarate. These women should be counseled to increase not only the amount of iron-rich foods (Table 10-8) in their diet but also the amount of protein. An increase in vitamin C may also aid iron absorption.

Although megaloblastic anemia due to folic acid deficiency is relatively uncommon in the United States, it does occur and must be considered in the differential diagnosis of any anemia encountered during pregnancy and puerperium. Folic acid deficiency can occur as a single deficiency state but is more commonly found in association with iron deficiency. Folic acid therapy very promptly produces a vigorous hematological response. Folic acid is commonly administered orally in doses of 1 mg or less.

Pica   Pica, a craving for unnatural foods or for nonfood items, such as clay, laundry starch, or ice, is seen in pregnant women and is often associated with iron-deficiency anemia. These substances usually replace other nutrients in the diet and can interfere with iron absorption.

Toxemia of pregnancy   Toxemia, or preeclampsia, is a pathological state specific to pregnancy in humans. It is diagnosed by a triad of symptoms: (1) generalized edema that may cause a sudden increase in weight gain, (2) proteinuria, and (3) blood pressure elevated above 140/90 or a systolic rise of 30 mmHg or a diastolic rise of 15 mmHg. Toxemia is more common among primiparas, adolescents (especially those under 15 years), and underweight women, in pregnancies with multiple fetuses, and in low-income populations. Eclampsia is the occurrence of one or more convulsions in a patient who has toxemia of pregnancy.

The role played by nutrition in the etiology of toxemia has been the subject of controversy for many years. Evidence in support of a nutritional etiology includes the high occurrence rate of toxemia among poor women and geographical patterns of toxemia coinciding with areas of low per capita income and high occurrence rate of nutritional disorders such as anemia. A specific nutritional deficiency, such as of protein or of a vitamin, has not been identified. Obesity is not considered a cause, and limiting weight gain does not prevent toxemia.

Another school of thought suggests that sodium causes or at least exacerbates toxemia as a consequence of its effects on fluid retention. Sodium and/or fluid restriction, with or without diuretics, will not prevent or cure toxemia. In fact, sodium restriction may actually exacerbate toxemia [35]. At present the best policy for preventing toxemia is comprehensive prenatal care, including education about a balanced diet that is adequate in nutrient and energy content, particularly for women entering pregnancy in poor nutritional status and with poor dietary habits. The RDAs (Table 4-1) provide a sound guide for planning and assessing the diet of pregnant women.

Adolescence Recent changes in the sexual behavior of teenagers in the United States are having an impact on the health care system. Zelnik et al. reported that one in five females have intercourse by the age of 16 and one in ten conceive before the age of 17. Over one-third of the females who are sexually active premaritally have a premarital pregnancy before reaching the age of 19, with one-third becoming pregnant by the age of 17 [36]. Girls are at increased biological risk when pregnancy occurs before cessation of growth. In the United States, the average age at menarche is 12.5 to 13 years. However, not until the age of 17 have the great majority of girls completed linear growth and achieved gynecological maturity [9]. The pregnant adolescent is also of major concern because of the psychological, educational, nutritional, and vocational difficulties that frequently complicate her situation. Generally, teenagers seek prenatal care later [37] and have fewer total visits than older women of childbearing age. Hence, their biological immaturity and the amount and frequency of prenatal care, as well as the overall life style of adolescence including food habits (see under "Eating Practices," below), place them at a greater risk.

In 1979, the Committee on Adolescence of the American Academy of Pediatrics stated that the two major complications in teenage pregnancy were preeclampsia and an excessive number of low-birth-weight infants [37]. All other potential ill effects of teenage pregnancy appear to be dependent on the social class of the teenager, rather than on adolescence itself, and on whether she has

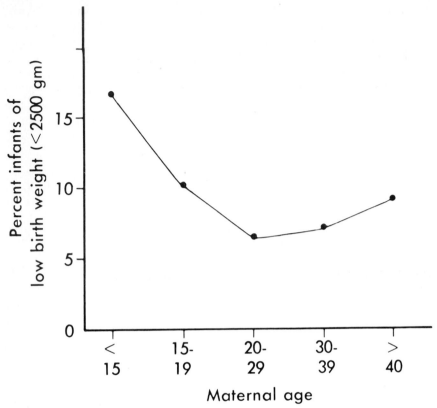

FIGURE 4-3
Incidence of low birth weight delivery in relation to maternal age. (*From Vital Statistics of the United States, Public Health Service, National Center for Health Statistics, 1978.*)

access to the health care system. The time interval between the onset of menses and conception is a risk factor because conception 2 years or less after onset of menses is associated with higher incidences of low birth weight, irrespective of social class (see Figure 4-3). The reported incidence of low-birth-weight infants born to teenage girls ranges from 6 to 20 percent. If gynecological age (time interval since menarche) rather than chronological age is used as a basis of comparison, data from different centers confirm a higher rate of low-birth-weight infants among young teenagers, irrespective of social class [38].

The most consistent, high-risk characteristic of adolescent pregnancy is toxemia. When other variables that correlate with poor nutrition, such as nonwhite race and poverty, are added, the incidence of toxemia is even higher. Anemia, another problem which is common in the pregnant adolescent, is associated with the amount of prenatal care received. Fetal pelvic disproportion and prolonged labor are other complications of teenage pregnancy. The pregnant adolescent is also at greater risk of having a baby with congenital malformations, especially of the central nervous system [39].

Very few studies have been done of the actual dietary intake of pregnant teenagers. The limited data reviewed by Weigley [40] indicate that the diets of pregnant adolescents are not adequate. In a well-controlled study of 18 pregnant teenagers in San Francisco, the nutrients most poorly supplied in the diet were calcium, iron, and vitamin A and the intake of calories was low as well [41]. In a larger study of 142 teenage pregnancies the young women showed considerable evidence of nutritional deficiency. Low blood levels of hemoglobin, vitamin B_6, niacin, folic acid, vitamin A, thiamine, and cobalamin were seen in from 13 to 58 percent of the patients [42].

Caffeine   During pregnancy, a woman consumes many foods and other substances which cross the placental barrier, enter the fetal circulation, and may possibly affect fetal development. Earlier animal studies indicated that caffeine is a teratogen [43] and more recent studies undertaken by the Food and Drug Administration in experimental animals have confirmed these findings [44]. Caffeine readily crosses the human placenta and enters the fetal circulation. The fetus and neonate appear to lack the enzyme or enzymes necessary to demethylate caffeine. In a recent study, 800 households were contacted and complete data were obtained on 489 pregnancies [45]. These data are presented in Table 4-4 and suggest that a high level of caffeine consumption (more than 600 mg or the equivalent of 8 cups of coffee daily) is associated with a high risk of fetal loss. In 1980, the Food and Drug administration advised as a precautionary measure that potentially pregnant women eliminate or limit their consumption of caffeine-containing products [44].

More recently, a group from Harvard examined the effects of coffee consumption in more than 12,000 women interviewed at the time of their hospitalization for delivery [46]. After controlling for smoking, alcohol consumption, and demographic characteristics such as age, race, education, and medical history, their analysis showed no relation between low birth weight or short gestation and heavy coffee consumption (> 4 cups per day). Furthermore, there was no excess of malformations among coffee drinkers. However, this study did not directly examine caffeine consumption, since information about consumption of soft drinks, cocoa, or caffeine-containing drugs was not obtained. On the other hand it did add to the data indicating that smoking is associated with poorer pregnancy outcome.

Health professionals can use the following approximations as a guide in advising patients:

Product	Caffeine, mg
Cup of coffee	75–155
Cup of tea	9–50
12-oz cola drink	30–65
Cup of cocoa	2–40
1-oz solid milk chocolate	6
OTC stimulant tablet	100–200

TABLE 4-4
OUTCOME OF PREGNANCY IN RELATION TO CAFFEINE CONSUMPTION

Daily caffeine consumption (estimate)	Number of households with pregnancies	Outcome of pregnancy			
		Spon-taneous abortion	Still-birth	Pre-mature birth*	Uncom-plicated delivery
⩾ 600 mg by woman	16	8	5	2	1 (6.3%)
> 600 mg by man, < 400 mg by woman	13	4	2	2 (1)	5 (38.5%)
300–450 mg by man, woman, or both	23	0	0	0	23 (100%)
< 300 mg by man, woman, or both	81	7	17	5 (3)	52 (64.2%)
None	356	33	38	6 (3)	279 (78.4%)

*Numbers in parentheses indicate deaths within 48 hours after birth.
Source: P. S. Weathersbee, L. K. Olsen, and J. R. Lodge, Caffeine and pregnancy, Postgrad. Med., 62:64, 1977.

Many noncola soft drinks, including "pepper drinks," may also contain added caffeine. For this reason, patients should be encouraged to read the labels. In addition, physicians should point out that many analgesic combinations, cold preparations, and stimulants contain caffeine.

Alcohol   Recent studies indicate that as little as 1 oz of alcohol per day may increase the risks of stillbirths, low birth weight, physical malformations, poor sucking ability, and numerous medical complications in the postnatal period [47]. The hazards of heavy maternal drinking and the "fetal alcohol syndrome" (FAS) are described in detail in Chapter 17.

LACTATION

"Satisfactory lactation represents the greatest nutritional stress imposed by a physiological process in the human body" [48]. Lactation allowances for nutrients have usually been determined by the factorial method as follows: Estimations are made of the nutrient content and the volume of the milk produced, with the addition of the physiological needs of the mother for synthesis of milk components; the efficiency of maternal absorption may also be incorporated into the calculation. The resulting value for each nutrient should then be added to the nonpregnant, nonlactating allowance (Table 4-1). Allowances for many nutrients during lactation are the same as during pregnancy, so the diet during pregnancy is a good basis for the diet during lactation.

Nutritional Requirements of the Lactating Mother

Energy and Protein   The Food and Nutrition Board's Committee on Recommended Dietary Allowances recommends that during lactation there be major increases in energy intake (500 kcal per day) and in protein (20 g per day). The additional energy requirements of lactation are proportional to the quantity of milk produced. Since human breast milk has an energy content of approximately 70 kcal/dl and the efficiency of conversion of maternal energy to milk energy is at least 80 percent [49], approximately 90 kcal are required for the production of 100 ml of milk. Thus nearly 800 kcal are required for the production of 850 ml of milk, the average daily output most expert committees have assumed. The basis of this value for average daily output is obscure, and it is not substantiated by measurements of actual milk outputs. Lower values are reported from a number of studies [50]. A mean value of 750 to 800 ml per day at 2 to 4 months postpartum seems typical of industrialized countries, while lower values are reported from developing countries. The RDA also presumes that at least 4 kg of body fat is laid down during pregnancy and is available to provide an additional 200 to 300 kcal per day [51]. If a mother continues to breast-feed beyond 3 months (so that these fat stores are then used up) or if she is breast-feeding more than one child or if her maternal weight is below the ideal weight for her height, her energy needs will be further increased.

English and Hitchcock compared the energy intake of 16 nursing women to 10 nonnursing women and found that the daily energy intake of breast-feeding mothers in the sixth to eighth postpartum week was 2460 kcal [52]. The energy intake of nonnursing mothers during the same postpartum period was 1880 kcal—a difference of 580 kcal per day. In another study, Thomson et al. found that lactating women ingested 2716 kcal per day and nonnursing mothers 2125 kcal per day—a difference of 591 kcal per day [49].

The protein content of human milk averages 1.2 percent. Again, if an average daily production of 850 ml is assumed, 850 ml contains 10 g of protein, and a higher level of production (1200 ml) contains 15 g of protein. The 20-g increment in the RDA for protein for lactating women assumes the production of 1200 ml and a 70 percent efficiency of dietary protein conversion to milk protein.

The increased energy and protein needs can be met with somewhat less than an additional quart of milk per day. This will not provide, however, the increased recommendation for ascorbic acid, folacin, vitamin E, zinc, etc. Hence, the intake of other foods such as citrus fruits, vegetable oil, and meat must be slightly increased.

Calcium   The calcium content of human milk is approximately 30 mg/dl. It is estimated that an infant obtains 250 to 300 mg per day during lactation. Since calcium absorption is far less than 100 percent efficient, an intake of 1200 mg is recommended to ensure sufficient absorption. If the maternal diet provides inadequate calcium, the calcium level of the milk will be maintained at the expense of the mother's skeleton. For women who cannot or will not take milk products, a supplement of at least 1 g of calcium daily is recommended to minimize the loss of bone calcium.

Other Minerals The iron requirement is not known but is assumed to be not substantially different from that of the nonpregnant woman. The iron content of milk is low, and amenorrhea during part of the lactation period would partially offset the iron needed for milk production. However, continued supplementation of the mother for 2 to 3 months after parturition is advised in order to replenish stores depleted by pregnancy. The zinc allowance for lactation is relatively higher than other minerals when compared to nonlactating allowances, but this value must be considered tentative in view of the limited knowledge of the role of zinc in human nutrition [7].

Vitamins An increased allowance is provided in the RDA for all vitamins during lactation. The breast milk content of ascorbic acid, thiamine, riboflavin, pantothenic acid, pyridoxine, biotin, folic acid, and vitamin B_{12} reflects maternal dietary intake. The vitamin D content of human milk is low and rickets has been observed occasionally in nursing infants. For this reason, vitamin D supplementation of nursing infants is frequently advised. Although the requirements for all vitamins are increased during lactation, these needs can be provided by a well-balanced diet. Hence nutritional supplements are usually unnecessary.

Fluids Approximately 87 percent of the volume of breast milk is water, and a generous fluid intake, probably close to 3 liters per day, is needed to avoid dehydration [7].

Nonnutritive Substances Found in Breast Milk

Chemicals other than nutrients readily enter breast milk; for some compounds breast milk is a route of excretion. Over 100 substances including caffeine, alcohol, morphine, marijuana, and oral contraceptive hormones are excreted in breast milk [53,54]. Care should be taken is prescribing medication for the lactating woman [55], and moderation in alcohol intake is appropriate. Excessive amounts of alcohol have been reported to cause a "pseudo-Cushing" syndrome, with excessive weight gain and poor growth in the infant [56].

In 1951, Laug et al. reported that dichlorodiphenyltrichloroethane (DDT) was present in human milk [57], and that observation was subsequently confirmed by authors in diverse parts of the United States. More recently, polychlorinated biphenyls (PCBs) have been detected in breast milk [58]. Both of these chemical contaminants have a high lipid solubility and gradually accumulate in the fat of breast milk. A clinical assessment of risk is difficult because to date no case reports of illness due to transmission of environmental chemicals through breast milk have appeared [59]. Pregnant and lactating women have been advised to avoid excessive weight loss which might mobilize these chemicals from fat stores and to avoid eating sport fish from contaminated waters, the only important source of PCBs remaining.

INFANCY AND CHILDHOOD

Both the Nutrition Committee of the Canadian Paediatric Society and the Committee on Nutrition of the American Academy of Pediatrics have strongly recommended breast-feeding for full-term infants, except in the few cases where specific contraindications exist [60]. A number of nutritional, immunological, economic, and psychological advantages can be cited for exercising this basic human physiological function. The Committee on Nutrition has also recommended that the introduction of solid foods and juices not begin until about the age of 4 to 6 months [61].

Despite these recommendations, recent surveys suggest that feeding practices in the United States vary widely depending on the population examined. A marketing research group found in a national survey that the percentage of infants breast-fed in the hospital increased from 24.7 percent in 1971 to 55.3 percent in 1980. Further, there was an increase in infants breast-fed for longer periods. Among infants 2 months old, breast-feeding increased from 13.9 percent in 1971 to 42.3 percent in 1980, while for infants 3 to 4 months old, the figures were 8.2 percent and 33 percent respectively [62]. Andrew and coworkers analyzed infant feeding practices in 270 families belonging to a prepaid group [63]. They found extensive use of commercially prepared infant formulas during the first months of life and the introduction of cow's milk into the diet at the age of 3 to 5 months. Only 10 percent of this population was breast-fed at the age of 3 months, and only 40 percent were given iron-supplemented formulas. Supplemental foods were given to all infants of less than 3 months. More recently, 22,211 mothers who gave birth at New York City private and city hospitals were studied. In municipal hospitals, where most of the maternity patients were low-income women, 82 percent planned to use infant formula. In private hospitals, the figure was 56 percent [64].

What accounts for this gap between the recommendations of "expert committees" and actual practice? Are physicians following the American Academy of Pediatrics' recommendations? Are mothers getting their nutritional advice from others? Do today's cultural attitudes and lifestyles discourage breast-feeding?

Although we do not know the answers to these questions, we have summarized briefly the following recommendations for infant-feeding practices:

1 The best food for the normal newborn infant is breast milk.

2 *Whole* cow's milk should not be a part of the diet for an infant under the age of 1 year.

3 Milk with reduced fat content should not be a part of the diet for an infant under the age of 1 year.

4 Vitamin and mineral supplementation may be required with some infant diets.

5 Solid foods should be introduced into the diet at the age of 4 to 6 months to support the normal infant's psychological, psychomotor, and educational development.

It must be borne in mind that information on the nutrient requirements of infants for specific nutrients is limited. The estimate of requirements is, for the most part, based on the intake of infants who have shown satisfactory growth and on the calculation of the probable nutrient intakes of breast-fed infants. The greater absorption and utilization of nutrients from breast milk, as compared to cow's milk, have led to adjustments of requirements when cow's milk is the basis of the infant's diet. However, requirements are known to vary with age, size, rate of growth, and level of activity, as well as with the composition of the diet. Thus, the recommendations should be considered tentative and should not be interpreted too strictly.

Infant Nutrient Requirements

Energy   Because infants have a high rate of heat loss due to their relatively large body surface area, their energy requirements for basal metabolism are high, approximately 55 kcal per kilogram of body weight. Another 35 kcal/kg is required for growth and 10 to 25 kcal/kg for activity, yielding a total daily energy requirement of 115 kcal/kg (48 kcal/lb) during the first 6 months of life (see Table 4-5). In the second 6 months of life, the energy requirement as a function of body weight gradually decreases to approximately 105 kcal/kg.

Fomon recommends that 7 to 16 percent of the calories be provided by protein, 30 to 55 percent by fat, and the remainder by carbohydrate [65]. During

TABLE 4-5
RECOMMENDED DAILY ENERGY AND PROTEIN
INTAKES FOR CHILDREN OF VARIOUS AGES

Age group	Energy, kcal/kg	Protein, g/kg
Infants		
0–0.5	115	2.2
0.5–1	105	2.0
Children		
1–3	100	1.8
4–6	85	1.5
7–10	85	1.2
Males		
11–14	60	1.0
15–18	42	0.8
Females		
11–14	48	1.0
15–18	38	0.8

Source: Food and Nutrition Board, Recommended Dietary Allowances, 9th ed., National Academy of Sciences, National Research Council, Washington, 1980.

the first few months of life, all energy intake can be provided by breast milk or infant formula. Breast milk contains about 70 kcal/dl and provides approximately 7 percent of its calories from protein, 55 percent from fat, and 38 percent from carbohydrate. Most commercial preparations of infant formula contain 67 kcal/dl (20 kcal/oz) with about the same distribution of energy-containing nutrients as breast milk.

Carbohydrate No requirement has been set for carbohydrate. Lactose, the natural sugar in both human and cow's milk, supplies 38 percent of the calories in human milk, and 27 to 29 percent of the calories in cow's milk. Most commercial infant formulas have carbohydrate added, so that 40 to 50 percent of the calories are supplied by lactose or other disaccharides. Lactose is important because it is the only dietary source of galactose for the infant. Galactose and glucose are needed for formation of cerebrosides and are vital components of myelin in nerve fibers and of collagen in connective tissue, cartilage, and bone. If other carbohydrates (glucose, sucrose, and fructose) are used in infant formulas, galactose can be synthesized from glucose in the liver.

Proteins and Amino Acids The National Research Council recommends a protein intake of 2.2 g/kg for infants during the first 6 months, declining to 2 g/kg from 6 months to 1 year (Table 4-5). Fomon and associates suggest that protein requirements expressed per unit of calories consumed would be more meaningful. They recommend a protein intake of 1.9 g per 100 kcal during the first 4 months of life and 1.7 g per 100 kcal for the remainder of the first year [66]. These values are similar to the American Academy of Pediatrics' Committee on Nutrition's recommendation that infant formulas provide a minimum protein concentration of 1.8 g per 100 kcal for a protein having a biological value equal to that of casein [67].

Nine amino acids (histidine, isoleucine, leucine, lysine, methionine, phenyl-alanine, threonine, tryptophan, and valine) are essential in infancy. Although there is evidence that infants can synthesize histidine, the amount may not be adequate to meet their physiological requirements.

Protein provides 7 percent of the calories in breast milk, in comparison to the 20 percent supplied by cow's milk protein. Qualitative differences exist as well. In human milk 80 percent of the protein is whey (mainly lactalbumin); the rest is casein. In cow's milk, the distribution is 18 percent and 82 percent respectively. The higher level of lactalbumin in human milk results in smaller and more flocculent curds in the infant's intestinal tract after exposure of the milk to hydrochloric acid in the stomach, resulting in easier digestion, greater absorption, and softer stools. Nitrogen absorption from human milk reaches 90 percent efficiency by the end of the second week of life [7]. Milk protein containing larger amounts of casein forms a tough hard-to-digest curd after exposure to hydrochloric acid in the stomach. "Humanized" formulas in which the ratio of casein to whey protein is adjusted to simulate human milk still have a profoundly different protein composition [68].

Fat   For the infant, fat is a significant source of energy; it is a vehicle for essential fatty acids and fat-soluble vitamins and contributes to the feeling of satiety through which the infant learns to regulate appetite. Fat provides 55 percent of the calories of human milk and slightly less in whole cow's milk. In commercial premodified infant formulas, fat provides from 35 to 50 percent of the calories. The Committee on Nutrition of the American Academy of Pediatrics [67] recommended that the Food and Drug Administration standard that a minimum of 15 percent of the calories in infant formulas be from fat should be raised to a minimum of 30 percent, with a maximum of 54 percent.

The cholesterol content of human milk ranges from 7 to 47 mg/dl, while cow's milk provides from 10 to 35 mg/dl [69]. Nonfat milk-based formulas contribute 1.4 to 3.3 mg/dl.

The Committee on Nutrition of the American Academy of Pediatrics recommends that 2.7 percent of the total calories be provided by linoleic acid, an important precursor of prostaglandins. Approximately 5 percent of the calories in human mik, 1 percent in cow's mik, and 10 percent in infant formulas are derived from this fatty acid [67]. When linoleic acid intake provided less than 0.5 to 1.0 percent of the caloric consumption of otherwise normal infants, they exhibited skin lesions typical of fatty acid deficiency (scaly skin) as well as growth impairment [11].

Concern about heart disease had led to controversy over whether children should consume unsaturated fat rather than saturated fat. Expert committees have agreed that for infants without familial hyperlipoproteinemia, such dietary restriction is not warranted during the first year of life [65].

Vitamins and Minerals   The RDAs for vitamins and minerals are shown in Appendix 8. The Committee on Nutrition of the American Academy of Pediatrics published recommendations in 1980 regarding vitamin and mineral supplement needs of normal infants and children [70] (see Table 4-6). These guidelines can be summarized as follows:

1 Newborn infants:
   a Vitamin K administration to all newborn infants is effective as prophylaxis against hemorrhagic disease of the newborn.
2 Breast-fed infants:
   a Vitamin and mineral supplementation generally is not required. However, if the mother's vitamin D nutrition has been inadequate and if the infant does not receive adequate ultraviolet light, supplements of 400 IU of vitamin D may be indicated.
   b Iron deficiency rarely develops before the age of 4 to 6 months because neonatal iron stores provide a major portion of iron needs during this period. Although breast milk contains only 0.5 mg of iron per liter, about half is absorbed in contrast to the much smaller portion absorbed from cow's milk or other foods. After the age of 6 months, the addition to the diet of iron-fortified cereal is probably desirable to supply adequate amounts of iron.

TABLE 4-6

GUIDELINES FOR USE OF SUPPLEMENTS IN HEALTHY INFANTS AND CHILDREN

Child	Multi-vitamin-multimineral	Vitamins			Mineral
		D	E	Folate	Iron
Term infants					
Breast-fed	0	±	0	0	±[a]
Formula-fed	0	0	0	0	0
Preterm infants					
Breast-fed[b]	+[b]	+	±[c]	±[b]	+
Formula-fed[b]	+[b]	+	±[c]	±[b]	+[a]
Older infants (after 6 months)					
Normal	0	0	0	0	±[a]
High-risk[d]	+	0	0	0	±
Children					
Normal	0	0	0	0	0
High-risk	+	0	0	0	0
Pregnant teenagers					
Normal	±	0	0	±	+
High-risk[e]	+	0	0	+	+

[a] Iron-fortified formula and/or infant cereal is a more convenient and reliable source of iron than a supplement.

[b] Multivitamin supplement (plus added folate) is needed primarily when calorie intake is below approximately 300 kcal per day or when the infant weighs 2.5 kg; vitamin D should be supplied at least until the age of 6 months in breast-fed infants. Iron should be started by the age of 2 months.

[c] Vitamin E should be in a form that is well absorbed by small premature infants. If this form of vitamin E is approved for use in formulas, it need not be given separately to formula-fed infants. Infants fed breast milk are less susceptible to vitamin E deficiency.

[d] Multivitamin-multimineral preparation (including iron) is preferred to use of iron alone.

[e] Multivitamin multimineral preparation (including iron and folate) is preferred to use of iron alone or iron and folate alone.

Note: +, a supplement is usually indicated; ±, a supplement is possibly or sometimes indicated; 0, a supplement is not usually indicated. Vitamin K for newborn infants and fluoride in areas where there is insufficient fluoride in the water supply are not shown.

Source: American Academy of Pediatrics Committee on Nutrition, Vitamin and mineral supplement needs in normal children in the United States, Pediatrics, 66:1015, 1980.

    c Fluoride supplementation in the breast-fed infant is controversial. Since supplemental fluoride would be expected to have a beneficial effect on unerupted teeth, the committee favored initiating fluoride supplements shortly after birth if the water supply contained less than 0.3 ppm of fluoride.

  3 Formula-fed infants:

    a Infants who consume amounts of iron-fortified commercial cow's milk formulas which are in keeping with the recommendations of the committee [67] do not need vitamin and mineral supplementation. Infants do not require supplementation during the latter part of the first year if formulas continue to be used in an appropriate combination with solid foods. After the age of 4 months, iron-fortified formulas and/or iron-fortified cereals are convenient sources of iron and preferable to the use of iron supplements.

4 Infants fed home-prepared evaporated milk or cow's milk formulas:

   a Home-prepared formulas are seldom used in the United States. The need for supplements with evaporated milk will depend on whether the preparation is fortified. Infants may need supplemental vitamins C and D. Supplemental iron should be started no later than at 4 months of age for term infants.

5 Older infants:

   a During the second 6 months of life, the normal infant may be on a diet of milk or formula, mixed feedings, and increased amounts of table food. Cow's milk, if used, should be fortified with vitamin D, and cereal should be fortified with iron. Other vitamin and mineral supplements are usually not required although it is important that the diet include an adequate source of vitamin C.

Fluid   The recommended allowance of water in infancy is 150 ml per 100 kcal per day [51]. Under ordinary circumstances, human milk and properly prepared infant formulas supply sufficient water. With increases in environmental temperature or during episodes of fever, vomiting, or diarrhea, infants should be offered additional fluids and watched carefully.

Infant Feeding Practices

The obvious food to supply the nutrients needed by the young infant is milk, and breast milk is the milk of choice. The obstetrician is the physician who can have a positive influence in the encouragement of breast-feeding. The most negative influences have been found to be discouragement by the obstetrician or by nursery nurses. Many pediatricians also have not encouraged breast-feeding, and this negative feeling has been transmitted to mothers [71].

Breast-Feeding   The past decade has seen an increase in breast-feeding, especially among better-educated women, on the basis of its being more "natural" and because of scientific support for its greater nutritional and health-promoting value. Among the advantages of breast milk are the following:

1 Breast milk is less likely to be associated with allergic manifestations in infants [72].

2 Breast milk contains readily absorbable iron; the iron in cow's milk formulas is less easily absorbed [73].

3 Zinc and perhaps other trace minerals are also more readily available from breast milk than from other milks [74].

4 Breast-fed infants have increased resistance to gastrointestinal and respiratory infections [60].

5 Breast-fed infants are less likely to overeat, since the infant determines the amount of milk consumed and is not influenced by subtle pressure from the feeder.

6 Breast milk has the additional advantages of being (*a*) sterile, (*b*) convenient, (*c*) available at the proper temperature and in the proper mixture, and (*d*) inexpensive.

7 Breast feeding is psychologically beneficial to infant and mother.

Tailor-made to meet the nutritional needs of the human infant during the first year, breast milk (Table 4-7) offers its carbohydrate as lactose, its fat as a mixture with a generous proportion of polyunsaturated fatty acids, and its protein largely as lactalbumin, a protein that the human infant can easily digest. Its vitamin contents are ample. Its calcium-phosphorus ratio (2:1) is ideal for the absorption of calcium, and both of these minerals and magnesium are present in amounts appropriate for the rate of growth expected in a human infant. Breast milk is also low in sodium. Iron absorption averages 49 percent from breast milk as compared with only 4 percent from fortified formula [73].

Breast milk also contains antibacterial agents. Lactoferrin, an iron-binding factor which prevents bacteria from getting the iron they need for growth, also directly kills some bacteria [75]. Breast milk also contains a factor that favors the growth of the "friendly" bacterium, *Lactobacillus bifidus,* in the infant's digestive tract so that other harmful bacteria cannot grow there.

During the first 2 or 3 days of lactation, the breasts produce colostrum, a premilk substance whose antibody content is even higher than the milk to come later. It also contains white blood cells to kill bacteria and viruses.

Bottle Feeding and Formulas   When a mother is unable or unwilling to breast-feed her infant, a number of substitute milks are available. When bottle-feeding is bacteriologically safe and nutritionally adequate and the mother warm and responsive to her infant's needs, the formula-fed infant thrives. Table 4-8 shows the content of some formulas commonly available in the United States. Changes are intermittently made in the content of these formulas, necessitating updating of information when precise values are required.

Most commercially prepared formulas contain cow's milk, which is modified to make it more suitable for infants as follows: Protein and solute contents are reduced; carbohydrate levels are increased with the addition of sucrose, lactose, or oligosaccharides; butterfat is replaced by vegetable oils; and vitamins and minerals are added. Since cow's milk is a poor source of iron, some formulas are fortified with iron. The energy density of the finished product is about 20 kcal/oz.

For infants who have conditions that contraindicate the use of cow's milk (milk allergy or lactose or galactose intolerance), the most commonly used products are soy milks. The most frequently used soy-milk formulas are constructed of protein isolated from soy meal and fortified with methionine, corn syrup, and/or sucrose and soy or vegetable oils to which vitamins and minerals have been added (Table 4-8).

Manufacturers market infant formulas as liquid concentrates that are

TABLE 4-7
AVERAGE NUTRIENT CONTENT OF MATURE HUMAN MILK AND WHOLE
COW'S MILK
(Per 100 ml)

	Mature human milk	Whole cow's milk
Energy, kcal	70	67
Water, g	87.5	87.5
Protein, g	0.9	3.5
Whey-casein ratio	80 : 20	20 : 80
Carbohydrate, g (source)	7.0 (lactose)	5.0 (lactose)
Fat, g	2.7–4.5	3.5
saturated, g	1.7–2.2	1.2
unsaturated, g	2.2–2.6	2.5
linoleic, %	10–15	4
Cholesterol, mg	14	11
Calcium, mg	34	120
Phosphorus, mg	15	95
Ca : P ratio	2.3	1.3
Iron, mg	0.05	0.04
Iodine, μg	3–6	5.2
Copper, μg	50	30
Magnesium, mg	3.5–4.0	12
Zinc, mg	0.1–0.5	0.4
Sodium, mg	16–19	52
Potassium, mg	50–55	148
Renal solute load	80	220
Oral solute load	250	263
Vitamin A activity, IU	190	149
Vitamin D activity, IU	2	42 (if fortified)
Vitamin E, mg	0.2	0.2
Vitamin K, μg	1.5	6
Ascorbic acid, mg	4–5	1.1
Thiamine, μg	16	31
Riboflavin, μg	36	175
Niacin equivalents, mg	0.1–0.2	0.1
Pyridoxine, μg	10–18	60
Pantothenic acid, mg	0.18–0.25	0.34
Vitamin B_{12}, μg	0.03	0.4
Folacin, μg	5.2	4–5.5

Sources: V. Beal, Nutrition in the Life Span, Wiley, New York, 1980; K. Brostrom, in Textbook of Pediatric Nutrition, R. M. Suskind (ed.), Raven, New York, 1981.

prepared for feeding by mixing equal amounts of the liquid with water. Ready-to-feed formulas that require no preparation and powdered formulas that are prepared by mixing 1 level tablespoon of powder and 2 oz of water are also available.

Home-prepared formula can also be made from a base of canned evaporated

TABLE 4-8
NUTRIENT COMPOSITION OF INFANT FORMULA
(Per 100 ml)

	Enfamil (Mead Johnson)	Similac (Ross Labs)	Isomil Ready-to-Feed (Ross Labs)
Source of protein	Nonfat milk	Nonfat milk	Soy protein isolate
Source of fat	Soy oil, coconut oil	Soy oil, coconut oil*	Coconut oil, soy oil
Source of carbohydrate	Lactose	Lactose	Corn syrup, sucrose
Energy:			
kcal/oz	20	20	20
kcal/dl	67	67	67
Protein, g	1.5	1.6	2.0
Fat, g	3.7	3.6	3.6
Carbohydrate, g	7.0	7.2	6.8
Vitamin A, IU	167.5	250.0	250.0
Vitamin D, IU	42.0	40.0	40.0
Vitamin E, IU	1.3	1.5	1.5
Ascorbic acid, mg	5.4	5.5	5.5
Vitamin B_1, μg	52.1	65.0	40.0
Vitamin B_2, μg	63.0	100.0	60.0
Niacin, μg	837.5	700.0	900.0
Vitamin B_6, μg	41.7	40.0	40.0
Vitamin B_{12}, μg	0.2	0.2	0.3
Folacin, μg	10.7	10.0	10.0
Sodium, mg (meq)	28.0 (1.2)	25.0 (1.1)	30.0 (1.3)
Potassium, mg (meq)	70.0 (1.8)	78.0 (2.0)	71.0 (1.8)
Chloride, mg (meq)	53.0 (1.5)	53.0 (1.5)	53.0 (1.5)
Calcium, mg (meq)	55.0 (2.7)	51.0 (2.6)	70.0 (3.5)
Phosphorus, mg (meq)	46.0 (2.7)	39.0 (2.3)	60.0 (2.9)
Iron, mg	0.2	Trace	1.2
Iodine, μg	6.9	10.0	15.0
Magnesium, mg	4.7	4.1	5.0
Zinc, mg	0.4	0.5	0.5
Renal solute, mOsm/liter	110	108	126
Osmolarity, mOsm/liter	262	262	230
Indications	Full-term infant	Full-term infant	For lactose intolerance

*Coconut and soy oil are used in Similac concentrates and Ready-to-Feed. Coconut and corn oil are used in Similac powder.

(not sweetened condensed) milk. One such formula calls for 13 oz of evaporated milk, 2 tbsp of corn syrup, and 18 oz of water. Evaporated milk is fortified with vitamin D but contains little ascorbic acid. Hence orange juice or a vitamin C supplement should be given to the infant. All of the formulas when properly prepared and adequately supplemented, provide the nutrients important for the infant in an appropriate caloric concentration and present a reasonable solute load for the normal full-term infant. Errors in dilution caused by lack of understanding of the proper method of preparation, improper measurements, or the belief of the parents that their child should have greater amounts of nutritious food can lead to problems.

Vitamin and Mineral Supplementation   It is difficult to make standard recommendations for all infants as to whether they should be given supplements of vitamins and/or minerals. Factors that influence the decision include the infant's birth weight and degree of maturity, the type of milk or formula being used, the use of iron-fortified cereal or formula, the presence of fluoride in the water supply and the amount of water consumed by the infant as water or in formula, the exposure of the infant to sunshine, and the inclusion of juices containing ascorbic acid. Table 4-6 shows the recent guidelines put out by the Committee on Nutrition of the American Academy of Pediatrics.

Introduction of Solid Food   The age of introduction of semisolid foods to infants in the United States declined from 1920, when these foods were seldom offered before the age of 1 year, to the period 1960–1970, when they were frequently offered in the first weeks and months of life. It is currently recommended that the feeding of semisolid food be delayed until the age of 4 to 6 months, when the extrusion reflex of early infancy has disappeared and the ability to swallow nonliquid foods has become established [61].

When solid foods are introduced, single ingredient foods should be chosen and started one at a time at weekly intervals in order to allow for an opportunity to identify food intolerances. Infant cereals, which provide additional energy and iron, are a good choice. Single-grain cereals, particularly rice, are usually well tolerated. Table 4-9 gives suggested guidelines for the introduction of semisolid foods.

Older Infants   During the second 6 months of life, the normal infant will be on a diet of breast milk or formula, mixed feedings, and increased amounts of table food. If the mother desires, breast-feeding can be continued during the second year of life. However, other foods should be included in the diet beginning at the age of 5 to 6 months. Some of these foods should be relatively rich in protein.

Although the American Academy of Pediatrics has recommended that formula-fed infants should continue to receive iron-fortified formulas through-out the first year of life, many infants receive homogenized cow's milk by the age of 5 to 6 months [76]. The enteric blood loss that can result from intakes of more than a quart of homogenized mik per day is felt to be one factor responsible for as much as 50 percent of the iron deficiency in infancy [77]. Amounts of homogenized milk consumed should be limited not only because of the potential for blood loss but because of the possibility that infants will reduce their intakes of semisolid foods which are good sources of iron.

TABLE 4-9

SUGGESTED AGES FOR THE INTRODUCTION OF SEMISOLID FOODS

Food	Age, months		
	4–6	6–8	9–12
Iron-fortified cereals for infants	Add		
Vegetables		Add strained	Gradually delete strained foods, introduce table foods
Fruits		Add strained	Gradually delete strained foods, introduce well-cooked chopped foods or canned foods
Meats		Add strained or finely chopped table meats	Decrease the use of strained meats, increase the varieties of table meats
Finger foods such as arrowroot biscuits, oven dried toast		Add those that can be secured with a palmar grasp	Increase the use of small-sized finger foods as the pincer grasp develops
Well-cooked mashed or chopped table foods, prepared without added salt or sugar			Add
Juice by cup			Add

Source: P. L. Pipes, Nutrition in Infancy and Childhood, 2d ed., Mosby, St. Louis, 1981.

Nutritional Status of Infants in the United States

There have been few studies that were broad-based enough to provide adequate data for accurate appraisal of the nutritional status of American infants. The Ten-State Nutrition Survey [22] focused on adults in poverty and near-poverty communities but did include 3700 children under the age of 6 years. The Health and Nutrition Examination Survey (HANES) [78] of 1971 to 1974 was more representative of the general population and included about 3500 children from birth to 18 years old. A preschool nutrition survey conducted from 1968 to 1970 studied about 3500 children aged 1 to 6 years [79].

Generally, these surveys did not indicate major nutrient deficiencies in young American children. More than 30 percent of the infants in the Ten-State Nutrition Survey had iron and vitamin C intakes which were less than two-thirds of the RDA for those nutrients, and anemia was identified in many. Few other nutritional problems were found; however, it was apparent that nutritional deficiencies were more prevalent among lower socioeconomic segments of the population.

A number of assistance programs including the Women, Infants, and

Children Supplemental Food Program (WIC), the Food Stamp Program, and the Child Nutrition Programs have been developed to increase the food-buying power of mothers who need it.

Special Concerns in Infant Feeding

Certain states in infants, such as low birth weight, food allergies, and failure to thrive, require special dietary considerations.

Low-Birth-Weight Infants   The daily energy requirements in proportion to body weight are higher for low-birth-weight infants. At the same time, their stomachs are smaller than normal for their age and hold less food. They should receive more frequent feedings to meet their high energy needs, and they may need more concentrated formulas to supply their energy and protein requirements. Initially, these infants may need to be fed by gavage through a nasogastric tube. Further information is available in pediatric texts [80,81].

Allergies   Food allergies are uncommon and frequently are diagnosed incorrectly. Manifestations include urticaria (hives), eczematous rash, respiratory symptoms, vomiting, and diarrhea. Because the symptoms may be non-specific, accurate diagnosis requires disappearance of the symptoms when the allergen is eliminated from the diet and reappearance of identical symptoms when the allergen is reintroduced on two or more occasions. Hypersensitivity to one of the proteins of cow's milk—lactalbumin, lactoglobulin, and casein—is encountered. Cow's milk globulins are the most frequent offenders. When solid foods are introduced—especially eggs, wheat, citrus fruit, and fish—susceptible infants experience allergic reactions. Only one new food should be introduced at a time; then, if there is any reaction, it will be easy to identify the cause.

Failure to Thrive   Decline in the slope of the growth curve (see growth charts in Chapter 1) is a sensitive, although nonspecific, indicator of an underlying problem. Failure to grow "normally" is a phenomenon associated with either infantile or maternal factors, some of which are poorly understood [82]. The problem can be due to inadequate intake caused by vomiting, refusal by an infant to consume food offered, inadequate calorie intake being offered, or excessive fecal loss associated with diarrhea. Many infants respond to supplemental feedings or to increased maternal milk production resulting from increased maternal calorie intake. Some researchers believe that "nonorganic failure to thrive" results from endocrinological changes in children who do not receive adequate nurturing [83]. When placed in an environment that provides adequate nurturing and stimulation, such as a foster home, the children consume greater quantities of food. Therapy for failure to thrive must be directed at correction of the underlying cause, be it organic (chronic gastroenteritis, congenital heart disease, etc.) or emotional (disturbed mother-child relationship).

Childhood

Three nutritional surveys indicate that nutritional deficiencies are not common among children in the United States [22,78,79]. Of the nutritional deficiencies found, iron deficiency and iron-deficiency anemia were the most common. Further, dental caries as a result of excessive intake of sweet foods, poor dental hygiene, and lack of dental care are common among all groups of children.

Growth is a major factor influencing the nutritional needs of developing infants and children. When nutrient and energy needs of children are expressed per kilogram of body weight, they are actually lower than those of infants. However, because children are larger, their absolute nutritional needs are actually increased. Appendix 8 shows the RDAs for children of different ages.

Additions to an infant's diet are selected according to the infant's readiness to handle them and his or her changing nutrient needs. Among the nutrients first needed beyond those provided by milk are iron and ascorbic acid. By the age of 1 year, an infant is able to eat food from all four food groups. Normal weight gain, tooth development, and health can be promoted by feeding a balanced diet, by avoiding empty-calorie foods, and by encouraging infants to learn to like a variety of foods. Extremes are unwise at this critical period of development.

After the age of 1, a child's growth rate slows and with it, the appetite. However, all essential nutrients continue to be needed in adequate amounts from foods having a high nutrient density. Milk remains important but should not exceed three servings per day because it is a poor source of iron and ascorbic acid.

Sometimes it is not realized how little food a young child actually needs. A child of average size and normal rate of development can manage only about 1 tbsp of each type of food served at each meal for each year of his or her age. For example, a 2-year-old can be expected to consume 2 tbsp of meat, 2 tbsp of vegetables, and 2 tbsp of fruit, in addition to a regular serving of milk or juice [84].

In general, the nutritional needs of children for vitamins, minerals, water, protein, carbohydrate, and fat are met if calorie needs can be met by a variety of foods. Certain children go on food binges or become food faddists. As long as these are short-lived, deficiencies do not develop. It is desirable for children to learn to like nutritious foods in all of the food groups. This liking seems to come naturally, although some children have trouble liking vegetables. Parents need to understand and support children in their food-related behavior so that eating habits are formed that are conducive to adequate nutrient intake and good health when they become adults.

Excellent accounts of the nutrition of children are the following:

Pipes, P. L.: *Nutrition in Infancy and Childhood,* 2d. ed., Mosby, St. Louis, 1981

Fomon, S. J.: *Infant Nutrition,* 2d. ed., Saunders, Philadelphia, 1974

Beal, V.: *Nutrition in the Life Span,* Wiley, New York, 1980

ADOLESCENCE

Nutritional Requirements

The adolescent of either sex passes through a rapid period of growth which is determined more by stage of maturation than chronological age. The stage of sexual maturation is closely linked with nutrient requirements [85]. Adolescence is a period in which the growth spurt is maximal; males may grow a maximum of 10 cm per year and females slightly less. In consequence, absolute demands for nutrients are great, although in proportion to body weight, the fastest growth actually occurs in the first 3 months of life. The weight of a 12-year-old child may increase in 1 year by 5 kg or more during this growth spurt, with no proportional increase in fat tissue. This represents a gain of 1 kg of protein and, therefore, 160 g of nitrogen (0.4 g per day). But dietary protein is available for growth only if there is adequate intake of energy as carbohydrate and fat. In order to meet these needs, healthy, physically active teenagers can have a food intake that may seem phenomenal to those responsible for feeding them.

RDAs for adolescents are not derived mainly from quantified metabolic studies, since few have been made, but rather by inference from adult data, with some reference to the results of nutritional surveys, which may identify nutrients for which the intake is most likely to be deficient. The important problems relate to iron deficiency and possibly low calcium intake. The RDA recognizes these by setting the daily iron intake at 18 mg for males and females between 11 to 18 years old and calcium (and phosphorus) at 1200 mg each.

Nutritional Problems

Eating Practices   Obtaining a satisfactory dietary history from an adolescent is frequently a formidable task. Their eating habits are erratic, and between-meal snacks constitute a large part of their total food intake. These snacks consist largely of foods and drinks that have a high content of phosphate, salt, and simple carbohydrates. In part, snacks are a means of satisfying an increased appetite, which is not always satisfied in the home, but social eating with the peer group and temporary rejection of adult precepts other than advertising and adult example play an important part. These types of eating habits result in unbalanced diets and an increased risk of dental caries of the permanent teeth. A life-long habit of excess consumption of calories or inadequate consumption of nutrients may be established, and the problem of dental caries may often be compounded by inadequate attempts at oral hygiene.

In spite of preventive legislation, habits of alcohol consumption may be formed in this age group. The early formation of these habits poses real dangers of abuse and overconsumption, because the influence of the family may be lacking, and peer-group pressures to consume alcohol, especially among boys, are very strong.

The most commonly occurring nutrient deficiency is of iron, and, contrary to widespread belief, this may occur in both sexes. It is most prevalent in females but is found in a significant number of 15-year-old males, especially in inner-urban communities and in black youths [86]. Iron-deficiency anemia has been observed also in young air force recruits in the United Kingdom [87].

While attempts to lose weight and to become slimmer are rare in adolescent males, most of whom tend to concentrate on increased stature and body build, in females these attempts are common and appear to be becoming commoner. Fortunately it is, or has been until now, a behavioral change which occurs after the growth phase is over, around the age of 16 to 17 years, so that stunting does not occur. But because of traditional, though false, beliefs about foodstuffs, some dietary components, such as bread and cereal, are specifically excluded and thus the dietary range of selection is limited and the intake of micronutrients may be significantly impaired [88].

Although the nutrient intakes of an appreciable number of girls may fall markedly below the recommended levels, signs of malnutrition do not appear for nutrients other than iron. Intakes of folacin and vitamin A have been observed to be low. Reduced calorie intake in part correlates with reduced physical activity. Concern has very reasonably been expressed [89] about decreased intake. Perhaps the most important consideration should be with regard to the teenage pregnancy and the risks of having an underweight (under 2500 g) newborn. A recent survey has shown a higher incidence of underweight offspring among mothers of lower socioeconomic class [90]. There may even be an increased incidence of birth defects in the offspring of undernourished mothers [91].

Finally, there may be important ethnic differences in diet, which, though evident at all ages, may have a special impact on teenagers. Black households consume less carbohydrate, calcium, iron, thiamine, and vitamin C and more fat than either white or Latin American households [92]. The family members of an urban, less-educated, black household appear in general to be at greatest risk of developing nutritional deficiencies.

Studies of taste preferences have shown that black subjects select for saltier taste than whites, and this is evident in 9- to 15-year old children [93]. Many believe that salt (sodium) consumption may be a factor in causing high blood pressure in susceptible individuals [94], though this is unproven (see Chapter 9). Despite this uncertainty, recommendations for reducing salt intake have merit as part of a "prudent diet," and this may be particularly important for young black people, since there is a higher prevalence of hypertension in blacks than in whites in the United States.

Obesity Overweight is an important expression of malnutrition in the adolescent. Theories of causation are discussed in Chapter 7. Overweight may be a persistence of early childhood obesity, or it may occur for the first time around or just after puberty and is likely to persist into adult life. It is associated with decreased physical activity [95] and is commoner in females.

Hyperlipidemia and atherosclerosis also may appear at around the time of puberty or slightly later [96,97] and are attributed to a faulty diet, to familial predisposition, and possibly to contributory factors such as smoking. It is generally believed that it is important to identify young people at risk. A dietary history and weight, height, and skin-fold measurements are the first steps to such recognition. A clinic visit or hospitalization of an adolescent for treatment of minor trauma, appendectomy, or orthopedic surgery, for example, provides the medical practitioner with the opportunity to identify young people at risk and to offer nutritional advice. The results of attempts at weight reduction are not, unfortunately, encouraging presently, though techniques of behavior modification are being developed and may offer the best chance of benefit.

Anorexia Nervosa   It has been stated that disorders of appetite are common around puberty and that food choices of adolescents appear bizarre to adults, especially parents. However, the most extreme expression of disordered appetite, anorexia nervosa, is rather uncommon, though according to some, it is becoming more common [98]. Among English schoolgirls aged 16 or over, the prevalance is 1 percent, and 1 in 250 over the age of 16 years develops the disease. Many more girls at some time during adolescence exhibit anorectic behavior, such as crash dieting to lose weight or using purgatives and vomiting after meals to lose weight. The disease also occurs in males but the rate is about 10 percent of all anorectics.

It is primarily a psychological disorder, in which the patient refuses to eat enough to maintain weight and may even adopt subterfuge to avoid ingesting and digesting food. It is most common between the ages of 15 to 25 years but may occur occasionally at a later age.

The disease is characterized by a marked loss of weight, including subcutaneous fat, so that subjects appear gaunt. The skin may be covered by fine hair (lanugo). The pulse is slow, the blood pressure is low, and skin temperature is low. In females secondary amenorrhea is invariably present. Subjects with the disease are restless, mentally alert, and surprisingly physically active.

Anemia is uncommon as is hypoalbuminemia, but both may occur. The urinary excretion of gonadotropins is low, and in females the urinary excretion of estrogens is markedly reduced as is that of testosterone in males. An intriguing phenomenon is the reversal of the normal diurnal pattern of plasma luteinizing hormone activity, so that it is low by day, and high by night.

An important complication is a low concentration of serum potassium, which is usually an index of induced vomiting and purgation and which may be associated with a fatal outcome.

Patients with anorexia nervosa appear to suffer from a distortion of the body image so that when asked to compare their images with the dimensions of an adjustable screen image, they give an overestimation of bust or waist by as much as 50 percent. Before the current trend in many young middle-class women to reduce their weight to the point of emaciation became manifest, anorexia nervosa stood out as a dramatic and unusual entity. Today, pressures to achieve a desirably slim figure have become increasingly eloquent, and the female patient with anorexia nervosa seems to be more a subject at one end of a spectrum which extends through extreme leanness to normal weight and beyond to obesity. An increasing number of young girls now adopt weight-reducing diets in their middle teens and even earlier. The desire to be thin is ascribed to fashion, although the reason why such a fashion has developed is not clear. It may be an expression of social liberation in the case of women. It is possible that fear of fatness is usually or always the driving force, but there is no reason why this fear should have become so intrusive, since the majority of girls do not develop anorexia nervosa. From reading a psychiatrist's account of many girls with the disease, one gains the impression that those with the disease derive great satisfaction from starving themselves, since starving themselves enhances their sense of self-efficacy, hunger becomes transformed into a pleasurable sensation, and their condition attracts wanted attention and concern [99]. It is also possible that anorexia nervosa, which is associated with a manifest effort on the part of those suffering from it to achieve prepubertal weight and body pattern, may represent denial of, fear of, or retreat from sexual maturity. The possible relationship between menarche and critical body mass [100] and the fact that amenorrhea is invariable in female anorexic subjects might support the latter belief. How well anorexia nervosa in the male fits a pattern similar to that in the female is unresolved and does not seem to be much addressed, lending some doubt to all current theories. It has been suggested that only obese males or those with major gender identity problems are likely to diet to the same extent as females with anorexia nervosa [101] and that the prognosis for males is not as good as that for females with the disease.

There is no consensus about treatment. There is fair agreement that the longer the duration of the disease, the poorer the prognosis. One reason given for this is that the patient becomes increasingly cut off from her or his peer group and its patterns of behavior and peer group pressures. If the disease persists for more than 10 years, the prognosis is very gloomy. An interesting feature, though not unexpected, is that parents of an anorectic child may become increasingly more anxious and depressed as their child responds to treatment, and the marital bonds are strained, which may provide yet another insight into the nature of the disease.

Overall mortality is about 5 percent of all patients. Causes of death are suicide and cardiac arrest resulting from an electrolyte imbalance associated with the starvation-dehydration-hypokalemia syndrome. Of interest is the apparent absence of increased intercurrent infection or of infection as a cause of death, which throws some doubt on undernutrition, as such, predisposing to reduced resistance to infection [102].

In North America the use of drugs to treat the disease is more evident than in Europe [103]. The drugs tried have included amitriptyline, cyproheptadine and L-dopa, but the results of such treatment are still uncertain. Both in the United States and the United Kingdom, behavioral techniques for restoring weight to normal are in use. A mean weight gain of 20 kg is the goal. Attempts are made to minimize the patient's preoccupation with his or her own weight control and to allow the patient to experience a gradual rekindling of the early pubertal process.

Individual and family psychotherapy are directed at problems of psychosocial and emotional growth, differentiation, and control [101]. Training in specific social skills and coping with sexual problems as they arise are combined with supportive treatment, which includes replacing any lack of essential nutrients early in treatment and continuing to do so until calorie intake has increased satisfactorily. Other papers may be consulted for a description of the basis of behavior modification techniques and the controversies that exist in this field [104,105].

Chronic Diseases The important complications of chronic, debilitating diseases such as rheumatoid arthritis, chronic nephritis, and inflammatory bowel disease at puberty and during the teenage years are retarded emotional and physical growth. The latter is now recognized as being almost always a consequence of depressed appetite leading to undernutrition, although in bowel disease, malabsorption may also be present [106]. Increasing efforts are now made to restore caloric intake and to achieve catch-up growth before fusion of the growing tips of the long bones (epiphyses) occurs and no further growth is possible. Deficiencies of specific nutrients, such as zinc, may also occur, and for such patients diets should be constructed which both stimulate appetite and achieve optimal nutritional content with supplementation, if necessary. In addition, too often young patients with many different types of chronic disease are left to their own devices instead of being actively encouraged to exercise within the limitations of their disability; such inactivity adds to anorexia.

Our experience with inflammatory bowel disease in children is that failure to grow at an acceptable rate despite optimal medical treatment is a major factor in making a recommendation for surgery, particularly for colectomy in ulcerative colitis.

MIDDLE AGE

Nutritional Requirements

The dietary needs of the healthy adult are currently regarded as being well defined and soundly based on a reliable foundation of research and measurements. Many nutritionists state that the important area in which progress must be made is the one that deals with why people eat what they do and how they may change eating habits which are nutritionally ill-advised to conform more frequently with eating habits which appear to be desirable.

A survey done by the U.S. Department of Agriculture in 1976 [107], revealed that approximately half of a random sample of the population had recently changed their eating habits because of concern about their health, some to avoid potential problems, others to alleviate existing ones. Many had responded to a physician's advice, which emphasizes the need for nutritionally knowledgeable physicians. The reasons given for change were obesity, hypertension, diabetes mellitus, and similar problems. But many had changed their diets for preventive reasons. Food consumption data support these changes. The recommendations of the U.S. Senate Select Committee [108] have provided in general a "prudent" diet to which many informed groups in the English-speaking world now subscribe, with some specific differences of opinion still unresolved.

Nutritional Problems

The major problems of nutrition in early and middle adult life are gradually developing obesity and nutrition-based preparations for old age.

Reduction in expenditure of energy with increasing age for all but heavy manual workers is a major factor in the development of obesity. Whether physical exercise has any specific protective value with regard to ischemic cardiovascular disease or osteoporosis is still controversial, although a good case can be made in the case of the former [109] and the effects of immobilization in accelerating net loss of mineral from bone at any age are well documented (see Chapter 13).

An increasing number of thoughtful people in western society reasonably question the widely accepted contemporary diet. They contend that in the past 10,000 years, agriculture and cattle herding have resulted in human beings adopting diets dissimilar to those previously used for 2 to 3 million years in two respects. The first change is that a major constriction in the variety of both vegetable and animal foods has occurred. Estimates have been made that several thousands of species of plants and several hundreds of species of animals were eaten by human beings before they adopted a pastoral life and that today their choices have become, by comparison, very restricted (Table 4-10).

The second change for western societies has been the increasing consumption of animal food. Paleoanthropologists now believe, on the basis of paleontological and archaeological evidence, that, at least in the main line or stream of human evolution, human beings were formerly hunter-gatherers, their diet being predominantly vegetable with an intermittent addition of flesh, similar to today's diet of the Hadza bushman of Tanzania or the Australian aborigine or the chimpanzee or baboon. Such a diet has a low calorie density; is high in fiber, low in salt, and low in animal protein and animal fat; lacks dairy products, including milk sugar or lactose (in fact, it lacks any sugar except a rare find of honey); and has little or no wheat gluten.

There is only one possible difficulty with this type of diet, namely, how did our ancestors maintain an adequate intake of essential amino acids, since the proteins of most single plant sources tend to be low in one or more amino acids essential for human beings, who must eat two sources of vegetable protein such as a legume and a cereal together, invoking what is called *complementarity*, if they are to obtain adequate essential amino acids from a pure vegetarian diet? This problem has obviously been overcome by the Nilotic and Australian bushmen, who eat the growing shoots of plants, which are an excellent and often overlooked source of good protein; some plants, such as the Ethiopian teff, provide an array of amino acids adequate for human needs.

TABLE 4-10
WORLD FOOD PRODUCTION

Vetetable products, $\times$ 10^6 metric tons		Animal foods, $\times$ 10^6 metric tons	
Wheat	360	Pork	42.5
Rice	320	Beef	42.0
Maize	300	Poultry	20.7
Potato	300	Lamb	5.4
Barley	170	Goat	1.4
Sweet potato	130	Buffalo	1.1
Cassava	100	Horse	0.7
Grapes	60		
Soybean	60		
Oats	50		
Sorghum	50		
Sugar cane	50		
Millets	45		
Banana	35		
Tomato	35		
Sugar beet	30		
Rye	30		
Peanut	20		

It is argued that some of the so-called diseases of western civilization may in small or large part be ascribed to a move away from the bushman's diet. It would be unwise to dismiss such ideas as faddist or alarmist. The matter is certainly one that should be addressed—but unfortunately the pressure of the increase in the world population and the need to provide more and more calories and protein through intensive farming techniques make our concerns about changes in the nutritional component of our ecology seem almost irrelevant. Unless it is arrested or modified, the move is toward more and more of fewer and fewer food choices, to many of which large numbers of the human races may not have had an opportunity to adapt by natural selection.

OLD AGE

Nutritional Requirements and Physiology of Aging

It is reasonably assumed, though with supporting evidence of variable quality, that metabolic changes are inevitable in the aging subject. Renal and pulmonary functions show marked deterioration, though, interestingly, similar impairment of the essential function of the gastrointestinal tract, namely absorption of nutrients, has not been well demonstrated, possibly in part because the system has not been subjected to a testing of the limits of its ability to function in the same way as have the kidneys, heart, or lungs and because, in youth, secretions

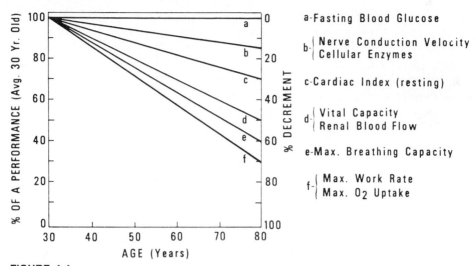

FIGURE 4-4

Age decrements in physiological performance. Average values for 30-year-old subjects taken as 100 percent. Decrements shown are schematic. (*From N. W. Shock, Energy metabolism, caloric intake and physical activity of the aging, in Nutrition in Old Age, L. A. Carlson (ed.), The Swedish Nutrition Foundation, Uppsala, 1972.*)

of enzymes and transport factors are produced in great excess. Figure 4-4 depicts some of the changes in physiological functions which occur with age [110].

Body composition also changes with age. The ratio of fat to lean body mass rises as lean body mass is lost. This has been shown to begin at the age of 25 years, by using radioactive potassium measurements [111], and it accelerates in later life. The major loss is of skeletal muscle. How much this phenomenon, especially the accelerated phase, is dependent on nutrient intake and on exercise, both of which are interdependent, is not known. The amount of muscle decreases from 45 percent of body weight in a young adult to 27 percent or less in a male over 70. With this change goes a gradual reduction in the basal metabolic rate.

Bone density likewise diminishes in most but not in all subjects. The change is perceptible rather late in life (see Chapter 13).

Whether these and other changes can be slowed by changes in diet or other components of lifestyle is not well worked out.

The turnover of muscle protein in old men is similar to that in young men, if an allowance is made for reduced muscle mass [112]. Fractional synthesis of albumin is the same at low levels of protein intake in old and in young men but fails to increase with increased protein intake in the old, unlike in the young, suggesting a low set point for albumin synthesis which is reflected in significantly lower serum albumin concentrations. There is some uncertainty whether higher levels of dietary protein intake are required to maintain nitrogen equilibrium in the old as compared with the young. The difference is probably small, and it seems unlikely that a strong argument can be made for attempting to avert some of the protein wasting of age by increasing the intake of protein alone or protein and calories, unless the diet is clearly inadequate in these respects, which in some subjects will be the case. The RDA, however, states that protein should constitute at least 12 percent rather than 10 percent of energy intake, and similar recommendations have been made elsewhere.

Approximately 10 percent of the population of North America is aged 65 years or more. The proportion and absolute numbers are steadily growing.

Dietary surveys in the United States and Britain have revealed marginal or inadequate intakes of a number of nutrients in groups of old people [22,113].

One important phenomenon is the remarkable individual variation in intake of food. Thus, a survey of elderly farmers revealed a daily calorie intake ranging from 2200 to 4200 kcal [114], and a study of elderly women in the London suburbs [115] revealed a range of intake of 1155 to 2931 kcal (mean = 1890 kcal) daily, and similarly low figures for low-income blacks of both sexes were found in the U.S. Ten-State Nutrition Survey [22]. Such discrepancies in intake are often masked by statements of the mean intake. At the lower end of the range the potential for deficiency of one or more essential nutrients is high, even if the diet conforms qualitatively to one of normal distribution. If some items, such as meat or fresh vegetables, are excluded for economic or idiosyncratic reasons, the possibility of deficiency is greater unless there is appropriate supplementation.

In practical terms, the healthy, active aged subject should be encouraged to eat well, choosing from a wide range of foodstuffs, and to maintain a constant weight. As physical activity and energy utilization fall, so energy intake should be reduced and the proportion of fruits, vegetables, and low-fat milk increased to prevent the development of nutrient deficiencies. There is no good case for supplementation with vitamins, although this is frequently done [116]. Measurements of nutrients in tissues have revealed low levels in some groups of old people but an associated clinical disease is rare or absent, and supplementation with ascorbic acid, thiamine, or riboflavin seems to effect no significant change [117,118].

However, superimposed disease such as infection, trauma, or surgery may precipitate clinical deficiency. In all old people, particularly those in whom diet is believed to have been poor, nutrient deficiency should be borne in mind in such circumstances. In the case of old people in institutions and those eating diets likely to be deficient in ascorbate, a case can be made for daily supplementation with 60 mg of ascorbic acid.

Occasionally scurvy is seen in old people living on a poor diet from which potatoes, fruit, and green vegetables have been excluded. Men are more prone to develop the disease.

Studies of tissue concentrations of trace elements have shown that all of them except chromium increase with age, which suggests that no supplementation with trace minerals is necessary. Opinion about calcium supplementation is divided. In areas where old people may be deprived of sunlight, deficiency of vitamin D may occur with a seasonal variation, and lower bone density may be related to this [119]. Old people living mainly, or wholly, indoors may benefit from drinking a glass of low-fat, vitamin D–fortified milk daily.

Iron-deficiency anemia is the commonest recognized deficiency in old people. It may be an expression of inadequate dietary iron intake, but by far the most frequent cause is loss of blood from the gastrointestinal tract. It must not be ignored, therefore, or dismissed as a physiological finding in the aged, which it is not. The stools should be examined repeatedly for occult blood, and if present, a diagnostic workup appropriate for the individual should be done. If dietary inadequacy of iron is established by patient history and by exclusion of blood loss or malabsorption, the deficiency can be overcome by dietary change and supplementation with oral iron.

The points to be emphasized in maintaining good nutrition in the elderly are anticipation of any social, psychiatric, and, if possible, physical factors (such as dentition) which may precipitate reduction of appetite or food intake; encouragement to exercise (dealing with minor physical problems such as the care of the feet); and provision of advice about choice and preparation of foods on an individual rather than group basis, emphasizing the need to make meals appetizing and to make some meals a social occasion. It has to be emphasized repeatedly that good feeding habits in old age, as is the case for all aspects of lifestyle, should be learned when young, and the nutritional components of preventive medicine cannot be adopted too early.

A unique longitudinal study of 141 elderly people in San Mateo County, California, is impressive in that the pattern of individual diets remained constant over the years; the major change was a significant reduction in the quantity eaten after the age of 75 years [120].

Inadequate Intake of Food

Physical Causes Old people are at greater risk than any other age group of developing nutritional deficiencies as a consequence of reduced food intake due to a physical disability. The cause may either be in some part of the gastrointestinal tract itself or affect some other system (Table 4-11).

With the gastrointestinal tract we include sense of smell and taste, which are major determinants of enjoyment of food. The threshold for food odors which underlies the savor of foods, may be 10-fold higher in subjects 65 years old or more [121]. A commonsense approach is to encourage consumption of well-seasoned and tasty food. If salt or sweet things are preferred, then they should not be proscribed, unless the subject is hypertensive or obese. The food eaten by old people is too often monotonous, unattractive in appearance, and tasteless. It is regrettable that packaged-food producers have not yet developed lines of savory food in appropriately sized portions to feed the elderly at a price they can afford.

After intercurrent infections old people may take several weeks to recover their sense of taste, and weight loss and general weakness may persist for many weeks.

TABLE 4-11
COMMON CAUSES OF REDUCED INTAKE
OF FOOD IN THE ELDERLY

Loss of smell and taste

Poor dentition or ill-fitting dentures

Lesions in mouth:
Sores
Glossitis
Lack of saliva

Dysphagia:
Incoordination of pharyngeal muscles
Esophageal spasm
Esophagitis
Stricture
Cancer of esophagus or stomach

Abdominal pain:
Ulcer of stomach or duodenum
Diverticular disease of colon

Others:
Depression
Constipation
Lack of exercise

Faulty dentition or ill-fitting dentures may deter those over 60 years old from eating because of discomfort and sometimes embarrassment. A sharp broken tooth may damage the tongue and cause a small but painful ulcer, which is quite likely to deter an older person from eating regularly. Good reparative dentistry or the provision of adequate dentures may result in improved eating habits.

The tongue may be sore because of iron deficiency due to undetected gastrointestinal bleeding or, rather rarely, because of B-group vitamin deficiency. Carcinoma of the tongue may develop as a painless ulcer, and the opinion of a specialist should be sought early if carcinoma is suspected; it rarely interferes with eating, at least in the early stages.

Difficulty in and sometimes pain on swallowing may be due to a neurological disease that causes incoordination of or incomplete movements of the muscles of swallowing, a condition which may occur sometimes after a stroke. This disability is however rather uncommon. Far more common is some degree of incoordination of the intrinsic muscles of the esophagus so that swallowing contractions are faulty or actual muscle spasm with pain occurs. This may be an intractable problem. Very hot or very cold solids or fluids should be avoided, as they frequently act as precipitating factors. If inflammation of the lower end of the esophagus is apparent on esophagoscopy, and especially if confirmed by tissue biopsy via the endoscope, then medical treatment, as described in Chapter 15, is begun. This sometimes improves the degree of esophagospasm. Occasionally surgery is necessary in intractable esophagitis to reduce acid gastric contents flowing back into the esophagus. Esophageal stricture may occur, usually but not always in the lower third of the esophagus, as a consequence of reflux esophagitis. The complaint of dysphagia may stem from a more serious and potentially lethal cause, such as cancer of the pharynx, esophagus, or stomach, and rarely from an aortic aneurysm or a growth inside the chest.

Old people are more likely to have peptic ulcer disease than the young. The main symptom is abdominal pain. However, there is no typical pattern. Pain may occur before ingesting food and may be temporarily relieved by food. The usual trigger for pain is the presence of unneutralized acid in the stomach or duodenum. Peptic ulcer is a common cause of blood loss into the gastrointestinal tract.

Gallbladder disease is a condition which may declare itself in the elderly by nausea with or without epigastric pain, though typically it is associated with pain in the upper abdomen on the right side after eating. Occasionally acute inflammation of the gallbladder may occur with fever but without localizing signs and present a major diagnostic dilemma in which there is risk of rupture of the gallbladder and bile peritonitis. Abdominal pain after meals, of a colic-like quality, may be due, on the other hand, to some inadequacy of blood supply to the small intestine, causing ischemia. This sometimes follows meals so regularly and is so unpleasant that selective injection of the arteries to the intestine with radiopaque material followed by cine x-ray studies is done in an attempt to locate a segmental narrowing of an artery. If the search is successful, the narrowed segment can sometimes be replaced with a graft. Diagnosis and treatment should not be delayed, since infarction of a segment of the small bowel may occur, a serious and life-threatening catastrophe.

Diverticulosis of the sigmoid part of the colon is common in the over 60 age group and is associated with attacks of pain in the left lower quadrant of the abdomen and with constipation. Constipation is indeed a major therapeutic problem in aging adults whether it occurs in the presence or absence of diverticular disease, especially if it is found on questioning to be of long duration. Although use of higher-fiber diets or addition of a bulk provider such as Metamucil is advocated, many patients do not tolerate either of these well and may need considerable and continuing encouragement to get over the initial unpleasant feeling of colonic dilatation. Sometimes increasing the patient's intake of water is effective; many old people reduce their water intake because they wish to reduce the frequency of getting up to void urine at night. They should be encouraged to drink larger quantities of water during the first part of the day.

Finally, painful hemorrhoids and anal fissures, which are increasingly common in old people, may discourage eating because of its inevitable consequences. Stool softening and local treatment should be used, as well as sitz baths, which are soothing and relieve pain.

Extragastrointestinal organic conditions which affect appetite are numerous. Those which need the most emphasis are the ailments of the feet and of the joints of the lower limbs which reduce physical activity. Particular attention should be given to keeping old people on their feet and to getting them to exercise regularly. Good podiatry is important. When activity declines, the need for energy is decreased. When intake falls below 2000 kcal per day, a standard mixed diet may become progressively inadequate for supplying nutrients such as iron, folacin, thiamine, pyridoxine, and ascorbic acid, unless the quality of the diet is changed from energy-rich foods to protective foods, such as low-fat milk, fruit, and vegetables, and the nutrient density of the diet is increased.

A far too common occurrence in old people, especially women, is fracture of the neck of the femur as a consequence of osteoporotic change which weakens the long bones. Fractures of this type may have a disastrous effect on mobility and precipitate an inactive life and a poor dietary intake from which there is often no recovery.

Congestive failure of the heart, which occurs in some old people, is a cause of anorexia and nausea. Careful treatment may produce marked improvement. Another organic problem, often overlooked, is postrenal uremia as a consequence of urethral obstruction by an enlarged prostate gland; such obstruction can now be removed by a relatively simple surgical procedure via the urethra, using either local anesthesia or light general anesthesia. This is well tolerated by even very old and frail men.

Psychosocial Causes   Mental disturbance is common in old people. It may assume many forms, of which depression, a sense of persecution, and varying degrees of dementia are the most common. The underlying causes are organic. Degenerative disease of the blood vessels to parts of the brain results in an impaired supply of oxygen and nutrients. Intrinsic biochemical disturbances may occur, though they have as yet been poorly characterized. Dramatic but rare examples are the dementia of pellagra due to niacin deficiency, or that seen in cobalamin deficiency. Depression and confusion from whatever cause may be significantly aggravated by adverse environmental factors, such as lack of human contacts, change to an unfamiliar environment, or intercurrent illness. In old people these factors can significantly impair good nutrition, often being compounded by ignorance, faulty knowledge of food, and lack of interest.

We lack the tools to modify significantly organic dementia, though it is possible to treat manic episodes. Endogenous depression may sometimes be treated effectively with antidepressant drugs, such as the so-called tricyclic agents and lithium salts.

In many old people attempts to relieve anxieties by discussion and reassurance and practical help with finances, housing conditions, and protection from harrassment may bring some improvement. A change of environment, such as moving to a home for the elderly, is not successful in many cases, since it may increase the sense of isolation by removing familiar landmarks, serving to add to disorientation, confusion, and anxiety.

The unavoidable truth is that too little planning for old age is done and effected at a stage when a person is capable of adapting to new surroundings and creating a reassuring personal environment. Such planning should include adequate provision for preparation of nutritious meals and establishing some human contacts and a pattern of interaction with younger members of the family. There are many texts on this subject which can be consulted.

Isolation comes with immobility or as a result of deafness, blindness, poverty, and neglect. Improvement may be achieved by providing hearing aids, spectacles, operations for cataracts and by increasing human contacts. Encouraging the person to eat with others, with the emphasis on the social aspects of a meal, should be attempted. Success requires effort and ingenuity.

Effects of Medications   Old people are likely to receive drugs continuously or intermittently for longer periods than any other age group. These drugs may produce adverse side effects, which are not necessarily dose-related, because of idiosyncrasy. Another cause is overdosage, which may occur as a result of an error or because dosage in relation to body weight has not been allowed for in a subject who is maintained on long-term medication and who is gradually losing weight. Another cause of an abnormal response to a drug, if it is bound wholly or partly to serum proteins, is a reduction in the concentration of serum albumin, which occurs commonly in the elderly. Overdosage may also result from an age-related increase in the serum half-life of some drugs [122].

Some medications produce anorexia. Fenfluramine, diethylproprion, and some amphetamines are used for that purpose. Biguanides such as phenformin (phenethylbiguanide) and metformin (dimethylbiguanide) are used as oral hypoglycemic agents in mild to moderately affected diabetics, who are often obese. Thus, these drugs may serve a dual purpose, but food intake must be carefully monitored.

An overdose of digoxin may cause anorexia and nausea. The problem with this drug is that the therapeutic index, or ratio (the quantitative difference between the effective dose and the toxic dose) is small, and since the aim of treatment is to produce the maximal effect in heart failure, some toxic side effects are almost always produced, usually early in the course of treatment. Using digoxin and some oral diuretics, such as furosemide, together may produce magnesium deficiency, because both induce loss of magnesium from the kidney [123].

Indomethacin and similar nonsteroid anti-inflammatory drugs produce anorexia and sometimes abdominal discomfort, dyspepsia, and nausea. Morphine may also induce anorexia, produce gallbladder symptoms, and cause nausea.

Cytotoxic drugs used in the treatment of different malignant conditions also have effects on appetite and create another cause of malnutrition in the already undernourished patient. Support of cancer patients receiving chemotherapy has become a special area of expertise. Parenteral feeding may have an important potential role. The problem to be resolved is whether improving nutritional status favors the host or the malignancy preferentially.

Need for Nutritional Information and Counseling

Social problems of large numbers of elderly Americans may be in part responsible for malnutrition. Low income, inability to afford food and transportation, poor facilities for preparation and cooking, and lack of dental care are well-recognized causes. Most states and local agencies have developed the means of providing assistance, currently under Title III legislation. This consists of a daily hot meal that is provided in local centers or at home. Home health aides are available in most areas, supported by private or public funds and supplied upon physician referral.

There is still need for repeated domiciliary advice about the purchase, storage, and preparation of foods, so that the nutrient content of the diet is optimal. Such advice is preferably given on a one-to-one basis and should be provided regularly. Such visits provide opportunities for discussions about oral hygiene, prevention of constipation, and any other relevant matters.

Current demands on medical resources by an aging population which is steadily increasing in numbers might be effectively reduced if much chronic disability which is related to faulty nutrition, among other factors, were to be prevented by earlier attention to diet.

REFERENCES

1 Hytten, F. E.: Nutritional aspects of human pregnancy, in *Maternal Nutrition during Pregnancy and Lactation,* H. Aebi and R. Whitehead (eds.), Hans Huber, Bern, Switzerland, 1980.

2 Jacobson, H. N.: Current concepts in nutrition, N. Engl. J. Med., 297:1051, 1977.

3 Task Force on Nutrition: *Assessment of Maternal Nutrition,* American College of Obstetrics and Gynecology, Chicago, 1978.

4 Committee on Nutrition of the Mother and Preschool Child, Food and Nutrition Board: *Laboratory Indices of Nutritional Status in Pregnancy,* National Academy of Sciences, Washington, 1978.

5 Bowering, J., A. M. Sanchez, and M. I. Irwin: A conspectus of research on iron requirements of man, J. Nutr., 106:985, 1976.

6 Hytten, F. E., and I. Leitch: *The Physiology of Human Pregnancy,* 2nd ed., Blackwell Scientific, Oxford, 1971.

7 Beal, V. A.: *Nutrition in the Life Span,* Wiley, New York, 1980.

8 Chesley, L. C.: Weight changes and water balance in normal and toxic pregnancy, Am. J. Obstet. Gynecol., 48:565, 1944.

9 Committee on Maternal Nutrition, Food and Nutrition Board: *Maternal Nutrition and the Course of Pregnancy: Summary Report,* National Academy of Sciences, Washington, 1970.

10 Oldham, H., and B. B. Sheft: Effect of caloric intake on nitrogen utilization during pregnancy, J. Am. Diet. Assoc., 27:847, 1951.

11 Hurley, L. S.: *Developmental Nutrition,* Prentice-Hall, Englewood Cliffs, N.J., 1980.

12 Pitkin, R. M., H. A. Kaminetzky, M. Newton, and J. A. Pritchard: Maternal nutrition. A selective review of clinical topics, Obstet. Gynecol., 40:773, 1972.

13 Irwin, M. I., and E. W. Kienholz: A conspectus of research on calcium requirements in man, J. Nutr., 103:1019, 1973.

14 Pitkin, R. M.: Nutritional support in obstetrics and gynecology, Clin. Obstet. Gynecol., 19:489, 1976.

15 Pitkin, R. M.: Calcium metabolism in pregnancy: a review, Am. J. Obstet. Gynecol., 121:724, 1975.

16 Felton, D. J. C., and W. D. Stone: Osteomalacia in Asian immigrants during pregnancy, Br. Med. J., 1:1521, 1966.

17 Raman, L., K. Rajalakshmi, K. A. V. R. Krishnamacheri, and J. G. Sastry: Effect of calcium supplementation to undernourished mothers during pregnancy in the bone density of the neonates, Am. J. Clin. Nutr., 31:466, 1978.

18 Lund, C. J., and J. C. Donovan: Blood volume during pregnancy. Significance of plasma and red cell volumes, Am. J. Obstet. Gynecol., 98:393, 1967.

19 Scott, D. E., J. A. Pritchard, and A. S. Saltin: Iron deficiency during pregnancy, in *Iron Deficiency,* L. Hallberg, H. G. Harweth, and A. Vannotti (eds.), Academic, London, 1970.

20 Puolakka, J.: Serum ferritin as a measure of iron stores during pregnancy, Acta Obstet. Gynecol. Scand., 95(suppl.):1, 1980.

21 Hemminki, E., and B. Starfield: Routine administration of iron and vitamins during pregnancy: review of controlled trials, Br. J. Obstet. Gynaecol., 85:404, 1978.

22 *Ten-State Nutrition Survey in the United States, 1968–1970, Highlights,* U.S. Department of Health, Education, and Welfare, Publication no. (HNS) 72-8134, U.S. Government Printing Office, Washington, 1972.

23 Committee on Nutrition: *Nutrition in Maternal Care,* American College of Obstetrics and Gynecology, Chicago, 1974.

24 Brown, J. E., H. N. Jacobson, L. H. Askune, and M. G. Peick: Influence of pregnancy weight gain on the size of infants born to underweight women, J. Obstet. Gynecol., 57:13, 1981.

25 Pitkin, R. M.: Risks related to nutritional problems in pregnancy, in *Risks in the Practice of Modern Obstetrics,* 2d ed., S. Aladjem (ed.), Mosby, St. Louis, 1975.

26 Eastman, N. J., and E. Jackson: Weight relationships in pregnancy. I. The bearing of maternal weight gain and pre-pregnancy weight on birth weight in full term pregnancies, Obstet. Gynecol. Surv., 23:1003, 1968.

27 Simpson, J. W., R. W. Lawless, and A. C. Mitchell: Responsibility of the obstetrician to the fetus. II. Influence of pregnancy weight and pregnancy weight gain on birth weight, Obstet. Gynecol., 45:481, 1975.

28 Tracy, T. A., and G. L. Miller: Obstetric problems of the massively obese, Obstet. Gynecol., 33:204, 1969.

29 Maternal weight gain and the outcome of pregnancy, Nutr. Rev., 37:318, 1979.

30 Niswander, K. R., and M. Gordon: *The Women and Their Pregnancies. The Collaborative Perinatal Study of the National Institute of Neurological Diseases and Stroke,* Saunders, Philadelphia, 1972.

31 Naeye, R. L.: Weight gain and the outcome of pregnancy, Am. J. Obstet. Gynecol., 135:3, 1979.

32 Burke, B. S.: Nutritional needs in pregnancy in relation to nutritional intakes as shown by dietary histories. Obstet. Gynecol. Surv. 3:716, 1948.

33 Chopra, J. G., E. Noe, J. Mathew, C. Dhein, J. Rose, J. M. Cooperman, and A. H. Luhby: Anemia in pregnancy, Am. J. Public Health, 57:857, 1967.

34 Wallerstein, R. O.: Iron metabolism and iron deficiency during pregnancy, Clin. Haematol., 2:453, 1973.

35 Pike, R., and H. Smiciklas: A reappraisal of sodium restriction during pregnancy, Int. J. Obstet. Gynecol., 10:1, 1972.

36 Zelnick, M., Y. J. Kim, and J. F. Kantner: Probabilities of intercourse and conception among U.S. teenage women, 1971 and 1976, Fam. Plann. Perspect., 11:177, 1979.

37 Committee on Adolescence: Statement on teenage pregnancy, Pediatrics, 63:795, 1979.

38 Zlatnik, F. J., and L. F. Burmeister: Low "gynecologic age": an obstetric risk factor, Am. J. Obstet. Gynecol., 128:183, 1977.

39 Butler, N. R., and E. D. Alberman: *Perinatal Problems,* Williams & Wilkins, Baltimore, 1969.

40 Weigley, E. S.: The pregnant adolescent, J. Am. Diet. Assoc., 66:588, 1975.

41 King, J. C., S. H. Cohenour, D. H. Calloway, and H. N. Jacobson: Assessment of nutritional status of teenage pregnant girls. 1. Nutrient intake and pregnancy, Am. J. Clin. Nutr., 25:916, 1972.

42 Kaminetzky, H. A., Langer, H. Baker, O. Frank, A. D. Thomson, E. D. Munves, A. Opper, F. C. Behrle, and B. Glista: The effect of nutrition in teen-age gravidas on pregnancy and the status of the neonate, Am. J. Obstet. Gynecol. 115:639, 1973.

43 Thayer, P., and P. Palm: A current assessment of the mutagenic and teratogenic effects of caffeine, CRC Crit. Rev. Toxicol., 3:345, 1975.

44 Caffeine and pregnancy, FDA Drug Bull., 10:18, 1980.

45 Weatherbee, P. S., L. K. Olson, and J. R. Lodge: Caffeine and pregnancy, Postgrad. Med., 62:64, 1977.

46 Linn, S., S. C. Schoenbaum, R. R. Monson, B. Rosner, P. G. Stubblefield, and K. J. Ryan: No association between coffee consumption and adverse outcomes of pregnancy, N. Engl. J. Med., 306:141, 1982.

47 Ouellette, E. M., H. C. Rosett, N. P. Rosman, and L. Weiner: Adverse effects on offspring of maternal alcohol abuse during pregnancy, N. Engl. J. Med., 297:528, 1977.

48 Hytten, F. E., and A. M. Thomsen: Nutrition of the lactating woman, in *Milk: The Mammary Gland and Its Secretion,* F. K. Kon and A. T. Cowie (eds.), Academic, New York, 1961.

49 Thomson, A. M., F. E. Hytten, and W. Z. Billewicz: The energy cost of human lactation, Br. J. Nutr., 24:565, 1970.

50 Rowland, M. G. M., A. A. Paul, and R. G. Whitehead: Lactation and infant nutrition, Br. Med. Bull., 37:77, 1981.

51 Food and Nutrition Board: *Recommended Dietary Allowances,* 9th ed., National Academy of Sciences, Washington, 1980.

52 English, R. M., and N. E. Hitchcock: Nutrient intakes during pregnancy, lactation and after the cessation of lactation in a group of Australian women, Br. J. Nutr., 22:615, 1968.

53 Knowles, J. A.: Excretion of drugs in milk - a review, J. Pediatr., 66:1068, 1965.

54 Arena, J. M.: Contamination of the ideal food, Nutr. Today, 5:8, Winter 1970.

55 Stirratt, G. M.: Prescribing problems in the second half of pregnancy and during lactation, Obstet, Gynecol. Surv., 31:1, 1976.

56 Binkiewicz, A., M. J. Robinson, and B. Senior: Pseudo-Cushing syndrome caused by alcohol in breast milk, J. Pediatr., 93:965, 1978.

57 Laug, E. P., F. M. Kunze, and C. S. Pickett: Occurrence of DDT in human fat and milk, Arch. Ind. Hyg. Occup. Hlth., 3:245, 1951.

58 Savage, E. P.: *National Study to Determine Levels of Chlorinated Hydrocarbon Insecticides in Human Milk: 1975–1976, and Supplementary Report to the National Milk Study: 1975–1976,* National Technical Information Service, Springfield, Va., 1977.

59 Rogan, W. J., A. Bagniewska, and T. Damstra: Pollutants in breast milk, N. Engl. J. Med., 302:1450, 1980.

60 Nutrition Committee of the Canadian Paediatric Society and the Committee on Nutrition: Breast-feeding, Pediatrics, 62:591, 1978.

61 Committee on Nutrition: On the feeding of supplemental foods to infants, Pediatrics, 65:1178, 1980.

62 Martinez, G. A., D. A. Dodd, and J. Samartgedes: Milk feeding patterns in the United States during the first 12 months of life, Pediatrics, 68:863, 1981.

63 Andrew, E. M., K. L. Clancy, and M. G. Katz: Infant feeding practices of families belonging to a prepaid group practice health care plan, Pediatrics, 65:978, 1980.

64 Community Nutrition Institute Weekly Rep., 11:7, Nov. 19, 1981.

65 Fomon, S. J.: Diet and atherosclerosis, in *Nutritional Disorders of Children: Prevention, Screening and Follow-up,* U.S. Department of Health, Education, and Welfare Publication no. (HSA) 76-5612, U.S. Government Printing Office, Washington, 1976.

66 Fomon, S. J., L. N. Thomas, L. J. Filer, T. A. Anderson, and K. E. Bergmann: Requirements for protein and essential amino acids in early infancy, Acta Paediatr. Scand., 66:17, 1977.

67 Committee on Nutrition: Commentary on breast-feeding and infant formulas, including proposed standards for formulas, Pediatrics, 57:78, 1976.

68 Lonnerdal, B., E. Forsum, and H. Hambraeus: A longitudinal study of the protein, nitrogen and lactose contents of human milk from Swedish well-nourished mothers, Am. J. Clin. Nutr., 29:1127, 1976.

69 Pipes, P.: Feeding babies in the 1980s, in *Contemporary Developments in Nutrition,* B. Worthington-Roberts (ed.), Mosby, St. Louis, 1981.

70 American Academy of Pediatrics, Committee on Nutrition: Vitamin and mineral supplement needs in normal children in the United States, Pediatrics, 66:1015, 1980.

71 Barness, L. A.,: Feeding children, in *Nutritional and Medical Practice,* L. A. Barness (ed.), Avi, Westport, Conn., 1981.

72 Bahna, S. L., and D. C. Heiner: Cow's milk allergy, Adv. Pediatr. 25:1, 1978.

73 McMillan, J. A., S. A. Landau, and F. A. Oski: Iron sufficiency in breast-fed infants and the availability of iron from human milk, Pediatrics, 58:686, 1976.

74 Eckhert, C. D., M. V. Sloan, J. R. Duncan, and L. S. Hurley: Zinc-binding. A difference between human and bovine milk, Science, 195:789, 1977.

75 Arnold, R. R., M. F. Cole, and J. R. McGhee: A bactericidal effect for human lactoferrin, Science, 197:263, 1977.

76 Fomon, S. J.: What are infants fed in the United States? Pediatrics, 56:350, 1975.

77 Woodruff, C. F., S. W. Wright, and R. Wright: The role of fresh cow's milk in iron

deficiency. II. Comparison of fresh cow's milk with a prepared formula, Am. J. Dis. Child., 124:26, 1972.

78 *Preliminary Findings of the First Health and Nutrition Examination Survey, U.S., 1971–1974,* U.S. Department of Health, Education, and Welfare: Publication no. (HRA) 77-1647, U.S. Government Printing Office, Washington, 1977.

79 Owen, G., and G. Lippman: Nutritional status of infants and young children: U.S.A., Pediatr. Clin. North Am., 24:211, 1977.

80 Fomon, S. J.: *Infant Nutrition,* 2d ed., Saunders, Philadelphia, 1974.

81 Barness, L. A.: Feeding the low-birth-weight infant, in *Infant and Child Feeding,* J. T. Bond et al. (eds.), Academic, New York, 1981.

82 American Academy of Pediatrics, Committee on Nutrition: Nutrition and lactation, Pediatrics, 68:435, 1981.

83 Thompson, R. G.: Nutritional considerations in the development and treatment of psychosocial dwarfism, in *Textbook of Pediatric Nutrition,* R. M. Suskind (ed.), Raven, New York, 1981.

84 Kreutler, P. A.: *Nutrition in Perspective,* Prentice-Hall, Englewood Cliffs, N.J. 1980, p. 529.

85 Heald, S. P.: New reference points for defining adolescent nutrient requirements, in *Nutrient Requirements in Adolescence,* J. I. McKigney and H. N. Munro (eds.), M.I.T., Cambridge, 1976.

86 Hepner, R.: General discussion, in *Nutrient Requirements in Adolescence,* J. I. McKigney and H. N. Munro (eds.), M.I.T., Cambridge, 1976.

87 Leonard, B. J.: Hypochromic anaemia in R.A.F. recruits, Lancet, 1:899, 1954.

88 Huenemann, R. L., L. R. Shapiro, M. C. Hampton, and B. W. Mitchell: A longitudinal study of gross body composition and body conformation and their association with food and activity in a teenage population, Am. J. Clin. Nutr., 18:325, 1966.

89 Dwyer, J.: Nutritional requirements of adolescence, Nutr. Rev., 39:56, 1981.

90 Doyle, W., M. A. Crawford, B. M. Laurance, and P. Drury: Dietary survey during pregnancy in a low-socioeconomic group, Hum. Nutr., 36A:95, 1982.

91 Susser, M., G. Saenger, and F. Marolla: *Famine and Human Development: The Dutch Hunger Winter, 1944/45,* Oxford, New York, 1975.

92 Adrian, J., and R. David: Impact of socioeconomic factors on consumption of selected food nutrients in the United States, Am. J. Agric. Econom., 58:31, 1976.

93 Desor, J. A., L. S. Greene, and O. Maller: Preferences for sweet and salty in 9- to 15-year-olds and adult humans, Science, 190:686, 1975.

94 Altschul, A. M., and J. K. Grommet: Sodium intake and sodium sensitivity, Nutr. Rev., 38:393, 1980.

95 Johnson, M. L., B. S. Burke, and J. Mayer: Relative importance of inactivity and overeating in the energy balance of obese high school girls, Am. J. Clin. Nutr., 4:37, 1956.

96 Enos, W. F., R. H. Holmes, and J. Beyer: Coronary disease among United States soldiers killed in action in Korea, J. Am. Med. Assoc., 152:1090, 1955.

97 McNamara, J. J., M. A. Molot, J. F. Stremple, and R. T. Cutting: Coronary artery disease in combat casualties in Vietnam, J. Am. Med. Assoc., 216:1185, 1971.

98 Crisp, A. H., R. L. Palmer, and R. S. Kalucy: How common is anorexia nervosa? A prevalence study, Br. J. Psychiatry, 128:549, 1976.

99 Bruch, H.: *The Golden Cage. The Enigma of Anorexia Nervosa,* Harvard, Cambridge, 1978.

100 Frisch, R. E.: Weight at menarche: similarity for well-nourished and undernourished girls at differing ages, an evidence of historical constancy, Pediatrics, 50:445, 1972.

101 Crisp, A. H., R. S. Kalucy, J. H. Lacey, and B. Harding: The long-term prognosis in anorexia nervosa: some factors predictive of outcome, in *Anorexia Nervosa,* R. A. Vigersky (ed.), Raven, New York, 1977.

102 Crisp, A. H.: Anorexia nervosa: "feeding disorder," "nervous malnutrition," or "weight phobia"? World Rev. Nutr. Diet., 12:452, 1970.

103 Vigersky, R. A. (ed.): *Anorexia Nervosa,* Raven, New York, 1977.

104 Agras, S., and J. Werne: Behavior modification, in *Anorexia Nervosa,* R. A. Vigersky (ed.), Raven, New York, 1977.

105 Bruch, H.: Perils of behavior modification in the treatment of anorexia nervosa, J. Am. Med. Assoc., 230:1419, 1974.

106 Kirschner, B. S., O. Voinchet, and I. H. Rosenberg: Growth retardation in inflammatory bowel disease, Gastroenterology, 75:504, 1978.

107 Jones, J. L.: Are health concerns changing the American diet? National Food Situation, NFS-159, U.S. Department of Agriculture, U.S. Government Printing Office, Washington, 1977.

108 U S Senate Select Committee on Nutrition and Human Needs: *Dietary Goals for the United States,* 2d ed., U.S. Government Printing Office, Washington, 1977.

109 Morris, J. N., M. G. Everitt, R. Pollard, D. P. E. Chave, and A. M. Semmence: Vigorous exercise in leisure-time: protection against coronary heart disease, Lancet, 2:1207, 1980.

110 Shock, N. W.: Energy metabolism, caloric intake and physical activity in aging, in *Nutrition in Old Age,* L. A. Carlson (ed.), The Swedish Nutrition Foundation, Uppsala, 1972.

111 Forbes, G. B., and J. C. Reina: Adult lean body mass declines with age; some longitudinal observations, Metabolism, 19:653, 1970.

112 Munro, H. N.: Nutrition and aging, Br. Med. Bull., 37:83, 1981.

113 *Nutrition and Health in Old Age The Cross Sectional Analysis of the Findings of a Survey Made in 1972/3 of Elderly People Who Had Been Studied in 1967/8,* Department of Health and Social Security, Report Health Social Subject no. 16, HMSO, London, 1979.

114 Durnin, J. V. G. A., and R. Passmore: *Energy, Work and Leisure,* Heinemann, London, 1967.

115 Exton-Smith, A. N., and B. R. Stanton: *Report on an Investigation into the Dietary of Elderly Women Living Alone,* King Edward's Hospital Fund, London, 1965.

116 Brin, M.: Vitamin needs of the elderly, Postgrad. Med., 63:155, 1978.

117 Brin, M.: Biochemical methods and findings in U.S. Surveys, in *Vitamins in the Elderly,* A. N. Exton-Smith and D. L. Scott (eds.), John Wright, Bristol, 1968.

118 Brocklehurst, J., L. L. Griffiths, G. F. Taylor, J. Mark, D. L. Scott, and J. Blackley: The clinical features of chronic vitamin deficiency, Gerontol. Clin., 10:309, 1968.

119 Smith, R. W., J. Rizek, B. Frame, and J. Mansour: Determinants of serum antirachitic activity, Am. J. Clin. Nutr., 14:98, 1964.

120 Steinkemp, R. C., N. L. Cohen, and H. E. Walsh: Resurvey of an aging population—14 years follow-up, J. Am. Diet, Assoc., 46:103, 1965.

121 Rivlin, R. S.: Nutrition and aging: some unanswered questions, Am. J. Med., 71:337, 1981.

122 Vestal, R. E., H. H. Norris, J. D. Tobin, B. H. Cohen, N. W. Shock, and R. Andres: Antipyrine metabolism in man: influence of age, alcohol, caffeine, and smoking, J. Clin. Pharmacol. 18:425, 1975.

123 Lim, P., and E. Jacob: Magnesium deficiency in patients on long-term diuretic therapy for heart failure, Br. Med. J., 3:620, 1972.

CHAPTER 5

CONTROVERSIES IN NUTRITION

CONTENTS

INTRODUCTION

During the last 20 years there has been an increased interest in foods and nutrition by the general public. This increased consciousness has provided an opportunity for the promotion of nutrition misinformation. Disregard for nutritional facts, medical science, and proven health measures is creating new problems in health education. Physicians and nutritionists constantly have to face the challenge of combating misinformation about inappropriate nutritional "therapies," food additives, and food safety.

Nutrition, a relatively young science, has been particularly prone to distortions by faddisms. In teaching nutrition, emphasis traditionally has been placed on the close association of good nutrition with health and poor nutrition with disease [1]. By capitalizing on people's fears (of food additives or pollution) and hopes (of freedom from disease, increased longevity, or improved reproductive ability), a number of individuals and quasi-professional organizations have created a multimillion-dollar business. In 1980 Americans spent an estimated $105 million on weight-loss fads alone [2].

Clinicians require knowledge, skill, and tact in dealing with patients who are deceived or deluded by various forms of misinformation. The following review discusses some of the more popular nutritional misconceptions and their potential hazards.

NUTRIENTS IN DISEASE THERAPY

It is evident that nutrition plays a role in the management of certain chronic disease states, e.g., diabetes, hypertension, and certain anemias. However, self-administration of specific nutrients as "cures" for specific diseases is a dangerous practice, especially when their use leads to avoidance of or delay in seeking appropriate medical advice [3].

Cancer

The relationship of cancer to nutrition and diet can be viewed from two perspectives: (1) diet as a factor in cancer causation and (2) nutritional treatment of the cancer patient. Various types of studies (epidemiological, animal, and case control) have suggested a number of associations between diet and cancer in humans, but there is as yet no proof of a direct cause-effect relationship. Caloric restriction, the type and amount of dietary fat, deficiencies of certain vitamins and minerals, and the protein and amino acid content of the diet all influence the induction or growth of tumors in animals. Diets that are deficient in certain amino acids are reported to have tumor-suppressing action, while others that are deficient in certain vitamins either enhance or suppress tumor development. Epidemiological studies in human populations have implicated high levels of fat or a lack of fiber in the diet as a risk factor in breast and colon cancer. Differences in diet may bring about the differences in the intestinal microflora which have been associated with variations in the incidence of cancer of the large bowel [4,5].

However, if the literature on dietary constituents and cancer incidence is reviewed, one finds contradictory arguments. It is important to remember that many dietary constituents vary together; diets high in energy are generally also rich in animal fat and protein, cholesterol, refined sugar, and food additives and low in dietary fiber and complex carbohydrates. Populations consuming such diets are often those of industrialized nations, in which the prevalence of pollution and other stresses may be high and the prevalence of physical fitness, infectious diseases, and parasites low. All of these factors as well as combinations of them may influence the etiology of cancer. Diet may play a modifying rather than causative role. More studies are needed to elucidate the mechanism(s) by which nutrition and diet influence carcinogenesis and to document associations between dietary practices and cancer.

At this point, what advice can the physician or health educator give the public? Cautious straddling of the fence, no matter how well intentioned and honest, is probably the main reason why the role of giving nutrition advice has devolved from the domain of legitimate science [6]. The public demands answers, and will look to anyone willing to give them, regardless of qualifications. At present, diets lower in total fat, refined sugar, certain additives, and total energy and higher in complex carbohydrates and fiber, together with maintenance of desirable body weight, are believed to reduce the incidence of specific cancers. These suggestions are much in line with the dietary goals suggested by the U.S. Senate Select Committee on Nutrition and Human Needs [7].

As of now, no nutrient, food, or special diet has been shown to cure or alleviate cancer. Ascorbic acid has attracted considerable attention as a result of the publication of a book by Pauling [8] and one by Cameron and Pauling [9], which advocate a daily ascorbic acid intake of 1 to 10 g. To date no properly designed, prospective, randomized study has been done to verify that large doses of ascorbic acid have beneficial effects in the treatment of cancers.

Several erroneously designated vitamins are alleged to provide a "cure" for cancer. Among these compounds are Laetrile (sometimes called "vitamin B_{17}" or amygdalin) and pangamic acid ("vitamin B_{15}").

Laetrile, which is derived from apricot kernels, is a cyanogenic glucoside consisting of glucose, benzaldehyde, and cyanide. It has been tested repeatedly in animals but has never been found to have any effect on cancer. Claims for its efficacy as a cancer cure are based on anecdotal evidence which lacks scientific support. The rationale for its use, namely the selective release of lethal amounts of hydrocyanic acid in tumor cells, is spurious [10]. In 1981 the National Cancer Institute concluded from a clinical trial of 156 patients that Laetrile offered "no substantial benefit" in curing cancer, slowing cancer's advance through the body, or ameliorating its symptoms [11].

Vitamin B_{15}, or pangamic acid, is frequently seen in advertisements for vitamin supplements. The substance consists of a variable mixture, which includes calcium gluconate, calcium chloride, dimethylglycine, D-gluconic acid 6-[bis-(1-methylethyl)]amino acetate, glycine, and diisopropylamine dichloroacetate. It is nutritionally worthless and is certainly not a vitamin. There is no proof that it is safe for human use, nor has any therapeutic benefit been demonstrated in scientifically acceptable studies, despite claims that it has value in the treatment of various diseases, including schizophrenia, hepatitis, and cancer. Herbert [12] has presented evidence that it may even be mutagenic. Finally, under the U.S. Food and Drug Administration regulations, it is illegal to promote pangamic acid as a dietary supplement.

Coronary Heart Disease (CHD)

The relationship of diet to risk of CHD has been substantiated (see Chapter 8). High intakes of foods rich in saturated fats, which can result in hypercholesterolemia in many people, is one of the demonstrated risk factors in CHD. Claims that some dietary factors, e.g., lecithin and large amounts of some vitamins—especially vitamins E and C—are effective in reducing the risk of ischemic heart disease are unproved.

Vitamin E

Vitamin E, sometimes referred to as "the vitamin in search of a disease," has been surrounded by controversy for years. Broad-based claims of relief from most heart ailments by use of large doses of vitamin E were made in the mid-1940s [13,14], and vitamin E continues to be promoted. In a controlled study of 38 patients with chronic chest pains and arteriosclerotic and hypertensive heart disease, 19 patients were given 300 mg of vitamin E and the other 19 patients a placebo, for an average of 16 weeks. No significant difference was reported between the groups as to chest pain, or the capacity of cardiac muscle or skeletal muscle to perform work. There have been 10 other studies reported, one-half of which were controlled. No positive effects of vitamin E were observed [15]. However, there are three special situations where large pharmacological doses of supplementary vitamin E have proved to be beneficial. Double-blind studies have shown that intermittent claudication, or calf pain when walking, can be relieved by treatment with large doses (400 mg or more) of vitamin E per day for at least 3 months [16,17]. Supplementary vitamin E may also be beneficial in cases of hemolytic anemia in newborn infants. Its use has also been recommended in cases of fat malabsorption, in postgastrectomy patients, and in patients with cystic fibrosis, liver cirrhosis, and obstructive jaundice [18]. There is no proof that it is beneficial in conditions such as muscle dystrophy, cancer, sexual dysfunction, or aging. Horwitt [19] has published a good evaluation of the clinical evidence that supports or refutes the various claims made for vitamin E.

Vitamin C

Claims have been made that large doses of vitamin C can aid in the regulation of cholesterol metabolism and help prevent atherosclerotic diseases. When hypercholesterolemic subjects whose vitamin C status was marginal were given large doses of vitamin C, their serum cholesterol levels decreased [20]. On the other hand, a later report by Gatenby-Davies and Newson [21] gave contrary results. The role of ascorbic acid in atherosclerosis remains unclear.

Since the publication of Linus Pauling's book *Vitamin C and the Common Cold* [22] enormous quantities of vitamin C have been consumed by the public. However, a number of controlled studies indicate that vitamin C does not prevent colds but may reduce the severity of the symptoms of the common cold [23]. Furthermore, the use of very high doses of vitamin C may be harmful to some individuals, particularly if it is taken for prolonged periods. Fortunately, the body has several physiological mechanisms which protect against the toxic effects of vitamin C megatherapy. First, the digestive tract has a limited capacity to absorb large quantities of vitamin C. Second, large doses (in excess of 2 g) produce an osmotic diarrhea that sweeps most of the excess vitamin out of the body. Third, when plasma levels rise above the renal threshold for vitamin C, urinary excretion greatly increases.

Also, it appears that when high serum levels of the vitamin are maintained, a catabolic enzyme is induced which destroys excess ascorbic acid. This explains not only the finding of normal plasma levels of ascorbic acid in persons taking large amounts of the vitamin but also the development of scurvy in persons who have abruptly reduced their intake after megavitamin supplementation [24]. When pregnant women ingest large amounts of vitamin C, their fetuses also induce this vitamin-destroying enzyme—so that the infant provided with only normal amounts of vitamin C develops scurvy soon after birth [24].

In diabetic patients, the greatest problem of high dosage with vitamin C is interference with tests for glycosuria. Large doses of ascorbic acid lower the urinary pH, and this may cause false-negative results for glucose with the popular dipstick and tape tests (such as Tes Tape, Clinistix, and Dextrostix). On the other hand, large doses of vitamin C give false-*positive* results with Clinitest reagent drops.

Ascorbic acid also interferes with the anticoagulant effects of warfarin and heparin. Ingestion of over 500 mg per day results in reduced levels of serum vitamin B_{12} [25]. One of the most serious toxic effects of vitamin C is that it contributes to kidney stone formation by promoting the urinary excretion of oxalates and urates [26,27].

Lecithin

There has been widespread interest in lecithin because of claims made by health food store operators that it lowers cholesterol and has a role in the treatment of CHD. Lecithin is a phospholipid (phosphatidylcholine) that is present in many foods, especially egg yolks and meat. Commercial preparations are made from soybeans. It can also be synthesized in the body from cholines, phosphates, and triglycerides. To date, there is no evidence that ingested supplementary lecithin is absorbed [28] or is efficacious in treating hyperlipidemia [29].

NATURAL AND SYNTHETIC FOODS

"Natural" and "Organic" Foods

Health, organic, and *natural* are words that appear frequently in advertisements and promotions for foods. It is impossible for consumers to know what these words really mean because there is little agreement as to their definition. Unfortunately, no federal agency or law defines these terms and certifies that food so labeled actually fits the description. The Federal Trade Commission (FTC) has been trying to propose definitions for use in advertising for a number of years, while the Food and Drug Administration (FDA) has yet to define these terms for labeling purposes. In 1981, after 6 years of deliberation, the FTC established a legal definition for "natural." A "natural" food may not contain artificial or synthetic ingredients and may not be more than "minimally processed." Minimal processing includes washing, peeling, canning, bottling or freezing, baking, and roasting. Foods such as ice cream and potato chips will qualify as natural under the new law so long as their ingredients are fully disclosed [30]. This term will not be officially adopted by the FTC until it has evaluated public comment and obtained Congressional approval—a process that could take years.

Generally, "organic foods" are taken to be those which are produced without chemical fertilizers, pesticides, or herbicides. The consumer has no way of knowing whether a product labeled organic is actually produced without the use of pesticides or chemical fertilizers, since there is rarely an inspection of farms claiming to raise products organically. "Health food" is a general term, which appears to encompass natural and organic foods. The term includes conventional foods which have been subjected to less processing than usual (such as unhydrogenated nut butters and whole-grain flours) and less conventional foods, such as brewer's yeast, pumpkin seeds, wheat germ, and herb teas [31].

The terms "no additives" and "no preservatives" are thought by many consumers to mean organic. Again, the meanings of these terms are determined by each manufacturer; some consider artificial flavors and both synthetic and natural colors to be additives, while others think *natural* colors should not be considered additives.

Ultimately, the value of a foodstuff to the consumer is determined by its nutritional content. The nutritional content not only depends on the composition of the raw materials but also on the changes that have occurred during processing, storage, and distribution. Nutritional losses occur whether a food is processed commercially or at home or is stored in an unprocessed state. There is no test that can differentiate organically grown products from similar commercial products. Long-term studies have failed to show that organically grown crops are nutritionally superior to those grown under standard agricultural conditions with chemical fertilizers [32]. If the soil is deficient in nutrients, the *yield* of the product, not the quality, is affected. Furthermore, organic fertilizers, e.g., manure and compost, cannot be absorbed per se by plants. Before the plant can take them in, they must be broken down by bacteria in the soil into *inorganic* elements. Thus the nutrients plants obtain from manure or chemical fertilizer are absorbed by the same path.

Organically grown foodstuffs cost more than their nonorganic counterparts [33]. The difference in cost (1⅓ to 2 times higher) for foods purchased in health food stores is of particular concern to low-income families, who may have to skimp on quantity or sacrifice other important items in order to afford health foods. There is no compelling evidence that the high cost of these products results in concomitant benefits to the consumer.

Claims or suggestions that certain foods or diets prevent or cure disease or provide other special health benefits are, for the most part, based on folklore and, sometimes, fabrication. Many consumers do not realize that the First Amendment to the United States Constitution exempts some kinds of statements about food and nutrition from federal regulation. Only if the label on a food product makes false or misleading claims can the FDA take action on the grounds that the product is mislabeled or misbranded. If false claims are made in advertisements or in other material promoting the product, the FTC may be able to take action.

Ultimately, the consumer is dependent on a careful reading of labels and on an assessment of the trustworthiness of the health food store proprietor for assurance that he or she is purchasing organic products.

Processed and Refined Foods

Over half the food Americans consume is processed [34]. The acceptance of processed or convenience foods has occurred over time, facilitated by several basic changes in lifestyle, including urbanization, an increased number of women in the work force, and smaller households. Refining has several purposes: to improve quality, shelf life, appearance, and taste; to eliminate undesirable components; and to provide greater convenience to the person who prepares meals.

Wheat is processed to yield white flour because whole-grain products have comparatively short shelf lives. Obviously, processing results in loss of several nutrients. However, processed foods are enriched to restore some of the nutrients that may be removed in preparation. For example, white flour is enriched with thiamine, riboflavin, niacin, and iron. The refining of sugar causes a similar loss of minute amounts of vitamins and minerals, so that to the food faddist, honey, brown sugar, or raw sugar is preferable, even though they provide little or no nutrient value other than calories and are more expensive. Because of the wide variety in the American food supply, those who wish to avoid refined foods can do so.

Food Additives

Concern about the safety of chemicals in the environment has led many consumers to believe that food additives are unnecessary chemicals added to foods by manufacturers in order to earn greater profits. However, additives play a necessary and beneficial role in the food supply. They contribute toward increasing and preserving the supply of food, improving and stabilizing nutritional value, and enhancing flavor, texture, and appearance.

The legal definition of food additives (which include natural substances such as spices, essential oils, enzymes, and even foods themselves) is exceedingly complex. It includes any substance or mixture of substances that becomes part of the food during production, processing, storage, or packaging. Additives are of two types: intentional and incidental. Intentional additives are added deliberately to maintain or improve nutritional value, to maintain freshness and product quality, to help in processing or preparation, or to make foods more appealing. Some examples include carrageenan, which makes ice cream thicker and prevents formation of ice crystals; starch, which thickens tomato sauce and gravies; and food colors. Incidental additives are present in foods in trace quantities as an unintentional result of some phase of production, processing, storage, or packaging. Some of these are pesticide residues, antibiotics fed to animals, mercury found in fish, and chemical substances that migrate from plastic packaging materials. Table 5-1 lists the general categories and functions of food additives.

Intentional food additives are further broken down into two groups: regulated food additives and GRAS ("generally recognized as safe"). In 1958, the Food Additive Amendment was enacted, according to which no additive could be used until it was proved safe. The burden of proof rested with the food manufacturer who was required by law to provide evidence that an additive was safe. The testing of an additive can take many years. First, it must go through a battery of chemical tests, and then it is tested on two species of laboratory animals, usually rodents and dogs. Finally, the FDA must approve its safety and regulate its use in food. In general, only one one-hundredth of the maximum amount of an additive that has been found *not* to produce any harmful effects in test animals is used. The Delaney Clause, a special provision of the 1958 legislation, states that a substance shown to cause cancer in animals or humans (regardless of the amount administered) may not be added to food in any amount.

Some additives are not subject to testing. The FDA classifies as GRAS "any substance of natural biological origin that has been widely consumed for its nutrient properties in the United States prior to January 1, 1958, without detrimental effects when used under reasonably anticipated patterns of consumption." Substances on the GRAS list include salt, sugar, corn syrup, and dextrose. In 1969, when the artificial sweetener cyclamate, a GRAS substance, was banned, the President ordered a reappraisal of all substances on the GRAS list. A committee of scientists called the Select Committee on GRAS Substances (SCOGS) began in 1972 to reevaluate additives that are GRAS.

Most additives on the list actually have been found safe. After completing the first scientific review of the 415 original ingredients on the list, this committee declared that 305 compounds are safe in their present uses and for foreseeable future uses. Another 68 are safe, at least at their present use level, and some substances were given conditional approval. Some, such as caffeine, were

TABLE 5-1
USE OF ADDITIVES

Additive	Purpose
Acidity and alkalinity agents	Increase or decrease acidity; increase intensity of flavor; improve texture of processed cheese
Anticaking agents	Ensure free flow of salts and powders such as powdered sugars
Bleaching and maturing agents	"Whiten" flour and some cheeses; change or "mature" the texture of flour to improve its baking qualities
Coloring agents	Intensify natural colors or impart new colors
Emulsifiers	Keep oil and water mixed, as in salad dressings; prevent fat-containing foods such as chocolate from separating from other ingredients; prevent whitish "bloom" from appearing on chocolate candy; improve texture in baked goods; can replace egg yolks
Firming agents	Prevent processed fruits from becoming mushy; used in pickles, canned peas, apples; also help to coagulate milk proteins in manufacture of some cheeses
Flavors and flavor enhancers	Impart flavors or increase intensity of flavors
Foaming agents	Keep foods such as whipped cream foaming as they emerge from container; put foam on top of hot chocolate mixes.
Foam inhibitors	Prevent foam from interfering with filling of containers such as foam on citrus fruit juice
Glazing agents	Maintain shiny surfaces on foods
Humectants	Absorb water and maintain correct "humidity" in foods; used in products such as shredded coconut and marshmallows
Leavening agents	Lighten (leaven) baked products
Nutrients	Vitamins, minerals, and protein added to improve nutritional quality of the food or to increase availability of nutrients that are hard to obtain in the diet, such as iron or iodine
Preservatives, antioxidants	Prevent food spoilage caused by microorganisms; prevent rancidity, discoloration
Sequestrants	Bind trace metals to prevent processes resulting in rancidity; prevent minerals from discoloring soft drinks; maintain color in mayonnaise, canned beans, salad dressings, other foods
Stabilizers and thickeners	Give foods a smooth texture; thicken beverages, jams, jellies, ice cream; prevent water from freezing into crystals

thought to need additional studies to answer unresolved questions. Others, such as salt and some modified starches, may have limits put on their use [35].

Controversial additives   A number of additives, chiefly nitrites, certain sweeteners, and coloring chemicals, have excited controversy and pose interesting problems of health policy.

Nitrites   Nitrites are a class of chemical additives that are relatively nontoxic themselves but which may interact with other chemicals or even with normal constituents of food to form carcinogens. Sodium nitrite is used to protect cured and smoked foods against contamination by bacteria, particularly *Clostridium botulinum*. This organism grows in an environment which contains little or no oxygen, and has been found in improperly prepared canned food and underprocessed vacuum-packed foods (for example, canned ham). Since the presence of the bacterium and the toxin it produces causes no detectable change in the appearance, taste, or odor of food, there is no way for the consumer to know that a food is contaminated. The toxin can be deadly, and food processors and the U.S. Department of Agriculture (USDA) are very concerned about preventing the growth of this bacterium. Sodium nitrite also flavors and colors cured meats. Nitrites are also found normally in the gastrointestinal tract, produced by the bacterial reduction of nitrates. Naturally occurring nitrites are found in some vegetables including spinach, cabbage, and beets. More than 80 percent of the nitrite entering the stomach comes from saliva [36]. Saliva in the salivary glands contains nitrate but not nitrite. Nitrite is produced from nitrate by oral microorganisms.

Secondary amines, which are found in certain foods, can react with nitrites to form nitrosamines. Some nitrosamines have been shown to cause cancer in laboratory animals. There is no direct evidence that nitrosamines are carcinogenic for humans. Vitamin C inhibits nitrosamine formation.

When nitrites and secondary amines are subjected to high temperatures—as when bacon is pan-fried or frankfurters grilled—the nitrosamine content of the meat increases greatly. Consequently the U.S. Department of Agriculture is requiring bacon manufacturers to decrease the nitrite used in processing (to 120 ppm) and to add sodium ascorbate or sodium erythroborate, substances that block nitrosamine formation. An alternative may be to buy bacon that has been precooked in a microwave oven. Cooking bacon by using microwaves protects it from *C. botulinum* growth, and thus its nitrite content can be reduced substantially [37].

Nitrite is added to some types of cured meats to confer a red color, as well as a flavor and consistency, to these products. Thus luncheon meat, salami, and sausage contain nitrites not to protect against botulism but for their flavor and color-producing qualities. As long as these products are kept refrigerated at a temperature below 4°C (40°F) at all times, they can be made without nitrite. Nitrite-free bacon and other meat products are available in some markets, but the traditional red color of bacon may be replaced in these products by a gray-brown hue.

In 1978, following the reports that nitrite *per se* causes tumors in rats, the

FDA and the U.S. Department of Agriculture announced that they would take steps to phase out its use. In 1980, the government agencies withdrew this proposed ban [38] after rejecting the studies [39] that led to the proposed ban. Unfortunately, American consumers were subjected to apparently unnecessary duress and anxiety during this period as the safety of nitrites was debated. The FDA also requested that the National Academy of Sciences (NAS) search the literature on nitrite and investigate alternative means of preserving meats. The first part of the National Academy of Sciences panel report was released in December 1981 and recommended that the amount of sodium nitrite in cured meats be reduced "to the extent that protection against botulism is not compromised" [40]. The second phase of the study, which will discuss possible alternatives to nitrite, will be released in 1982.

Artificial and Alternate Sweeteners Experts estimate that Americans eat or drink more than 5 million pounds of saccharin a year—about three-fourths of it in diet beverages, the rest in coffee, tea, and dietetic foods. Saccharin is also added to many drugs and oral hygiene products to improve taste, particularly of those intended for children.

Concern about the possible carcinogenicity of saccharin initially arose as a result of animal experiments. The most persuasive evidence was derived from a study showing an increased incidence of bladder cancer in rats exposed to saccharin in utero and then weaned to a saccharin-rich diet [41]. A ban on the use of saccharin was proposed by the FDA in 1977 but never implemented because Congress voted delays in its implementation.

Several groups of investigators have also examined epidemiological evidence for increased incidence of bladder cancer in people who have consumed saccharin. Some investigators have reported an increased incidence in saccharin users; others could identify no relationship. As in the rat studies, the experimental method used in all of these investigations has also been criticized.

Two recent studies which were designed to avoid much of this criticism have been reported by Morrison and Buring [42] and by Hoover and Strasser from the National Cancer Institute [43]. Both studies concluded that saccharin is, at worst, a weak carcinogen which does not greatly increase the risk of bladder cancer. However, these researchers did not investigate other possible ill effects of artificial sweeteners, nor cancer in organs other than the bladder. In a New England Journal of Medicine editorial [44], Robert Hoover, of the National Cancer Institute, also pointed out that these studies did not investigate the effect of in utero exposure—an important question because of the widespread use of saccharin by women in their childbearing years. He also expressed concern about the increased use of artificial sweeteners by children and adolescents, who consume much greater doses per kilogram of body weight than adults. Dr. Hoover concluded by stating:

> When all the evidence of toxicity is weighed against the lack of objective evidence of benefit, any use by nondiabetic children or pregnant women, heavy use by young women of childbearing age, and excessive use by anyone is ill-advised and should be actively discouraged by the medical community.

He called "heavy use" the equivalent of drinking more than four cans of dietetic beverage per day. Table 5-2 gives the saccharin content of some "sugar-free" foodstuffs.

The concern about saccharin would diminish if other sweeteners could be used. In 1981, the FDA approved the synthetic dipeptide aspartame (L-aspartyl-L-phenylalanine methyl ester), developed by G.D. Searle and Company for use as a tabletop sweetener and as an ingredient in dry food products [45]. Aspartame is marketed to food industries under the brand name Nutra-Sweet; the tabletop version is Equal. Carbonated beverages were not included in the original food-additive petition to the FDA because aspartame tends to lose its sweetening capacity in liquids after 6 months of unrefrigerated shelf life. Aspartame may have a more widespread use than simply being a substitute for saccharin. Other possibilities include the sweetening of foods and beverages that normally contain relatively high levels of sucrose or corn syrup, since aspartame tastes like sugar and does not have the metallic aftertaste of saccharin.

The FDA's approval of aspartame was somewhat unexpected. Although submitted to FDA in 1973 and approved for use in 1974, objections to aspartame have kept the compound in regulatory limbo. A public board of inquiry was convened in January 1980, to resolve scientific arguments that had been raised against aspartame.

The principal question was whether the amino acid components of the compound—either by themselves or in combination with another common amino acid, glutamic acid—could cause brain lesions or brain tumors if ingested at high levels. In late 1980, the board of inquiry gave qualified disapproval of aspartame. The FDA, however, reviewed all the data, plus additional tests from Japan that were concluded after the board's decision, and approved aspartame.

Fructose, sorbitol, and xylitol are also being used with greater frequency as sweeteners. The caloric content of these sweeteners is the same as sucrose (table sugar) on a weight basis, and so they have no benefit for overweight persons. However, fructose and xylitol are sweeter than sucrose, so that less is required to

TABLE 5-2
SACCHARIN CONTENT OF SOME "SUGAR-FREE" FOODSTUFFS

Product	Saccharin content
Diet Pepsi	125 mg per 12 fl oz
Tab	110 mg per 12 fl oz
Sugar-free Sprite	86 mg per 12 fl oz
Diet 7-Up	88 mg per 12 fl oz
Alba '77 fit & frosty mix	4.2 mg per fl oz
Sugar twin	14.1 mg per tsp
Sweet 'n Low	20 mg per tsp
Sucaryl liquid	7.6 mg per $\frac{1}{8}$ tsp

obtain the sweetness level of sucrose. They are not without their own problems. Consuming large amounts of sorbitol or fructose (30 to 50 g) daily may result in abdominal cramping and diarrhea. Feeding studies done in several animal species have indicated that chronic ingestion of xylitol may be associated with tumor induction and other pathology. For more details, see the reviews by Brunzell [46] and Olefsky and Crapo [47]. Thus, it appears that the ideal sweetener has yet to be found.

Colors   Of all the additives, food coloring is perhaps the hardest to justify as necessary, even though color for some products is a useful means of identification. For example, strawberry color and strawberry flavor go together. Most foodstuffs are not artificially colored, but approximately 10 percent of foods do contain color additives. More than half of all food colors consumed are found in soft drinks. The rest are found in gelatin and pudding mixes, bakery goods, cereal, and snack foods.

Food coloring chemicals fall into one of three categories: (1) synthetic organic compounds (the FD&C colors), (2) mineral or synthetic inorganic colors (iron oxide, for example), and (3) natural coloring of either vegetable or animal origin (vegetable or fruit juices or color extracts). For clarification, it should be noted that there are both natural and synthetic coloring agents for food. However, when coloring is added to a food, the coloring is described as "artificial." Here the word *artificial* refers strictly to color that has been added over and above that which may be present naturally. The added food coloring may be either natural or synthetic.

Color additives find uses not only in foods but also in drugs, cosmetics, and medical devices. The 1960 Color Additives Amendment to the Federal Food, Drug, and Cosmetic Act provided for separate listings of the uses for which colors could be safely employed. Thus, for example, a given color might be approved for external drugs and cosmetic use but not approved for food use or ingested drug use.

Color additives are officially designated as either "subject to certification" (synthetic colors that are required to be batch-certified) or "exempt from certification" (mostly "natural" colors that may be used without batch certification).

Surprisingly, there are relatively few synthetic color additives approved for use in the United States. There are only six synthetic food colors that are "permanently" approved for *food* use (see Table 5-3). Red No. 40 is now under indictment as a possible carcinogen. The FDA has been reviewing the safety of Red No. 40 since 1976, when Red No. 2 was outlawed and Red No. 40 became the most widely consumed food coloring in the United States. Denmark and Mexico are the only other countries that permit use of Red No. 40 in food. Yellow No. 5 (tartrazine) has been identified as an allergen affecting an estimated 100,000 U.S. residents [48]. In July 1980, the FDA moved to require food and drug manufacturers to label all products containing FD&C Yellow No. 5, effective July 1, 1981 [49].

Little concern about safety has heretofore been expressed about colors

TABLE 5-3
APPROVED SYNTHETIC FOOD COLORS

Official and (common) name	Permitted uses
FD&C Blue No. 1 (Brilliant Blue FCF)	General, including dietary supplements
Orange B	Casing of surfaces of frankfurters and sausage, up to 150 ppm
Citrus Red No. 2	Skins of oranges not intended for processing, up to 2 ppm in whole orange
FD&C Red No. 3 (erythrosine)	General, including dietary supplements
FD&C Red No. 40 (Allura Red AC)	General, including dietary supplements
FD&C Yellow No. 5 (tartrazine)	General, including dietary supplements

Source: Code of Federal Regulations, Title 21, U.S. Government Printing Office, Washington, 1979.

exempt from certification (see Table 5-4). Many of these, by practical experience rather than by toxicological examination, have been assumed to be safe. Undoubtedly, the popular belief that "natural is good" has added to this lack of scrutiny. Furthermore, the precise chemical characterization of these colors is impracticable. These colorants are obtained by chemical extraction, heat treatment, steeping, or drying of natural materials or, in some cases, by chemical synthesis. Now, however, attention is being drawn to these colorants. The Food and Agriculture Organization (FAO) and the World Health Organiza-

TABLE 5-4
COLOR ADDITIVES EXEMPT FROM CERTIFICATION

Algae meal, dried	Grape skin extract
Annatto extract	Iron oxide, synthetic
β-Apo-8'-carotenal	Juice, fruit
Beets, dehydrated (beet powder)	Juice, vegetable
Canthaxanthin	Paprika
Caramel	Paprika oleoresin
β-Carotene	Riboflavin
Carrot oil	Saffron
Cochineal extract, carmine	Tagetes (Aztec marigold)
Corn endosperm oil	meal and extract
Cottonseed flour, cooked,	Titanium dioxide
toasted, partially defatted	Turmeric
Ferrous gluconate	Turmeric oleoresin

tion (WHO) of the United Nations have ruled that any additive, natural or synthetic, must undergo chronic toxicity studies in various animal species over a period of 2 years before it becomes eligible for approval [48]. In the United States, the FDA cyclic review program will permit an assessment of all food colorants [50].

Additives and Hyperkinesis   Hyperactivity is a poorly defined combination of symptoms, primarily behavioral, that has been estimated to have a prevalence of between 3 and 20 percent in all school children in the United States. The lack of a precise definition and the heterogeneity of classifications have led to confusion; terms such as hyperactivity, hyperkinesis, minimal brain dysfunction, and learning disabilities have all been used, and attempts by professional groups to narrow the definitions have been unsuccessful. Behavioral characteristics include short attention span, easy distractibility, impulsive behavior, overactivity, resistance to discipline, restlessness, emotional lability, and learning disabilities [51]. The male-female ratio has been reported to range in various groups of children from 4:1 to 10:1. The usual therapy is treatment with central nervous stimulants, such as methylphenidate (Ritalin) or amphetamines.

Food intake was proposed as a cause of hyperactivity by Feingold [52]; he implicated artificial colorings and flavorings, antioxidant preservatives such as butylated hydroxytoluene (BHT) and butylated hyroxyanisole (BHA), and salicylates occurring naturally in oranges, apples, plums, peaches, berries, tomatoes, apricots, cucumbers, and almonds. He stated that improvement in nearly 50 percent of his subjects could be accomplished by dietary changes.

The Feingold hypothesis evolved from anecdotal clinical and parental observations, not from double-blind control studies. Two conferences organized to review available data recommended carefully controlled studies to test the hypothesis [53,54]. Two experimental methodologies have been employed to evaluate the evidence: dietary crossover studies and specific challenge experiments. In dietary crossover studies, hyperactive children are assigned randomly to one of two different experimental diets, the Kaiser-Permanente (K-P) diet (or modification thereof) or a diet disguised to look like the Feingold diet but containing the food additives under question. The children remain on a single diet for several weeks after which they are "crossed over" to the other diet so that the behavior of the same subjects on the two different diets can be compared. Behavior is observed by parents and/or teachers and/or trained observers. Tests of learning ability and other psychological functions are also sometimes administered. In one study of this type [55], the behavior of the children on the K-P diet appeared to improve according to the teachers but not according to the parents. In a study by Harley et al. [56] parents, not teachers, were the only ones who noticed a change. In both studies the *sequence* in which the diets were fed influenced the results, with behavior improving when the control diet was offered first followed by the K-P diet but not when the diets were introduced in the reverse order.

Specific challenge experiments are designed to minimize the possibility of placebo effects on the children's observed behavior. Children who demonstrate measurable behavioral improvement on the K-P diet are randomly assigned to either a challenge or a control group and are then crossed over to the other group, thus allowing each child to serve as his own control. Most challenge experiments have tested artificial food colors [57–59]. On the basis of the cumulative evidence, the National Advisory Committee on Hyperkinesis and Food Additives, assembled by the Nutrition Foundation, concluded that "the studies already completed provide sufficient evidence to refute the claim that artificial food colorings, artificial flavorings, and salicylates produce hyperactivity and/or learning disabilities" [60]. More recently, a 13-member committee convened by the National Institutes of Health concluded that the link between certain food additives and hyperactivity remains unconfirmed [61].

Clearly, all hyperkinesis is not caused by food additives, and most hyperkinetic children are not helped by an additive-free diet. Hence, it appears there is no justification for sweeping changes in foods or in the diets of children.

A number of questions remain. As stated in an editorial by Bierman and Furukawa [62] they are: How can one identify the child who might be sensitive to food additives? What are the risks of the diet? (The original Feingold diet, since modified, was very deficient in vitamin C.) Are these risks greater than the risk of medication? Does the correction of hyperkinesis, by any means, make the child a better student or ultimately a more functional adult? Since the Swanson and Kinsbourne study [58] suggests a possible dose effect, is there a safe limit for food color additives?

None of these questions can yet be answered. Meanwhile, the physician must help the hyperkinetic child and his or her anxious parents. Presumably, there can be no physical harm in eliminating food additives as long as a nutritionally sound diet, acceptable to the child, can be provided. Consultation with a registered dietitian may be needed to determine accurately whether a sound diet is indeed being provided. On the other hand, there is virtually no knowledge about the potential psychological harm that could result from a child being forced to consume a diet different from his or her peers. As is often the case in medicine, the physician must make a clinical judgment for each individual child without all the facts being available.

DIETS

Fad Weight-Reduction Diets

The humorist Art Buchwald once suggested that the word *diet* comes from the verb *to die* [63]. Anyone whose commitment to weight loss has made them the victim of hunger pangs, headaches, fatigue, or boredom might agree. Most overweight people have discovered that losing weight—and maintaining that lower weight—is no easy matter. Effective and sustained weight reduction must be achieved in a regular, orderly fashion on a diet adequate in all required nutrients but low in calories. Effective weight loss also involves a change in eating habits.

The public appears not only to be vitally interested in weight reduction but also to be quick to believe in and to buy books on fad diets, drugs that suppress appetite, and reducing gadgets. Most of these measures slenderize only one's pocketbook. Some may introduce health complications of their own. Dieting and weight reduction have become an industry worth billions of dollars. Each year the best-seller list includes at least one book on fad diets written by a self-styled expert promising "quick weight loss," "inches off," or "diet revolution." The diets discussed below *are not recommended* for a variety of reasons including the following:

1 The recommended calorie intake is so low as to preclude ingestion of adequate amounts of all the essential nutrients.

2 The proportions of energy nutrients—fat, carbohydrate, and protein—are suspect; a diet very low in carbohydrates, for example, can cause ketosis.

3 The diet emphasizes one food or a small number of foods and hence prevents the intake of a variety of foods containing adequate amounts of all essential nutrients.

4 The diet appeals to the emotions of an individual by making illogical promises, such as the loss of a large number of pounds within a limited time, weight loss without making decisions, the ability to "eat all you want and still lose weight," etc.

5 Follow-up care and weight maintenance, once ideal weight is achieved, are lacking.

6 The basis of the diet is partially or totally without scientific foundation.

Low-Carbohydrate Diets   The most popular low-carbohydrate diet is Dr. Atkins' "diet revolution" [64], which is neither new nor revolutionary. This diet is similar to those advocated earlier in *The Drinking Man's Diet* [65] and *Calories Don't Count* [66], and the concept dates back at least 100 years to William Banting, a coffin-maker, who successfully lost weight by excluding bread and potatoes and who wrote the first book on dieting and weight loss, *A Letter on Corpulence*. Since protein in the diet is limited by the fact that most high-protein foods are less than 40 percent protein, this diet is actually a high-fat diet. The diet at first excludes virtually all carbohydrates and later permits a gradual increase to no more than 40 g per day. Restriction of carbohydrate to under 100 g results in the synthesis of glucose from protein. Furthermore, carbohydrate is necessary for the complete oxidation of fat. In the absence of sufficient carbohydrate, acetyl-CoA molecules (intermediary products in fat metabolism) accumulate and condense, forming ketone bodies, and these accumulate in the blood, causing ketosis (a desirable state according to Dr. Atkins), and disturb the acid-base balance of the body. He further claims that many calories are lost daily in the urine and breath as ketones and as other incompletely oxidized metabolites, that the diet stimulates secretion of a "fat-mobilizing hormone," that the mobilized fat is readily converted to carbohydrate, thereby keeping the blood sugar "at an even level." Atkins claims this book represents his experiences with 10,000 patients. However, he has not published his work in medical journals, which would allow his findings to be properly evaluated by peer review.

Most diets that promote ketosis are likely to produce fatigue, dehydration, and, in some instances, nausea and vomiting, especially in persons who attempt to remain physically active. This type of diet may cause an appreciable hyperuricemia, which can precipitate an attack of gout. The starvation-like state induced by a low-carbohydrate ketogenic diet stimulates release of free fatty acids (FFA) into the plasma; in patients with cerebrovascular and coronary artery disease, increased FFA may induce cardiac arrhythmias [67]. This type of diet is not recommended because of the health hazards associated with ketosis and the increased intake of saturated dietary fat and cholesterol. Other essential nutrients such as vitamin C and minerals and fiber are not supplied in amounts sufficient to meet body needs. The American Medical Association has published a detailed critique of this type of diet [68], essentially showing that it is without scientific merit.

The Stillman diet, described in *The Doctor's Quick Weight Loss Diet* [69], is also known as the "water diet." It specifies the types but not the amount of foods which are permitted. It basically restricts carbohydrate and is rich in protein and animal fat. The diet consists of low-fat cheeses, lean meat, fish, poultry, eggs, and eight glasses of water a day. Neither milk nor visible fats are permitted.

This diet is not recommended for the same reasons as Dr. Atkins' diet—it has a ketosis-producing effect, it is practically limited to protein and fat, and it is higher in fat than the average diet. Its nutritional inadequacies include low intakes of vitamins A and C, thiamine, iron, and fiber.

The Scarsdale diet [70], created by the late Dr. Herman Tarnower, is essentially a low-carbohydrate, low-calorie, low-fat, high-protein diet. It consists of a single week of menus. There are five variations to accommodate epicurean, budget, vegetarian, and international tastes, in addition to the basic plan. The dieter chooses one regimen and for 2 weeks eats exactly the foods prescribed for each meal. However, the amounts to be eaten are not specified.

At the end of 2 weeks, the dieter switches to a "keep trim diet" for another 2 weeks. This diet, designed for weight maintenance, has a greater range of allowed foods and even permits a cocktail or a glass of wine with dinner. Because of its low-carbohydrate (about 50 g) content, this diet is also ketogenic. Additional constraints on fluid intake, which is limited to black coffee or tea, both diuretics in themselves, and on the use of salt favor diuresis. Much of the weight loss which occurs on the diet is water loss. The diet is vague as to the quantity of foods to be eaten; low in milk, breads, and cereals; and low in iron, vitamin A, calcium, and riboflavin. This diet has been described as minimally effective [71] and as dangerous to use without medical supervision [72].

Protein-Sparing Modified Fast Diets   There are several variations of the protein-sparing modified fast diet which utilize powdered and liquid formulas and which are undertaken without medical supervision. They are different from the "protein-sparing modified fast" prescribed for patients and supervised by physicians with special expertise in metabolism [73]. The variations of this type of diet include the following:

- The consumption of 9 to 12 oz of lean meats and fish per day, with black coffee or tea
- The use of a liquid protein formula by itself or of a liquid or powdered protein formula mixed with water, club soda, fruit juices, or other liquids
- The use of liquid protein beverages in combination with one or two meals
- The use of a liquid protein beverage as the sole "food"

Most of these protein products are hydrolysates of collagen or gelatin and are of extremely low nutritional quality. Some are fortified with a limited number of essential amino acids, vitamins, and minerals, and most are nutritionally incomplete. There are a few products that contain high-quality protein derived from meat, milk, or soy. The amount of protein formula used in any of the above situations ranges anywhere from 4 to 10 oz a day. Vitamin and mineral supplements are prescribed with all of these variations, and at times other medications, such as hormones, may be prescribed. The liquid and powdered proteins are marketed under many brand names (Prolinn, P-86, Ultrathin, NaturSlim, and Slim Fast) and have varied formulas [74].

The best known diet in this category is described in Dr. Robert Linn's *The Last Chance Diet* [75]. This diet is a fast supplemented with a protein source, Prolinn, which sells for $12 to $15 a quart. Such fasts are dangerous in that they may induce ketosis, hypokalemia, and other complications. During the fast, vitamin and mineral supplements, potassium, and folic acid are also prescribed, with at least 2 qt of noncaloric fluids a day. Gradually, food is introduced during a refeeding phase, but the Prolinn powder must still be consumed twice a day. Intakes of vitamin A, riboflavin, thiamine, iron, and calcium are inadequate.

The dangers of this diet are well documented. By June 1978, 58 deaths associated with very low caloric, high-protein diets had been reported; 16 of these deaths occurred among women aged 23 to 51 who showed no evidence of underlying medical problems that could have caused their deaths [76].

This diet is not recommended and should never be self-prescribed. Likewise, over-the-counter purchase of liquid or powdered protein is to be strongly discouraged. Individuals who want to lose up to 50 lb should not use this regimen, which was originally conceived for the massively obese (individuals more than 50 percent above ideal body weight).

The Cambridge diet, developed by Dr. Alan Howard of Cambridge University, England, involves drinking a flavored powder, the "Ultimate Diet, a complete and delicious food that actually melts off fat virtually as fast as complete fasting," mixed with water three times per day. By following this diet one consumes 330 kcal per day which consists of 31 g of high biological value protein from milk, 44 g carbohydrate from sugars, and 2 g of fat, plus the RDA for all known vitamins and minerals. Headquartered in Monterey, California, the Cambridge Plan International operates through a pyramid sales structure in which "patrons" are encouraged to become product "counselors" who, in turn, recruit other participants. The program has enjoyed considerable success in the western United States [77].

It is feared that this diet plan is too closely related to the aforedescribed liquid-protein diets popular in the 1970s, although the quality of protein is higher. The amount of protein is less than that recommended for semistarvation therapy of obesity [73]. Randall B. Lee, executive director of the American Society of Bariatric Physicians, reports that several participants have been hospitalized for cardiac irregularities suspected of stemming from electrolyte imbalances associated with the diet [77]. All experts agree that diets of less than 800 kcal a day should not be attempted without frequent medical supervision which includes appropriate laboratory evaluation at regular intervals [78].

The Beverly Hills Diet   *The Beverly Hills Diet* [79] occupied the number one spot on the hardcover best-seller list for many weeks in late 1981. A paperback version, which will probably top the list again, has appeared as well. This book combines a number of totally bizarre statements about nutrition and uses a regimen of eating vast amounts of fruits—to be eaten in a set pattern—and little other food. In fact, as pointed out by Mirkin and Shore [80], the diet's initial 11-day only-fruit regimen can result in severe diarrhea, with potentially life-threatening consequences (including fluid loss and irregularities of heart rhythm). For the first weeks, the diet is extremely low in protein, as well as calcium, iron, and some B vitamins.

The book is full of misinformation so bizarre that it would be humorous, except that so many people seem to believe it. The author, Judy Mazel, claims that certain combinations of food clog your stomach's enzyme system and prevent the food from being digested. As a result, the undigested food turns into fat! This runs contrary to conventional scientific principles of nutrition as does the statement that enzymes in fruit make hard-to-digest foods less fattening. The enzymes in fruit do nothing to help break down food in the stomach and intestines. Mazel also claims that potatoes, if eaten with meat, ferment into vodka in the stomach and cause intoxication! Fermentation does not occur in the healthy stomach, and when it does, in cases of gastric outlet obstruction, ethanol is not produced in appreciable quantities!

Skim Milk and Bananas Diet   This diet guarantees quick weight loss—half pound per day—and consists solely of skim milk and bananas. Of course, weight loss can be achieved on this monotonous diet because the caloric intake is limited (5 cups milk and 4 bananas total 948 kcal). This diet is not recommended, since it has nutrient inadequacies (vitamin A, niacin, and iron) and promotes unreasonable eating habits.

The Grapefruit Diet   Another name for this diet is the "10-day, 10-pounds-off diet." The premise of this diet is that grapefruit eaten before each meal acts as a "catalyst" to burn body fat and thereby causes hastened weight loss. This claim has no support from a biochemical standpoint and cannot be substantiated. Weight loss occurs as a result of low calorie intake rather than from eating grapefruit. This diet is not recommended because it is based on false premises, its low carbohydrate level promotes ketosis, and it does not provide enough food from the milk and bread and cereal groups.

Recommended Weight-Reduction Diets

Some diet plans do satisfy the criteria for a good dietary regimen (see Table 5-5).

Slim Chance in a Fat World, by Drs. Richard B. Stuart and Barbara Davis [81], offers several food plans, each with a specific energy level (usually 1200 kcal for women, more for men). These plans satisfy all nutrition needs and provide a lot of information about behavior modification and for planning a good diet and exercise program.

Eating Is Okay by Drs. H. A. Jordon, L. S. Levitz, and G. M. Kimbrell [82], offers a "behavioral control diet" which contains about 1500 kcal and if followed closely, will meet all nutritional needs. This is a self-administered course in behavioral modification rather than just a weight-loss diet. The dieter learns how to make long-term changes in eating styles. The value of exercise is stressed.

Other books outlining similar self-directed methods of dietary change include: *Learning to Eat: Behavioral Modification for Weight Control,* by J. M. Ferguson, Bull Publishing, Palo Alto, 1976; and *Permanent Weight Control,* by Drs. Michael and Katherine Mahoney, Norton, New York, 1976.

TABLE 5-5
CRITERIA THAT A WEIGHT-CONTROL DIET SHOULD MEET

1 It must be deficient only in energy.

2 It should contain a wide variety of foods to ensure adequate amounts of all essential nutrients.

3 It should educate the dieter about proper nutrition and include behavior modification techniques that will help the dieter maintain weight loss.

4 It should reduce energy intake to a point where there is a slow but steady weight loss (1 to 2 lb per week).

5 It should be based on sound scientific and biochemical facts.

6 It must be palatable and provide for a variety of foods.

7 It must have no medical risks or serious metabolic side effects.

8 It should be economical and not require the purchase of special products.

9 It should be adaptable to a variety of lifestyles and circumstances, e.g., following a vegetarian diet or eating in restaurants or at friends' homes.

The "Pritikin diet," from *Live Longer Now: The First One Hundred Years of Your Life,* by N. Pritikin [83] is extremely low in fat (about 10 percent of total calories) and is also low in sugars, salt, margarine, oils, and beef. Skim-milk dairy products, fruits, vegetables, breads, and cereals are emphasized. At 1400 kcal per day, it meets the requirements for essential nutrients, although it is slightly low in iron. In practice, this diet is so restrictive that many people cannot comply. Pritikin has popularized the regimen as a cure for heart disease, but to date, evidence supporting this claim is lacking.

Weight Watchers (Weight Watchers International, Manhasset, New York) is a self-help group which enrolls members in chapters all over the world. It is staffed by paid employees who follow a centrally conceived program developed under professional auspices and monitored for effectiveness. Meetings are held weekly to reinforce motivation and to give psychological support by group interaction. The Weight Watchers diet is restricted in calories but adequate in all essential nutrients. The program also has a strong behavioral component and emphasizes nutrition education.

Diets for Athletes

A Harris poll conducted in 1979 indicated that 41 percent of Americans get no exercise at all, 44 percent are somewhat active, and only 15 percent are seriously involved in regular exercise [84]. Among the last group, nutrition is an important topic of conversation and, unfortunately, food faddism is widespread. Two reasons have been suggested for this. First, coaches and athletes are under great pressure to win at all costs, and second, athletes have a tremendous desire to believe in almost anything that will give them a competitive advantage [85].

Popular among athletes are various ergogenic, or work-enhancing, dietary aids: glucose and dextrose, honey, bee pollen, gelatin, lecithin, wheat germ oil, yeast powder, phosphates, and vitamins [86]. While it is recognized that any one of the above may confer psychological benefit to the athlete, their ergogenic benefits are all without scientific documentation.

In general, the nutritional needs of a physically active person are similar to those of the more sedentary individual, the difference being the increased energy and water requirements associated with more activity. A nutritionally adequate diet can be achieved quantitatively by following the Recommended Dietary Allowances (RDA), based on the individual's age, sex, and activity level [87]. Although the RDAs are standards for population groups rather than for individuals, the needs of most healthy individuals will not exceed them. In practical terms, the athlete can follow the "basic diet plan" outlined by Smith [88]. This plan consists of two servings daily from the milk group, two from the protein-rich group, four from the cereal group, and four from the fruit and vegetable group. Such a basic diet supplies only 1200 to 1500 kcal per day, whereas an athlete may need two or three times this amount of energy. While the energy deficit can be erased by eating additional helpings from any of the four groups, much of the additional energy is best provided by complex carbohydrates, which are found in such foods as vegetables, pastas, and bread— foods that also provide fiber, trace elements, vitamins, and minerals. When energy requirements approach 5000 kcal per day, five or six meals a day may be preferred to three meals a day. Also the demand for thiamine (0.5 mg per 1000 kcal) increases proportionately to the output of energy [89]. Some athletes whose energy needs are very high, e.g., 5000 kcal per day, may have difficulty in consuming enough complex carbohydrates to meet this energy requirement. They may have to supplement their diet with refined carbohydrates (to some nutritionists' horror!). Because fat is a less readily available source of energy and because it has almost unlimited storage in the body, there is no rationale for increasing the fat content of the diet. In fact, high-fat diets, by creating a condition of acidosis, may adversely affect performance [86].

In a normal mixed diet, carbohydrates provide about 45 percent of the calories; in a carbohydrate-rich diet, as much as 70 percent of the energy comes from carbohydrates. Such high-carbohydrate diets are better able to provide the energy required for sustaining physical performance for long periods [90]. During prolonged exercise at less than full (submaximal) effort (e.g., distance running or cross-country skiing), most energy is derived from the oxidation of fat. As the intensity of exercise (e.g., sprinting) increases, the athlete's metabolism changes from predominantly aerobic to anaerobic. This shift, combined with other complex metabolic signals, causes the body to oxidize carbohydrates more and fat less.

The onset of exhaustion is thought to reflect the depletion of glycogen stored in the muscles and liver [91]. Unlike stores of fat, glycogen stores are limited. A 70-kg man has approximately 50,000 to 100,000 kcal of energy stored as fat but only 1000 to 1400 kcal stored as carbohydrate in the form of muscle and liver glycogen [92].

Carbohydrate Loading Carbohydrate loading is a technique used by many athletes to increase muscle glycogen stores for prolonged, exhaustive exercise. It is usually accomplished in three phases. In the first phase, the muscles are depleted of their glycogen stores by prolonged exercise to exhaustion and by consumption of a low-fat, high-protein, low-carbohydrate diet for 3 days. Carbohydrate intake is limited to less than 100 g per day. Fatigue, irritability, and/or nausea may be present during this time. This sets the stage for a rebound of muscle glycogen to above normal levels, sometimes to as much as 100 percent above normal levels.

During the second phase, the diet contains adequate protein and fat but most of the energy is provided by carbohydrate, 275 to 450 g per day. Most of the carbohydrate intake consists of complex carbohydrates, such as breads, cereals, fruits, and vegetables. Sugar, candy, honey, and soft drinks are not advised in carbohydrate loading. Total energy intake in the first and second stages is the same, but exercise is not recommended during the second stage in order to conserve the glycogen stores.

The third phase is on the day of the athletic event. The athlete may eat anything he or she wishes. In order that the stomach and upper intestine be empty at the time of competition, the pre-event meal is eaten 3 to 4 hours before the activity.

Carbohydrate loading should be used only for endurance events and preferably only a few times a year. It should not be used by children or pregnant women. The technique makes tremendous demands on the muscles. For shorter events, the first phase can be omitted and the second phase followed in order to fill, but not to supersaturate, the glycogen stores.

Protein Supplementation The myth that athletes need protein supplements persists and is hard to dispel. The suggested adult RDA for protein is 0.8 g per kilogram of body weight; younger children and teenagers may require 1.3 to 1.5 g/kg. Protein supplements are advisable only if daily dietary needs are not met.

A high-protein diet may have several negative aspects. First, this diet leads to increased urea production, increased obligatory urine volume, and greater losses of salt, which enhance the chance of dehydration during activities that increase sweating. Second, a high-protein diet can be expensive, while providing the body with little available energy.

Fluid and Electrolyte Replacement Perhaps the most critical nutrient for the athlete is water. The risk of dehydration is greatest in nonacclimated athletes. Consequently, the combination of heat and humidity poses the greatest risk of dehydration injury. Athletes who must maintain a certain weight to participate in their sport, e.g., wrestling and boxing, should also be warned of the risks of dehydration. These individuals often subject themselves to intermittent periods of starvation and dehydration.

To prevent dehydration, the athlete should drink enough fluids to maintain preexercise weight. Each pound of body weight lost during activity should be replaced by 14 to 16 oz of water or other fluids. Cold drinks offer the advantages of emptying more rapidly from the stomach and, at the same time, enhancing body cooling. Loss of only 3 percent of body weight through dehydration may seriously hinder athletic performance.

When an athlete incurs considerable sweat loss, sodium and chloride may be depleted. Adequate salting of food normally replenishes these electrolytes. Salt tablets should be avoided, since they may draw body fluids into the alimentary tract and cause cramping, nausea, and vomiting.

Athletes training for marathon or ultradistance (50 to 100 miles) events may incur not only loss of sodium and chloride but also depletion of potassium, magnesium, and other essential minerals. Emphasis on rehydration and diet can assist these athletes. In most sports, electrolyte levels can be regulated by eating a balanced diet. If commercial electrolyte replacement fluids are used during endurance events, they should be diluted because of their high glucose content [93].

Vitamin Supplements Most nutritionists agree that vitamin supplementation is not necessary for athletes who consume a balanced diet. However, vitamin supplementation is common among athletes. Excess water-soluble vitamins are not stored in the body, and thus are rapidly excreted in the urine once tissue levels are saturated. The fat-soluble vitamins are retained and stored in the body. Chronic excessive intakes of vitamins A and D may produce toxic effects. Although it may be advisable under certain conditions to increase the vitamin intake for an athlete, this need is normally met when the total energy content of a nutritionally balanced diet is increased.

The text by McArdle et al. [94] is recommended for further information on nutrition and exercise.

HOW TO RECOGNIZE FOOD QUACKERY

The essence of quackery—a word derived from *quacksalver,* meaning literally "to boast of a cure"—is self-advertisement of the ability to cure disease. Jarvis [95] has defined food quackery as "the practices of someone who, because of avoidable ignorance, delusion, misconception, or intent to deceive, makes excessive claims or promises for the value of a nutritional substance or dietary practice to prevent, alleviate, or cure a disease, extend life span, or improve physical or mental performance."

As shown in Table 5-6, one identifying feature of a food quack is the use of meaningless credentials. Quacks are salespersons who use personal appeal, sincerity, and enthusiasm to sell products that they are suggesting. Additional clues that suggest probable misinformation or fraudulent claims are given in Table 5-7. It is not always easy to recognize a quack. The quack wears the cloak of science; he or she talks in "scientific terms" and cites scientific references.

Oftentimes the quack can operate beyond the arm of the law. The FDA *can* take action if foods, drugs, cosmetics, or medical devices sold in interstate commerce are misbranded or include false or misleading claims in their labeling. The agency can also act against such products if they are dangerous or in the case of drugs ineffective, and against products that are sold before they comply with certain premarket requirements. Products that may be in violation of the law can be seized only after the FDA goes to court and only if the products are sold in interstate commerce [63].

Anyone can state, in any medium of his or her choice, any false, misleading, or deceptive health information he or she chooses. The First Amendment (freedom of speech) protects him or her from the consequences of the harm he or she does unless the false information is on the label of a product or the fraud occurs in the course of a provable doctor-patient relationship [96]. Thus, the FDA, which can act against misleading labels, has no jurisdiction over misleading books.

The Federal Trade Commission (FTC) is empowered to act against false and misleading advertisement but only if the product (or advertising) has first moved across state lines. Usually the FTC acts against gross violations but does not take action against subtle forms of misleading information. For effective policing the FTC would have to monitor all newspapers, magazines, and other publications that carry advertising plus all the radio and television stations. In fact, two people spend half their time checking advertising [97].

TABLE 5-6
INDIVIDUALS WHO ARE SOURCES OF QUESTIONABLE
NUTRITION INFORMATION

---

1 Holders of degrees in fields other than nutrition, dietetics,
or related areas who identify themselves as nutritionists.
Suspect degrees include the following:
Certified herbologist (C.H.)
Certified Nutritionist
Doctor of Chiropractic (D.C.)
Doctor of Naturopathy (N.D.)
Registered Healthologist (R.H.)

2 Holders of degrees from institutions which are not
approved (although they may be *authorized*) by the
states in which they operate.

3 Holders of mail-order Ph.D.s or other "advanced"
degrees.

4 Those without appropriate educational credentials who pro-
claim themselves "nutritionists" or "nutritional counselors."

5 Those who receive direct financial gain from the nutritional products they are suggesting (i.e., proprietors of
"health" food stores and those who sell dietary supplements).

6 Anyone convicted of nutrition fraud.

7 Book authors, publishers, and broadcasters who present in-
accurate nutrition information. All of these sources should
be evaluated for the accuracy of the information they present.

Source: Nutritional misinformation and food faddism, An American
Dietetic Association Newstars broadcast, June 4, 1981.

The U.S. Postal Service can take action against anyone who uses the mail to defraud. Proving a violation in court, however, has often been difficult and time-consuming. Even if an offender is convicted, he or she may merely pay a fine and move elsewhere. The need for consumer awareness becomes even more important in the face of the limited success of governmental efforts.

People become food faddists for many different reasons. It may result from misinformation, as an outgrowth of deeply held philosophical beliefs, or from a health neurosis. According to Jarvis, most people who are immersed in faddism can be placed in one of two categories—the "deceived" and the "deluded" [98]. The deceived and the deluded can be differentiated on the basis of how they react when faced with substantive evidence that their beliefs are wrong. The deceived will change, the deluded will not.

For physicians and health practitioners, dealing with faddist patients requires skill and tact. Success often depends more on how one meets their emotional needs than on one's scientific or academic credentials. Being informed about the popular or contemporary fads enhances one's credibility. Condemnation of a fad by a physician or health practitioner out of ignorance or unwillingness to investigate its claims reinforces the notion of "establishment bigotry," which is a

TABLE 5-7
CLUES THAT SUGGEST PROBABLE NUTRITION
MISINFORMATION OR FRAUDULENT CLAIMS

1 Use of testimonials and case histories to support specific nutritional therapies

2 Magazine articles that promote nutrients or products advertised in the publication

3 Claims of effortless exercise and dietless reducing plans

4 Assertions that food from supermarkets is unhealthy and only food or products from "health" food stores are safe and healthful

5 General recommendations for nutrient supplementation far exceeding current RDAs

6 Reports of research in articles or books written only for the general public and not submitted for critical peer review to scientific or medical journals

7 Claims that natural vitamins are more effective than synthetic ones

8 Use of hair analysis as a primary method of detecting nutritional problems

9 Assertions that the American Medical Association, the Food and Drug Administration, the government, or organized medicine has suppressed the person's work

10 Unusual methods of nutritional assessment, such as psychic testing, muscle testing, pendulums, or pulse testing for food allergies

11 Instant computerized nutritional evaluations where nutrient supplements are sold

12 Routine use of enemas, colonics, or other detoxification programs

Source: Nutritional misinformation and food faddism, An American Dietetic Association Newstars broadcast, June 4, 1981.

powerful weapon in the hands of health quacks. Attention must be given to more than just providing nutritional facts. Faddism is often based on deeply held beliefs and values which are emotional expressions of health consciousness and a desire for wholesomeness. When debunking ideas, such as honey is "natural" and "good," while white sugar is "artificial" and "bad," credit should be given to the merit that the idea *appears* to have; this avoids the appearance of being against the basic ideals.

REFERENCES

1 McBean, L. D., and E. W. Speckmann: Food faddism: a challenge to nutritionists and dietitians, Am. J. Clin. Nutr., 27:1071, 1974.
2 Economics of food faddism, Nutrition & the M.D., 7:5, April 1981.

3 Bruch, H. J.: The allure of food cults and nutrition quackery, J. Am. Diet. Assoc., 57:316, 1970.

4 Wynder, E. L.: Nutrition and cancer, Fed. Proc., 35:1309, 1976.

5 Alcantara, E. N., and E. W. Speckmann: Diet, nutrition and cancer, Am. J. Clin. Nutr., 29:1035, 1976.

6 Oace, S.: Diet and cancer, J. Nutr. Educ., 10:106, 1978.

7 U.S. Senate Select Committee on Nutrition and Human Needs: *Dietary Goals for the United States,* 2d ed., U.S. Government Printing Office, Washington, December 1977.

8 Pauling, L.: *Vitamin C, the Common Cold and the Flu,* Freeman, San Francisco, 1976.

9 Cameron, E., and L. Pauling: *Cancer and Vitamin C,* Linus Pauling Institute of Science and Medicine, Menlo Park, Calif., 1979.

10 Young, V. R., and P. M. Newberne: Vitamins and cancer prevention: issues and dilemmas, Cancer, 47:1226, 1981.

11 Sun, M.: Laetrile brush fire is out, scientists hope, Science, 212:758, 1981.

12 Herbert, V.: Pangamic acid ("vitamin B_{15}"), Am. J. Clin. Nutr., 32:1534, 1979.

13 Vogelsang, E., and E. V. Shute: Effect of vitamin E in coronary disease (letter), Nature, 157:772, 1946.

14 Shute, W. E., and H. J. Taub (eds.): *Vitamin E for Ailing and Healthy Hearts,* Pyramid, New York, 1972.

15 Institute of Food Technologists, Expert Panel on Food Safety and Nutrition: Vitamin E, Nutr. Rev., 35:57, 1977.

16 Haeger, K.: Long time treatment of intermittent claudication with vitamin E, Am. J. Clin. Nutr., 27:1179, 1974.

17 Williams, H. T. G., D. Fenna, and R. A. MacBeth: Alpha-tocopherol in the treatment of intermittent claudication, Surg. Gynecol. Obstet., 132:662, 1971.

18 Binder, H. J., and H. M. Spiro: Tocopherol deficiency in man, Am. J. Clin. Nutr., 20:594, 1967.

19 Horwitt, M. K.: Therapeutic uses of vitamin E in medicine, Nutr. Rev., 38:105, 1980.

20 Ginter, E., I. Kajaba, and O. Nizer: The effect of ascorbic acid on cholesterolemia in healthy subjects with seasonal deficit of vitamin C, Nutr. Metab., 12:76, 1970.

21 Gatenby-Davies, J. D., and J. Newson: Ascorbic acid and cholesterol levels in pastoral peoples in Kenya, Am. J. Clin. Nutr., 27:1039, 1974.

22 Pauling, L.: *Vitamin C and the Common Cold,* Freeman, San Francisco, 1970.

23 Anderson, T. W.: New horizons for vitamin C, Nutr. Today, 12:6, 1977.

24 Toxicity of vitamin C megadoses, Nutrition & the M.D., 7:3, October 1980.

25 Herbert, V., and E. Jacob: Destruction of vitamin B_{12} by ascorbic acid, J. Am. Med. Assoc., 230:241, 1974.

26 Dykes, M. H., and P. Meier: Ascorbic acid and the common cold, J. Am. Med. Assoc., 231:1073, 1975.

27 Briggs, M. H., P. Garcia-Webb, and P. Davies: Urinary oxalate and vitamin-C supplements, Lancet, 2:201, 1973.

28 terWelle, H. F., C. M. vanGent, W. Dekker, and A. F. Willebrands: The effect of soya lecithin on serum lipid values in type II hyperlipoproteinemia, Acta Med. Scand., 195:267, 1974.

29 Hodges, R. E.: Vitamins, lecithin and additives, in *Nutrition, Lipids and Coronary Heart Disease,* R. Levy et al. (eds.), Raven, New York, 1979.

30 When is a food "natural"? Nutr. Notes, 17:21, 1981.

31 American Academy of Pediatrics Committee on Nutrition: Nutritional aspects of vegetarianism, health foods, and fad diets, Pediatrics, 59:460, 1977.

32 Seelig, R. A.: It's "organic"!...so what? United Fresh Fruit and Vegetable Association Monthly Supply Letter, January 1977.

33 Jukes, T. A.: The organic food myth, J. Am. Med. Assoc., 230:276, 1974.

34 Traub, L. G., and D. D. Odland: Convenience food as home prepared: cost, yield, and quality, *National Food Review,* no. 4, U.S. Department of Agriculture, Economics, Statistics, and Cooperative Services, Washington, 1978.

35 GRAS food additives probably are safe, Chem. Eng. News, 59:17, Jan. 12, 1981.

36 CAST weighs risks and benefits of using nitrite in cured meats, Food Prod. Dev., 12:89, 1978.

37 Mattson, P.: Bacon precooked by microwaves offers the potential of lowering nitrosamine levels, Food Prod. Dev., 12:47, 1978.

38 Smith, J. R.: Nitrites: FDA beats a surprising retreat, Science, 209:1100, 1980.

39 Newberne, P. M.: Nitrite promotes lymphoma incidence in rats, Science, 204:1079, 1979.

40 Community Nutrition Institute Weekly Report, 11:2, Dec. 17, 1981.

41 *Toxicity and Carcinogenicity Study of Orthotoluene Sulfonamide and Saccharin,* Canadian National Health and Welfare Department, Health Protection Branch, 1977.

42 Morrison, A. S., and J. E. Buring: Artificial sweeteners and cancer of the lower urinary tract, N. Engl. J. Med., 302:537, 1980.

43 Hoover, R. N., and P. H. Strasser: Artificial sweeteners and human bladder cancer, Lancet, 1:837, 1980.

44 Hoover, R.: Saccharin—bitter after taste? N. Engl. J. Med., 302:573, 1980.

45 Smith, R. J.: Aspartame approved despite risks, Science, 213:986, 1981.

46 Brunzell, J. D.: Use of fructose, xylitol, or sorbitol as a sweetener in diabetes mellitus, Diabetes Care, 1:223, 1978.

47 Olefsky, J. M., and P. Crapo: Fructose, xylitol, and sorbitol, Diabetes Care, 3:390, 1980.

48 Little, A. C.: The eyes have it, J. Am. Diet. Assoc., 77:688, 1980.

49 Community Nutrition Institute Weekly Report, 9:6, February 12, 1981.

50 Roberts, H. R.: *Food Additives in Food Safety,* H. R. Roberts (ed.), Wiley-Interscience, New York, 1981.

51 Ross, D. M., and S. A. Ross: *Hyperactivity: Research, Theory, Action,* Wiley, New York, 1976.

52 Feingold, B. F.: *Why Your Child is Hyperactive,* Random House, New York, 1975.

53 The National Advisory Committee on Hyperkinesis and Food Additives: *Report to the Nutrition Foundation,* The Nutrition Foundation, New York, 1975.

54 Interagency Collaborative Group on Hyperkinesis: *First Report of the Preliminary Findings and Recommendations,* U.S. Department of Health, Education, and Welfare, Washington, 1975.

55 Connors, C. K., C. H. Goyette, D. A. Southwick, J. M. Lees, and P. A. Andrulis: Food additives and hyperkinesis: a controlled double-blind study, Pediatrics, 58:154, 1976.

56 Harley, J. P., R. S. Ray, L. Tomasi, P. L. Eichman, C. G. Mathews, R. Chun, C. S. Cleeland, and E. Traisman: Hyperkinesis and food additives: testing the Feingold hypothesis, Pediatrics, 61:818, 1978.

57 Harley, J. P., C. G. Mathews, and P. Eichman: Synthetic food colors and hyperactivity in children: double-blind challenge experiment, Pediatrics, 62:975, 1978.

58 Swanson, J. M., and M. Kinsbourne: Food dyes impair performance of hyperactive children on a laboratory learning test, Science, 207:1485, 1980.

59 Weiss, B., J. H. Williams, S. Margen, B. Adams, B. Caan, L. J. Citron, C. Cox, J. McKibben, D. Ogar, and S. Schultz: Behavioral responses to artificial food colors, Science, 207:1487, 1980.

60 The National Advisory Committee on Hyperkinesis and Food Additives: *Final Report to the Nutrition Foundation,* The Nutrition Foundation, New York, 1981.

61 Diet/hyperactivity link remains unconfirmed, Chem. Eng. News, 60:11, 1982.

62 Bierman, C. W., and C. T. Furukawa: Food additives and hyperkinesis: are there nuts among the berries? Pediatrics, 61:932, 1978.

63 Editors of Consumer Reports Books: *Health Quackery,* Consumers Union, Mt. Vernon, N.Y., 1980.

64 Atkins, R. C.: *Dr. Atkins' Diet Revolution,* David McKay, New York, 1972.

65 Jameson, G., and E. Williams: *The Drinking Man's Diet,* Cameron, San Francisco, 1964.

66 Taller, H.: *Calories Don't Count,* Simon and Schuster, New York, 1961.

67 Dr. Atkins' diet revolution, Med. Lett., 15:41, 1973.

68 American Medical Association Council on Foods and Nutrition: A critique of low-carbohydrate ketogenic weight reduction regimens, J. Am. Med. Assoc., 224:1415, 1973.

69 Stillman, I. M., and S. Baker: *The Doctor's Quick Weight Loss Diet,* Dell, New York, 1967.

70 Tarnower, H., and S. S. Baker: *The Complete Scarsdale Medical Diet,* Rawson, Wade Publishers, New York, 1978.

71 The Scarsdale diet, Nutrition & the M.D., 6:1, October 1980.

72 Dwyer, J.: Sixteen popular diets, in *Obesity,* A. J. Stunkard, (ed.), Saunders, Philadelphia, 1980.

73 Bistrian, B.: Clinical use of a protein-sparing modified fast, J. Am. Med. Assoc., 240:2299, 1978.

74 After the "last chance" diet, Consumer Rep., 43:92, 1978.

75 Linn, R.: *The Last Chance Diet,* Bantam, New York, 1977.

76 Liquid protein and sudden cardiac deaths. An update, FDA Drug Bull., May-June 1978.

77 Community Nutrition Institute Weekly Report, 11:6, Dec. 3, 1981.

78 Potpourri, Am. Diet. Assoc. Courier, 21:13, 1982.

79 Mazel, J.: *The Beverly Hills Diet,* Macmillan, New York, 1981.

80 Mirkin, G. B., and R. N. Shore: The Beverly Hills diet, J. Am. Med. Assoc., 246:2235, 1981.

81 Stuart, R. B., and B. Davis: *Slim Chance in a Fat World,* Research Press, Champaign, Ill., 1972.

82 Jordon, H. A., L. S. Levitz, and G. M. Kimbrell: *Eating Is Okay,* Rawson Associates Publishers, New York, 1976.

83 Pritikin, N.: *Live Longer Now: The First One Hundred Years of Your Life,* Grosset & Dunlap, New York, 1974.

84 Time Magazine, 116:140, Feb. 5, 1979.

85 Nutrition and human performance, Dairy Council Digest, 51:13, 1980.

86 Williams, M. A.: *Nutritional Aspects of Human Physical and Athletic Performance,* Charles C Thomas, Springfield, Ill., 1976.

87 Food and Nutrition Board: *Recommended Dietary Allowances, 1980,* National Academy of Sciences, Washington, 1980.

88 Smith, N. J.: *Food for Sport,* Bull Publishing, Palo Alto, Calif., 1976.

89 Statement by The American Dietetic Association: Nutrition and physical fitness, J. Am. Diet. Assoc., 76:437, 1980.
90 Consolazio, C. F., and H. L. Johnson: Dietary carbohydrate in work capacity, Am. J. Clin. Nutr., 25:85, 1972.
91 Askew, W.: Nutrition for top sports performance, Dietetic Currents, Ross Laboratories, 8:12, May-June 1981.
92 Astrand, P. O., and K. Rodahl: *Textbook of Work Physiology*, McGraw-Hill, New York, 1970, pp. 19, 445–488.
93 Hagerman, G. R.: Nutrition in part-time athletes, Nutrition & the M.D., 7:1, August 1981.
94 McArdle, W. D., F. Katch, and V. L. Katch: *Exercise Physiology*, Lea & Febiger, Philadelphia, 1981.
95 Jarvis, W. T.: Food quackery is dangerous business, Nutr. News, 43:1, 1980.
96 Herbert, V.: The health hustlers, in *The Health Robbers,* S. Barrett and G. Knight (eds.), George F. Stickley, Philadelphia, 1976.
97 Deutsch, R. M.: *The New Nuts Among the Berries,* Bull Publishing, Palo Alto, Calif., 1977.
98 Jarvis, W. T.: Coping with food faddism, Nutrition & the M.D., 6:1, October 1980.

CHAPTER 6

DRUG-NUTRIENT INTERACTIONS

CONTENTS

INTRODUCTION

Increasing recognition of the possibility of both antagonistic and synergistic interactions between drugs has led to the development of monitoring systems to provide information about the potential dangers of such interactions before the patient has been put at risk. Similar systems must in the future be developed to deal with drug-nutrient interactions. Computerized data systems, such as the one in use at Stanford for drug interactions, can have a role in this development. Proliferation of therapeutic drugs and increasing efforts to provide adequate nutritional support of both the acute and chronically sick are good reasons for giving special attention to the possibilities of drug-nutrient interactions.

Presently, many drugs are in use which are known to have potentially harmful side effects. These side effects range from depression of appetite to inhibition of absorption of specific nutrients by the small intestine to derangement of specific metabolic processes, which may be an essential part of the therapeutic efficacy of the drug but which may also have an adverse effect on the host's metabolism. Some antibacterial and many antineoplastic agents behave in this way.

Some of these effects have been recognized for a long time. Other drugs, which have been in use for decades, have been discovered only in recent years to possess a potentially harmful effect on nutritional status. Some of those to be introduced in the future may display similar, unsuspected side effects. Others may exert an effect which becomes clinically overt only when the patient commences a therapeutic regimen which imposes a further strain on a shared system. An example of this is the patient maintained on warfarin anticoagulants who, when treated in addition with oral antibiotics for an intercurrent infection, develops a bleeding diathesis because the intestinal flora, some of which synthesize vitamin K, have been inhibited by the antibiotic. The potential for similar complications is great and has not been systematically explored. If a patient has a background of chronic alcoholism with liver damage and nutrient deficiencies or of cancer, particularly of the gastrointestinal tract, the complications may be more severe and sometimes lethal.

At present, the complexities of nutrient synthesis by bacteria and molds in the human small and large intestines and the extent to which any such nutrients may be absorbed by the host are conjectural. We would be foolish to ignore their potential importance and the possible consequences of interfering with the flora for any periods of time exceeding a few days.

The mode and degree of utilization of trace elements from our diets are equally uncertain. It is highly likely that if we use, for instance, oral chelators of divalent cations, these create a risk of depriving the body not only of copper, iron, and zinc but also of many other trace elements as well.

Clearly the duration of administration of a drug or drugs and the dosage are of great importance in this context. As a general rule, no therapy should be prolonged a day longer than necessary. However, anticonvulsants, anticoagulants, and chelators (including some antacids), have all to be used for long periods during the lives of many patients. Their side effects may have important nutritional consequences, and it may be necessary to devise special precautionary regimens, such as brief interruptions in dosage of the drug and special efforts to prevent depletion of nutrients.

Old people tend increasingly to require maintenance therapies for long periods. Some of these may have quite profound effects on appetite, bowel function, or metabolism and thus influence nutritional status.

Other significant factors of which it is important to be aware are differences among patients in the way each handles a particular drug in terms of absorption, utilization, degradation, and excretion.

Another risk inherent in some drugs is that they may be significant sources of constituents, intake of which either has already been rigorously controlled or is undesirable. Sodium and potassium are particularly important in the setting of acute medicine. Some patients may be allergic to traces of protein present in excipients, such as cornstarch, and may require appropriately different drug formulations.

Another aspect of drug-food interactions is that the rate and amount of absorption of oral medications may be significantly affected by the relation of the ingestion of the drug with the timing and the nature of meals. Efficacy of drugs may vary consequently. Food may act as a physical block to absorption. Gastric emptying times are determined by the size and content of meals so that the rate of presentation of a drug to the absorptive surface of the small intestine may vary with different meals. Some dietary components may react with a drug (milk inhibits tetracycline absorption, whereas fat enhances the absorption of the antifungal agent griseofulvin) or influence pH so that the drug's absorption is enhanced or inhibited.

Oral drugs, which must be absorbed quickly to attain a therapeutic plasma level in order to relieve a symptom, should be given on an empty stomach. Unfortunately, most drugs of this sort, such as aspirin, are gastric irritants and should be taken with food. Many are listed in Table 6-1. Some drugs are destroyed at low pH and should therefore be taken when gastric acid secretion has not been stimulated by food (Table 6-2). For the same reason, they should not be given with juices or acidic beverages, but with water.

TABLE 6-1
DRUGS TO BE TAKEN WITH FOOD

Aminophylline	Phenylbutazone
Aminosalicylic acid	Salicylazosulfapyridine
Aspirin	Prednisone
Chlorpromazine	Tolbutamide
Hydrochlorthiazide	Triamterene
Indomethacin	Trihexiphenidyl
Iron	

TABLE 6-2
DRUGS TO BE TAKEN ½ HOUR
BEFORE MEALS (ACID-LABILE)

Ampicillin	Penicillamine
Cloxacillin	Penicillin G
Erythromycin	Tetracycline
Lincomycin	

Of all the commonly used drugs which may interfere both with nutrient status and with the way in which other drugs are absorbed, metabolized, or excreted, ethanol is the most important. However, it is fully discussed in a separate chapter (Chapter 17) and will not be considered here in detail.

In conclusion, it must be emphasized that it is of importance in clinical medicine that thought be given to the nutritional state of a patient when any medications are recommended, be they prescription or over-the-counter.

ADVERSE EFFECTS OF DRUGS DUE TO EXCIPIENTS (VEHICLES)

In several diseases, restriction of sodium intake has a valuable role in treatment. Examples are hypertension, cirrhosis and ascites, and the nephrotic syndrome. The daily maximal sodium intake in such subjects may be set at 20 to 40 mcq. The use of ampicillin, carbenicillin, or methicillin sodium may reverse a satisfactory state of sodium restriction. Alka-seltzer, Metamucil, and some antacids such as Bisodol and Maalox are also strongly contraindicated because of their sodium content (see Table 9-2).

In renal failure, potassium overload is a threat to life and must be avoided. Effersyllium, Bromo-seltzer, and penicillin G contain significant amounts, and disasters have occurred, almost unbelievably, with potassium-containing salt substitutes (see Table 9-5).

DRUG-NUTRIENT INTERACTIONS

General Considerations

Some of the mechanisms which underlie these interactions of drugs and nutrients are listed in Table 6-3. Others will be alluded to in the account which follows. The list in Table 6-3 is not intended to be exhaustive; it is designed to be of practical value to the prescribing physician as a checklist.

The most frequently used therapeutic drugs which are likely to affect nutritional status are antacids, diuretics, and some antibiotics. Chelating agents, such as cholestyramine and penicillamine, may produce disturbances of nutritional status, but they are used so often in patients whose metabolism is already

TABLE 6-3
MECHANISMS OF DRUG-NUTRIENT INTERACTIONS

	Example	
Mechanism	**Drug**	**Nutrient**
Reduction in solubility	Antacids	Iron
	Aluminum and calcium antacids	Phosphate
	Tetracycline	Calcium, magnesium, iron, zinc
Destruction of nutrient	Antacids	Thiamine
Malabsorption		
Nonabsorbed solvent	Mineral oil	Fat-soluble vitamins A, D, E, and K
Bile acid precipitation	Cholestyramine, kanamycin, neomycin	Fats, fat-soluble vitamins
Mucosal change	Colchicine, neomycin	Cations, fat-soluble vitamins, cobalamin
	p-Aminosalicylic acid	Cobalamin, fat
	Anticonvulsants*	Folacin
Metabolic interference	Methotrexate	Folacin
	Anticonvulsants	Vitamin D (inhibition of 25-hydroxylation)
	Isoniazid	Pyridoxal 5-phosphate
Renal excretion	Salicylates, indomethacin	Niacin, ascorbic acid
	Corticosteroids	Zinc
	Thiazides	Sodium, potassium
	Penicillamine	Pyridoxine

*Mechanism remains in doubt.

disturbed that their specific effects may pass undetected. Antineoplastic drugs produce fundamental disturbances, which are reflected in impaired protein synthesis, cell turnover, and disrupted metabolic pathways, but in patients with cancer, their effects may be masked by nutrient deficiencies already present as a consequence of impaired appetite and hepatic involvement and sometimes of malabsorption, gastrointestinal bleeding, and abnormal loss of protein into the gastrointestinal tract.

Drugs Affecting Appetite

Disturbance of Taste Some drugs have an unpredictable effect on taste, producing impaired or enhanced taste or unpleasant taste sensations. Penicillin, lincomycin, penicillamine, griseofulvin, and cholestyramine may behave in this way. Antihistaminics, which are used to suppress symptoms of allergies, especially those of the respiratory tract, and which are also used as mild sedatives in older people, have atropine-like side effects and make the mouth dry. This may result in reduced intake of food.

Anorectic (Appetite-Depressing) Drugs   A valuable rule in clinical practice is to question any patient complaining of change of appetite or significant change of weight about therapeutic drugs to determine whether the onset of the complaint coincided with the introduction of some medication or change in the dose of some medication.

At one time, *d*-amphetamines had widespread use as anorectic drugs to treat obesity. Increasingly rigorous control has reduced their legal use, but there is a large illegal consumption by adolescents as analeptics and mood elevators. Chronic, dangerously low intake of food may be a consequence of suppression of appetite. Other drugs with similar effects are diethylproprion, fenfluramine, and mazindol; these may cause irritability, insomnia, increased pulse rate, elevated blood pressure, and sometimes frank psychosis.

Digoxin may cause anorexia, and in older people, who are more likely to be receiving digoxin, this may be an important cause of loss of appetite and loss of weight. Further, as weight loss continues, an unchanged dosage may have an increasingly toxic effect. Digoxin and its congeners have a small therapeutic index, or ratio. As a consequence, most patients receiving maintenance treatment will, at some time, develop toxic symptoms because of the practice of increasing the dose until toxicity appears and then reducing the dose sufficiently for the symptoms to disappear. Optimal dosage is thus achieved.

Nonsteroidal anti-inflammatory drugs, such as indomethacin and phenyl butazone, almost without exception produce upper gastrointestinal symptoms, including dyspepsia and anorexia, in the majority of subjects. They should always be taken with food.

Analgesics may depress appetite. The opium alkaloids, especially morphine, have such an effect. Antineoplastic drugs, such as cyclophosphamide and 5-fluorouracil, may also produce anorexia, which is usually transient but sometimes may persist. The effect may summate with anorexia already present as a consequence of malignant disease.

Estrogen preparations in too large dosage sometimes induce anorexia; in our experience, these are an important cause of anorexia in perimenopausal women.

Nausea   Digoxin is one of the important causes of nausea, especially so in older people. Estrogens and nonsteroid anti-inflammatory agents are other widespread causes. Opium alkaloids, especially morphine, have an emetic effect in some subjects. Chemotherapeutic agents used in malignant disease may also induce nausea and vomiting, but their effect is usually short-lived, as is the case with radiotherapy, which in some respects they mimic.

Bulk   Some subjects, particularly older people, do not tolerate bulky intestinal contents, so that increasing fiber in the diet may induce a sense of bloating and discomfort and may depress appetite. Enthusiastic use of bran, Metamucil, or other bulk producers must be tempered with caution.

Constipation   Constipation is a common cause of anorexia in the aged. Hence any drugs which tend to constipate may be associated with loss of appetite. Codeine, morphine, and other analgesics, even aspirin, may have this effect. Oral iron preparations may constipate. If powerful analgesics have to be used, it is sound practice to give regular doses of milk of magnesia to preclude constipation.

Drugs Which Enhance Appetite   Some drugs, such as the oral hypoglycemic agents tolbutamide and chlorpropamide, which are sulfonylureas, increase appetite. This may be due to stimulation of insulin secretion. Cyproheptadine, a serotonin antagonist, also increases appetite and has a hypoglycemic effect.

In depressed subjects, antidepressants, such as phenothiazines and benzodiazepines, may stimulate appetite when they relieve depression and agitation.

Some patients respond to treatment with corticosteroids, particularly in large doses, by developing voracious appetites.

One danger in the use of all corticosteroids is stimulation of appetite, resulting in increased energy intake and obesity. Such a possibility must be anticipated, and advice from a dietitian should be given to patients of whatever age before commencing therapy. Switching to a diet of low caloric density is usually the best strategy.

Malabsorption

Changes in the Intestinal Lumen   Many therapeutic drugs inhibit the absorption of nutrients from the small intestine. The mechanisms of their actions fall into several categories. Some disturb the milieu of the intestinal lumen. Aluminum and calcium antacids inhibit absorption of phosphorus by forming insoluble phosphates in the lumen. All antacids raise the intragastric pH, which permits increased destruction of dietary thiamine and the conversion of ferrous iron, which is well absorbed, to ferric iron, which is poorly absorbed.

In recent years, ascorbic acid (vitamin C) in daily doses of 500 mg to 10 g has been recommended as prophylaxis against respiratory infections and malignant disease. Such doses far exceed the absorptive capacity of the gut and cause an osmotic diarrhea. In addition, they markedly enhance the absorption of any inorganic iron present in the stomach and upper part of the small intestine, so that concern has been expressed about the possibility of iron overload. No cases of such overload have yet been reported, but it has been reported that large amounts of ascorbic acid will destroy dietary cobalamin (vitamin B_{12}) [1]. There is a possibility that some signs of deficiency of cobalamin may result from ingesting 500 mg or more of ascorbate daily, including polymorphonuclear hypersegmentation, but to date anemia has not been reported [2].

Antibiotics such as neomycin and kanamycin form insoluble precipitates with bile acids, and the absorption of fats and the fat-soluble vitamins A, D, and K is impaired. Chelating agents, such as cholestyramine, have a similar effect. In consequence the absorption of calcium and magnesium may also be inhibited because these cations form insoluble soaps with the excess fat in the lumen of the bowel, and deficiencies may occur. Cholestyramine also binds to folacin and to gastric intrinsic factor, so that the absorption of folacin and cobalamin may be impaired [3]. It also appears to bind inorganic iron and to inhibit its absorption.

Mineral oil, still used by many older people as a laxative, is known to dissolve fat-soluble nutrients, which are then excreted from the colon and not absorbed. In consequence, rickets and osteomalacia have occurred because of deficiency of vitamin D [4].

Phenolphthalein, a widely used cathartic, may produce "intestinal hurry" and a secretory diarrhea. Its habitual use may be associated with deficiencies of vitamin D and calcium; potassium depletion may also occur and depress mucosal absorption [5]. Unexplained potassium depletion is frequently found to be due to laxative abuse.

Some broad-spectrum antibiotics, given orally, inhibit the growth of bacteria in the lower part of the small bowel and colon. In consequence synthesis of some nutrients may be impaired. The only known effect of importance is the destabilization of therapy with warfarin anticoagulants, because the endogenous vitamin K supply from the gut is reduced.

Neomycin forms complexes with bile salts and appears also to inhibit the action of pancreatic lipase, both of which effects tend to inhibit formation of micelles and thus the absorption of lipids and lipid-soluble substances.

Changes in the Intestinal Wall   Many drugs damage the intestinal mucosa or inhibit its transport mechanisms and thus interrupt the absorptive process.

Colchicine interferes with absorption of fat, increases the fecal excretion of sodium, potassium, and nitrogen [6], and inhibits the absorption of cobalamin [7].

Methotrexate, a folacin antagonist, and some other antineoplastic drugs, such as cyclophosphamide, induce inhibition of mucosal cell turnover. Severe disturbances of intestinal absorption and ulceration of the surface of the intestine may occur. Brush-border enzymes, such as disaccharidases, are lost, so that malabsorption of carbohydrates, as well as of fat, fat-soluble vitamins, folacin, and cobalamin, occurs.

p-Aminosalicylic acid (PAS), an antituberculous drug, inhibits absorptive processes in the ileum and may induce steatorrhea. It also interferes with the absorption of cobalamin. The mechanism is not fully understood but appears to be due to a block of the ileal enterocyte [8].

Other drugs which cause derangement of mucosal function are neomycin (which thus impairs absorption in three ways) and anticonvulsant drugs such as phenobarbital and diphenylhydantoin, which may inhibit both the synthesis of the vitamin D–dependent, calcium-transporting protein in the small-intestinal enterocyte and some part of the mechanism responsible for intestinal absorption of folacin.

Actinomycin D and mithramycin inhibit calcium absorption by blocking the action of 1,25-dihydroxycholecalciferol on the intestinal mucosal cell, so that calcium-transporting protein is not synthesized.

The foregoing are some examples which may have clinical importance. For an exhaustive source of information, *Drug-Induced Nutritional Deficiencies* by Roe [9] is recommended.

Disturbed Metabolism

Significant disturbance of the metabolic activity of various tissues may occur as a consequence of prolonged exposure to certain drugs, and these changes may affect the way in which nutrients that share the same pathways behave. Many drugs, important examples of which are ethanol (which must be considered both a drug and a nutrient), phenytoin, barbiturates, tolbutamide, and warfarin, induce hepatic microsomal enzymes when given for long periods. Increased activity of these enzymes may in turn accelerate the rate of degradation of any of these drugs when administered alone, and also of such compounds as vitamin D. Thus phenytoin may depress absorption of calcium both by a direct effect on the intestinal enterocyte and by enhancing the intrahepatic destruction of vitamin D.

There is some evidence that a similar mechanism may in part explain the low levels of serum and red cell folacin associated with long-term anticonvulsant therapy [10].

Conversely, ethanol, in high dosage in a subject who is not a chronic alcohol abuser, may acutely inhibit hepatic microsomal enzymes. The rate of clearance of many drugs is therefore reduced after exposure to alcohol. This is the recognized mechanism for increased toxicity of barbiturates when taken with alcohol. Drugs such as disulfiram (Antabuse), metronidazole (Flagyl), chlorpropamide, and tolbutamide (see Table 17-3 for others) block the oxidation of ethanol if ethanol is ingested while any of these drugs is present in the body in significant concentration. In consequence, acetaldehyde accumulates and may produce symptoms of severe nausea and flushing.

Another important interaction is that of drugs which inhibit the enzyme monoamine oxidase (pargyline, tranylcypromine, phenelzine sulfate). These are all used as antidepressants and occasionally as hypotensive agents. The monoamine oxidase pathway is an important one for degrading biologically active amines, such as norepinephrine and also tyramine. Normally tyramine, which is contained in several foods (Table 6-4), is metabolized in the intestinal wall and liver and does not appear in the bloodstream. However, the combination of a monoamine oxidase inhibitor and ingestion of a tyramine-containing food such as cheese may result in a marked increase of tyramine in the blood, which may cause severe hypertension and sometimes strokes or death.

Oral contraceptives, usually a combination of ethinyl estradiol, or its methyl

TABLE 6-4
FOODS CONTAINING TYRAMINE
(Contraindicated When Monoamaine Oxidase
Inhibitors Are Used)

Hard cheeses	Sour cream and yogurt
Aged soft cheeses:	Liver
Camembert	Pickled herring
Stilton	Salami
Gruyere	

ester, and a progestin, induce some of the metabolic changes associated with pregnancy. Thus circulating plasma triglyceride and cholesterol concentrations are elevated [11], circulating ceruloplasmin and copper are raised, and plasma zinc concentration is lower than normal.

In spite of sporadic reports to the contrary, it does not appear that use of oral contraceptives induces consistent changes in serum folacin concentrations [9, 12].

The ascorbic acid content of leukocytes and platelets is reduced in women taking oral contraceptives [13], but there seems to be no clinical significance and the reason is not known, though it has been suggested that it is related to increased ceruloplasmin, which is an ascorbate oxidase.

The effect of contraceptive steroids on pyridoxine metabolism is controversial. The controversy is believed to be due in part to the use of different methods to estimate pyridoxine and to differences in interpretation by different investigators. Tryptophan conversion to niacin metabolites is dependent on pyridoxine. The estrogen component of contraceptive preparations induces increased urinary excretion of kynurenine and xanthurenic acid [14], following a loading dose of tryptophan. However, it is debatable whether women taking oral contraceptives should also take pyridoxine supplements, since there has been no well-documented clinical evidence of signs or symptoms of deficiency. The possibility that depression associated with use of oral contraceptives is due to deranged pyridoxine metabolism has been suggested [15] but is currently unproven.

Increased plasma vitamin A concentrations are found in women taking oral contraceptives [16]. The reason for this is unknown.

The antituberculous drug isoniazid is believed to form a compound, isoniazid pyridoxine hydrazone, with pyridoxine and induce pyridoxine deficiency, which is often of clinical significance in patients receiving the drug [17]. The most important complication is a peripheral motor and sensory neuropathy. This is dose-related and occurs in subjects who are "slow acetylators," i.e., who detoxify isoniazid by acetylation in the liver at a relatively low rate. Supplements of pyridoxine provide adequate treatment.

L-Dopa interacts with pyridoxine in a way that is not well understood. Large doses of pyridoxine impair the antiparkinsonian effect of L-dopa, but this effect is probably insignificant when ingestion of pyridoxine is on the order of 2 mg per day, the normal dietary intake. The current explanation is that large amounts of pyridoxine accelerate the extracerebral decarboxylation of L-dopa to dopamine, so that reduced amounts of L-dopa are available to those parts of the brain (corpus striatum) in which dopamine concentrations are abnormally low in Parkinson's disease.

Methotrexate is a folacin antagonist which is used in the treatment of leukemia, some other malignant diseases, and psoriasis. It binds to the enzyme dihydrofolate reductase, displacing folate, so that increased urinary excretion of the vitamin occurs after administration of methotrexate [18] and synthesis of tetrahydrofolate is depressed. Megaloblastic changes may occur in the bone marrow, but frank anemia is uncommon. Continuous dosage with methotrexate causes damage and consequent fibrosis of the liver, which is dose-related.

Changes in Renal Excretion

Some drugs have significant effects on the functions of the kidneys. Some diuretics such as furosemide and ethacrynic acid inhibit calcium reabsorption by the renal tubule, and increased urinary calcium loss results. By contrast, thiazide diuretics stimulate tubular reabsorption of calcium and may occasionally cause hypercalcemia. These drugs have a similar effect on magnesium excretion. Since digoxin and other cardiac glycosides also augment the renal clearance of calcium and magnesium, their use in combination with furosemide or ethacrynic acid may result in calcium and magnesium depletion. There is also a possibility of zinc depletion [19].

Both salicylates and indomethacin increase the renal excretion of ascorbic acid, but this is probably due to inhibition of tissue uptake. Both plasma and leukocyte ascorbate concentrations may be low in salicylate users.

Penicillamine enhances the renal excretion of both zinc and copper, and there have been cases of zinc deficiency reported in patients with rheumatoid arthritis who are being treated with penicillamine [20].

Other examples of drugs affecting the excretion of nutrients are known, and it must be expected that many more will be described. A sound policy in therapeutics must be to use any drug for as short a period as possible to achieve the required effect and, when long-term use is essential, to review the possibility of potential effects on nutritional status.

METABOLISM OF DRUGS IN THE MALNOURISHED PATIENT

It is very likely that protein-calorie deficiencies have an effect on the ways in which many drugs are metabolized. Since many hospitalized patients are depleted of protein and calories, the possibility of significantly altered responses to drugs in such patients should be considered. Unfortunately, very little is known about these matters in humans, and the results of animal experiments are not necessarily applicable to clinical situations. Most current knowledge is derived from studies of children with kwashiorkor. Drugs bound to plasma proteins may be more active in states of hypoalbuminemia, since the ratio of bound to unbound drug is likely to be lower. The binding of digoxin [21] and salicylates [22] is reduced in kwashiorkor, and a similar change in the distribution of barbiturates probably occurs.

Another important change in protein-calorie deficiency is impairment of the microsomal oxidizing enzyme system in the liver. It has been shown that the half-life of drugs such as antipyrine when administered intravenously may be prolonged [23].

The implications are clear. A demonstrated example may be the slower decline of chloramphenicol levels in the plasma of undernourished children [24].

This is a subject in which a great deal of research should be done.

DRUGS AND LACTATION

The past 25 years have seen increases in the practice of breast-feeding and in the number of prescription and over-the-counter medications. Regularly updated knowledge about which drugs in the maternal system appear in breast milk is essential.

In general, a large number of drugs present in the blood achieve detectable concentrations in milk. Factors which affect concentration are the amount and patterns of concentration in the blood, frequency of dosage, the ionization of the drug in the blood, its lipid solubility, and the ability of the mammary glands to actively secrete it. Some drugs may accumulate and achieve higher than calculated blood concentrations if maternal renal function is impaired. It is worth emphasizing that, when prescribing for a lactating woman, it is better to assume that any drug may enter breast milk unless there is reliable evidence to the contrary. There are now large amounts of accumulated data about drugs and nursing, but much of the information is based on studies of small groups or isolated case reports.

Only in exceptional circumstances should nursing mothers take any drugs, since the effect of so many on the suckling infant is not known. This is even true of alcohol, the concentration of which in breast milk is approximately the same as in maternal blood. The risk presented by the presence of alcohol in breast milk, in terms of inducing damage in the suckling infant or a tendency to alcohol abuse in later life, is unknown.

Anticoagulants

Anticoagulants present a special problem, since women are liable to develop deep vein thromboses in the perinatal period and may require treatment with anticoagulants for weeks or months. Heparin does not gain access to milk, but it cannot be used for prolonged treatment [25].

The coumarins (warfarin) appear in breast milk but in very low concentrations [26]. Bishydroxycoumarin, or dicumarol, was administered to 125 nursing mothers; no changes in the prothrombin times of the infants were noted, nor were any hemorrhages seen in them [27]. There is one report of hematoma formation in a surgical scar, following repair of an inguinal hernia in a nursing infant whose mother was taking phenindione, an oral anticoagulant [28]. It would appear that warfarin is probably a safe medication if continuing anticoagulants must be given, but the mother should be informed and should make the decision whether to continue breast-feeding.

Anticonvulsants

Barbiturate administration to a nursing mother is rarely reported to be associated with drowsiness in the infant [29], and hydantoinates, such as phenytoin (Dilantin), when ingested by the mother, have not been shown to affect nursing infants [30]. Carbamazepine (Tegretol) may appear in breast milk in very small amounts [31].

The best advice to an epileptic mother maintained on anticonvulsants and determined to breast-feed is to do so unless her infant appears abnormally drowsy. If the infant is a first-born, monitoring by a pediatrician is indicated.

Hypotensive Drugs

Propranolol (Inderal) is excreted in breast milk in very small amounts, and its use is believed not to be contraindicated [32]. Chlorthalidone (Hygroton) achieves higher concentrations in milk and is contraindicated [33]. Thiazides appear in milk; chlorothiazide (Diuril) does so in low concentration and is deemed to be harmless [34]. Digoxin appears not to gain access to breast milk.

Antibiotics

Antibiotics present a special problem. Chloramphenicol (Chloromycetin), which appears in breast milk in only very small amounts, is contraindicated because of the possibility of irreversible depression of formation of blood cells in the bone marrow, were the infant to be affected. No such instances are known to have been reported, possibly because the number of susceptible individuals is very small (about 1 in 30,000). Metronidazole (Flagyl) is also contraindicated. It does have access to milk, and it has been shown to be carcinogenic in rats [35].

Ampicillin, when taken by nursing mothers, is believed to have caused diarrhea and candidiasis in the infant [36]. In general, since penicillins have been shown to sensitize suckling infants, their use should be restricted to the patient in whom they are essential.

Nalidixic acid (Neg Gram) has been reported to produce a hemolytic anemia in the suckling infant of a mother with some renal failure [37], and sulfonamides in breast milk may cause hemolytic anemia in infants with glucose-6-phosphate dehydrogenase deficiency [38].

Tetracyclines have been contraindicated in the nursing mother by some, but there does not seem to be good evidence that they are absorbed from breast milk. Their use probably does not create a hazard.

Antithyroid Drugs

All antithyroid drugs are contraindicated, including radioactive iodine, which is concentrated by the mammary gland and may destroy the infant's thyroid gland and increase the risk of thyroid cancer developing in later life [39].

Thiouracil (and probably propylthiouracil) may achieve concentrations in maternal milk sufficiently high to produce inhibition of the infant's thyroid function [40].

Narcotics and Sedatives

Narcotics and sedatives gain access to milk in varying concentrations. Morphine is present in only very small amounts, but propoxyphene (Darvon) is excreted in milk and may achieve a pharmacological effect [41]. Methadone is reported to enter breast milk in pharmacologically significant amounts, and chloral hydrate may do likewise. Diazepam (Valium) taken by a nursing mother may induce lethargy and weight loss in the infant [42].

Lithium

Lithium is reported to achieve concentrations in breast milk sufficient to produce hypotonia, hypothermia, cyanosis, and electrical abnormalities in the heart of suckling infants [43], and its use is contraindicated in breast-feeding.

Likewise, it seems advisable to avoid use of anticancer drugs by the nursing mother. The decision fortunately has rarely to be made. Use of cyclophosphamide has been reported to be associated with bone-marrow depression in a nursing infant [44]. Little is known about other similar agents, presumably because lactation and malignant neoplastic disease are infrequently associated.

In conclusion, it is probably wisest to counsel nursing mothers to take no drugs. If medication is essential, then breast feeding should probably be terminated if there is any doubt about an effect on the infant in the light of current knowledge. There will be some instances where the mother and the health professional must arrive at a decision after careful examination of potential risks and available options.

The reader is referred for more information to D. C. March, *Handbook: Interactions of Selected Drugs with Nutritional Status in Man*, The American Dietetic Association, Chicago, 1976; D. A. Roe, *Drug-Induced Nutritional Deficiencies*, Avi, Westport, Conn., 1976; and J. N. Hathcock and J. Coons (eds.), *Nutrition and Drug Interactions*, Academic, New York, 1978.

REFERENCES

1 Herbert, V., and E. Jacob: Destruction of vitamin B_{12} by ascorbic acid, J. Am. Med. Assoc., 230:241, 1974.
2 Hines, J. D.: Ascorbic acid and vitamin B_{12} deficiency, J. Am. Med. Assoc., 234:24, 1975.
3 Coronato, A., and G. B. J. Glass: Depression of the intestinal uptake of radio-vitamin B_{12} by cholestyramine, Proc. Soc. Exp. Biol. Med., 142:1341, 1973.

4 Sinclair, L.: Rickets from liquid paraffin, Lancet, 1:792, 1967.

5 Cummings, J. H., G. E. Sladen, D. F. W. James, M. Sarner, and J. J. Misiewicz: Laxative-induced diarrhoea: A continuing clinical problem, Br. Med. J., 1:537, 1974.

6 Race, T. F., I. C. Paes, and W. W. Faloon: Intestinal malabsorption induced by oral colchicine. Comparison with neomycin and cathartic agents, Am. J. Med. Sci., 259:32, 1970.

7 Webb, D. I., R. B. Chodos, C. Q. Mahar, and W. W. Faloon: Mechanism of vitamin B_{12} malabsorption in patients receiving colchicine, N. Engl. J. Med., 279:845, 1968.

8 Palva, I. P., O. Heinivaara, and M. Mittila: Drug-induced malabsorption of vitamin B_{12}. III. Interference of PAS and folic acid in the absorption of vitamin B_{12}, Scand. J. Haematol., 3:149, 1966.

9 Roe, D. A.: *Drug-induced Nutritional Deficiencies*, Avi, Westport, Conn., 1976.

10 Maxwell, J. D., J. Hunter, D. A. Stewart, and R. Williams: Folate deficiency after anti-convulsant drugs: an effect of hepatic enzyme induction?, Br. Med. J., 1:297, 1972.

11 Wynn, V., J. W. H. Doar, G. L. Mills, and T. Stokes: Fasting serum triglyceride, cholesterol, and lipoprotein levels during oral contraceptive therapy, Lancet, 2:756, 1969.

12 Spray, G. H.: Oral contraceptives and serum folate levels, Lancet, 2:110, 1968.

13 Briggs, M., and M. Briggs: Oral contraceptives and vitamin nutrition, Lancet, 1:1234, 1974.

14 Brown, R. R., D. P. Rose, J. M. Price, and H. Wolf: Tryptophan metabolism as affected by anovulatory agents and vitamin B_6 in metabolism of the nervous system, Ann. N.Y. Acad. Sci., 166:44, 1969.

15 Adams, P. W., V. Wynn, D. P. Rose, M. Seed, J. Folkand, and R. Strong: Effect of pyridoxine hydrochloride (vitamin B_6) upon depression associated with oral contraception, Lancet, 1:897, 1973.

16 Gall, I., C. Parkinson, and I. Croft: Effect of oral contraceptives on human plasma vitamin A levels, Br. Med. J., 2:436, 1971.

17 Vilter, R. W.: The vitamin B_6–hydrazide relationship, Vitam. Horm., 22:747, 1964.

18 Swenseid, M. E., A. L. Swanson, S. Miller, and F. H. Bethell: The metabolic displacement of folic acid by aminopterin. Studies in leukemia patients, Blood, 7:302, 1952.

19 Wester, P. O.: Zinc during diuretic treatment, Lancet, 1:578, 1975.

20 Multicentre Trial: Controlled trial of D($-$)penicillamine in severe rheumatoid arthritis, Lancet, 1:275, 1973.

21 Buchanan, N., L. A. van der Walt, and B. Strickwold: Pharmacology of malnutrition. III. Binding of digoxin to normal and kwashiorkor serum, J. Pharmaceut. Sci., 65:915, 1976.

22 Eyberg, C., G. P. Moodley, and N. Buchanan: The pharmacology of malnutrition. Part 1. Salicylate binding studies using normal serum/plasma and kwashiorkor serum, S. Afr. Med. J., 48:2564, 1974.

23 Narang, R. K., S. Mehta, and V. S. Mathur: Pharmacokinetic study of antipyrine in malnourished children, Am. J. Clin. Nutr., 30:1979, 1977.

24 Mehta, S., H. K. Kalsi, S. Jayaraman, and V. S. Mathur: Chloramphenicol metabolism in children with protein-calorie malnutrition, Am. J. Clin. Nutr., 28:977, 1975.

25 Levine, W. G.: Anticoagulant, antithrombotic, and thrombolytic drugs, in *The Pharmacological Basis of Therapeutics,* 5th ed., L. S. Goodman and A. Gilman (eds.), Macmillan, New York, 1975.

26 de Sweit, M., and P. J. Lewis: Excretion of anticoagulants in human milk, N. Engl. J. Med., 297:1471, 1977.

27 Brambel, C. E., and R. E. Hunter: Effect of dicumarol on nursing infants, Am. J. Obstet. Gynecol., 59:1153, 1950.

28 Eckstein, H. B., and B. Jack: Breast-feeding and anticoagulant therapy, Lancet, 1:672, 1970.

29 Tyson, R. M., E. A. Shrader, and H. H. Perlman: Drugs transmitted through breast milk; barbiturates, J. Pediatr., 13:86, 1938.

30 Mirkin, B. L.: Diphenylhydantoin: Placental transport, fetal localization, neonatal metabolism, and possible teratogenic effects, J. Pediatr., 78:329, 1971.

31 Niebyl, J. R., D. A. Blake, J. M. Freeman, and R. D. Luffe: Carbamazepine levels in pregnancy and lactation, Obstet. Gynecol., 53:139, 1979.

32 Anderson, P. O., and F. J. Saltzer: Propanolol therapy during pregnancy and lactation, Am. J. Cardiol., 37:325, 1976.

33 Mulley, B. A., G. D. Parr, W. K. Pace, R. M. Rye, J. J. Mould, and N. C. Siddle: Placental transfer of chlorthalidone and its elimination in maternal milk, Eur. J. Clin. Pharmacol., 13:129, 1978.

34 Werthmann, M. W., Jr., and S. V., Knees: Excretion of chlorthiazide in human breast milk, J. Pediatr., 81:731, 1972.

35 Update: drugs in breast milk, Med. Lett., 21:21, 1979.

36 Williams, M.: Excretion of drugs in milk, Pharmaceut. J., 217:219, 1976.

37 Belton, E. M., and R. V. Jones: Haemolytic anaemia due to nalidixic acid, Lancet, 2:691, 1965.

38 Brown, A. K., and N. Cevic: Hemolysis and jaundice in the newborn following maternal treatment with sulfamethoxypyridazine (Kynex), Pediatrics, 36:742, 1965.

39 Bland, E. O., M. F. Docker, J. S. Crawford, and R. F. Farr: Radioactive iodine uptake by thyroid of breast-fed infants after maternal blood volume measurements, Lancet, 2:1039, 1969.

40 Williams, R. H., G. A. Kay, and B. J. Jandorf: Thiouracil; its absorption, distribution, and excretion, J. Clin. Invest., 23:613, 1944.

41 Coty, C. S., and G. P. Giacoia: Drugs and breast milk, Pediatr. Clin. N. Am., 19:151, 1972.

42 Patrick, M. J., W. J. Tilstone, and P. Reavey: Diazepam and breast feeding, Lancet, 1:542, 1972.

43 Tunnessen, W. W., Jr., and C. G. Hertz: Toxic effects of lithium in newborn infants: a commentary, J. Pediatr., 81:804, 1972.

44 Amato, D., and J. S. Niblett: Neutropenia from cyclophosphamide in breast milk, Med. J. Aust., 1:383, 1977.

OBESITY

CONTENTS

INTRODUCTION

Despite the social stigma of being obese, the adverse effects of obesity on health, and the proliferation of new diets and treatments for obesity, the condition itself shows no sign of going away. In fact, many investigators believe that the prevalence of obesity is actually increasing in the United States. According to the Health and Nutrition Examination Survey (HANES), adults examined during the years 1971 to 1974 weighed more, on the average, than those examined from 1960 to 1962 [1]. It is generally recognized that in many persons obesity is associated with significant increases in morbidity and mortality from such diseases as hypertension, diabetes, coronary heart disease, and gallbladder disease and that mortality from these diseases is reduced following weight reduction [2]. What is more disturbing is that investigators know neither what causes obesity nor how best to treat it. The many theories as to the cause of obesity apparently have little basis in fact. Discouragingly few people lose weight with any diet, drug, or other treatment, and those who do lose weight are likely to regain it later.

The simplest definition of *obesity* is an excessive amount of body fat. It must be distinguished from *overweight*, which refers to an excess of body weight relative to height. A muscular professional football lineman is at a weight for his height which may be clearly excessive in a physically inactive man. For most situations, overweight and obesity are used synonymously, although they are not identical.

Obesity is probably best assessed by the visual judgment of an experienced observer. If a man, woman, or child looks fat when undressed, he or she is probably obese. The most objective quantitative methods for estimating body fat content are those which measure total body potassium (^{40}K), total body water with deuterium oxide (D_2O) or tritiated water (^3H_2O), or body density by underwater weighing. Although these methods have a firm theoretical basis and provide a good estimate of adiposity, they cannot be applied on a widespread clinical basis or in population surveys, since they are time-consuming and require specialized skills and specially equipped laboratories.

Measurement of subscapular and triceps skin-fold thicknesses with calipers is the simplest objective way to assess body fat (see Chapter 1). On the basis of population studies, it has been suggested that a triceps skin-fold thickness

TABLE 7-1

PREVALENCE OF OVERWEIGHT*

Age	Percentage of men deviating from desirable weight by:		Percentage of women deviating from desirable weight by:	
	10–19%	20% or more	10–19%	20% or more
20–74	18.1	14.0	12.6	23.8
20–24	11.1	7.4	9.8	9.6
25–34	16.7	13.6	8.1	17.1
35–44	22.1	17.0	12.3	24.3
45–54	19.9	15.8	15.1	27.8
55–64	18.9	15.1	15.5	34.7
65–74	19.1	13.4	17.5	31.5

*Estimated from regression equations of weight to height for men and women aged 20 to 29 years, obtained from U.S. Health and Nutrition Examination Survey, 1971 to 1974 (HANES I).
Source: G. A. Bray, Obesity in America, U.S. Department of Health, Education, and Welfare Publication no. (NIH) 79-359, 1979.

greater than 23 mm in men and 30 mm in women should be defined as obesity [3]. The weight/height^2 index (body mass index), in which metric units are used, is the best anthropometric measurement using height and weight. A nomogram for obtaining the body mass index is shown in Figure 7-5. Simpler yet are tables of "desirable," "ideal," or "best" weight, which represent the weight ranges associated with longevity that are derived from pooled life insurance data on mortality. The Fogarty modifications of the Metropolitan Life Insurance Company data used in the Recommended Dietary Allowances [4] are given in Appendix 2, Table 4.

Obesity, then, is defined as some arbitrarily determined deviation from a standard of the type described above. In the case of desirable weight, obesity is often considered to be a weight 20 percent or more above the mean of the desirable weight range for adults of a given sex and height. If life insurance criteria of relative weight are applied to the HANES data for 1971 to 1974, 14 percent of men and 24 percent of women aged 20 to 74 are 20 percent or more overweight (Table 7-1).

EPIDEMIOLOGY

Obesity can be correlated with many epidemiologic variables, such as age, sex, race, religion, socioeconomic status, national origin, and number of generations who have lived in one country or region. In the United States, the strongest correlation with obesity is with social class; Stunkard has pointed out that every social factor studied has been correlated with obesity [5].

Social Factors

The first evidence of how the large-scale social environment influences obesity was obtained by the Midtown Manhattan Study, a comprehensive survey of the epidemiology of mental illness [6]. The population studied consisted of 110,000 adults aged 20 to 59 who lived in an area which was selected because it housed persons at both ends of the socioeconomic scale. A cross section of 1660 persons was studied by interview in their homes.

The study showed a striking association of socioeconomic status with obesity, especially among women [7]. Socioeconomic status was rated by a simple score based on occupation, education, weekly income, and monthly rent. Figure 7-1 shows the strong inverse relation between socioeconomic status and obesity. Fully 30 percent of women of lower socioeconomic status were obese, compared with 16 percent of those of middle status and no more than 5 percent of the upper status group.

Among men, the differences between social classes were similar, but to a lesser extent. Of men of lower socioeconomic status, for example, 32 percent were obese, compared with 16 percent of men in the higher socioeconomic group. The socioeconomic status of the parents when the respondents were 8 years old was also examined. Figure 7-1 shows that the association between the social class of the respondents' parents and the respondents' obesity was also strong.

Other variables examined in the Midtown Study were social mobility, the number of generations of family members born in the United States, and ethnic and religious affiliations. Obesity was more prevalent among subjects moving downward in the social scale (22 percent) than it was among those who remained

FIGURE 7-1
Decreasing prevalence of obesity with increase in socioeconomic status (SES). (*From P. B. Goldblatt, M. E. Moore, and A. J. Stunkard, J. Am. Med. Assoc., 192:1039, 1965.*)

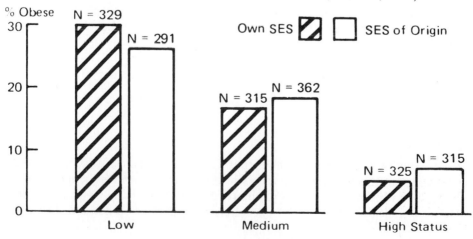

in the social class of their parents (18 percent), and it was far more prevalent than among those who were moving upward socially (12 percent) [7]. The number of generations of the family that had lived in the United States was also strongly linked to obesity. Of first-generation respondents, 24 percent were overweight; the prevalence fell to 22, 6, and 4 percent for successive generations.

The presence of nine different ethnic groups in the Midtown Study permitted assessment of the influence of ethnicity on obesity [8]. The strongest evidence of this influence was found among persons of lower socioeconomic status. When only lower-class respondents were considered, Hungarians and Czechs showed a prevalence of 40 percent and fourth-generation Americans, the least obese group, showed a prevalence of only 13 percent.

Religious affiliation is another social factor linked to obesity [9]. The greatest prevalence of obesity was found among Jews, followed by Roman Catholics and Protestants. Among Protestants, the pattern was further defined: Baptists were most obese, with decreasing prevalence in Methodists, Lutherans, and Episcopalians.

This relationship of social factors with obesity seems characteristic of western urban affluent societies, since similar findings have been reported in London [10]. In contrast, mean body weight or skin-fold thickness (not obesity) is associated directly with increased socioeconomic class in developing countries. Among adults in India, Latin America, and Puerto Rico and among children in south China and the Philippines, an increasing standard of living is associated with increasing mean body weight or skin-fold thickness [5].

Age

The second strongest correlation is with age. Obesity affects individuals of all ages, from infancy to old age. It increases in frequency from young adult life to middle age, but whether it is more frequent in later life depends on whether allowance is made for the reported decrease in lean body mass with aging. If this is taken into account and obesity is defined on the basis of percent body weight as fat, obesity would appear to increase in frequency throughout the life of the American population. Whether increased obesity with age is inevitably concomitant with the aging process or whether it is the product of a sedentary lifestyle is not yet clear.

Race

A correlation between obesity and certain racial groups has also been reported. Black women are at greater risk than white women. But the reverse is true for male adults; white men suffer more obesity than do black men. Thus, the nature of the relationship between race and obesity remains to be defined. It should also be noted that differences between races disappear when the groups are of the same socioeconomic level.

Sex

Obesity may occur in either sex, but it is usually more common in women. Obesity is likely to occur after pregnancy, when women increase their adipose tissue stores for the later demands of lactation. Many women gain more than is necessary and retain part of this weight, becoming progressively obese with each succeeding child. Twenty-four months from the onset of pregnancy, a woman will be, on the average, 5 to 7 lb heavier than if she had not been pregnant [11].

ETIOLOGY AND PATHOGENESIS

Although the overall mechanism in the development of obesity is an imbalance in energy intake versus energy expenditure, its underlying cause is not understood. Much research has been undertaken to assess the importance of a number of factors which are thought to contribute to the imbalance, and a discussion of some of these follows.

Heredity

Although there are several animal strains in which obesity is an inherited trait, no such pattern has been established in humans. While it is true that obese parents often have obese children [12], factors of lifestyle and attitude toward food undoubtedly play a role in the etiology of the observed familial pattern. Additional evidence linking obesity with genetics is provided by studies showing that identical twins, even when raised in different homes, tend more often to have similar weights than do fraternal twins, even if the latter are raised together in the same environment [13]. Withers found overweight of parents to be more highly correlated with overweight in natural children than in adopted ones [14]. However, Garn et al. found adoptive parent-child pairs to have fatness similarities comparable to those of biological parent-child pairs [15].

One factor in the development of obesity that has been related to heredity is the body type (somatotype) passed down from parents to children. Somatotyping is a physical anthropological classification of physique, based on body size and proportion. The *endomorph* has a relatively large body and short arms and legs. The *mesomorph* has a large muscular chest that dominates over the abdomen; body joints are prominent. The *ectomorph* has a relatively small body, slender, delicate bone structure, and long arms and legs (see Figure 7-2). Seltzer and Mayer found obese adolescent girls were more endomorphic but also somewhat more mesomorphic and considerably less ectomorphic than nonobese girls from a similar population [16]. A group of 94 obese women were also

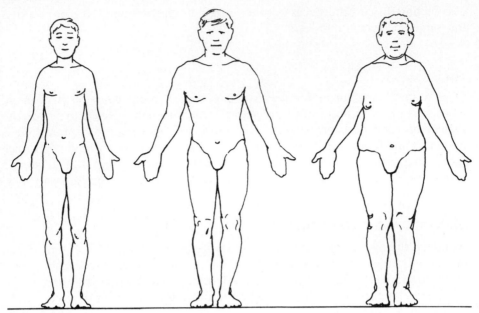

FIGURE 7-2
Extreme ectomorph, extreme mesomorph, and extreme endomorph.

studied with similar results [17]. Apparently, obesity is rare in some body-build types and very prevalent in others. Body build is inherited, although the genetic mechanism is not clear.

Physical Activity

Activity and obesity are related. There is evidence suggesting that relative inactivity is a cause of obesity. A study of obese and nonobese adolescent girls which used motion picture sampling while subjects swam or played tennis, reported that the obese were far less active than the nonobese, even during supervised exercise periods [18].

Mayer et al. studied the relation between caloric intake, body weight, and physical work in an industrial male population [19]. A group of over 200 adult workers 5 feet 2 inches to 5 feet 4 inches tall, who worked in a mill in West Bengal, was divided according to the physical demands of their jobs, which ranged from sedentary to very heavy work, into five classes. As shown in Figure 7-3, body weight was inversely proportional to the level of job activity, but caloric intake showed a biphasic distribution, with higher consumption by the most active and the most sedentary, suggesting that the increased weight

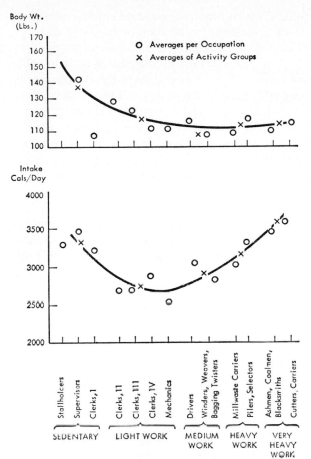

FIGURE 7-3
Body weight and caloric intake as a function of physical activity in man. (*From J. Mayer, Overweight, Causes, Cost, and Control, Prentice-Hall, Englewood Cliffs, N.J., 1968.*)

observed in the least active class was due as much to the lack of activity as to the increased caloric consumption.

In another study of 95 sedentary male office workers degree of overweight, as estimated by skin-fold measurements, correlated inversely with the time spent in and level of strenuousness of leisure time activities [20]. Curtis and Bradfield found that obese housewives spent less time in moderate energy-requiring activities and more time in sitting or light activities than did a comparable group who were not obese [21].

It is apparent from the studies reviewed that voluntary energy expenditure is reduced in many obese individuals. The simultaneous observation of decreased activity and obesity in these individuals does not, however, confirm the hypothesis that the inactivity causes the obesity. Equally valid may be the conclusion that the increased weight, which requires increased energy utilization for the same level of activity, leads to voluntary inhibition of excessive activity.

Another aspect of activity in obesity is the relationship of activity to appetite. In a normal person, an increase in appetite follows an increase in activity. This explains why the weight of most adults is relatively constant. Energy balance is most difficult to achieve, however, when energy expenditure is low, as is the case all too often in the American population. In experiments with laboratory rats, Mayer and collaborators studied the variation of food intake with exercise on a treadmill. They found that rats exercised 1 or 2 hours daily did not eat more than did the unexercised rats; indeed, they ate somewhat less (Figure 7-4). From 2 hours onward, increased duration of exercise was accompanied by increased food intake, up to a duration of exercise which represented the peak that the rats could endure. Within the range of "normal activity," appetite apparently is a sensitive and reliable mechanism for equating energy intake to energy expenditure. These observations in experimental animals may have some application to humans, since it has been shown that increased exercise in obese children does not generally increase their food intake and is therefore an effective weight control measure [22].

FIGURE 7-4
Food intake and body weight as functions of duration of exercise in normal adult rats. (*From J. Mayer, N. B. Marshall, J. J. Vitale, J. H. Christensen, M. B. Mashayekhi, and F. J. Stare, Am. J. Physiol., 177:544, 1954.*)

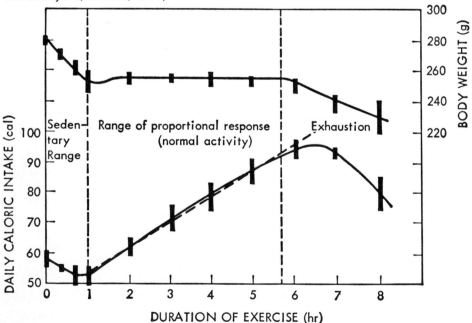

Endocrine Status

While attempts have been made to associate obesity with disturbances of the endocrine system, especially the thyroid, very few cases of obesity are caused by an underactive thyroid. Furthermore, hypothyroidism responds to hormone replacement therapy. Most endocrine abnormalities associated with obesity, including the hyperinsulinism observed in some subjects, appear to be a consequence rather than a cause of the obese condition, for they diminish following weight loss.

Diet Composition

Composition of diet is a prominent etiologic factor in experimental animals; it may also play a role in the development of human obesity. When rats are fed a high-fat diet, most strains are unable to regulate caloric intake appropriately and ingest more energy-producing food than is needed. The animals accumulate fat and become grossly obese. Whether the increasing fat consumption observed in most developed western nations and the increase in corpulence in these societies are manifestations of a similar phenomenon is not clear.

Neural Factors in the Control of Food Intake

The development of obesity in rats following experimental damage to the hypothalamus [23] has dominated thinking about the regulation of feeding. According to this view, feeding is initiated by a lateral hypothalamic (LH) "feeding center," whose activity reflects the energy state of the organism; it is terminated by the inhibitory action of a ventromedial hypothalamic (VMH) "satiety center." VMH activity, in turn, is modulated by postprandial satiety signals. In addition to controlling food intake, the VMH and LH centers appear to be critical in the long-term regulation of body weight. More recent work suggests that there are many variables in feeding behavior, and the description of a mechanism in the hypothalamus alone will not adequately explain the neural regulation of energy intake [24,25]. Other brain structures also participate in feeding behavior. Hypothalamic obesity has been reported in humans, but it is extremely rare. The major factors producing hypothalamic damage are trauma, malignancy, and inflammatory disease involving the hypothalamus. Excessive appetite (bulimia) may ensue.

Adipocyte Development and Metabolism

Expansion of adipose tissue is achieved in only two ways: through an excessive storage of triglyceride in preexisting adipose cells (adipose cellular hypertrophy) or in newly formed adipose cells (adipose cellular hyperplasia). It has been claimed that there are two patterns of human obesity, based on the cellular character of the expanded adipose depot: hyperplastic, with increased adipose-cell number and normal or increased cell size, and hypertrophic, with increased cell size alone. To date, the one factor which best differentiates hypercellular from hypertrophic obesity is the time of life at which obesity begins; hypercellular obesity is associated with an onset prior to adulthood, hypertrophic with adult onset [26].

Studies in humans have shown that adipose cell number is determined early in life. In the nonobese, two periods of adipose cell proliferation have been identified: in the first 2 years of life, and again just prior to puberty. Hirsch and Knittle presented evidence that both the number and size of adipocytes were greater in obese children than in nonobese children, and they demonstrated that (lifelong) grossly obese humans characteristically have an increased number as well as size of adipocytes [27]. After weight reduction, adipocytes shrink but hypercellularity remains fixed. Studies by Sims et al. suggest that adult-onset obesity represents an increase in the size but not the number of adipocytes [28].

The theory that has evolved from these observations is the following: Overfeeding in early life will cause excessive hyperplastic growth of adipose tissue as well as increased lipid accumulation within each cell. The increase in cell number persists throughout life; even though weight reduction may occur later as a consequence of loss of lipid from the cells, the adipocyte count remains constant. They persist, waiting to be refilled with fat as soon as energy intake exceeds energy output.

This theory is not universally accepted. If accepted, it has profound implications with regard to the effects of infant and childhood feeding practices on the subsequent development of obesity. Evidence has been presented to indicate that infant obesity is correlated with obesity in childhood [29,30] and that childhood obesity predisposes to obesity in adult life [31,32]. However, studies done in England indicate that most fat babies become lean during childhood and that obese people who were obese in infancy constitute only a small portion of the total number of obese adults [33]. Many other factors, including social class, education, parental weight, and gender, are related to adult weight [32,34]. In summary, the data suggest that some obese children become obese adults but that most adult obesity does not originate in childhood.

Thermogenesis

It is often claimed that there are obese persons who find it difficult to maintain normal body weight because they have such low energy requirements that even normal intakes of energy result in obesity. Studies have shown there to be a twofold difference in energy intake between individuals, despite apparently similar patterns of physical activity [35]. Furthermore, Sims and Horton showed that lean individuals who ingested 2 to 3 times their daily normal energy intake over a period of 3 to 5 months, while following their usual routine, increased their weight by only 10 to 12 percent [36]. Two groups of prison volunteers, following a similar protocol, gained approximately double the amount of weight at double the rate, reaching an average of 26 percent above their initial lean weight [37]. Experiments in nonruminant animals and in humans have shown that the efficiency of carbohydrate use is considerably higher when food intake is below the level required for maintenance than when it is above that level [38]. These observations, together with the first law of thermodynamics, suggest that one or more processes exist in which excess energy is dissipated in the form of heat and that the control of the rate of these processes permits maintenance of normal body weight. Miller has suggested that individual variation in the capacity to produce heat unassociated with basal metabolic rate or physical work (thermogenic response) may explain these observations [39].

Brown fat (brown adipose tissue), which is found in many cold-adapted animals, hibernators, and the neonates of many species, including human beings, may be the site of the thermogenic response. It is generally accepted that heat production in mammals varies, but there is controversy about the factors which cause this variation. It has been shown in cold-adapted animals that nonshivering thermogenesis is mediated by the sympathetic nervous system [40]. In vivo measurements indicate that brown fat (only 1 to 2 percent of body weight in the cold-adapted rat) can account for up to 68 percent of nonshivering thermogenesis [41]. The significance of diet-induced thermogenesis remains controversial. However, Rothwell and Stock demonstrated diet-induced thermogenesis in brown fat in voluntarily overfed rats [42]. Whether a defect in thermogenesis or in brown adipose tissue predisposes some individuals to obesity is not known; more direct methods must be developed for studying local tissue heat production in humans.

In genetically obese *ob/ob* mice, there are two components in the deposition of body fat: hyperphagia and increased metabolic efficiency [43]. Metabolic efficiency in energy utilization is the major factor responsible for obesity when animals are kept at 20°C. These *ob/ob* mice may provide a model for studying the link between metabolic rate and obesity. Preobese and obese *ob/ob* mice also have a defective thermogenic response to cold [44]. The *ob/ob* mouse will die at 4°C, despite its insulating layer of fat. A defect in nonshivering thermogenesis can be monitored by measuring the thermogenic response to maximum doses of noradrenaline. The *ob/ob* mouse exhibits only half the response of its lean litter mate. These studies in mice have their human counterparts. Jung et al. found the rise in resting metabolic rate of obese women and "postobese" women (women who had lost weight) after noradrenaline infusion to be half that seen in lean subjects [45]. The defective thermogenic response of the obese women conforms with reports of their enhanced susceptibility to body cooling [46]. The defect in the women seems to be unrelated to energy intake; two obese women who were deliberately fed a high-energy diet (40 kcal per kilogram of ideal body weight) for 7 days before testing responded to noradrenaline in a manner similar to that after 3 weeks on a diet providing one-third as much energy per day. The physiological basis for these observations has not yet been established. However, Newsholme has proposed that a "futile cycle" in muscle at the fructose-6-phosphate–fructose-1,6-diphosphate step of glycolysis may be involved in heat production [47].

CLINICAL MANIFESTATIONS

Although limitations are recognized in the data, life insurance statistics show an association between obesity and decreased longevity. Furthermore, obesity aggravates or predisposes individuals to a number of clinical problems (Table 7-2). Generally, the frequency and severity of medical complications are proportional to the degree of obesity.

Extreme adiposity in the thoracic and abdominal regions can interfere with the mechanics of ventilation to the extent that cardiorespiratory failure occurs. This is referred to as Pickwickian syndrome and is characterized by alveolar hypoventilation associated with extreme obesity. Hypoxia, secondary polycythemia, pulmonary hypertension and, eventually, cor pulmonale with cardiopulmonary failure ensue. Many of these abnormalities can be reversed by weight loss. Although the full-blown syndrome is seen only in grossly obese adults, milder mechanical pulmonary abnormalities can be seen with lesser degrees of obesity.

There is a strong association between hypertension and obesity. The mechanism by which obesity causes hypertension is uncertain, but peripheral vascular resistance is usually normal, while blood volume is increased. A large portion of the increased death rate of obese individuals may be a direct or indirect consequence of hypertension, e.g., cerebrovascular accidents.

An association between obesity and hyperlipoproteinemia has also been observed, suggesting that obesity may influence lipid metabolism. The best studied and clearest association is between obesity and hypertriglyceridemia. Increased triglyceride levels are due to increased hepatic, very low density lipoprotein (VLDL) production, with no defect in the removal of VLDL from plasma. Obesity has been less closely associated with increased plasma levels of cholesterol. Obesity is a serious risk factor for the development of coronary artery disease and stroke. Most of the risk imparted by obesity is mediated through the associated hypertension, hyperlipoproteinemia, and diabetes.

The National Commission on Diabetes has reported that the factor most

TABLE 7-2
SOME COMPLICATIONS ASSOCIATED WITH OBESITY

Respiratory difficulties	Gallbladder disease
Hypertension	Menstrual irregularities
Insulin resistance	Toxemia of pregnancy
Hyperlipidemia	Orthopedic problems

strongly associated with the prevalence of adult-onset diabetes in the United States is the degree and duration of obesity [48]. Eighty to ninety percent of adult-onset diabetics are more than twenty percent overweight. The close association between obesity, abnormal carbohydrate metabolism, and diabetes has been recognized for many years, but the nature of this relation is poorly understood. In some patients obesity appears to be part of the syndrome of diabetes mellitus, but in many instances obesity seems to be acting as a primary factor, somehow inducing abnormalities in carbohydrate metabolism and insulin secretion which may or may not be manifestations of the diabetic syndrome. Weight loss by obese patients usually ameliorates the diabetic state.

Obesity is associated with increased rates of pancreatic insulin secretion and increased concentrations of insulin in the blood, both in the basal state and in response to glucose. The explanation most commonly advanced for this is "insulin resistance," i.e., the decreased ability of insulin to influence glucose uptake and metabolism in the insulin-sensitive tissues of the obese individuals. It is postulated that insulin resistance in the target tissues (liver, skeletal muscle, and adipose tissue) leads first to hyperglycemia and second to hyperinsulinemia.

Gastrointestinal symptoms are frequent in the obese and are usually nonspecific (bloating, dyspepsia). Diaphragmatic hernias may become symptomatic. Fatty liver is common. The incidence of cholesterol-rich gallstones is strikingly related to the degree of obesity, especially among women.

Women who are obese tend to have irregular menses and increased morbidity associated with pregnancy and again after childbearing ceases. The incidence of toxemia of pregnancy and hypertension is increased. Obstetric risk is higher, and later in life there is an increased incidence of uterine fibroids and endometrial cancer [49].

A number of bone and joint diseases are greatly benefited by weight reduction, which decreases the pressure on the damaged structures and facilitates mobility. For example, osteoarthritis is more common and severe in the obese, and the intervertebral and weight-bearing joints benefit from weight reduction.

DIAGNOSIS

Obesity is a disorder which is frequently overlooked by the physician, who may be preoccupied with one of its many complications. A routine practice of weighing patients and examining them for evidence of excessive fat would help initiate treatment as an early, optimal stage.

History

A careful medical history can serve as a screening tool for the identification of factors which place patients at risk for developing medical complications of obesity or which may help implement therapy. The following areas should receive special attention:

1 Usual body weight
2 Recent significant weight gain or loss
3 Previously recorded height and weight
4 Chronic diseases
   a Diabetes mellitus
   b Hypertension
   c Hyperlipidemia
   d Coronary heart disease
   e Circulatory problems or heart failure
5 Usual eating habits
6 Alcohol intake
7 Results of previous attempts at weight reduction

The history of the patient helps delineate the pattern of weight gain and allows differentiation between early- and late-onset obesity. Though seldom present, medical diseases associated with obesity, such as Cushing's syndrome and Prader-Willi syndrome, should be excluded. Identification of medical complications of obesity (Table 7-2) may motivate the patient to follow the plan of therapy.

Physical Examination

Complicated examinations usually are not necessary to determine the presence of obesity. The appearance of the naked patient is usually a reliable enough means for the experienced clinician to make a diagnosis of obesity. Quantitative anthropometric measures including height, weight, circumference of waist, and skin-fold measurements should also be assessed.

The Fogarty modifications of the Metropolitan Life Insurance tables of standard height/weight [1] express a central weight and range of acceptable weight (Appendix 2, Table 4). If overweight (weight in excess of average) is marked, obesity (excessive fatness) is present. For moderate degrees of overweight, obesity may not be obvious. College football linemen are generally overweight but they are generally not obese. Conversely, some extremely sedentary persons can be obese without being markedly overweight. The degree of overweight can be expressed several ways. Weight (W) and height (H) can be related by several ratios such as the W/H, W/H^2 (body mass index), and $H/\sqrt[3]{W}$ (ponderal index), using metric units for weight and height.

None measures body fat very well, since the correlation of these indexes with body fat measured by densitometry determinations is between 0.7 and 0.8 [11]. The body mass index has the best correlation with body fat and is shown in Figure 7-5.

From a practical point of view, the most widely used criterion for obesity is measurement of skin-fold thickness using calipers (for details see Chapter

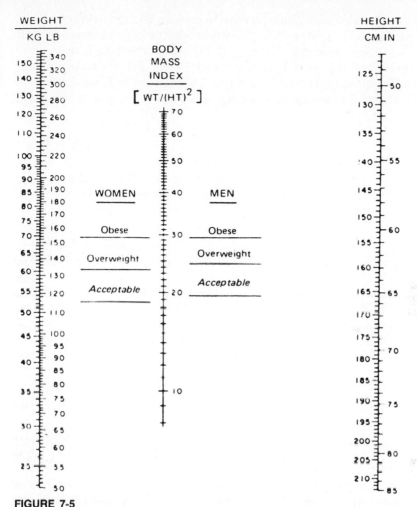

WEIGHT

KG LB

HEIGHT

CM IN

BODY
MASS
INDEX

$[WT/(HT)^2]$

WOMEN

MEN

Obese

Overweight

Acceptable

Obese

Overweight

Acceptable

FIGURE 7-5
Nomogram for body mass index. [*From G. A. Bray (ed.), Obesity in America,
U.S. Department of Health, Education, and Welfare, Publication no. (NIH) 79–
359, 1979, p. 6, fig. 2.*]

1). Subcutaneous fat is thought to account for about 50 percent of total body fat,
although the constancy of this proportion in extremely obese individuals has not
been clearly established [50]. Skin-fold thickness measured at such sites as the
biceps, the triceps, and the subscapular or suprailiac area has been shown to
provide a very reliable estimate of obesity [51]. The work of Seltzer et al.
indicates that for obese individuals the triceps skin fold, which is the easiest to
measure, is also the most representative of body fatness [52]. Data collected on
various groups show that skin-fold measurements represent a continuum within
certain limits and are independent of height. It is difficult and arbitrary to

determine where on this continuum obesity begins. In the United States Ten-State Nutrition Survey of 1968 to 1970, obesity in adults was defined as a fat fold greater than the 85th percentile (Table 1-4) [53]. This standard is nearly the same as that earlier suggested by Seltzer and Mayer [3]. Butterworth and Blackburn used a normal standard of 12.5 mm for male and 16.5 mm for female triceps skin-fold measurements in assessing malnutrition among hospitalized adult patients [54].

Biochemical Tests

There are no biochemical tests presently used to assess obesity. However, an evaluation for the complications that are known to be frequently associated with obesity (diabetes mellitus, hyperlipidemia, etc.) may be in order.

Physiological Tests

There are ways to measure body fat more accurately. In one, densitometry, the weight of the body in and out of water is compared (with allowances made for the air retained by the lungs). Another approach is to use dilutional techniques: body water is measured by the distribution of tritiated water, or "cell mass" is determined by quantifying the amount of naturally occurring potassium isotope (^{40}K) in the body. These techniques remain research methods and are described in some detail by Grande [50].

MANAGEMENT

General Comments

Any experienced practitioner, whether a physician or a nutritionist, knows the complexities of treating the obese. To date these problems have not been satisfactorily resolved, probably because "obesity" is not a simple problem but many problems with many possible causes—genetic, metabolic, psychologic, socioeconomic, and cultural—which are lumped together and treated as a single disease entity. The traditional approach has relied on the concept that no one violates the basic laws of thermodynamics, i.e., if energy intake in food and drink is greater than energy output, body fat will be stored. To lose excess fat, negative energy balance must be achieved by a decrease in caloric intake, or an increase in caloric expenditure, or some combination of both.

A number of circumstances contribute to successful weight reduction. Both the patient and the therapist should evaluate the patient's situation before the patient attempts weight reduction, for unless there is a reasonable possibility of success, it may be better not to attempt it. The most important ingredient for success is a well-motivated patient with a reason that is meaningful to him or her for losing weight. The reason must be the patient's, not the therapist's or anyone else's, and it must be significant enough to enable the patient to sustain the therapy to its desired end. Another important ingredient is the emotional stability to undertake the self-discipline of behavioral change [55]. Even for the most stable individuals, there are times in their lives when stability is difficult; at such times weight reduction should not be undertaken. When a patient is in the early stages of obesity, there is a greater possibility of success. The task does not seem so monumental, and results are visible earlier. Success is more likely if the patient has developed obesity as an adult rather than as a child. Juvenile obesity is especially refractory to treatment. Also a patient with no previous history of attempting to lose weight but failing or of regaining weight that had been lost is more likely to succeed.

There are also a number of essential points which the patient must comprehend. First, he or she needs to understand that it is the loss of *fat* which is the desired goal, not just the loss of weight. The objective is not to lose weight as quickly as possible and then return to old patterns, but rather *to change the intake and activity habits*. The rate of weight loss is less important than a continuing movement in the right direction. Second, the patient should be instructed in some elementary, physiological principles with regard to appetite, exercise, the expenditure of energy, and the energy content of foods. Misconceptions about "quick weight-loss regimens" or "slimming foods," often acquired from popular books and papers, must be overcome. A dietitian or a similarly trained health professional can be of tremendous help to the physician in assisting the patient to cope with the planned therapy.

Dietary Management

There are many kinds of effective reducing diets. People most likely to have long-term success in weight reduction prefer a simplified pattern which they can follow easily with a few simple instructions. Most reducing diets which lead to long-term weight loss share certain characteristics:

1 Caloric intake less than energy expenditure
2 Satisfaction of all nutrient needs except calories
3 Adaptation to tastes and habits of the patient
4 Provision of satiety for a patient, leaving him or her with a sense of well-being and a minimum of fatigue
5 Adaptation to family and/or restaurant menus
6 Suitability for use over a long period of time
7 Education of patient in food choices and retraining of eating habits, so that with suitable caloric addition the diet may become a *pattern for lifetime eating*

The goal of dietary treatment is to redress caloric imbalance by reducing energy intake. This requires an initial assessment of the energy requirements of the patient. Energy requirements can be estimated by a number of methods, and the reader is referred to Appendix 2 for details. The amount of energy needed to *maintain* body weight can be estimated by multiplying the individual's ideal body weight (see Appendix 2, Table 4) in kilograms by 30 kcal for a sedentary individual, 35 kcal for a moderately active individual, and 40 to 45 kcal for a markedly active individual. For example, a woman whose ideal body weight should be 55 kg and who is sedentary should consume approximately 1650 kcal per day (55 kg × 30).

The next step is to determine a reasonable level of caloric restriction. If a caloric deficit of 500 kcal per day is maintained for 7 days, 3500 kcal must be provided from body energy stores to maintain energy supplies. Since 1 lb of fat tissue contains approximately 3500 kcal, a caloric deficit of 500 kcal per day will produce the loss of 1 lb of fat tissue each week. It is important to remember that the catabolism of stored body fat may not register immediately as a loss in weight. Each 100 g of fat oxidized produces 112 g of water. Excretion of this water is essential before weight loss occurs [11].

For most people food intake in the range of 1000 to 1200 kcal per day is generally most appropriate. The question naturally arises whether more severe caloric restriction would be better. Studies with diets containing less than 800 kcal suggest that little extra fat is catabolized [56,57]. Severe caloric restriction appears to produce a reduction in basal metabolic rate to conserve energy. This reduction can amount to 15 to 20 percent of prediet caloric needs [11]. Furthermore, it has been shown that the additional weight loss achieved by total starvation over that achieved by a 800-kcal balanced diet is due to selective loss in lean body mass rather than fat mass [58].

The distribution of nutrients in a weight reduction diet should be "balanced," meaning that no single food or nutrient predominates. "Unbalanced diets," including the "low-carbohydrate diet" and diets in which one food predominates, such as the grapefruit diet, the banana diet, the ice cream diet, and the hard-boiled-egg diet, are usually monotonous, making compliance a problem. Moreover, these diets may be nutritionally inadequate if continued for a prolonged period. A balanced diet, consisting of a *variety* of foods and containing no less than 12 to 14 percent protein, approximately 30 to 35 percent fat, and the rest carbohydrate (with sucrose restricted to a low level), is preferable.

Total nutrient needs can be met by developing an individualized diet pattern based on the exchange system discussed in Chapter 2. An energy-restricted diet can usually be planned to meet vitamin and mineral requirements. However, if the individual is eating 1000 kcal per day or less or if the individual on the energy-restricted diet is a growing child, vitamin and mineral supplementation is advisable.

The exchange lists described in Chapter 2 are tools to help patients plan their own diets. The total desired calorie level can be divided into a suggested number of servings from each exchange list and distributed into a pattern of meals and snacks. On a daily basis the consumption of one or two milk exchanges should be encouraged, along with adequate amounts of fruits and vegetables. The number of meat and bread exchanges may be adjusted to the preference of the patient. A larger number of meat exchanges will make the diet higher in protein and fat and lower in carbohydrate than if the number of meat exchanges were kept to a minimum and more choices were made from the bread list. The daily carbohydrate level of the diet should probably not go below 100 g. The minimum daily protein level should probably be about 70 g. Table 7-3 shows diet patterns using the exchange lists for a 1200-kcal diet, and Table 7-4 shows sample menus using the exchange lists.

One disadvantage of the exchange system is that it provides no information for monitoring alcohol intake, which may represent 10 percent of daily calories in some individuals. A second disadvantage is that it fails to provide information about sugar (sucrose) when it is the predominant item in a food (e.g., soft drinks) or when it is added to beverages such as tea or coffee. Exchange substitutions for high-sugar-content foods (Tables 2-3 and 2-4) and alcoholic beverages (Table 2-7) have been shown to help in patient education. Sugar and alcohol, which provide only energy, can be exchanged for fruits, which are important sources of vitamins, minerals, and fiber.

Education of the patient about the caloric content of various foods in different size portions is essential not only to the success of the weight reduction program but also to the success of the subsequent maintenance program. Food models can demonstrate the size of the portions. Expressions such as "average size" potato or "average serving" of lean meat are understood to mean widely different sizes by various individuals. A small scale and a measuring cup are

TABLE 7-3
DIET PATTERNS FOR A 1200-kcal DIET

Exchange group	Total daily exchanges	Protein, g	Fat, g	Carbo-hydrate, g	Energy kcal
Option 1					
Milk	2	16		24	160
Meat	9	63	27		495
Bread	2	4		30	140
Vegetable	4	8		20	100
Fruit	3			30	120
Fat	4		20		180
Total		91	47	104	1195
Option 2					
Milk	2	16		24	160
Meat	6	42	18		330
Bread	4	8		60	280
Vegetable	3	6		15	75
Fruit	3			30	120
Fat	5		25		225
Total		72	43	129	1190

TABLE 7-4
SAMPLE MENUS FOR 1200-kcal WEIGHT REDUCTION DIET

Option 1	Option 2
Breakfast	
½ cup orange juice	½ small banana
1 soft boiled egg	1 cup puffed wheat
1 slice whole wheat toast	1 cup skim milk
1 tsp margarine	Coffee, black
1 cup skim milk	
Coffee, black	
Lunch	
3 oz sliced chicken	½ cup low-fat cottage cheese
1 medium tomato, sliced with	1 medium tomato, sliced
lettuce leaves	½ cup asparagus
1 tbsp French dressing	2 slices whole wheat bread
½ cup spinach	2 tsp margarine
1 cup skim milk	1 small orange
1 small fresh apple	Coffee or tea
Coffee or tea	
Dinner	
5 oz baked sole	4 oz roast beef
1 small baked potato with	1 small baked potato with
2 tbsp sour cream	2 tbsp sour cream
½ cup summer squash	½ cup cooked carrots with
1 tsp margarine	2 tsp margarine
	¾ cup strawberries
Snack	
1 medium fresh peach	1 cup skim milk

helpful aids for portion control and for making the patient aware of the amount of food eaten. Some individuals use these aids for "counting calories," measuring the weight or volume of food eaten and using the calorie values of food as obtained from a calorie guide to calculate energy intake. Once individuals become accustomed to counting calories, some use it as a primary technique for controlling and monitoring their weight loss.

Along with diet composition, frequency of meals has received some attention. Many obese individuals eat little or no breakfast, often a late lunch, and tend to eat most of their food in one meal, usually in the late afternoon or in the evening [59]. Some investigators have suggested that excessive weight, increased serum cholesterol, and reduced glucose tolerance are more common among those who eat three or fewer meals daily than among those who eat more often. Pattern of food intake, however, has no effect on accelerating or retarding weight loss in subjects on a hypocaloric diet [60]. Generally, eating three or more meals and snacks each day will mitigate the problem of excessive hunger. Although the long-term data are inadequate, it appears that eating three or more balanced meals each day is preferable to eating one or two times per day.

Starvation or Fasting

Undoubtedly the fastest way to lose body weight is by total starvation. The metabolic changes that take place during fasting include decreases in blood glucose and insulin levels and an increase in serum free fatty acids during the first few days. These levels then stabilize and ketosis develops. As the body adapts to starvation, it uses fat as the major fuel, with the brain using ketones. The need for glucose, which is supplied by gluconeogenesis using amino acids from lean body tissue as substrates, gradually decreases, and loss of nitrogen diminishes. However, some protein continues to be lost. Side effects which may accompany this regimen include nausea, headaches, and hypotensive episodes. Management of these complications rarely causes any significant problem, but some instances of severe complications due to cardiovascular disturbances have been described. Electrolyte imbalances, vitamin deficiencies, and ketoacidosis have also occurred. In fact, the literature contains reports of a few deaths in obese patients on starvation regimens. Because of such complications, patients should be hospitalized during prolonged starvation to ensure that sufficient amounts of fluids, electrolytes, and vitamins are given and that bodily functions are closely monitored.

The prognosis for the long-term maintenance of the reduced weight achieved by fasting for periods of 2 months or more is not good. Johnson and Drenick followed 121 patients for 7.3 years and found that fasting-induced weight losses were maintained by only 50 percent of the group within 2 to 3 years, and by the end of the follow-up period, less than 10 percent weighed less than they had originally [61]. Since no food is consumed during the period of fasting, it is difficult to change the original eating habits that produced excessive weight gain in the first place, and weight may be easily regained if previous eating patterns are resumed.

An alternative to total fasting is a protein-sparing modified fast. This reducing regimen involves daily ingestion of 0.6 to 1.4 g protein per kilogram of ideal body weight, as lean meat, fish, or fowl. These diets reduce the loss of nitrogen, and ketosis is less pronounced than in starvation. However, there is no satisfactory evidence that the loss of protein is stopped completely. In the recent past, the use of a proteolytic digest of collagen ("liquid protein") was widespread until a series of 59 deaths among women on this diet was reported. The Center for Disease Control, Atlanta, Georgia, has released data on some of the women who died. Autopsy showed abnormalities of the myocardium with premortal evidence of cardiac arrhythmias. Because of this experience with liquid protein diets, it would appear judicious for very low calorie diets to contain some carbohydrates as well as protein. Diets containing only protein should remain under investigational status only. Furthermore, starvation or a modified fast is not recommended as a routine therapeutic procedure because (1) excessive loss of lean body tissue occurs early in starvation, (2) hospitalization, which is recommended for these regimens, is expensive, and (3) the long-term results do not justify the cost since most patients regain weight. It would appear that the treatment of obesity by prolonged starvation, if it is to be undertaken at all, should be restricted to a select few patients with severe obesity in whom a rapid weight loss appears to be vital.

Physical Activity

The value of physical activity and exercise in the prevention of obesity and in the treatment of moderately obese people in otherwise good health is well established [62]. The energy requirements of human beings can be divided into three components: requirement for basal metabolism, heat losses due to the thermic effects of food, and energy needs for physical activity. Since basal metabolism is not subject to significant changes and thermic effects are small (not more than 10 percent of the caloric value of ingested food), the only aspect of expenditure amenable to manipulation is physical activity. Exercise is the major variable in energy expenditure. The caloric expenditure in exercise is proportional to the duration of exercise; it is also proportional to the weight of the subject, so that an obese person will use up proportionally more calories to perform the same task than will a thin person. For example, a 54-kg (119-lb) man who runs 1.5 miles in 15 minutes will use 114 kcal, while another man weighing 100 kg (200.5 lb) and running at the same pace will expend 219 kcal.

Table 2 in Appendix 2 summarizes levels of physical activity (adapted from the Recommended Dietary Allowances). The lowest level of activity is approximately 1.0 kcal per minute. Thus, if a 70-kg man sleeps for an entire 24 hours, only 1680 kcal will be expended. Very light activity (i.e., the level at which people spend much of their time) consumes between 1.2 to 2.5 kcal per minute. Light activity increases this to 2.0 to 4.9 kcal per minute, whereas moderate activity ranges from 4.0 to 7.9 kcal per minute and heavy activity from 6.0 kcal per minute upward. Few people spend much of their time involved in physical activity at this latter level.

While very obese patients should not start to exercise suddenly, it is a good idea to start them walking every day and to increase the duration and eventually the intensity of the exercise as their weight reduction progresses. Advantage should be taken of every opportunity for walking, stair climbing, etc., to increase mobility in patients used to automobiles, elevators, and a multitude of laborsaving devices.

Exercise does not increase voluntary food intake until it has reached a certain critical duration and intensity, depending on the individual. Furthermore, exercise can also decrease body fat. Several studies in college-age students showed that during periods of exercise that consisted of walking and slow jogging, obese women showed a reduction in body weight and a decrease in skin-fold thickness [63,64]. Boileau et al. showed that a program with exercise carried on during weekdays by obese college men reduced body fat and produced a small reduction in body weight [65]. Thus, for college-age students, it is clear that a program of mild to moderate physical activity, consisting of jogging and walking on a treadmill, can reduce body fat, increase lean body mass, and decrease body weight without other dietary control.

Drug Treatment

At present there is no entirely acceptable, safe, and effective pharmacological agent for treating obesity. Because weight loss is difficult to achieve, and even more difficult to maintain, pharmaceutical agents have been used to promote weight reduction. It should be stated at the outset that these drugs are generally unsatisfactory in the long run and that they should be used only under the supervision of a physician.

The drugs which have been used to treat obesity fall into several categories. The first group is appetite suppressants; the compounds most used for this purpose are amphetamines. While they do cause appetite depression, the anorectic effect is relatively short-lived, and they produce serious side effects including addiction, insomnia, and excitability. One amphetamine, fen-fluramine, appears to exert a depressive effect on the central nervous system, producing drowsiness rather than excitability in its users.

A second group comprises calorigenic agents, of which thyroid hormone is the most important example. Both thyroxine (T_4) and triiodothyronine (T_3), when administered in sufficiently high doses, will reduce body weight. However, the weight loss consists primarily of lean body mass, and there are considerable hazards associated with the use of thyroid hormones in treating obesity, including palpitations, tachycardia, elevated systolic pressure, sweating, and negative calcium and nitrogen balance. Thyroid hormones should be used only for obese patients in whom hypothyroidism can be clearly documented [66].

A third, less important group of drugs consists of agents postulated to increase fat mobilization. This action has been alleged for human chorionic gonadotropin (HCG). Simeons introduced a regimen of HCG in conjunction with a 500-kcal diet in 1954 [67]. However, Simeons could not dissociate the weight loss attributable to HCG from that caused by the severe restriction of dietary energy. Several recent clinical trials have provided unequivocal evidence that this drug is no more effective than are placebo injections [68,69].

Surgery

An increasingly common approach to weight loss in the morbidly obese, i.e., those more than 100 lb above ideal weight, is surgical treatment. Two types of surgery are used: gastric bypass or stapling, and intestinal bypass. Gastric bypass is a reversible operation patterned after subtotal gastric resection that excludes about 90 percent of the stomach. It restricts the amount of food that can be eaten at one time; therefore less total food is consumed, and weight is thereby lost. Weight loss after this procedure has been comparable to that achieved after intestinal bypass operations but without the complications.

Intestinal bypass surgery excludes a major portion of the small intestine and thus reduces the absorbing surface by up to 90 percent. In the original procedure, a short section of the jejunum was anastomosed to the colon, thereby bypassing the entire ileum and most of the jejunum. Extremely severe diarrhea, with electrolyte imbalance, was a frequent side effect, and this procedure has been succeeded by more moderate jejunoileostomies. One of two procedures is now generally performed. In an end-to-side bypass, approximately 14 inches of proximal jejunum is anastomosed to the distal ileum, leaving only 4 inches of terminal ileum above the ileocecal valve and the ascending colon. The second procedure, in which the proximal jejunum is joined to the cut end of the ileum, is called an end-to-end bypass. Either of these operations results in a 16- to 22-foot-long loop of intestine, which is either sutured closed or anastomosed to the transverse section of the colon. The patients apparently lose weight, in variable amounts, because of decreased intestinal absorption, loss of nutrients in the feces, and decreased food intake. However, most patients are unable to reach their ideal weight after surgery. For further discussion see Chapter 15.

A number of clinical problems and complications from intestinal bypass commonly occur. There is a 3 to 6 percent mortality rate associated with the surgical procedure itself. Nausea and diarrhea are major problems. There is a decrease in the intestinal absorption of fat, protein, carbohydrates, vitamins (particularly vitamins B_{12}, A, and E), and minerals (most notably potassium, calcium, and magnesium). A serious side effect is fatty liver. Lithocolic acid, a breakdown product of unabsorbed bile acids in the colon, has been suggested as a possible hepatotoxic factor [70]. Protein insufficiency has also been implicated, but the evidence to support either of these hypotheses is weak.

As the number of patients having an intestinal bypass has increased, the enthusiasm for this procedure has declined. The mortality from this form of therapy far exceeds that of all other forms of treatment for obesity. However, it does appear that the quality of life for the obese patient who has had an intestinal bypass is improved. It should be cautioned that (1) this procedure seems indicated only for those in whom the obesity itself is life-threatening, (2) long-term follow-up is essential, and (3) nutritional deficiency states must be watched for and vigorously treated. A comprehensive symposium on jejunoileostomy for obesity has been published recently [71].

Behavior Modification

Presently behavior modification is the treatment modality receiving the most attention. Rather than focusing on presumed underlying causes of the obesity problem, the various behavior modification procedures are symptom-oriented and aimed at teaching obese people how to modify their behavior in relation to food consumption. The theory behind behavior modification is that both normal and abnormal behaviors follow the same laws of learning, i.e., Pavlovian classical conditioning, operant or trial-and-error learning, and imitation learning. These learning principles therefore can be applied in the extinction of maladaptive behaviors and in the learning of new, more adaptive behavior patterns. The targets of treatment are such behavior as overeating, eating high-caloric foods, snacking between meals, and reduced levels of physical activity.

The basic principles of the behavior modification approach can be described under the ABCs of eating. A stands for *antecedent*. The antecedent events that trigger eating are very important. Eating might be stimulated by turning on the television set, passing a pizza parlor, or hearing the noon whistle blow. B is the *behavior* of eating: the rate and frequency with which an individual eats and the actual act of eating. C is the *consequence* of eating, the feelings an individual has about it.

Before therapy begins, obese patients are asked to keep a detailed record of their activities in relation to eating and food. Such things as time of eating, place of eating, physical position when eating, social aspects of the situation, activities associated with eating, perceived degree of hunger, perceived mood, foods selected, and amount consumed, both in terms of volume and of calories, are recorded.

These records are then scrutinized, and intervention is planned on the basis of the maladaptive behavior. For example, the individual who eats rapidly is instructed to put the fork down between each bite of food; for the individual who eats when bored, activities are substituted to fill the void. Reinforcement for appropriate behavior is the final component of the behavior modification program and is carried out in a number of ways. One, known as the *contingency contract*, establishes a system of rewards for appropriate behavior. Family participation is used, especially in the case of children, and each member is instructed on how to respond to the individual.

An obese person may choose to consult a professional therapist, or he or she may choose to follow a self-directed program. There are numerous books that individuals can follow to establish a behavior modification program for themselves or, as lay leaders of behavior modification groups, for others [72,73]. In some programs nutritionists are trained by a behavioral psychologist before acting as therapists [74]. Considerable nutrition information can be built into these programs so that the participants can become knowledgeable about a number of food and nutrition topics.

Significant weight loss and superior maintenance after treatment with behavior techniques have been accomplished by some researchers, in comparison with reports of insufficient weight loss or regaining of lost weight following traditional therapy [75,76]. However, recently Mahoney and Mahoney have cautioned: "The fact that behavioral strategies are more effective than others does not imply they are therefore very effective. We remain a long distance away from any semblance of justification for complacency in weight regulation.

Significant poundage losses are still in the minority and long-term maintenance has been seldom examined" [77].

PREVENTION

Recently, Kannel and Gordon from the Framingham Study wrote:

> The earlier in life obesity is established and the more pronounced it is, the more resistant it is to treatment. Based on existing evidence of the efficacy of treatment of long-standing pronounced obesity, it must be classed as one of the less tractable diseases. For this reason, it is better *prevented* [emphasis added] than cured. It would be most helpful if the medical profession were to develop a sense of urgency about obesity, so when the disease is beginning or when it first appears, action would be taken immediately, as it is for a lump in the breast or for a high blood sugar [78].

Wherever possible, good medical practice stresses prevention rather than treatment. Of infants in the 90th percentile of weight or higher, 36 percent become overweight adults. In contrast, only 14 percent of those who are average or below average in weight as infants become obese adults [79]. The extent to which fatness runs in families should provide the pediatrician with a rationale for early institution of an adequate regimen of dietary instructions and exercise for likely candidates for overweight. The fact that most obese adolescents become obese adults further emphasizes the need for attention to weight problems at an early stage.

Prevention of obesity should begin with the education of the present generation for the benefit of the following generation. New mothers and fathers need sound nutrition information both before and after the birth of their children. Especially to be encouraged is the avoidance of concentrated sweets and fats, enthusiasm for exercise, and the use of food for nutritional purposes only, rather than as a reward for good conduct or a substitute for affection.

CASE STUDY

A 17-year-old student was referred to a nutrition outpatient clinic for help in weight reduction. The patient lost her right leg 3½ years before in an automobile-pedestrian accident and had not successfully adapted to a prosthesis. She had a family history of obesity (both parents were overweight, as were her three siblings). The patient weighed approximately 160 lb at the time of her accident. Within 2½ years she had gained 105 lb. She then joined a health spa and lost 75 lb during the subsequent 6 months. Her weight then plateaued at 194 lb. She gets around in a wheel chair or an automobile outfitted with hand controls. On physical examination the patient was found to be 5 feet 4 inches tall, weighed 194 lb, and otherwise appeared healthy. Blood pressure was recorded at 118/80 and triceps skin fold at 37 mm. No laboratory values were available.

Food intake was calculated to be 800 kcal per day (35 percent carbohydrate,

40 percent fat, and 25 percent protein). The patient stated that she took one multivitamin per day and usually ate two or three small meals per day.

Study Questions

1 What is the patient's estimated ideal weight?

2 Does the history of the patient provide any clues as to the cause of her obesity?

3 Should there be a change in physical activity? Explain.

4 Should the present diet be changed in terms of energy intake? What should the proportions be of protein, carbohydrate, and fat in her diet?

REFERENCES

1 Bray, G. A.: Overview, in *Obesity in America,* G. A. Bray (ed.), U.S. Department of Health, Education, and Welfare Publication no. (NIH) 79-359, 1979.

2 Dublin, L. I., and H. H. Marks: Mortality among insured overweights in recent years, Trans. Assoc. Life Insur. Med. Dir. Am., 35:935, 1952.

3 Seltzer, C. C., and J. Mayer: A simple criterion of obesity, Postgrad. Med., 38:A101, 1965.

4 Food and Nutrition Board: *Recommended Dietary Allowances,* 9th ed., National Academy of Sciences, Washington, 1980.

5 Stunkard, A. J.: Obesity and the social environment: current status, future prospects, in *Obesity in America,* G. A. Bray (ed.), U.S. Department of Health, Education, and Welfare, Publication no. (NIH) 79-359, 1979.

6 Srole, L., T. S. Langer, and S. T. Michael: *Mental Health in the Metropolis: the Midtown Manhattan Study,* McGraw-Hill, New York, 1962.

7 Goldblatt, P. B., M. E. Moore, and A. J. Stunkard: Social factors in obesity, J. Am. Med. Assoc., 192:1039, 1965.

8 Stunkard, A. J.: Environment and obesity: recent advances in our understanding of the regulation of food intake in man, Fed. Proc., 27:276, 1968.

9 Stunkard, A. J.: Obesity and social environment, in *Recent Advances in Obesity Research:1,* A. Howard (ed.), Newman, London, 1975.

10 Silverstone, J. T., R. P. Gordon, and A. J. Stunkard: Social factors in obesity in London, Practitioner, 202:682, 1969.

11 Bray, G. A.: *Major Problems in Internal Medicine, The Obese Patient,* vol. IX: Saunders, Philadelphia, 1976.

12 Garn, S. M., and D. C. Clark: Trends in fatness and the origins of obesity, Pediatrics, 57:443, 1976.

13 Mayer, J.: Genetic factors in human obesity, Postgrad. Med., 37:A103, 1965.

14 Withers, R. J. S.: Problems in the genetics of human obesity, Eugen. Rev., 58:81, 1964.

15 Garn, S. M., P. E. Cole, and S. M. Bailey: Effect of parental fatness levels on the fatness of biological and adoptive children, Ecol. Food Nutr., 7:91, 1977.

16 Seltzer, C. C., and J. Mayer: Body build and obesity—who are the obese? J. Am. Med. Assoc., 189:677, 1964.

17 Seltzer, C. C., and J. Mayer: Body build (somatotype) distinctiveness in obese women, J. Am. Diet. Assoc., 55:454, 1969.

18 Bullen, B. A., R. B. Reed, and J. Mayer: Physical activity of obese and nonobese adolescent girls appraised by motion picture sampling, Am. J. Clin. Nutr., 14:211, 1964.

19 Mayer, J., P. Roy, and K. P. Mitra: Relation between caloric intake, body weight, and physical work. Studies in an industrial male population in West Bengal, Am. J. Clin. Nutr., 4:169, 1966.

20 Marr, J. W., J. Gregory, T. W. Meade, M. R. Alderson, and J. N. Morris: Diet, leisure activity, and skinfold measurements of sedentary men, Proc. Nutr. Soc., 29:17A, 1970.

21 Curtis, D. E., and R. B. Bradfield: Long-term energy intake and expenditure of obese housewives, Am. J. Clin. Nutr., 24:1410, 1971.

22 Seltzer, C. C., and J. Mayer: An effective weight control program in a public school system, Am. J. Public Health, 60:679, 1970.

23 Tepperman, J., J. R. Brobeck, and C. N. H. Long: A study of experimental hypothalamic obesity in the rat, Am. J. Physiol., 133:468, 1941.

24 Sutin, J.: Neural factors in the control of food intake, in Obesity in Prospective, part 2, G. A. Bray (ed.), U.S. Department of Health, Education, and Welfare Publication no. (NIH) 75-708, 1975.

25 Rodin, J.: Pathogenesis of obesity: energy intake and expenditure, in Obesity in America, G. A. Bray (ed.), U.S. Department of Health, Education, and Welfare Publication no. (NIH) 79-359, 1979.

26 Salans, L. B., S. W. Cushman, and R. E. Weismann: Studies of human adipose tissue: adipose cell size and number in nonobese and obese patients, J. Clin. Invest., 52:929, 1973.

27 Hirsch, J., and J. L. Knittle: Cellularity of obese and nonobese human adipose tissue, Fed. Proc., 29:1516, 1970.

28 Sims, E. A., E. S. Horton, and L. B. Salans: Inducible metabolic abnormalities during development of obesity, Ann. Rev. Med., 22:235, 1971.

29 Eid, E. E.: Follow-up study of physical growth of children who had excessive weight gain in the first 6 months of life, Br. Med. J., 2:74, 1970.

30 Asher, P.: Fat babies and fat children, Arch. Dis. Child., 41:672, 1966.

31 Lloyd, J. K., O. H. Wolf, and W. S. Whelan: Childhood obesity: a long-term study of height and weight, Br. Med. J., 2:145, 1961.

32 Charney, E., H. C. Goodman, M. McBride, B. Lyon, and R. Pratt: Childhood antecedents of adult obesity, N. Engl. J. Med., 295:6, 1976.

33 Poskitt, E. M. E., and T. J. Cole: Do fat babies stay fat? Br. Med. J., 1:7, 1977.

34 Weil, W. B.: Current controversies in childhood obesity, J. Pediatr., 91:175, 1977.

35 Edholm, O. G., J. M. Adams, M. J. R. Healy, H. S. Wolff, R. Goldsmith, and T. W. Best: Food intake and energy expenditure of army recruits, Br. J. Nutr., 24:1091, 1970.

36 Sims, E. A. H., and E. S. Horton: Endocrine and metabolic adaptation to obesity, Am. J. Clin. Nutr., 21:1455, 1968.

37 Sims, A., R. F. Goldman, C. M. Gluck, E. S. Horton, P. C. Kelleher, and D. W. Rowe: Experimental obesity in man, Trans. Assoc. Am. Physicians, 81:153, 1968.

38 Blaxter, K. L.: Methods of measuring the energy metabolism of animals and interpretation of results obtained, Fed. Proc., 30:1436, 1970.

39 Miller, D. S.: Energy balance and obesity, in Obesity, W. A. Burland, P. D. Samuel, and J. Yudkin (eds.), Churchill, Livingstone, Edinburgh, 1974.

40 Himms-Hagen, J. A.: Cellular thermogenesis, Ann. Rev. Physiol., 38:315, 1976.

41 Foster, D. O., and M. L. Frydman: Nonshivering thermogenesis in the rat. II. Measurements of blood flow with microspheres point to brown adipose tissue as the dominant site of the calorigenesis induced by noradrenaline, Can. J. Physiol. Pharmacol., 56:110, 1978.

42 Rothwell, N. J., and M. J. Stock: A role for brown adipose tissue in diet-induced thermogenesis, Nature, 281:31, 1979.

43 Trayhurn, P., P. L. Thurlby, C. J. H. Woodward, and W. P. T. James: Thermoregulation in genetically obese rodents: the relationship to metabolic efficiency, in *Animal Models of Obesity,* M. F. W. Festing (ed.), MacMillan, London, 1979.

44 Trayhurn, P., P. L. Thurlby, and W. P. T. James: Thermogenic defect in pre-obese ob/ob mice, Nature 266:60, 1977.

45 Jung, R. T., P. S. Shetty, W. P. T. James, M. A. Barrand, and B. A. Callingham: Reduced thermogenesis in obesity, Nature, 279:322, 1979.

46 Anderson, J., A. Short, and M. Yaffe: The relationship between physiological and psychological measurements in obesity, in *Recent Advances in Obesity Research: 1,* A. Howard (ed.), Newman, London, 1975.

47 Newsholme, E. A.: A possible metabolic basis for the control of body weight, N. Engl. J. Med., 302:400, 1980.

48 *National Commission on Diabetes Report,* vol. 3, part 1, U.S. Department of Health, Education, and Welfare Publication no. (NIH) 76-1021, 1975.

49 Rimm A. A., and P. C. White: Obesity: its risks and hazards, in *Obesity in America,* G. A. Bray (ed.), U.S. Department of Health, Education, and Welfare Publication no. (NIH) 79-359, 1979.

50 Grande F.: Assessment of body fat in man, in *Obesity in Perspective,* part 2, G. A. Bray (ed.), U.S. Department of Health, Education, and Welfare Publication no. (NIH) 75-708, 1975.

51 Durnin, J. V. G. A., and J. Womersley: Body fat assessed from total body density and its estimation from skinfold thickness: Measurements of 481 men and women, aged from 16-72, Br. J. Nutr., 32:77, 1974.

52 Seltzer, C. C., R. F. Goldman, and J. Mayer: The triceps skinfold as a predictive measure of body density and body fat in obese adolescent girls, Pediatrics, 36:212, 1965.

53 Frisancho, A.: Triceps skinfold and upper arm muscle size norms for assessment of nutritional status, Am. J. Clin. Nutr., 27:1052, 1974.

54 Butterworth, C. E., and G. L. Blackburn: Hospital malnutrition, Nutr. Today, 10:8, 1975.

55 Young, C. M., K. Berresford, and N. S. Moore: Psychologic factors in weight control, Am. J. Clin. Nutr., 5:186, 1957.

56 Buskirk, E. R., R. H. Thompson, L. Lutwak, and G. D. Whedon: Energy balance of obese patients during weight reduction: influence of diet restriction and exercise, Ann. N.Y. Acad. Sci., 110:918, 1963.

57 Blondheim, S. H., N. A. Kaufman, and M. Stein: Comparison of fasting and 800-1000 calorie diet in obesity, Lancet, 1:250, 1965.

58 Bierman, E. L.: Obesity, in *Textbook of Medicine,* 15th ed., P. B. Beeson, W. McDermott, and J. B. Wyngaarden (eds.), Saunders, Philadelphia, 1979.

59 Huenemann, R. L.: Food habits of obese and nonobese adolescents. Postgrad, Med., 51:99, 1972.

60 Bortz, W. M., A. Wroldsen, B. Issekutz, and K. Rodahl: Weight loss and frequency of feeding, N. Engl. J. Med., 274:3, 1966.

61 Johnson, D., and E. Drenick: Therapeutic fasting in morbid obesity, Arch. Intern. Med., 137:1381, 1977.

62 Mayer, J.: *Overweight: Causes, Cost and Control,* Prentice Hall, New York, 1968.

63 Moody, D. L., J. Kollias, and E. R. Buskirk: The effect of a moderate exercise program on body weight and skinfold thickness in overweight college women, Med. Sci. Sports, 1:75, 1969.

64 Moody, D. L., J. H. Wilmore, R. N. Girandola, and J. P. Reyce: The effects of a jogging program on the body composition of normal and obese high school girls, Med. Sci. Sports, 4:210, 1972.

65 Boileau, R. A., E. R. Buskirk, D. H. Horstman, J. Mendex, and W. C. Nicholas: Body composition changes in obese and lean men during physical conditioning, Med. Sci. Sports, 3:183, 1971.

66 Rivlin, R. S.: Drug therapy, N. Engl. J. Med., 292:26, 1975.

67 Simeons, A. T. W.: The action of chorionic gonadotropin in the obese, Lancet, 2:946, 1954.

68 Greenway, F. L., and G. A. Bray: Human chorionic gonadotropin (HCG) in the treatment of obesity: a critical assessment of the Simeons Method, West. J. Med., 127:461, 1977.

69 Stein, M. R., R. E. Julius, C. C. Peek, W. Henshaw, J. R. Sawicki, and J. J. Deller: Ineffectiveness of human chorionic gonadotropin in weight reduction: a double-blind study, Am. J. Clin. Nutr., 29:940, 1976.

70 Drenick, E. J., F. Simmons, and J. F. Murphy: Effect on hepatic morphology of treatment of obesity by fasting, reducing diets, and small bowel bypass, N. Engl. J. Med., 282:289, 1970.

71 Faloon, W. W.: Symposium on jejunoileostomy for obesity, Am. J. Clin. Nutr., 30:1, 1977.

72 Stuart, R. B., and B. Davis: *Slim Chance in a Fat World,* Research Press, Champaign, Ill., 1972.

73 Ferguson, J. M.: *Learning to Eat, Leader's Manual and Student's Manual,* Bull Publishing, Palo Alto, Calif., 1975.

74 Paulsen, B. K., R. N. Lutz, W. T. McReynolds, and M. B. Kohrs: Behavior therapy for weight control: long-term results of two programs with nutritionists as therapists, Am. J. Clin. Nutr., 29:880, 1976.

75 Stuart, R. B.: Behavioral control of overeating, Behav. Res. Ther., 5:357, 1967.

76 Penick, S. B., R. Filion, S. Fox, and A. J. Stunkard: Behavioral modification in the treatment of obesity, Psychosom. Med., 33:49, 1971.

77 Mahoney, M. J., and K. Mahoney: *Permanent Weight Control,* Norton, New York, 1976.

78 Kannel, W. B., and T. Gordon: Physiological and medical concomitants of obesity: The Framingham Study, in *Obesity in America,* G. A. Bray (ed.), U.S. Department of Health, Education, and Welfare Publication no. (NIH) 79-359, 1979.

79 Anderson, A. E., and S. Margolis: Eating disorders: obesity and anorexia nervosa, in *The Principles of Medicine,* 20th ed., A. M. Harvey et al. (eds.), Appleton Century Crofts, New York, 1980.

CHAPTER 8

CORONARY HEART DISEASE

CONTENTS

INTRODUCTION

Coronary heart disease (CHD) is the leading cause of death in the United States. Although its incidence has been dropping during the past 15 years, in 1976 it was responsible for close to 650,000 deaths [1] and an additional 188,623 cardiovascular deaths were due to stroke. Not only is it a disease that affects older people; it is also an important cause of premature death and disability in middle age. Clinical manifestations of CHD develop in about 20 percent of men under the age of 60. A quarter of them die within 3 hours of the onset of symptoms. Another quarter die in the first few weeks after a heart attack. Advances in intensive hospital care are not likely to reduce mortality from sudden deaths. The prevalence of CHD in the United States is 10 times that in Japan, which enjoys the lowest rate in the modern industrialized world. If we wish to achieve these low rates, we must think in terms of *preventing* rather than curing the underlying disease.

Epidemiological studies have helped to define apparent biological, demographic, and social differences between normal and coronary-prone individuals. Habits or traits which appear to be associated with *risk* for CHD are called *risk factors*. Although some 37 variables have been correlated with CHD [2], three major risk factors have been identified: total plasma cholesterol level, systolic and diastolic blood pressure, and cigarette consumption.

Arteriosclerosis is a general term for degenerative diseases of the large and medium-sized arteries, which result in loss of elasticity (sclerosis) and thickening of the arterial wall. *Atherosclerosis,* one type of arteriosclerosis, is characterized by the accumulation of lipids (primarily cholesterol) as atheromatous plaques at sites at which damage to the intimal lining of the artery has occurred and by subsequent accumulation of fibrous tissue. As these plaques increase in size, they may impede blood flow through the affected arteries or they may become detached into the circulation and obstruct smaller vessels, leading in each case to ischemia (deprivation of blood supply). Tissue damage may be generalized, or it may be more prominent in certain organs or locations—heart, kidney, brain, lungs, and extremities—where it induces specific clinical syndromes. Although death or morbidity resulting from atherosclerosis is most apparent from the fifth decade of life on, autopsy studies of young soldiers [3] show that the lesions are established by the age of 25 years. In this chapter, CHD will be emphasized because of its high incidence and because of the direct implications of dietary management in prevention and treatment.

EPIDEMIOLOGY

Epidemiological studies have been crucial in identifying risk factors that are correlated with the subsequent development of clinical CHD. However, one must distinguish risk factors from causal factors. The fact that two events tend to occur together certainly does not establish a causal relation between them;

neither does it exclude one. The noncommittal term *risk factor* avoids the question of whether these characteristics are causative agents, intervening variables, early manifestations of disease, or secondary indications of an underlying disturbance. Further, of the factors identified as being associated with the increased rate of atherosclerosis, none is believed to be solely responsible. Most diseases are not the result of a single cause but represent instead a combination of necessary and permissive conditions that disturb the homeostasis of a living organism. The risk factors for atherosclerosis can be separated into (1) inherent or endogenous factors and (2) environmental factors (see Table 8-1). Of the inherent factors some such as age, gender, and heredity are factors over which we have no control, while others like diet and exercise are theoretically more amenable to change.

Endogenous Risk Factors

Age As with many chronic diseases the incidence rate for atherosclerotic disease increases with age.

Sex Except for age, being male is one of the best-documented and strongest risk factors for *coronary* heart disease, but not for other forms of atherosclerotic disease [4]. The sex differential in CHD is most marked in whites. Despite the attractiveness of the hypothesis that the estrogenic hormones of the female are responsible for relative protection from coronary atherosclerosis, it has become clear that exogenous estrogen administration does not protect the male. Neither does it appear that exogenous estrogen, as in oral contraceptives, adds to the natural protection of the female. Females have slightly lower levels of three

TABLE 8-1
RISK FACTORS FOR CORONARY HEART DISEASE

Endogenous	Exogenous
Major risk factors	
Total plasma cholesterol Elevated blood pressure	Smoking cigarettes
Minor risk factors	

Age
Sex
Family history or genetics
Diabetes mellitus
Obesity
Personality type
	Diet: Total fat, saturated fat,
	  cholesterol, carbohydrate, sugar,
	  fiber, alcohol
	Physical activity
	Psychosocial stress

major risk factors (serum cholesterol, blood pressure, and cigarette smoking) between the menarche and the menopause, but lower levels of these risk factors do not seem sufficient to account for the differences in CHD [5].

Family History   There is evidence that CHD tends to aggregate among blood relatives [6]; however, the evidence implicating genetic factors in CHD is not very satisfactory except in the rare cases of familial hypercholesterolemia (see discussion under "Hyperlipidemia," below). Serum lipid levels and blood pressure come under both genetic control and environmental influences. Families share habits and attitudes as well as genes. No definitive studies have looked at such factors as parental age at death, or other genetic tags, in terms of prediction of new CHD or death.

The physician should be alert to the age of onset of CHD in a family. If a man sustains a myocardial infarction before the age of 40 and there is a history of heart attack or sudden death before the age of 40 in other male members of his family, it is reasonable to suspect that his family has an inherited lipoprotein defect. Lipid patterns of his children and wife should be evaluated; if his wife has hyperlipidemia, their children will be at increased risk. However, a bad family history can be considerably discounted by the physician if an individual is found to be at the low end of the distribution of primary risk factors.

Hyperlipidemia   Hyperlipidemia is elevation of serum cholesterol or triglycerides, or both. Total serum cholesterol concentration has long been recognized as the strongest and most consistent risk factor for atherosclerotic disease other than age and sex. Hyperlipidemia may occur as a secondary manifestation of another disease, e.g., diabetes mellitus or hypothyroidism, or it may result from dietary extremes or a rare hereditary disorder. Cholesterol, triglycerides, and phospholipids are carried in the plasma, bound to specific proteins. These lipoproteins vary as to the amount of protein and fat they contain and can be identified according to their density and/or electrophoretic mobility. Figure 8-1 shows the classification of the lipoproteins: chylomicrons, low-density lipoproteins (LDL), very low density lipoproteins (VLDL), and high-density lipoproteins (HDL). Table 8-2 gives the normal limits of plasma lipids and lipoproteins.

Chylomicrons are the largest and the lightest of the lipoproteins. Their principal component is triglyceride derived entirely from exogenous (dietary) fat. The remaining components are cholesterol, phospholipid, and protein. Chylomicrons are synthesized in the intestine and transport dietary triglycerides from the intestinal mucosa via the thoracic duct to the tissues; the chylomicron remnants are ultimately cleared by the liver.

VLDL is synthesized by the liver and small intestine from free fatty acids, carbohydrates, glycerol, and 2-carbon fragments of other dietary components. They carry endogenous triglycerides.

Intermediate low-density lipoprotein (ILDL) is an intermediate in the conversion of VLDL to LDL. ILDL is present in minute amounts in healthy

TABLE 8-2

PLASMA LIPID AND LIPOPROTEIN CONCENTRATIONS IN NORMAL SUBJECTS*

Age, Years	Sex	Total cholesterol mg/dl	Triglyceride mg/dl	VLDL cholesterol† mg/dl	LDL cholesterol† mg/dl	HDL cholesterol mg/dl	No. of subjects
0–19	M	72±34	61±34	9±7	108±33	49±11	43
	F	179±33	73±34	11±8	108±10	53±12	38
20–29	M	183±37	73±32	11±8	111±30	53±11	41
	F	179±35	62±29	12±10	115±31	52±9	37
30–39	M	210±33	78±39	21±13	143±27	48±11	50
	F	204±37	67±48	14±10	119±31	58±13	32
40–49	M	230±55	90±41	21±9	128±28	49±10	67
	F	217±35	80±42	14±9	130±24	62±14	44
50–59	M	240±48	104±45	29±8	152±22	47±15	28
	F	251±49	83±46	23±8	147±36	59±15	41
Suggested "normal" limits‡‡							
0–19		120–230	10–140	5–25	50–170	30–65 (M)	
						30–70 (F)	
20–29		120–240	10–140	5–25	60–170	35–70 (M)	
						35–75 (F)	
30–39		140–270	10–150	5–35	70–190	30–65 (M)	
						35–80 (F)	
40–49		150–310	10–160	5–35	80–190	30–65 (M)	
						40–85 (F)	
50–59		160–330	10–190	10–40	80–210	30–65 (M)	
						35–85 (F)	

*Population sample is derived from subjects with no evidence of metabolic disease or family history of hyperlipoproteinemia whose triglycerides were < 200 mg/dl; all samples obtained 12 to 14 hours after evening meal. Values in upper half of table represent mean ± standard deviation.
†Obtained on smaller number of patients, varying from 13 to 27 in number.
‡Based on 95 percent fiducial limits calculated for small samples; all values rounded to nearest 5 mg. (It should be noted that, for practical purposes, differences between sexes have been ignored except for HDL concentrations.)

Source: D. S. Fredrickson, N. Engl. J. Med., 276:151, 1967.

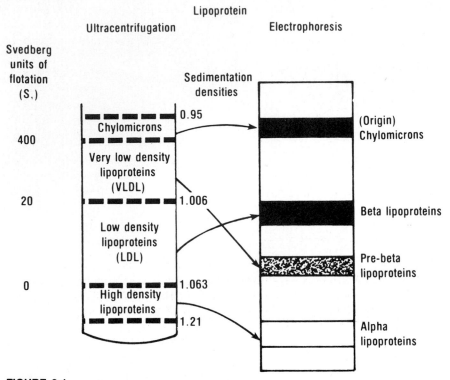

FIGURE 8-1
Classification of blood lipoproteins by ultracentrifugation and lipoprotein electrophoresis. (*Adapted from W. P. Castelli and R. F. Moran, Hum. Pathol., 2:153, 1971.*)

persons and in hyperlipoproteinemic patients other than those with type III abnormality, in which ILDLs are greatly increased.

LDL is a degradation product of the breakdown of VLDL by the liver. About 60 percent of total serum cholesterol is contained in LDL.

HDL originates in the liver but is independent of VLDL function. HDL transports cholesterol out of the tissues.

There is some disagreement among researchers and practitioners as to what constitutes a normal or desirable serum cholesterol level. Hyperlipidemia is said to be present when an individual's plasma cholesterol and/or triglyceride levels exceed the 95th percentile for his or her respective age and sex distribution [7]. Such definitions are continuous, and since risk of CHD is linearly related to cholesterol levels, no cutoff point separates subjects at risk from subjects free from risk. However, the use of cutoff points to classify subjects with specific types of hyperlipidemia has the advantage of focusing attention (1) on especially high risk subjects and (2) on certain genetically determined hyperlipidemias.

Hypertriglyceridemia has also been associated with increased prevalence of CHD [8]. However, none of the evidence indicates that triglyceride levels contribute information on CHD risk independently of the other associated risk factors, such as plasma cholesterol, obesity, sedentary lifestyle, hypertension, or impaired glucose tolerance [9].

The terms *hyperlipidemia, hypercholesterolemia,* and *hypertriglyceridemia* do not indicate which lipoproteins are elevated. Hence, it is desirable to translate hyperlipidemia into hyperlipoproteinemia. In 1967, Fredrickson, Levy, and Lees proposed a classification of hyperlipoproteinemia that was based on the quantitative assessment of the lipoproteins. Originally, five types were described, and more recently one of these types has been subdivided into two. The classification is as follows [10]:

Type I: Increased chylomicrons
Type IIa: Increased LDL
Type IIb: Increased LDL and VLDL
Type III: Increased ILDL
Type IV: Increased VLDL
Type V: Increased chylomicrons and VLDL

Each hyperlipoproteinemia may be secondary to a variety of diseases, in which case the treatment is primarily directed to the underlying disease [11]. Each may also occur as a primary, sometimes genetically determined abnormality. *Only a small percentage of all patients with CHD have a true inborn error of lipid metabolism* responsible for elevation of lipids. In the great majority of cases of CHD the lipid abnormality is probably acquired. A summary of the types of hyperlipoproteinemia is given in Table 8-3. Types I, III, and V are very uncommon. Individuals with many of the features of type II (hypercholesterolemia) or type IV (hypertriglyceridemia) are more commonly seen.

High-Density Lipoprotein Recently, epidemiological studies have firmly established that there is a very strong *negative* correlation between plasma HDL cholesterol levels and the risk of CHD [12,13]. The correlation holds in men and in women, and it holds at any level of LDL cholesterol; that is, it is an independent predictor. In fact, the power of the HDL level as a negative predictor is even greater than the power of the LDL level as a positive predictor [14]. The mechanism for this protective relationship is unknown. Miller and Miller hypothesized that HDL transports cholesterol from peripheral tissues to the liver for catabolism and excretion [12]. The recent reports that physical activity and weight loss increase HDL levels are provocative and will stimulate further exploration [15,16].

Hypertension The risk of developing CHD is strongly related to the level of blood pressure. As with plasma cholesterol there is no clearly defined cutoff point below which the blood pressure can be defined as "normal." The lower the blood pressure, the lower the risk. This is true for men and woman at all ages.

Diabetes Mellitus Cardiovascular disease, particularly atherosclerotic disease, remains a major health hazard for the diabetic. Diabetics have higher

TABLE 8-3
TYPES OF HYPERLIPOPROTEINEMIA

Features	Type I	Type IIa	Type IIb	Type III	Type IV	Type V
Incidence	Very rare	Common	Common	Relatively uncommon	Common	Uncommon
Lipoprotein abnormality	↑ Fasting chylomicrons	↑ LDL	↑ LDL ↑ VLDl	↑ ILDL	↑ VLDL	↑ Fasting chylomicrons ↑ VLDL
Plasma cholesterol	Normal or ↑	↑	↑	↑	Normal or ↑	Normal or ↑
Plasma triglycerides	Greatly ↑	Normal	↑	↑	↑	↑ or greatly ↑
Clinical signs	Lipemia retinalis Eruptive xanthomas Hepatospleno-megaly Abdominal pain Childhood expression	Tendon and tuber-ous xanthomas Xanthelasma Juvenile corneal arcus Accelerated coronary atherosclerosis Severe cases detected in childhood		Palmar, tuberous, and tendon xanthomas Accelerated atherosclerosis	Abnormal gluose tolerance Hyperuricemia Accelerated coronary vessel disease Detected in adults	Lipemia retinalis Eruptive xanthomas Hepatospleno-megaly Hyperglycemia Hyperuricemia
Inheritance, if primary	Recessive Deficiency in lipoprotein lipase	Dominant, sporadic		Recessive	Dominant, sporadic	Dominant, sporadic
Secondary causes	Diabetic acidosis Hypothyroidism Insulin-dependent diabetes Dysgamma-globulinemia	Hypothyroidism Nephrosis Obstructive liver disease Porphyria Excess dietary cholesterol		Diabetes mellitus* Hypothyroidism Renal insuf-ficiency	Diabetes mellitus Nephrosis Pancreatitis Glycogen storage disease	Pancreatitis Alcoholism Nephrosis

*Secondary causes are rare in type III hyperlipoproteinemia.

serum lipids, especially triglycerides, than do nondiabetics, but the differences do not account for the increased risk of atherosclerotic disease. Impaired glucose tolerance, even in the absence of overt diabetes, has also been associated with CHD [17]. Neither insulin nor oral hypoglycemic agents protect diabetics from the increased risk of atherosclerotic disease. This is discussed at greater length in Chapter 11.

Obesity   The role of obesity in atherosclerotic disease remains uncertain, despite the nearly universal recommendation that obesity should be avoided in order to reduce risk of atherosclerotic disease. Obesity appears well-established as a risk factor for hypertension and diabetes, and it undoubtedly influences atherosclerosis indirectly through these mechanisms, but in their absence, no clear association of obesity with either atherogenesis or atherosclerotic disease has been demonstrated.

Personality Type   Many people believe that the behavioral and emotional aspect of life is related to CHD. Meyer Friedman and Ray H. Rosenman, authors of *Type A Behavior and Your Heart,* believe that people can be categorized as type A, or coronary-prone, and type B, or non-coronary-prone [18]. Type A behavior is characterized by striving for achievement, competitiveness, a feeling of time urgency, and excesses of drive and hostility. Type B individuals are not so characterized and are more easygoing. It should be emphasized that this behavior pattern is not the same as "stress." It represents neither a stressful situation nor a distressed response, but rather a style of behavior with which some persons habitually respond to circumstances that arouse them. Jenkins reviewed 23 studies and found all but one supported the association of at least some part of the type A behavior pattern with the incidence or prevalence of coronary disease [19]. However, the data remain highly controversial and are not accepted by many cardiologists.

Environmental Factors

Cigarette Smoking   Cigarette smoking has repeatedly been shown substantially to increase the risk of cardiovascular disease. Several large-scale studies in the United States and Britain show that male cigarette smokers are from 1.5 to 2.5 times more likely to die from CHD than nonsmokers [20,21].

Physical Activity   Several studies have shown an inverse relationship between the degree of physical activity required at work and risk of CHD. The studies of London bus drivers and conductors showed that the conductors, who climbed up and down the stairs in double-decker buses, had a lower CHD incidence than the less physically active bus drivers, who sat at the wheel all day [22]. However, the bus drivers were more obese on entry into their occupation. There is some question as to the selective forces that determine the type of job a person chooses; e.g., a man who is less "fit" and who is at greater risk of CHD for other reasons may choose to enter a less active occupation.

In affluent societies where CHD is most common, few jobs require much physical activity. Hence the amount of physical activity expended in leisure time discriminates more active individuals from less active individuals. Morris et al. attempted to mitigate the occupational selection problem by a prospective study of CHD in civil servants in sedentary occupations who were allocated to any one of five categories of leisure-time exercise habits. The results, adjusted for age and smoking habits, indicated a significantly lower rate of new CHD in those who took part in endurance activity involving peaks of 7.5 kcal per minute of energy expenditure [23].

Two epidemiologic studies in the United States have investigated the inverse relationship of vigorous exercise and risk of heart attack among 6300 San Francisco longshoremen [24] and 17,000 Harvard University alumni [25]. These projects obtained and analyzed detailed information about dockworkers' energy output on the job and the physical characteristics and exercise patterns of college men in student days and later life. Table 8-4 shows age-adjusted rates and relative risk of first heart attacks among Harvard alumni in a 6- to 10-year follow-up, presented according to differences in physical exercise. The one-third who reported climbing fewer than 50 steps per day were at 25 percent increased risk of heart attack over those who climbed more. Results were similar for the one-fourth who walked fewer than five blocks daily as compared to those who walked more. There was no difference in risk for those who played light sports as compared to those who played no sports at all. On the other hand, the 59 percent of men who did not play strenuous sports were at 38 percent greater risk than those who did. A complete physical activity index constructed from the energy equivalents required to walk, climb stairs, and play at specific sports showed that 60 percent of the alumni expended less than 2000 kcal weekly and were at 65 percent higher risk of heart attack than their classmates who were more active.

There have been studies that failed to show an association between physical activity and CHD risk. These negative results may, in part, result from the difficulties of accurate classification of degree of physical activity. For example, the study of sedentary civil servants and the study of Harvard alumni suggested a "threshold" effect; i.e., only vigorous activity appeared to be protective. Failure to appreciate this phenomenon may have accounted for negative results in other studies.

More recently, HDL cholesterol, as a measure of HDL, was found to be elevated in cross-country skiers and marathon runners [26,27]. Investigators have debated whether this is a self-selection phenomenon; i.e. lean athletic persons naturally have higher HDL levels and are attracted to long-distance competitive sports, or whether increased physical activity somehow changes body metabolism, producing a rise in HDL. That exercise per se may be a causal factor in producing HDL elevations is suggested by studies of medical students in New Orleans [28] and Air Force officers [29] in whom an increase in HDL

TABLE 8-4

AGE-ADJUSTED RATES AND RELATIVE RISKS OF FIRST HEART ATTACK (HA) AMONG HARVARD ALUMNI IN A 6-10-YEAR FOLLOWUP, BY MEASURES OF PHYSICAL ACTIVITY

Physical activity	% man-years	No. with HA	HA per 10,000 man-years	Relative risk of HA	p
Stairs climbed daily:					
< 50	33	222	56.5	1.25	0.008
≥ 50	67	329	45.1		
Blocks walked daily:					
< 5	23	140	57.8	1.26	0.016
≥ 5	77	385	45.7		
Light sports activity					
No	76	288	59.8	1.08	0.501
Yes	24	102	55.3		
Strenuous sports activity					
No	59	390	54.1	1.38	0.001
Yes	41	148	39.3		
Weekly energy expenditure, kcal:					
< 2000	60	307	57.9	1.64	< 0.001
≥ 2000	40	122	35.3		

Source: R. S. Paffenberger, Jr., Countercurrents of physical activity and heart attack trends, in Proceedings of the Conference on the Decline in Coronary Heart Disease Mortality, R. J. Havlik and M. Feinleib (eds.), U.S. Department of Health, Education, and Welfare Publication no. (NIH) 79-1610, 1979.

levels was observed after they entered exercise programs. These observations have been extended to men with CHD. Moderate exercise (walking or jogging 2.8 km three times per week for 13 weeks) produced an increase in the HDL-cholesterol levels with no notable changes in weight, diet, serum triglycerides, or plasma LDL cholesterol [30]. Erkelens and coworkers showed that HDL-cholesterol levels were higher in patients with CHD who exercised and that in a longitudinal study the HDL levels rose with physical activity [31]. That there is an inverse correlation between HDL levels and incidence of CHD has previously been discussed (see discussion under "High-density Lipoprotein").

The evidence in humans that exercise may protect against CHD is indirect. Recent direct evidence from studies with monkeys showed that conditioning with treadmill exercises produced a reduction in atherosclerotic involvement, a reduction of lesion size (intimal thickening), suppression of collagen accumulation in lesions, and widening of coronary artery lumina, even when the monkeys consumed an atherogenic diet. Serum total cholesterol was the same in both exercised and nonexercised monkeys; however, HDL cholesterol was significantly higher, and total triglyceride (LDL plus VLDL triglyceride) was much lower in the exercise group [32].

The hypothesis that exercise elevates HDL-cholesterol levels, resulting in protection from coronary artery disease, is an attractive theory, but it remains unproven. The balance of evidence indicates that a sedentary lifestyle is likely to be harmful. A program of regular physical activity, provided it is begun prudently, is likely to be beneficial and without risk. Not only may it be protective with respect to CHD, but it is likely to help control obesity and create a sense of well-being. For these reasons, although definitive proof of the beneficial effects is lacking, promotion of physical activity should be included in any health education program for the prevention of CHD.

Psychosocial Stress It has long been believed by many clinicians and lay people that psychosocial factors, including stress, are important in the genesis of CHD, and much epidemiological evidence has been presented to support this notion. Two reviews by Jenkins cited findings from more than 200 papers, the majority of which reported a relationship between CHD and such psychological or social variables as education, religion, income, occupation, social mobility, and stressful life events [19]. "Stress" is possibly an important risk factor for CHD; however, quantification of stress remains a problem in these studies.

Diet The importance of plasma cholesterol levels in the development of CHD has led to a search for the factors that determine serum cholesterol levels in individuals and populations. Dietary factors have long been thought to play a major role in influencing plasma cholesterol levels.

In 1908, Ignatowski, investigating the effects of animal protein from meat, milk, and eggs in rabbits, observed intimal lesions of the aorta that resembled those of human atherosclerosis [33]. Anitschkow in 1913 traced the effects of these foods to cholesterol by feeding rabbits the pure chemical dissolved in vegetable oil and producing identical lesions [34]. These observations were later extended to dogs, swine, pigeons, and rats. However, today it is known that in most animals except primates the lipoprotein profile is different from that of humans. Man has more LDL and less HDL than laboratory animals. The study of rhesus monkeys, which showed that atherosclerotic lesions developed during 17 months of high-cholesterol feeding and regressed after feeding cholesterol-free chow for 40 months, was an important advance [35].

Associations between diet, serum cholesterol, and atherosclerotic disease in humans were suggested during World War II, when food rationing in northern Europe led to lowered total caloric intakes, a higher proportion of carbohydrate calories, and a reduced proportion of all dietary fats as well as cholesterol. Although the data have many shortcomings, it is generally agreed that mortality from atherosclerotic disease decreased abruptly in the early years of the war and rose after cessation of hostilities.

These observations were then followed by a number of epidemiological studies which suggested that populations with a low incidence of atherosclerosis tend to consume diets high in vegetables and populations with an increased prevalence of atherosclerosis tend to consume a fat-rich diet high in dairy products, meat, and eggs. In international comparisons there were also strong correlations between CHD and sucrose intake, protein intake, and per capita income, as well as other factors. In the view of the authors, the strongest case can be made for the relationship between saturated fat and CHD; however, a number of other nutrients have been implicated, and the data relating to them will be briefly reviewed.

Dietary Fat There is no evidence, either observational or experimental, that conclusively demonstrates a causative relationship between dietary fat per se and human atherosclerotic disease. The linkage between disease causation and dietary fat intake in humans is an indirect one. Keys first suggested that differences in incidence of CHD between different countries correlated with differences in fat intake of their populations. In the Seven Countries Study, based on prospective observations of 18 populations in 7 countries (Finland, Greece, Italy, Japan, the Netherlands, the United States, and Yugoslavia), investigators compared the incidence of heart disease over a 10-year period among 12,000 men who were between 40 and 59 years of age at the beginning of the study [36]. As shown in Figure 8-2, mean rates of heart disease varied four fold, with the highest rates in the United States and Finland and the lowest in

FIGURE 8-2
Shaded bars represent the average percentage of total dietary calories provided by saturated fatty acids. Solid bars represent the 5-year incidence of CHD. (*From A. Keys, ed., Circulation, 41 (suppl. 1):1, 1970.*)

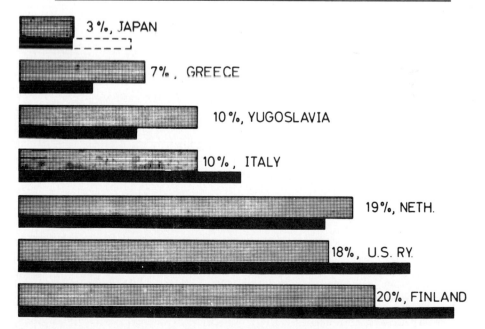

MEN 40-59, % DIET CALORIES PROVIDED BY SATURATED F.A.

3%, JAPAN

7%, GREECE

10%, YUGOSLAVIA

10%, ITALY

19%, NETH.

18%, U.S. RY.

20%, FINLAND

NARROW, SOLID BARS SHOW CHD INCIDENCE RATE

Japan. The rates were significantly correlated with the serum cholesterol concentration and also with the saturated fat intake of the populations (see Table 8-5). Other components of the diets, which included total calories, total fat, monounsaturated and polyunsaturated fats, and total protein, were not significantly correlated with incidence of heart disease.

Individuals from populations that have a characteristically low plasma cholesterol level, who migrate to an area in which the population has a characteristically high plasma cholesterol level, acquire an elevated cholesterol level [37]. A comparison of saturated fat consumption, blood lipids, and coronary-event rates in indigenous Japanese, migrant Japanese in Hawaii, and migrant Japanese in Los Angeles reveals parallel increases in all three.

Studies of individuals within a single population reveal a paradox. Such studies have consistently failed to detect a relationship between individual intake of saturated fat, the level of plasma cholesterol, and risk of CHD. The Framingham Study reported that no statistical relationship between any of the measured dietary components (saturated fat, cholesterol, sucrose, or energy) and serum cholesterol could be shown [38]. The explanation for this finding may be that the dietary intake patterns are very similar in all socioeconomic groups in the United States.

Within the United States, several studies have compared various types of vegetarians with their meat-eating counterparts [39,40]. Vegetarians (lacto-ovo-vegetarians as well as strict vegetarians) whose diets are low in cholesterol and

TABLE 8-5
DIETARY FAT, SERUM CHOLESTEROL, AND 10-YEAR CORONARY HEART DISEASE (CHD) MORTALITY RATE, MEN ORIGINALLY AGE 40–59, SEVEN COUNTRY STUDY*

Cohort	Total fat, % calories	Saturated fat, % calories	Polyun-saturated fat, % calories	Serum cholesterol Median	Serum cholesterol 90th percentile	10-year mortality CHD	10-year mortality All
Greece	36	7	3	201	258	9	57
Yugoslavia	31	5	5	171[†]	219[†]	12[†]	105[†]
Italy	26	9	3	198	253	21	126
Rome (railroad workers)	—	—	—	207	260	22	75
United States (railroad workers)	40	18	5	236	294	57	115
Finland	37	20	3	259	323	65	167
Netherlands	40	18	5	230	291	44	125

*Keys, A. (ed.): Coronary heart disease in seven countries, Circulation 41: Suppl. 1, 1970.
†Excludes Belgrade and Slavonia.
Source: J. Stamler, in Nutrition, Lipids and Coronary Heart Disease, R. Levy et al. (eds.), Raven, New York, 1979.

saturated fat but relatively high in polyunsaturated fats and plant sterols have lower plasma cholesterol levels and a lower prevalence of CHD; they also fail to show the increase in plasma cholesterol level with age that is regularly seen in nonvegetarians in developed societies.

Cholesterol   Comparisons of population groups have shown a strongly positive correlation between the intake of dietary cholesterol, total plasma cholesterol, LDL-cholesterol levels, and atherosclerotic disease mortality. Because intake of cholesterol is always associated with intake of fat (especially saturated fats), similar positive correlations occur with total fat, animal fat, and saturated fat. Thus, it is impossible to identify an independent effect of dietary cholesterol per se from epidemiological studies.

Carbohydrates   Some epidemiological data have related the increased death rates from CHD in industrialized nations to an increased dietary intake of carbohydrate, particularly of sucrose. Yudkin reviewed patterns and trends in carbohydrate consumption throughout the world and concluded that wealthier nations with the highest death rates from CHD consume the most sugar [41]. However, countries with high per capita consumption of sugar also have high per capita consumption of saturated fat and high CHD rates. Partial correlation analysis shows that when sugar is held constant, CHD is highly correlated with per capita consumption of saturated fats, but when fat is constant, there is no significant correlation between sugar in the diet and the initial CHD incidence rate [42]. Yudkin's analysis also has notable gaps; his comparison did not include Cuba and Venezuela, the Latin American countries having the highest sugar intakes and low CHD rates. In contrast, the epidemiological data suggest that if starch, a complex carbohydrate, has any effect on CHD, it is a beneficial one. Countries where the intake of starch is high tend to have low rates of CHD.

Fiber   Fiber is a generic term for substances that are generally regarded as indigestible or nonnutritive. Although even this definition is open to debate, fiber is generally understood to be plant residues. *Dietary fiber,* the skeletal remains of plant cells that are resistant to hydrolysis by human digestive enzymes, includes cellulose, hemicellulose, pectin, and the noncarbohydrate lignin. *Crude fiber* (data for which are given in most food composition tables) is a measurement of the residue of plant food after extraction with acid, alkali, water, alcohol, and ether and is not the same as dietary fiber [43]. Crude fiber includes lignin and cellulose. Burkitt has hypothesized that a diet deficient in fiber is one of the causes of many diseases of western civilization, including CHD [44,45]. Trowell was the first to show that rural Africans with a high intake of dietary fiber have low blood cholesterol levels and a low incidence of heart disease. As the African has become semiurbanized, the incidence of CHD has increased; it is highest in the urban African [44]. During the African's migration through successive steps toward urbanization, the quantity of dietary fiber ingested has decreased. However, many other concomitant changes in dietary intake and lifestyle have occurred, including increased consumption of meat, saturated fat, and cholesterol. Hence, epidemiological data linking CHD and lack of dietary fiber are circumstantial at best. Apart from the African, no other races have been so closely observed, and no real attempt to quantify differences in fiber intake at the international level has been reported.

Alcohol   A few recent studies have associated modest alcohol consumption with reduced risk of CHD [46]. Of particular interest is the observation that such alcohol intake, while also increasing levels of VLDL, may promote increased levels of HDL. However, excessive alcohol intake can produce cardiomyopathy and is associated with much morbidity and an overall excess mortality, so that these new observations must be treated with caution.

EFFECTS OF DIET ON PLASMA LIPID CONCENTRATIONS

Dietary Fats, Sterols, and Triglycerides: Composition

Cholesterol is the most abundant of the animal sterols, and it is the only one absorbed in appreciable amounts by the intestine. It is synthesized exclusively by animal tissues, which, together with other animal products such as milk and eggs, form the main source of cholesterol in our diet. The cholesterol content of some common foods is summarized in Table 8-6.

Human plasma cholesterol is carried primarily in LDL and to a lesser extent in HDL and VLDL. Plasma cholesterol is derived from two sources and is eliminated by one main pathway. One source is the diet, which may contribute about 500 mg per day to the total body cholesterol pool of the average American. The absorbed cholesterol enters the plasma and is directly additive to the amount derived from body synthesis, approximately 500 to 1000 mg per day. In the steady state, cholesterol intake is balanced by its excretion in the bile, which contains both the neutral sterol cholesterol and its acidic derivatives, the bile acids, formed by the hepatic catabolism of cholesterol. Most of the bile acids are reabsorbed in the terminal ileum; hence an average of 700 to 1000 mg sterol is eliminated each day.

In the American population, with the exception of a fall in cholesterol concentration at puberty, there is a steady rise in cholesterol concentration until a maximum is reached at about the age of 55 to 60. At the age of 21, the mean plasma cholesterol concentration is approximately 180 mg/dl. After the age of 25, on the typical American diet, this value will predictably rise to between 200 and 250 mg/dl. The effect of dietary feeding of cholesterol is an extremely complex question and is discussed later in this chapter in conjunction with the effect of intake of saturated and polyunsaturated fats.

Plant sterols represent a relatively minor constituent of the diet unless one intentionally consumes large amounts, e.g., in a medication that contains β-Sitosterol. β-Sitosterol competes with cholesterol for intestinal absorption. When ingested in large quantities, it can reduce plasma cholesterol levels.

The simple fats or triglycerides consist of triesters of fatty acids that are found in most foods, although insignificant amounts occur in fruits, grain products, and most vegetables. Naturally occurring fatty acids are primarily long unbranched hydrocarbon chains (saturated, monounsaturated, or polyunsaturated) with an

TABLE 8-6
CHOLESTEROL CONTENT OF COMMON MEASURES OF SELECTED FOODS

Food	Amount	Cholesterol, mg
Milk: skim, fluid, or reconstituted dry	1 cup	5
Cottage cheese, uncreamed	$\frac{1}{2}$ cup	7
Lard	1 tbsp	12
Cream, light table	1 oz	20
Cottage cheese, creamed	$\frac{1}{2}$ cup	24
Cream, half and half	$\frac{1}{4}$ cup	26
Ice cream, regular, approximately 10% fat	$\frac{1}{2}$ cup	27
Cheese, cheddar	1 oz	28
Milk, whole	1 cup	34
Butter	1 tbsp	35
Oysters, salmon	3 oz, cooked	40
Clams, halibut, tuna	3 oz, cooked	55
Chicken, turkey (light meat)	3 oz, cooked	67
Beef, pork, lobster, chicken, turkey (dark meat)	3 oz, cooked	75
Lamb, veal, crab	3 oz, cooked	85
Shrimp	3 oz, cooked	130
Heart, beef	3 oz, cooked	230
Egg	1 yolk or 1 egg	250
Liver: beef, calf, hog, lamb	3 oz, cooked	370
Kidney	3 oz, cooked	680
Brains	3 oz, raw	> 1700

Source: R. M. Feeley, P. E. Criner, and B. K. Watt, J. Am. Diet. Assoc., 61:134, 1972.

even number of carbon atoms. There are variations in their chain length, in the number of double bonds in the carbon chain, and in the structural configuration of the molecule, i.e., cis versus trans isomerism. Fatty acids can be classified into three groups: saturated, monounsaturated, and polyunsaturated. At room temperature, the short-chain fatty acids of less than 10 to 11 carbon atoms are liquid, whereas the long-chain hydrocarbons are solid. Myristic ($C_{14:0}$), palmitic ($C_{16:0}$), and stearic ($C_{18:0}$) acids are the most abundant saturated fatty acids found in foods as triglycerides. Saturated fats are found predominantly in animal products, such as the fat of beef, pork, lamb, and poultry and in dairy products. Some vegetable fats, including coconut, palm kernel, and cashew nut oils, cocoa butter (which is a fat in chocolate), and, to some extent, hydrogenated vegetable shortenings, are predominantly saturated. Monounsaturated fatty acids contain a single double bond; by far the most common of these in nature is oleic acid ($C_{18:1}$). The composition of some commonly used fats is given in Table 8-7.

TABLE 8-7
DIETARY SOURCES OF FAT AND RELATIVE AMOUNTS OF SATURATED AND
UNSATURATED FATTY ACIDS

	Amount	Total fat, g	Saturated fat, g	Unsaturated fat	
				Oleic, g	Linoleic, g
Meats:					
Sirloin steak, fat and lean, broiled	3 oz	27	13	12	1
Sirloin steak, lean, broiled	3 oz	6	3	3	Trace
Ground beef, regular, broiled	3 oz	17	8	8	Trace
Ground beef, lean, broiled	3 oz	10	5	4	Trace
Ham, fat and lean, roasted	3 oz	19	7	8	2
Lamb, leg roast, fat and lean	3 oz	16	9	6	Trace
Veal, fat and lean, roasted	3 oz	9	5	4	Trace
Chicken, white meat, broiled	3 oz	3	1	1	1
Tuna, oil-packed	3 oz	7	2	1	1
Dairy products:					
Milk, 3.5% fat	1 cup	9	5	3	Trace
Milk, fortified low fat	1 cup	5	3	2	Trace
Cream, 12%	1 tbsp	3	2	1	Trace
Butter	1 tbsp	12	6	4	Trace
Cheese, cheddar	1 oz	9	5	3	Trace
Cheese, cream	1 oz	11	6	4	Trace
Egg, large	1	6	2	3	Trace
Yogurt	1 cup	4	2	1	Trace
Ice cream, 10% fat	1 cup	14	8	5	Trace
Vegetable fats:					
Margarine, regular	1 tbsp	12	2	6	3
Margarine, special	1 tbsp	11	2	4	4
Mayonnaise	1 tbsp	11	2	2	6
Oils					
Safflower	1 tbsp	14	1	2	10
Corn	1 tbsp	14	1	4	7
Soybean	1 tbsp	14	2	3	7
Cottonseed	1 tbsp	14	4	3	7
Peanut	1 tbsp	14	3	7	4
Olive	1 tbsp	14	2	11	1
Coconut	1 tbsp	14	12	1	Trace
Avocado, 3$\frac{1}{8}$-in diameter	1	37	7	17	5
Peanut butter	1 tbsp	8	2	4	2
Peanuts	$\frac{1}{2}$ cup	36	8	15	10
Cashews	$\frac{1}{2}$ cup	32	5	22	2
Walnuts, English	$\frac{1}{2}$ cup	38	2	13	18

Source: Nutritive Value of Foods, Home and Garden Bulletin no. 72, U.S. Department of Agriculture, 1971.

The degree of unsaturation affects the chemical reactivity of a fatty acid and its glyceride. At room temperature, all the common unsaturated fatty acids are liquid. These fatty acids exist as either cis or trans isomers because of the presence of double bonds in the molecule. Most naturally occurring unsaturated fatty acids occur in the cis form, but trans isomers are also found in small quantities. Relatively large quantities of fatty acids are converted from the cis form to the trans form as a result of heating or hydrogenation. This change occurs in the preparation of certain margarines.

Polyunsaturated fats can be partially hydrogenated by hydrogen gas in the presence of nickel or platinum as a catalyst. This hydrogenation reaction transforms liquid vegetable oil into solid cooking fat. In this process, the double bonds take up hydrogen, which yields a partially saturated product. The most abundant naturally occurring polyunsaturated acids are linoleic ($C_{18:2}$), linolenic ($C_{18:3}$), and arachidonic ($C_{20:4}$) acids. These fatty acids are sometimes referred to as *essential fatty acids,* since they cannot be synthesized in the body in quantities adequate to meet metabolic needs.

Direct Metabolic Experiments

The mass of observational data summarized under "Epidemiology" is supplemented by studies in which diet has been adjusted in groups of individuals. These studies show that plasma cholesterol levels can be readily lowered by means of reduction of dietary saturated fat and cholesterol intake; this has been achieved in both institutionalized and free-living populations and in normal and hypercholesterolemic subjects [47,48]. Both primary prevention trials of apparently healthy men and secondary prevention trials of men who have already had a myocardial infarct or other evidence of disease, in which the amount of dietary saturated fat and/or cholesterol is diminished, leave no doubt that plasma cholesterol concentrations fall, but effects on CHD morbidity and mortality are equivocal.

Effect of Dietary Fat on Plasma Lipids The relationship between the consumption of dietary fats and the concentration of plasma lipids and lipoproteins is complex. Furthermore, since 1 g of fat provides 9 kcal of energy, fat represents a major source of energy in the diet. The typical American derives about 40 to 45 percent of his or her calories from fat.

There have been multiple, detailed, direct metabolic studies in humans on the effects of dietary saturated and polyunsaturated fatty acids on plasma cholesterol. Before 1952, the total fat content of the diet was considered to be the controlling factor in determining blood cholesterol concentrations. In that year Kinsell reported that animal fats raised plasma cholesterol, while vegetable fats lowered it [49]. Keys later found that, gram for gram, saturated fats were twice as effective in raising the blood cholesterol as polyunsaturated fats were in lowering it, while monounsaturated fats had no effect [50]. Keys et al. [51]

empirically derived the following expression for relating dietary polyunsaturated and saturated fats to changes in plasma cholesterol:

$$\Delta Y = 1.35(2\Delta S - \Delta P)$$

where ΔY = change in plasma cholesterol concentration, mg/dl
       S = amount of saturated triglyceride expressed as a percentage of total dietary calories
       P = amount of polyunsaturated triglyceride expressed as a percentage of total dietary calories

In the few studies that have strictly tested the interaction of dietary cholesterol and degree of saturation of dietary fat, the addition of cholesterol to a saturated fat diet of healthy normolipidemic adults has led to a slightly larger increase in plasma cholesterol level than when cholesterol was added to a polyunsaturated fat diet [52].

Truswell has summarized what is known about the contribution of individual fatty acids in dietary triglycerides (Table 8-8) [53]. In general, saturated fatty acids have a stronger elevating effect than the cholesterol-lowering effect of linoleic acid, but the effect of saturated fats is mainly due to palmitic acid, which is more abundant in dietary fats than myristic acid. Chain length thus partly determines the activity. Saturated fatty acids containing 10 carbons or less and medium-chain triglycerides (MCTs), though saturated, do not increase plasma cholesterol, and, surprisingly, stearic acid has less elevating effect than palmitic acid.

Sinclair proposes that the high ratio of certain nonessential to essential fatty acids (non-EFA:EFA) in the body is the most important factor in atherosclerotic

TABLE 8-8
EFFECTS OF DIFFERENT DIETARY FATTY ACIDS ON PLASMA CHOLESTEROL, AS DEMONSTRATED IN ACUTE EXPERIMENTS IN HUMANS

Dietary fatty acid	Plasma cholesterol
Medium-chain triglycerides, $C_{8:0}$ to $C_{10:0}$	0
Lauric, $C_{12:0}$	↑
Myristic, $C_{14:0}$	↑↑
Palmitic, $C_{16:0}$	↑↑
Stearic, $C_{18:0}$	?↑
Oleic, $C_{18:1}$	0
Linoleic, $C_{18:2}$	↓
Other polyunsaturated	↓

Source: Adapted from A. S. Truswell, Bibl. Nutr. Dieta, 25:53, 1977.

disease and coronary thrombosis [54]. Medium-chain saturated fatty acids (lauric and myristic, as in coconut oil) are strongly atherogenic but do not greatly affect the thrombotic tendency of blood. The thrombotic tendency is increased by long-chain fatty acids (palmitic and stearic) and reduced by linoleic acid ($C_{18:2}$) and its derivative, arachidonic acid ($C_{20:4}$), and by linolenic acid ($C_{18:3}$) and its derivatives, and long-chain highly unsaturated fatty acids ($C_{20:5}$ and $C_{22:6}$) present in fish oils.

Effect of Dietary Cholesterol on Plasma Lipids Dietary studies in humans have produced much conflicting and often confusing evidence. Some of the early studies were misinterpreted because cholesterol was not fed in a form suitable for absorption. Cholesterol must be dissolved in other fats in order to be absorbed. A recent comprehensive review concluded that in healthy adults who are normolipidemic by United States standards, plasma cholesterol concentration increases as cholesterol intake increases within the range of 0 to 600 mg per day [55] (see Figure 8-3). For each additional 100 mg dietary cholesterol per 1000 kcal, estimates of the average increase in plasma cholesterol vary from 3 to 12 mg/dl. Dietary cholesterol above about 600 mg per day produces no additional effect in most persons. Further, the response tends to be greater if dietary cholesterol is combined with saturated fat. Few hyperlipidemic subjects have been studied, but available data indicate that their responses to dietary cholesterol are more variable. No estimate of an average response for persons with any specific type of hyperlipidemia can be made.

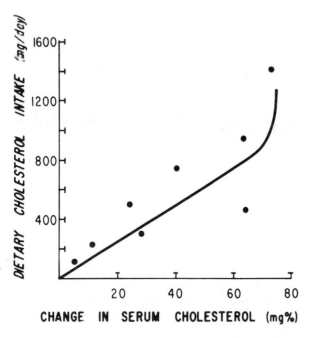

FIGURE 8-3
The effects of different intakes of dietary cholesterol levels in humans. The base-line data in all instances were virtually cholesterol-free. (*From C. J. Glueck and W. E. Connor, Am. J. Clin. Nutr., 31:727, 1978.*)

In most diets, the intake of cholesterol and saturated fat is closely linked, and most diets designed to control hyperlipidemia include reduction of both components. However, the independent contribution of dietary cholesterol to hypercholesterolemia may be important with regard to a specific food, namely, egg yolks. Eggs (about 250 mg cholesterol per yolk) contribute about 46 percent of the total cholesterol, but only 4 percent of total fat and 3 percent of saturated fat, to the average American diet [55].

Effect of Dietary Carbohydrate on Plasma Lipids   It has been shown that carbohydrate, in substantial quantities, influences serum lipids, particularly triglycerides [56]. Palumbo et al. reported that 2 g of simple carbohydrate per kilogram of body weight had no effect on serum triglycerides, but diets containing 4 g of simple carbohydrate (predominantly sucrose) were associated with a significant rise in serum triglycerides that was greater in CHD patients than in normal controls [57]. However, the elevation in triglycerides was short-term (a few days or weeks), and the amount of sugar consumed was greater than that usually eaten. Further, as pointed out elsewhere, the independent contribution of serum triglycerides to the risk of CHD is conjectural.

Dietary carbohydrates have been shown to have less effect on serum cholesterol than on triglycerides. In isocaloric experiments in which sucrose was substituted for starches (for 23 percent of dietary energy), there was no effect on plasma cholesterol in healthy subjects. This is more than the average sucrose consumption in western industrial countries. When sucrose is 34 percent of total energy, plasma cholesterol levels increased 5 percent [58].

Effect of Dietary Fiber on Plasma Lipids   Hypotheses and controversies regarding dietary fiber were featured at the Fifth Annual Marabou Symposium: Food and Fiber, held in 1977 [59]. Specific studies of the effect of dietary fiber on blood lipid levels have neither proved nor disproved Burkitt's hypothesis that the amount of fiber in the diet is related to the incidence of CHD in a population [45]. Studies in humans have also been hampered by an imprecise definition of dietary fiber and by the failure to distinguish between its constituents in experimental studies. However, there appears to be a pattern of results from experiments stimulated by this hypothesis [60,61]. In humans with normal blood cholesterol levels, rolled oats, Bengal gram (chick pea), and pectin are hypocholesterolemic, whereas wheat fiber, cellulose, and lignin are not. The mechanism by which dietary fiber acts on cholesterol has not been established. One suggested mechanism involves the binding and excretion of bile salts [62]. This action would reduce cholesterol absorption and increase its turnover. However, additional research is necessary to further define dietary fiber and clarify its relationship to serum lipids and CHD.

Effect of Alcohol on Plasma Lipids   The effects of alcohol vary with the frequency with which and the amounts in which it is consumed, and with individual sensitivity, etc. Moderate social drinking can double plasma trigly-cerides acutely; there is a smaller effect on cholesterol [63]. In groups of alcoholics, triglycerides are significantly elevated but total cholesterol is not [64]. Alcoholics tend also to have high HDL levels. The association between alcohol and HDL was first recognized by Johansson and Laurell [65]. Berg and Johansson, in a subsequent study, monitored the effects of beer (60 g of ethanol per day) on healthy students over a period of 5 weeks and noticed a slow but significant climb in plasma HDL [66]. They later found HDL cholesterol was increased to over 200 mg/dl in chronic alcoholics after drinking bouts [67]. Still unresolved is the significance of alcohol-induced hyperlipidemia as a risk factor in CHD.

PATHOGENESIS

The normal artery wall contains three layers: the intima which consists of a single continuous layer of endothelial cells; the media, which consists of only smooth muscle cells; and the adventitia, which is an admixture of collagen, elastic fibers, smooth muscle cells, and fibroblasts. Atherosclerosis is apparently multifactorial in its origin and progression, and a number of theories have been proposed to explain this. Endothelium seems to be important in determining the rate of entrance of circulating materials, including lipoproteins, into the blood vessel wall and in maintaining the nonthrombogenicity of the vascular surface. Smooth muscle cells elaborate the extensive connective tissue matrix of the arterial wall and metabolize those circulating components which gain entrance to the vessel wall. Alterations in the functional or structural integrity of the endothelial lining are thought to be an early event in the pathogenesis of atherosclerosis. Consequences of endothelial changes include increased throm-bogenicity and increased entrance of circulating plasma components, including lipoproteins, into the blood vessel wall. Platelet adhesion and aggregation quickly follow; platelets contain a mitogen which can stimulate smooth muscle proliferation in vitro. Increased connective tissue synthesis is also closely linked to cell proliferation. Specific stimuli at the cellular level for increased synthesis of connective tissue protein have not been identified. With loss of endothelial integrity it is assumed that an increased influx of lipoprotein occurs, which may result in progressive accumulation of lipids by the vascular smooth muscle cells. The capacity of the smooth muscle cells to balance catabolism of lipoproteins and synthesis of lipids may determine their susceptibility to intracellular lipid accumulation. If ingress of substrate exceeds egress of the product, lipid accumulation results. It is possible that many "risk factors" exert an influence on this influx-efflux balance. For example, the relationship between LDL and HDL levels and risk of disease may derive at least in part from the putative role attributed to LDL of carrying cholesterol to the cell and to HDL of carrying cholesterol away from the cell [68]. However, the mechanisms by which risk factors exert their influence at the cellular level await identification.

CLINICAL MANIFESTATIONS

No symptoms of atherosclerosis appear until atheromatous plaques obstruct the lumen of a blood vessel and cause ischemia or infarction with death of a tissue. In the coronary arteries this results in angina pectoris (due to transient localized myocardial ischemia) or myocardial infarction and, possibly, sudden death. In the arteries of the neck and circle of Willis it results in stroke—either transient ischemic attacks due to platelet microemboli or full-blown permanent damage with infarction of brain tissue. In the leg arteries, atherosclerosis causes claudication and gangrene, and in the renal arteries it may produce hypertension and poor renal function.

DIAGNOSIS

History

The history should carefully review the cardiovascular system, and a complete family history should be obtained in which the presence or absence of familial hypercholesterolemia, hypertriglyceridemia, diabetes mellitus, hypertension, and obesity is ascertained, as well as the presence or absence of heart disease. A dietary history, including the usual pattern of food intake and estimates of the frequency of consumption of various types of food, may assist in determining factors contributing to hyperlipidemia.

Physical Examination

Clinical findings which suggest that a patient should undergo further lipid studies include the following:

1 *Xanthelasma:* Deposit of lipid, primarily cholesterol, in soft tissue surrounding the eye (Color Figure 16).

2 *Arcus senilis or arcus corneae:* Deposition of cholesterol on the posterior surface of the cornea adjacent to the limbus. It appears as a faint blue-gray opacity which may be almost invisible in individuals with blue or green pigmentation of the iris but is readily apparent in those who have dark-brown pigmentation of the iris. Arcus senilis is very common in individuals in their seventies or eighties, but when it is found in people less than 40 years old, it has much greater significance.

3 *Tendinous xanthoma:* Lipid deposits consisting primarily of cholesteryl ester, which are found on extensor tendons of hands and on the Achilles tendon.

4 *Tuberous or eruptive xanthomas:* Small red-orange elevations; can be found on face, buttocks, mucous membranes, elbows, and knees (Color Figure 17).

5 *Plantar of palmar xanthoma:* Yellowish lipid deposits seen in creases of palm or digital creases (Color Figure 18).

6 *Hepatomegaly:* Enlargement of the liver.

7 *Obesity:* Although obesity does not contribute directly to CHD, it may be accompanied by an elevation of the arterial blood pressure or by diabetes mellitus, both of which are associated with the development of CHD.

Biochemical Tests

There is no blood test for atherosclerosis; however, practically all patients with myocardial infarction, as defined by electrocardiographic and enzyme changes, have coronary atherosclerosis. For the purposes of a careful lipid appraisal, a profile consisting of plasma total cholesterol, HDL cholesterol, and triglycerides is sufficient in most cases. The blood sample should be obtained after a 12- to 14-hour fast, and it should be stored at 4°C. The measurement should be done when the subject is in a steady state—i.e., stable weight, no acute illness within the previous 4 to 6 weeks, no medications (especially hypolipidemic agents or hormones), and a regular diet for at least 2 weeks prior to sampling. Pregnancy, myocardial infarction, and stress can be expected to affect lipid levels. The presence of a creamy layer at the top of the sample after storage at 4°C overnight identifies the presence of chylomicrons. This observation suggests either a nonfasting subject or an abnormality that should be investigated. Cloudiness, or turbidity, of the plasma without evidence of chylomicrons is caused by increased concentration of triglycerides, which are carried by the VLDL. Clear plasma may contain an elevated concentration of cholesterol, which is carried by the LDL. LDL cholesterol can be estimated from the following formula [69]:

$$\text{LDL cholesterol} = \text{total cholesterol} - \text{HDL cholesterol} - \tfrac{1}{5}\,\text{triglyceride}$$

"Normal" values of lipid and lipoprotein concentrations are listed in Table 8-2. However, these normal values are arbitrary and would be better designated "average" values. Lower values may be more desirable. In adults under 55 years of age, a cholesterol concentration greater than 250 mg/dl or a triglyceride concentration greater than 200 mg/dl clearly indicates hyperlipidemia sufficient to require attention by the physician to the items listed in Table 8-9.

If the patient's plasma cholesterol or triglyceride levels are elevated, it is desirable to do a lipid profile by electrophoresis. The underlying cause of hyperlipidemia may be metabolic, genetic, or secondary to another disorder. If hyperlipidemia is secondary to another disease, then treatment of the underlying disease must be attempted. No further treatment of lipid elevation should be undertaken until the basic disorder has been controlled. Potential causes of hyperlipidemia include dietary excess, diabetes mellitus, hypothyroidism, pancreatitis, dysproteinemia, nephrosis, hepatobiliary diseases, and alcoholism. Therefore, measurements of blood levels of glucose, thyroxin, thyroid-stimulating hormone, blood urea nitrogen, creatinine, bilirubin, and alkaline phosphatase are indicated.

Physiological Tests

In addition to a routine electrocardiogram, assessment of electrocardiographic changes induced during standardized exercise is a relatively simple noninvasive aid to the diagnosis of coronary atherosclerosis. Another technique which demonstrates the presence of atherosclerosis is cardiac angiography. Angiographic visualization of deformity in the lumen of the vessel remains the best

TABLE 8-9
FACTORS TO CONSIDER IN PATIENTS WITH HYPERLIPIDEMIA

Genetic disorders

Family history of hyperlipoproteinemia
History of pancreatitis or recurrent abdominal pain

Secondary hyperlipidemia	
Biliary obstruction	Dysproteinemias (multiple my-
Dietary factors:	eloma, lupus erythematosus)
Kilocalories (recent weight	Hypothyroidism
gain)	Nephrotic hypoproteinemia
Saturated fats	Multiple myeloma
Cholesterol	Nephrotic hypoproteinemia
Alcohol	Uncontrolled diabetes mellitus
Drugs producing hyperlipi-	Uremia
demia:	
Oral contraceptives	
Estrogens	
Glucocorticoids	

presumptive test of silent atherosclerosis. In this procedure a radiopaque medium is injected into the circulatory system through a catheter passed into the heart, and a cine-angiogram is made. The angiogram shows where arteries are blocked, how extensive the blockage is, and how the heart is functioning. Coronary angiography permits visualization and assessment of arteries as small as 0.5 mm in diameter.

MANAGEMENT

Since there is no single cause of hyperlipidemia, there is no single all-encompassing treatment; however, diet is the cornerstone of therapy. Often no other treatment is necessary. Lipid concentrations should be followed after treatment is started. If after several weeks the therapy is ineffective, then it must be modified. The diet should be continued if additional therapy, such as lipid-lowering drugs, are added to the regimen.

Dietary Management

A single dietary approach to all forms of hyperlipidemia, including reduced intake of energy, cholesterol, and saturated fats, is appropriate for most patients. The degree of dietary restriction should be proportional to the degree of hyperlipidemia. However, the point cannot be overemphasized that the diet must be tailored and modified to the individual patient. It is essential to bear in mind the medical history and other factors that may require modification of the diet (e.g., presence of hypertension, patient's food likes and dislikes). The dietary prescription must be explained to a patient in terms of food products and serving sizes. Since the diet is effective only as long as the patient complies, it must not be too extreme; that is, it must be practicable. A dietitian can play an important role in interpreting the prescription and in adapting it to the individual and his family.

Control of personal habits, especially cigarette smoking, should also be stressed. Physical activity should be increased gradually by provision of some form of regular exercise, such as swimming, bicycling, tennis, jogging, or any other activity compatible with the patient's physical condition and personal inclinations. The abrupt adoption of a program of vigorous exercise may have serious, even fatal, consequences.

Appropriate regimens are selected from the following elements:

1 Restriction of dietary cholesterol to reduce elevated LDL levels. Dietary cholesterol is found exclusively in foods containing animal fat. Examples of foods especially rich in cholesterol are egg yolks, dairy products (cheese and whole milk), and organ meats (liver and kidney) (see Table 8-6).

2 Reduction of saturated fat intake, and substitution of polyunsaturated fats. The polyunsaturated-saturated fat ratio (P:S) is raised to about 2.0. In calculating the P:S ratio, the total grams of linoleic acid in the diet are divided by the total grams of saturated fatty acids.

$$P:S = \frac{\text{linoleic acid (g)}}{\text{saturated fatty acid (g)}}$$

Polyunsaturated vegetable oils are substituted for solid shortening in cooking, and a polyunsaturated margarine is used in place of butter. Certain vegetable fats such as palm oil and coconut oil are rich in saturated fats and should be avoided (see Table 8-7).

3 A program of weight reduction for obese subjects, followed by a weight maintenance program.

4 A decrease in or the elimination of alcohol intake. This is an important and sometimes vital element for treatment and control of hypertriglyceridemia.

Specific dietary guidelines for each type of primary hyperlipoproteinemia have been suggested by Fredrickson et al. and are available from the National Heart and Lung Institute (see Table 8-10) [70]. Sample menus for the more commonly occuring hyperlipoproteinemias, IIa, IIb, and IV, are shown in Tables 8-11 to 8-13.

Drug Therapy

Drug therapy should not be undertaken until the effectiveness of the diet has been tested. Six weeks of diet therapy are desirable, during which time serum lipid values should be recorded at regular intervals. If there is no appreciable

TABLE 8-10
SUMMARY OF DIETS FOR HYPERLIPOPROTEINEMIAS TYPES I TO V

	Type I	Type IIa	Type IIb and Type III	Type IV	Type V
Diet prescription	Low fat (25–35 g)	Low cholesterol; PUF increased	Low cholesterol Approximate calorie breakdown: 20% protein 40% fat 40% CHO	Controlled CHO Approximately 45% of calories Moderately restricted cholesterol	Restricted fat (30% of calories) Controlled CHO (50% of calories) Moderately restricted cholesterol
Calories	Not restricted	Not restricted	Achieve and maintain "ideal" weight, i.e., reduction diet if necessary	Achieve and maintain "ideal" weight, i.e., reduction diet if necessary	Achieve and maintain "ideal" weight, i.e., reduction diet if necessary
Protein	Total protein intake is not limited	Total protein intake is not limited	High protein	Not limited other than control of patient's weight	High protein
Fat	Restricted to 25–35 g	Saturated fat intake limited; PUF intake increased	Controlled to 40% of calories (PUF recommended in preference to saturated fats)	Not limited other than control of patient's weight (PUF recommended in preference to saturated fats)	Restricted to 30% of calories (PUF recommended in preference to saturated fats)
Cholesterol	Not restricted	As low as possible; the only source of cholesterol is the meat in the diet	Less than 300 mg (the only source of cholesterol is the meat in the diet)	Moderately restricted to 300–500 mg	Moderately restricted to 300–500 mg
Carbohydrate	Not limited	Not limited	Controlled, concentrated sweets are restricted	Controlled, concentrated sweets are restricted	Controlled, concentrated sweets are restricted
Alcohol	Not recommended	May be used with discretion	Limited to 2 servings (substituted for CHO)	Limited to 2 servings (substituted for CHO)	Not recommended

Note: PUF, polyunsaturated fat; CHO, carbohydrate.
Source: D. S. Fredrickson, R. I. Levy, M. Bonnel, and N. Ernst, Dietary Management of Hyperlipoproteinemia, U.S. Department of Health, Education, and Welfare, National Heart and Lung Institute, Bethesda, Md., 1973.

TABLE 8-11
SAMPLE MENU FOR ADULT WITH TYPE IIa HYPERLIPOPROTEINEMIA (1700 to 2000 kcal)

Daily food plan	

1 pt or more skim milk
Cooked poultry, fish, or lean
  meat (with fat trimmed off)
5 servings vegetable and fruit,
  including:
    1 serving citrus
    1 serving dark-green or
      deep-yellow vegetable
	7 or more servings whole-
	  grain or enriched bread
	  or cereal
	1 or more servings potato,
	  rice, etc.
	Allowed fat
	Allowed desserts and
	  sweets

Sample menu pattern	

Breakfast:
  Citrus fruit or juice
  Cereal
  Toast
  Allowed fat
  Jelly and sugar
  Skim milk
  Coffee or tea, if desired
	Dinner:
	  Poultry, fish, or lean meat
	  Potato or substitute
	  Vegetable
	  Bread
	  Allowed fat
	  Fruit or allowed dessert
	  Skim milk

Lunch:
  Poultry, fish, or lean meat
  Potato or substitute
  Vegetables
  Bread
  Allowed fat
  Fruit or allowed dessert
  Skim milk
	Between-meal snack:
	  Fruit
	  Skim milk

change in the lipid levels, then the addition of drug therapy should be considered.

Table 8-14 lists the drugs which may be used for the treatment of hyperlipoproteinemia. They fall into two categories: (1) drugs that decrease lipoprotein production and (2) drugs that increase lipoprotein catabolism. Nicotinic acid and clofibrate (Atromid-S) belong to the first group. Clofibrate has also been shown to enhance the catabolism of VLDL. Cholestyramine (Questran), colestipol, D-thyroxine (Choloxin), and probably sitosterol (Cytellin) belong to the second group. All of these drugs have been approved by the Food and Drug Administration for use as hypolipidemic agents [10].

Long-term therapy with a drug should be contingent upon a marked reduction in plasma lipid levels. The criterion for this should be a reduction of approximately 15 percent in lipid levels within 4 to 6 weeks. Patients should also be monitored for potential drug toxicity.

TABLE 8-12

SAMPLE MENU FOR ADULT WITH TYPE IIb HYPERLIPOPROTEINEMIA (2000 kcal)

Daily food plan	
2 servings poultry, fish, or lean meat (with fat trimmed off)	8 servings bread, cereal, etc.
	15 servings allowed fat
	3 servings fruit
3 servings skim milk	Vegetables as desired

Sample menu pattern	
Breakfast:	Dinner:
1 serving citrus fruit or juice	1 serving poultry, fish, or lean meat
2 servings cereal or toast	2 servings potato or substitute
3 servings allowed fat	Vegetables
1 serving skim milk	2 servings bread
Lunch:	6 servings allowed fat
1 serving poultry, fish, or lean meat	1 serving fruit
1 serving potato or substitute	1 serving skim milk
Vegetables	
2 servings bread	
6 servings allowed fat	
1 serving fruit	
1 serving skim milk	

PREVENTION

Probably no other contemporary topic in human nutrition stimulates more controversy than the variety of dietary recommendations being made to the entire American population by various government agencies, health agencies, consumer groups, and health-food advocates. Within a framework of suggestive, but not unequivocal, scientific proof that dietary modification will prevent CHD, physicians must examine the issues for which facts are incomplete and opinions differ.

Epidemiological studies have provided a basis for a preventive approach to CHD. First, they have established that the rate of the disease is not a fixed characteristic of populations; second, they have shown that it is possible to predict the occurrence of the disease in advance; and third, they have pointed to potentially reversible causes [71]. Identified major risk factors for CHD include age, sex, hypercholesterolemia, hypertension, cigarette smoking, and diabetes mellitus. Less certain risk factors include obesity, hypertriglyceridemia, lack of physical activity, and personality type [72].

Age-adjusted mortality from CHD increased 19 percent in the United States from 1950 to 1963 [73]. In 1964, the surgeon general of the U.S. Public Health

TABLE 8-13

SAMPLE MENU FOR ADULT WITH TYPE IV HYPERLIPOPROTEINEMIA (1800 kcal)*

Daily food plan	
2 servings poultry, fish, or lean meat (with fat trimmed off)	Allowed fat
	6 servings fruit
2 servings skim milk	Vegetables as desired
8 servings bread, cereal, etc.	

Sample menu pattern	
Breakfast:	Dinner:
2 servings citrus fruit or juice	1 serving poultry, fish, or lean meat
2 servings cereal or toast	1 serving potato or substitute
Allowed fat	Vegetables
1 serving skim milk	2 servings bread
Lunch:	Allowed fat
1 serving poultry, fish, or lean meat	2 servings fruit
1 serving potato or substitute	1 serving skim milk
Vegetables	
2 servings bread	
Allowed fat	
2 servings fruit	

*Limit skim milk, breads, cereals, etc., and fruit as designated. This diet controls only carbohydrate foods. If patient is not able to follow this relatively free diet (an indication might be weight gain), a more strictly controlled diet may be prescribed.

Service warned of the health hazards of cigarette smoking and the American Heart Association recommended a change in the general American diet by limiting the intake of saturated fat and cholesterol [74,75]. A decline in mortality from CHD, the leading cause of death, started in the same year these warnings were issued, and it has continued [76].

Since 1964, there has been a decline in per capita consumption of tobacco (Table 8-15), particularly among middle-aged and older males who are at high risk of death from CHD [77]. Cigarettes containing lower amounts of tar and nicotine may also have reduced their risk. During the same time, however, smoking habits among women have not been consistent with the decline in CHD mortality. Generally, more women are now smoking, and among those who do smoke, daily cigarette consumption has increased. Since 1964, there has also been a decline in per capita consumption of animal fats and oils, butter, liquid milk, cream, and eggs, with an associated increase in consumption of vegetable fats and oils (Table 8-15).

TABLE 8-14
HYPOLIPIDEMIC DRUGS

Drug and dosage	Used to treat elevated levels of:	Drug-nutrient interactions	Side effects
Nicotinic acid, 3–6 g/day	ILDL, VLDL, LDL	Excessive vaso-dilation and hypotensive effects of gan-glionic blocking agents	Flushing, nausea, diarrhea, fatty liver
Clofibrate, 2 g/day	ILDL, VLDL	Increases hypo-prothrombin effect of coumarin	Nausea, diarrhea
Cholestyramine, 12–32 g/day	LDL	Decreased absorption of digitalis, fat-soluble vitamins	Nausea, constipation
Colestipol, 15–30 g/day		Decreased ab-sorption of warfarin, vita-min K	Steatorrhea
D-Thyroxine, 4–8 mg/day	LDL, ILDL	Increased coumadin effect	Increased metab-olism, cardio-toxicity
Sitosterol, 30 ml four times a day	LDL	—	Nausea, diarrhea

The fact that two events occurred together does not establish a causal relation between them. Certainly, other factors, such as better control of hypertension, coronary-care units, improved cardiovascular surgical procedures, and exercise programs, may have contributed to the decline. However, it can be suggested that reduced smoking by men and change in diet had a major role in reversing the trend in coronary mortality.

Hence, the evidence in toto related to CHD suggests that a more moderate diet will lessen the impact of CHD. There are no reasons to believe that such a diet will impose nutritional risks. The authors therefore suggest the following elements for a CHD-prevention regimen:

1 Avoid obesity.
2 Do not smoke cigarettes, and if you smoke a pipe or cigar, do not inhale.

TABLE 8-15

CHANGE IN PER CAPITA CONSUMPTION IN THE UNITED STATES BETWEEN 1963 AND 1975

Product	Change
Tobacco products	−22.4%
Fluid milk and cream	−19.2%
Butter	−31.9%
Eggs	−12.6%
Animal fats and oils	−56.7%
Vegetable fats and oils	+44.1%

Source: W. J. Walker, N. Engl. J. Med., 297:163, 1977.

3 Find some exercise that you enjoy and indulge in it.

4 Eat less animal and dairy fat.

5 Avoid abuses of alcohol, sugar, and other sweets.

Of necessity, recommendations for dietary modification in an entire population group blanket a heterogeneous group of "hypercholesterolemic" subjects. Glueck et al. suggested that risk can be individualized by measurement of fasting plasma cholesterol, HDL cholesterol, and triglyceride [72], which allows estimation of LDL cholesterol [78]. This procedure allows identification of the approximately 1 in 250 Americans with familial hypercholesterolemia who usually require diet and drug treatment [79]. Specific identification could also be made of the approximately 30 percent of Americans with a plasma cholesterol equal to or greater than 250 mg/dl. Hypercholesterolemic patients at higher risk due to elevated LDL cholesterol could be separated from those having elevated HDL cholesterol. Quantification of blood lipids would be particularly important for children, since atherosclerosis begins early in life, long before there is any suspicion of CHD, and prevention must be the best solution to this major public health problem.

CASE STUDY

A 39-year-old plumber was admitted to the hospital with complaints of fatigability and lethargy and for evaluation of possible liver disease. The past history revealed that the man had been a heavy beer drinker (½ to 1 case per day) for 17 years until he stopped drinking 3 years previously. He had a family history of diabetes mellitus, and 3 years earlier had a record of increased liver function tests (SGPT and alkaline phosphatase).

On physical examination the man was found to be 6 feet 7 inches tall and to weigh 260 lb. He appeared healthy and had no enlargement of his spleen or liver on x-ray scan. Blood pressure was recorded at 130/90. Significant laboratory data include the following:

Serum cholesterol	166 mg/dl
Serum triglycerides	686 mg/dl
SGOT (serum aspartate aminotransferase)	60 units/liter
SGPT (serum alanine aminotransferase)	48 units/liter
Alkaline phosphatase	174 units/liter
Glucose tolerance test:	
Fasting	100 mg/dl
½ hour	196 mg/dl
1 hour	124 mg/dl
2 hours	114 mg/dl
3 hours	53 mg/dl

The patient's food intake was 3600 kcal per day (51 percent carbohydrate, 38 percent fat, and 11 percent protein), and he stated that he drank six to nine soft drinks per day. He does not smoke.

Study Questions

1 What risk factors for CHD did the patient have?

2 Describe the presumptive type of hyperlipoproteinemia in this case.

3 How would a plasma lipoprotein electrophoretic analysis aid in the diagnosis?

4 What type of dietary counseling would you suggest for this patient? Is it critical that the type of hyperlipoproteinemia be identified in order to advise him about his diet?

REFERENCES

1 *Report of the National Heart, Lung and Blood Institute Working Group on Heart Disease Epidemiology,* U.S. Department of Health, Education, and Welfare Publication no. (NIH) 79–1667, 1979.

2 Strasser, T.: Atherosclerosis and coronary heart disease: the contribution of epidemiology, WHO Chron., 26:7, 1972.

3 Enos, W. F., J. C. Beyer, and R. H. Holmes: Pathogenesis of coronary disease in American soldiers killed in Korea, J. Am. Med. Assoc., 158:912, 1955.

4 McGill, H. C., Jr., and M. P. Stern: Sex and atherosclerosis, in *Atherosclerosis Reviews,* vol. 4, A. M. Gotto and R. Paoletti (eds.), Raven Press, New York, 1978.

5 McGill, H. C., Jr.: Risk factors for atherosclerosis, Adv. Exp. Med. Bio., 104:273, 1978.

6 Bloor, C. M.: Hereditary aspects of myocardial infarction, Circulation, 39(suppl. 4):130, 1969.

7 Lipid Research Clinic Program Epidemiology Committee: plasma lipid distribution in selected North American populations: the LRC Program Prevalence Study, Circulation, 60:427, 1979.

8 Brown, D. F., S. H. Kinch, and J. T. Doyle: Serum triglycerides in health and in ischemic heart disease, N. Engl. J. Med., 276:947, 1965.

9 Rifkind, B. M., R. S. Goor, and R. I. Levy: Current status of the role of dietary treatment in the prevention and management of coronary heart disease, Med. Clin. North Am., 63:911, 1979.

10 Levy, R. I., J. Morganroth, and B. M. Rifkind: Treatment of hyperlipidemia, N. Engl. J. Med., 290:1295, 1974.

11 LaRosa, J. C.: Secondary hyperlipoproteinemia, in *Hyperlipidemia: Diagnosis and Therapy,* B. M. Rifkind and R. I. Levy (eds.), Grune & Stratton, New York, 1977.

12 Miller, G. J., and N. E. Miller: Plasma high density lipoprotein concentration and development of ischaemic heart disease, Lancet, 1:16, 1975.

13 Gordon, T., W. P. Castelli, M. C. Hjortl, W. B. Kannel, and T. R. Dawber: High density lipoprotein as a protective factor against coronary heart disease, Am. J. Med., 62:707, 1977.

14 Steinberg, D.: The rediscovery of high-density lipoprotein: a negative risk factor and atherosclerosis, Eur. J. Clin. Invest., 8:107, 1978.

15 Wood, P. D., W. Haskell, H. Klein, S. Lewis, M. P. Stern, and J. W. Farquhar: The distribution of plasma lipoproteins in middle-aged male runners, Metabolism, 25:1249, 1976.

16 Wilson, D. E., and R. S. Lees: Metabolic relationships among the plasma lipoproteins. Reciprocal changes in the concentration of very low and low density lipoproteins in man, J. Clin. Invest., 51:1051, 1972.

17 Epstein, F. H., T. Francis, Jr., N. S. Hayner, B. C. Johnson, M. O. Kjelsberg, J. A. Napier, L. D. Ostrander, Jr., M. W. Payne, and H. J. Dodge: Prevalence of chronic disease and distribution of selected physiologic variables in a total community, Tecumseh, Michigan, Am. J. Epidemiol., 81:307, 1965.

18 Friedman, M., and R. H. Rosenman: *Type A Behavior and Your Heart,* Knopf, New York, 1974.

19 Jenkins, C. D.: Recent evidence supporting psychologic and social risk factors for coronary disease, N. Engl. J. Med., 294:987, 1033, 1976.

20 Doll, R., and A. B. Hill: Mortality in relation to smoking: ten years' observation of British doctors, Br. Med. J., 1:1399, 1964.

21 Kahn, H. A.: *The Dorn Study of Smoking and Mortality among U.S. Veterans,* National Cancer Institute Monograph no. 19, Bethesda, Md., January 1966.

22 Morris, J., J. Heady, P. Raffle, C. Roberts, and J. Parks: Coronary heart disease and physical activity of work, Lancet, 2:1053, 1953.

23 Morris, J. N., S. P. W. Chave, C. Adams, C. Sirey, and L. Epstein: Vigorous exercise in leisure time and the incidence of coronary heart disease, Lancet, 1:333, 1973.

24 Paffenbarger, R. S., and W. E. Hale: Work activity and coronary heart mortality, N. Engl. J. Med., 292:545, 1975.

25 Paffenbarger, R. S., A. L. Wing, and R. T. Hyde: Physical activity as an index of heart attack risk in college alumni, Am. J. Epidemiol., 108:161, 1978.

26 Enger, S. C., K. Herbjornsen, J. Erickssen, and A. Fretland: High density lipoproteins and physical activity: the influence of physical exercise, age and smoking on HDL-cholesterol and the HDL/total cholesterol ratio, Scand. J. Clin. Lab. Invest., 37:251, 1977.

27 Wood, P. D., W. L. Haskell, M. P. Stern, S. Lewis, and C. Perry: Plasma lipoprotein distribution in male and female runners, Ann. N.Y. Acad. Sci., 301:748, 1977.

28 Lopez, S. A., R. Vial, L. Balart, and G. Arroyave: Effect of exercise and physical fitness on serum lipids and lipoproteins, Atherosclerosis, 20:1, 1974.

29 Hoffman, A. A., W. R. Nelson, and F. A. Gross: Effect of an exercise program on plasma lipids of senior Air Force officers, Am. J. Cardiol., 20:516, 1967.

30 Streja, D., and D. Mymim: Moderate exercise and high-density lipoprotein-cholesterol, J. Am. Med. Assoc., 242:2190, 1979.

31 Erkelens, D. W., J. J. Albers, W. R. Hazzard, R. C. Fredrick, and E. L. Bierman: High-density lipoprotein-cholesterol in survivors of myocardial infarction, J. Am. Med. Assoc., 242:2185, 1979.

32 Kramsch, D. M., A. J. Aspen, B. M. Abramowitz, T. Kreimendahl, and W. B. Hood, Jr.: Reduction of coronary atherosclerosis by moderate conditioning exercise in monkeys on an atherogenic diet, N. Engl. J. Med., 305:1483, 1981.

33 Ignatowski, A.: Ueber die Wirkung des tierischen Eiweisses auf die Aorta und die parenchymatosen Organe der Kaninchen, Virchow's Arch. Pathol. Anat. Physiol., 198:248, 1909.

34 Anitschkow, N., and S. Chalatow: Ueber experimentelle Cholesterinsteatase und ihre Bedeutung für die Enstehung einiger pathologischer Prozesse, Centralbl. Allg. Pathol. Anat., 24:1, 1913.

35 Armstrong, M. L., E. D. Warner, and W. E. Connors: Regression of coronary atheromatosis in Rhesus monkeys, Cir. Res., 27:59, 1970.

36 Keys, A. (ed.): Coronary heart disease in seven countries, Circulation, 41(suppl. 1):1, 1970.

37 Keys, A., N. Kimura, A. Kusukawa, B. Bronte-Steward, N. Larsen, and M. H. Keys: Lessons from serum cholesterol studies in Japan, Hawaii, and Los Angeles, Ann. Intern. Med., 48:83, 1958.

38 Kannel, W. B.: The disease of living, Nutr. Today, 6:27, May-June 1971.

39 Sacks, F. M., W. P. Castelli, A. Donner, and E. H. Kass: Plasma lipids and lipoproteins in vegetarians and controls, N. Engl. J. Med., 292:1148, 1975.

40 Burslem, J., G. Schonfeld, M. A. Howard, S. W. Weidman, and J. P. Miller: Plasma apoprotein and lipoprotein lipid levels in vegetarians, Metabolism, 27:711, 1978.

41 Yudkin, J.: Patterns and trends in carbohydrate consumption and their relation to disease, Proc. Nutr. Soc., 23:149, 1964.

42 Keys, A.: Sucrose in the diet in coronary heart disease (letter to the editors), Atherosclerosis, 18:352, 1973.

43 *Official Methods of Analysis—Association of Official Analytical Chemists,* 12th ed., W. Horwitz (ed.), Association of Official Analytical Chemists, Washington, 1975.

44 Trowell, H.: Ischemic heart disease and dietary fiber, Am. J. Clin. Nutr., 25:926, 1972.

45 Burkitt, D. P., A. R. P. Walker, and N. S. Painter: Dietary fiber and disease, J. Am. Med. Assoc., 229:1068, 1974.

46 Castelli, W. P., J. T. Doyle, T. Gordon, C. G. Hames, M. C. Hjortland, S. B. Hulley, A. Kagan, and W. J. Zukel: Alcohol and blood lipids. The cooperative lipoprotein phenotyping study, Lancet, 2:153, 1977.

47 Blackburn, H.: Diet and mass hyperlipidemia. A public health view, in *Nutrition, Lipids and Coronary Heart Disease,* R. I. Levy et al. (eds.), Raven, New York, 1979.

48 *Diet-Heart Review Panel: Mass Field Trials of the Diet-Heart Question,* American Heart Association Monograph no. 28, 1969.

49 Kinsell, L. W., J. Partridge, L. Boling, S. Margen, and G. P. Michaels: Dietary modification of serum cholesterol and phospholipid levels, J. Clin. Endocrinol., 12:909, 1952.

50 Keys, A., J. T. Anderson, and F. Grande: Prediction of serum-cholesterol responses of man to changes of fat in the diet, Lancet, 2:959, 1957.

51 Keys, A., J. T. Anderson, and F. Grande: Serum cholesterol response to changes in diet. I. Iodine value versus 2S-P, Metabolism, 14:747, 1965.

52 Glueck, C. J.: Appraisal of dietary fat as a causative factor in atherogenesis, Am J. Clin. Nutr., 32:2637, 1979.

53 Truswell, A. S.: Dietary fat and cholesterol metabolism, Bibl. Nutr. Dieta, 25:53, 1977.

54 Sinclair, H.: Dietary fats and coronary heart disease, Lancet, 1:414, 1980.

55 McGill, H. C.: The relationship of dietary cholesterol to serum cholesterol concentration and to atherosclerosis in man, Am. J. Clin. Nutr., 32:2664, 1979.

56 Albrink, M.: Triglyceridemia, J. Am. Diet. Assoc., 62:626, 1973.

57 Palumbo, P. J., E. R. Broines, R. A. Nelson, and B. A. Kottke: Sucrose sensitivity of patients with coronary-artery disease, Am. J. Clin. Nutr., 30:394, 1977.

58 Truswell, A. S.: Diet and plasma lipids—a reappraisal, Am. J. Clin. Nutr., 31:977, 1978.

59 Fifth Annual Marabou Symposium: Food and Fiber, Nutr. Rev., 35:1, 1977.

60 Palumbo, P. J., E. R. Briones, and R. A. Nelson: High fiber diet in hyperlipemia, J. Am. Med. Assoc., 240:223, 1978.

61 Truswell, A. S.: Food fiber and blood lipids, Nutr. Rev., 35:51, 1977.

62 Kritchevsky, D., and J. A. Story: Fiber, hypercholesterolemia and atherosclerosis, Lipids, 3:366, 1978.

63 Taskinen, M. R., and E. A. Nikkila: Nocturnal hypertriglyceridemia and hyperinsulinemia following moderate evening intake of alcohol, Acta Med. Scand., 202:173, 1977.

64 Sirtori, C. R., E. Agradi, C. Mariani, N. Canal, and L. Frattola: Alcoholic hyperlipidemia, Lancet, 2:820, 1972.

65 Johansson, B. G., and C. B. Laurell: Disorders of serum alpha-lipoproteins after alcoholic intoxication, Scand. J. Clin. Lab. Invest., 23:231, 1969.

66 Berg, B., and B. G. Johansson: Prolonged administration of ethanol to healthy volunteers, 3. Effects on parameters of liver function, plasma lipid concentrations and lipoprotein patterns, Acta Med. Scand., 194(suppl. 552):13, 1973.

67 Johansson, C. G., and A. Medhus: Increase of plasma alpha-lipoproteins in chronic alcoholics after acute abuse, Acta Med. Scand., 195:273, 1974.

68 Wolinsky, H.: Atherosclerosis, in *Textbook of Medicine,* 15th ed., P. B. Beeson, W. McDermott, and J. B. Wyngaarden, (eds), Saunders, Philadelphia, 1979.

69 Fridewald, F. T., R. I. Levy, and D. S. Fredrickson: Estimation of plasma low density lipoprotein cholesterol concentration without use of the preparative ultracentrifuge, Clin. Chem., 18:499, 1972.

70 Fredrickson, D. S., R. I. Levy, M. Bonnell, and N. Ernst: *Dietary Management of Hyperlipoproteinemia,* U.S. Department of Health, Education, and Welfare, National Heart and Lung Institute, Bethesda, Md., 1973.

71 Marmot, M. G.: Epidemiological basis for the prevention of coronary heart disease, Bull. WHO, 57:331, 1979.

72 Glueck, C. J., F. Mattson, and E. L. Bierman: Diet and coronary heart disease: another view, N. Engl. J. Med., 298:1471, 1978.

73 Walker, W.: Changing United States life-style and declining vascular mortality: cause or coincidence? N. Engl. J. Med., 297:163, 1977.

74 *Smoking and Health: Report of the Advisory Committee to the Surgeon General of the Public Health Service,* Public Health Service Publication no. 1103, U.S. Department of Health, Education and Welfare, 1964.

75 Committee on Nutrition, *Diet and Heart Disease,* American Heart Association, New York, 1964.

76 Proceedings of the Conference of the Decline in Coronary Heart Disease Mortality, R. J. Havlik, and M. Feinleib (eds.), Department of Health, Education, and Welfare Publication no. (NIH) 79–1610, 1979.

77 Kleinman, J. C., J. J. Feldman, and M. A. Monk: Trends in smoking and ischemic heart disease mortality, in *Proceedings of the Conference on the Decline in Coronary Heart Disease Mortality,* R. J. Havlik and M. Feinleib (eds.), Department of Health, Education, and Welfare Publication no. (NIH) 79–1610, 1979.

78 Castelli, W. P., J. T. Doyle, T. Gordon, C. G. Hames, M. C. Hjortland, S. B. Hulley, A. Kagan, and W. I. Zukel: HDL cholesterol and other lipids in coronary heart disease: the cooperative lipoprotein phenotyping study, Circulation, 55:767, 1977.

79 Glueck, C. J., and W. E. Connor: Diet—coronary heart disease relationships reconnoitered, Am. J. Clin. Nutr., 31:727, 1978.

HYPERTENSION

CONTENTS

INTRODUCTION

Hypertension, or *high blood pressure,* is defined as levels of systolic and/or diastolic blood pressure which are causally associated with the occurrence of ill health or death. Hypertension is associated with coronary heart disease, stroke, congestive heart failure, renal disease, and visual impairment as well as with a shortened life span. Although there is no sharp dividing line between normal and elevated blood pressure, in an adult hypertension is frequently defined as a pressure greater than or equal to 160/95 mmHg. Even within the so-called normal range of blood pressure, higher levels are associated with more illness [1]. Williams et al. [2] have proposed that a more appropriate definition of hypertension may be the following:

Women at any age	160/95 mmHg
Men above the age of 45	140/95 mmHg
Men below the age of 45	130/90 mmHg

If hypertension is defined as a diastolic blood pressure exceeding 95 mmHg and a systolic blood pressure of at least 160 mmHg, the magnitude of the problem is evident from the findings of the U.S. Public Health Service Health and Nutrition Examination Survey [3] (1971–1974), which are based on a representative sample of 7796 persons who were examined. The following are estimates of the prevalence of hypertension:

Total adults, aged 18–74	23.2 million
Prevalence rates	
(per 100 population):	
White men	18.5
White women	15.7
Black men	27.8
Black women	28.6

Kaplan has suggested that in the course of a week, an average practitioner will see 20 to 40 patients with hypertension [4]. In 1976, it was estimated that a substantial majority of the approximately 24 million hypertensive individuals in the United States had undetected, untreated, or inadequately treated high blood pressure. Recently, however, as a result of extensive educational programs by a number of private and government agencies, the number of undiagnosed and/or untreated patients has been substantially reduced. This has been suggested as one of the factors contributing to the recent decline in cardiovascular mortality [5].

Patients with hypertension for which a specific organic cause cannot be found are said to have *primary, essential,* or *idiopathic hypertension.* Approximately 85 to 90 percent of all hypertension is this kind. Undoubtedly this group represents a spectrum of diseases which includes as yet undefined forms of secondary hypertension. *Secondary hypertension* is due to definable causes, such as renal disease, hyperaldosteronism (excessive secretion of aldosterone by the adrenal cortex) or pheochromocytoma (a tumor of the adrenal glands which produces large amounts of epinephrine and norepinephrine), or coarctation of the aorta.

Primary hypertension can be treated with a combination of drugs, diet modification, weight control, and stress management. This chapter focuses on nutritional aspects of essential hypertension, because of the role of diet in the prevention and treatment of essential hypertension.

EPIDEMIOLOGY

Population studies have indicated that elevations of blood pressure are associated with family history, advancing age, obesity, being black, oral contraceptive use, endocrine disorders including diabetes and Cushing's syndrome, excessive alcohol intake, small family size, less formal education, inactivity, psychological stress, uterine fibroids, and excessive sodium intake [6–9]. When all these factors are placed in perspective, it appears that in a population of patients with essential hypertension, heredity and sodium intake play the most important roles.

Genetic Studies

Family studies have consistently shown aggregation among family members for both systolic and diastolic blood pressure, while studies of twins and adopted children indicate that familial aggregation is due to heredity rather than to shared environmental factors [10]. A study of monozygotic and dizygotic twins indicated that monozygotic twins have higher correlations for both systolic and diastolic blood pressures than other relatives [11]. The Montreal Adoption Survey was a cross-sectional study of French-Canadian families that had at least one adopted child of the same ethnic origin. The correlation of blood pressure scores between parents and natural children is highly significant for systolic and diastolic pressures, and correlation between pairs of natural children is significant. However, the correlation between parents and adopted children, as well as that between pairs of adopted children, is not statistically significant. It is estimated that the level of an individual's blood pressure is determined about 50 percent by genetic factors [12]. Additional support for a strong genetic role in humans is provided by studies of diastolic blood pressure in individuals of African ancestry which indicate that an excess of hypertension in blacks is due, at least in part, to common genetic factors [13].

Sodium Intake

Since sodium intake seems to be the major environmental factor, data relating sodium to hypertension will be reviewed in detail. The main source of dietary sodium is sodium chloride (NaCl) or table salt; sodium represents 40 percent by weight of the salt molecule. The association between sodium and hypertension is not a new discovery; it was suggested as long ago as 2300 B.C. by a Chinese physician [14]. Epidemiological studies of several societies have shown a correlation between chronically high salt intake and the prevalence of hypertension (see Figure 9-1). Eskimos, who ingest an average of 30 meq of sodium per

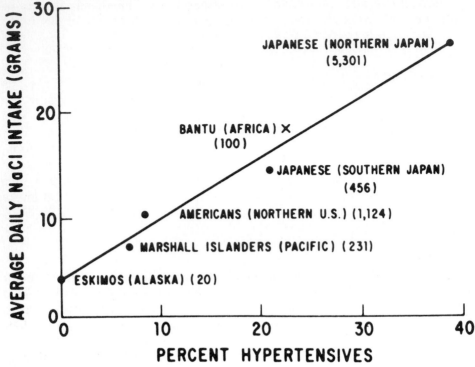

FIGURE 9-1
Comparison of the prevalence of hypertension among various populations according to their average salt (NaCl) intake. Number of persons studied in parentheses. •, derived from Meneely and Dahl [16]; ×, derived from Isaacson et al. [15]. (*From R. L., Weinsier, Prev. Med., 5:7, 1976.*)

day, are virtually free of hypertension; some Japanese farmers ingest an average of 500 meq of sodium per day, and 40 percent of them over 40 years old are hypertensive. Average salt consumption in the United States is 150 to 200 meq of sodium per day, and there is a 20 percent prevalence of hypertension among adults over 40 years of age. Isaacson et al. [15] studied 100 Bantu subjects and added another point of correlation to Figure 9-1, which is derived from the earlier studies of Meneely and Dahl [16]. Additional studies have supported Meneely and Dahl's findings. When blood pressure and salt intake were compared in two ethnically similar Polynesian populations by Prior et al., the prevalence of hypertension was greater with increasing age in the group averaging an intake of 120 to 140 meq of sodium per day than in the group averaging 60 meq per day [17].

Conversely, Prior and Evans noted that natives in small villages in New Guinea had virtually no hypertension and that blood pressures in old men were no higher than those in young men [18]. This demonstrated that blood pressure does not *necessarily* rise with advancing age. International epidemiologists have found a number of populations in which blood pressure tends to remain low throughout life; the table that follows lists several such groups.

Africa	Congo pygmies
	Kalahari bushmen
	Kenyan nomads
America	Cuna Indians (Panama)
Australasia	New Guinea highlanders
	Pacific atoll Polynesians
	Aborigines (Australia)

All are remote, rural tribal groups living hard, simple lives and consuming a low-sodium diet. However, genetically similar natives nearly always developed their share of hypertension whenever they moved to modern cities, where salt intake is greater. Shaper reported that when Samburu warrior-herdsman were tending their herds and eating 50 meq sodium daily, they had very little hypertension [19]. However, when they were drafted into the Army of Kenya, they began eating an army ration providing 308 meq of sodium daily. This sudden increase in sodium intake did not bring on a great rise in blood pressure during the first year, but beginning with the second year of high salt intake, blood pressures rose progressively (Table 9-1).

These populations studies can be summarized as follows: Areas with very high salt intakes have a high incidence of hypertension. Areas with low salt intake (less than 70 meq sodium daily) have a very low incidence of hypertension, and blood pressure does not rise with advancing years. Furthermore, a low intake of salt (70 meq sodium daily) is apparently compatible with vigorous health.

Studies of correlations between salt intake and blood pressure within a population have given conflicting results. Dahl conducted a pilot study among

TABLE 9-1

WEIGHT AND BLOOD PRESSURE CHANGES IN NOMADIC SAMBURU AFTER ENTERING KENYAN ARMY

	Excess over controls	
Interval from entry	Weight	Blood pressure, mmHg
6 months	17%	Nil
2 years	6%	8/0
6 years	11%	12/4

Source: G. Rose, Postgrad. Med. J., 53 (suppl. 2):139, 1977; adapted from Shaper [19].

1346 Brookhaven National Laboratories employees. The employees were classified according to their salt intake as follows:

Low intake: Never adds salt to food
Average intake: Adds salt after tasting if insufficiently salty
High intake: Customarily adds salt before tasting.

One hundred and five persons were found to be hypertensive. Those classified as having a low salt intake were found to be unlikely to have hypertension (one case), whereas those classified as having a high salt intake were significantly more hypertensive (61 cases) than would have been predicted by chance alone [20].

In a more recent study [21], a correlation coefficient of +0.69 was found between casual systolic blood pressure and 24-hour urinary sodium excretion. Other studies attempting to compare salt habits and hypertension of groups within the U.S. population have not borne out these correlations. Dawber and his colleagues [22] failed to find a correlation in the Framingham Study between blood pressure and daily salt intake. Langford and Watson [23] found none among black females in Mississippi. Limitations in these data include (1) the crude methods used to assess salt ingestion over the years (1- or 2-day samples of dietary intake determined from a dietary history or sodium excretion in a 24-hour urine sample) and (2) the relatively small sample size. Furthermore, an association between hypertension and salt ingestion may be difficult to establish in an American population in which, regardless of stated salting practices, most individuals are exposed to a generous sodium intake from childhood as a result of the widespread use of salt in commercially prepared foods.

The observations that salt and hypertension show close correlations between different populations but not within one society may be explained by the presence of other predisposing factors. For example, hereditary susceptibility [24,25], interacting with high sodium intake, may be the shared mechanism by which essential hypertension develops. In addition, potassium intake is generally low in high-sodium-intake populations [26]. Although sodium-potassium equilibrium is tightly regulated in mammals, there is evidence that the effects of excessive sodium intake on hypertension can be modified by dietary potassium [27]. The role of the sodium-potassium ratio in hypertension needs to be further evaluated.

EXPERIMENTS RELATING SODIUM TO HYPERTENSION

Human Studies

The evidence relating salt intake to hypertension in humans is indirect and derives from three types of observations:

1 Effects of salt restriction on blood pressure
2 Effects of high salt administration on blood pressure
3 Effects of salt elimination by diuretics on blood pressure

Effects of Sodium Restriction on Blood Pressure   It is well-established that reduction of dietary sodium in hypertensive individuals produces a lowering of blood pressure. The first demonstration that hypertension could be successfully treated involved the use of a drastically low sodium (10 meq per day) rice and fruit diet [28]. Kempner observed improvement in almost two-thirds of 500 patients. A later clinical trial by the British Medical Research Council in 1950 confirmed Kempner's studies [29]. Grollman and his colleagues [30] observed a marked decrease in blood pressure of six patients with essential hypertension who were treated with a more liberal diet containing 22 meq sodium daily. Dahl [31] further emphasized the importance of dietary sodium in a 7-month study of an obese hypertensive woman. During the first month the patient received a daily diet containing 10 g sodium chloride (170 meq sodium), with adequate calories to maintain her admission weight. After the first month, calories were restricted but a daily intake of 10 g sodium chloride was continued. The patient lost 25 kg body weight over the next 4½ months, with no fall in blood pressure. After 5½ months of observation, low sodium chloride intake (4 to 6 meq sodium) was started and, simultaneously, her caloric intake was increased to maintain her present weight. Only after sodium chloride was restricted did blood pressure fall (see Figure 9-2). However, Reisen et al. [32] recently reported that weight reduction exerts an independent effect on hypertension and that weight reduction is associated with a decrease in blood pressure.

More recently a study from New South Wales [33] revealed a small but significant fall in diastolic blood pressure in hypertensive outpatients advised to reduce their salt intake to 70 to 100 meq sodium per day. The 31 borderline hypertensive patients with diastolic blood pressure between 95 and 109 mmHg were treated for 2 years, and the results were compared to an untreated control group and a drug-treated group. Salt restriction reduced diastolic blood pressure by 7.3 ± 1.6 mmHg, a result similar to that in patients treated with antihypertensive drugs. Additional important observations in this study were (1) that the maximum fall in blood pressure took place only after a prolonged period of treatment (2 years) and (2) that the 24-hour urinary sodium excretion fell from a mean value of 195 meq per day to 157 meq per day in these patients. The latter value, of course, includes some patients who clearly adhered to the salt-restricted diet and others who clearly did not. Stricter adherence to the diet might have caused further falls in blood pressure.

Effects of High Sodium Administration   There is good evidence that very high sodium intake will increase the level of blood pressure. In a recent study at Indiana University, 800 meq sodium per day was fed to normotensive human volunteers. They showed a significant rise in blood pressure, body weight, and potassium excretion [34]. The increase was even greater when the subjects were given 1500 meq sodium per day. McDonough and Wilhelmj [35] fed 637 meq sodium daily to a single normotensive subject for 23 days and observed an increase in systemic blood pressure. McQuarrie et al. [36] administered from 835 to 1043 meq of sodium daily to diabetic children. They noted 30 to 50 percent increases in both systolic and diastolic blood pressures above control values.

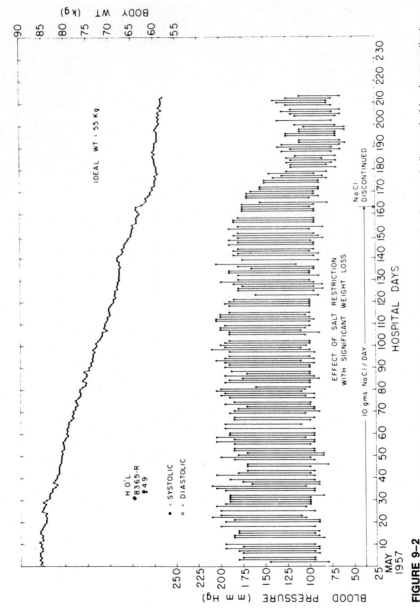

FIGURE 9–2

Effect of salt (NaCl) restriction in an obese patient. During the first month on the metabolic ward, this obese patient was on salt and calories sufficient to maintain her admission weight. After the first month, caloric restriction was started but salt continued. Over 4½ months, she lost approximately 25 kg body weight, with no fall in blood pressure. After 5½ months of observation, during which time her blood pressure had remained unchanged, a low-salt regimen was started and, simultaneously, her caloric intake was increased to maintain weight. Only after salt was restricted did her blood pressure fall (*P*<0.01). (*From L. K. Dahl, Am. J. Clin. Nutr., 25:231, 1972.*)

More relevant perhaps are salt-feeding experiments at the University of Iowa [37]. When young normotensive human subjects were fed 400 meq sodium for 4 weeks, their forearm blood flow increased, their forearm vascular resistance went down, and their blood pressure did not change. When the same procedure was applied to subjects with borderline hypertension, their forearm vascular resistance went up instead of down, and arterial blood pressure rose. These mild hypertensives responded completely differently to a dietary salt load. Extracellular fluid volume increased in both groups, but only the borderline hypertensive showed a rise in blood pressure and peripheral resistance.

Effects of Salt Elimination by Diuretics   Diuretic agents, such as thiazides, which facilitate the renal excretion of sodium, definitely reduce blood pressure in the majority of patients with essential hypertension [38,39]. Concomitant high salt intake (350 meq sodium per day) can prevent this lowering of blood pressure [26], while the combination of salt restriction and diuretics produces a statistically significantly greater blood presure reduction than either treatment alone [40].

Animal Studies

In humans, one can state only that there is a statistical correlation between salt intake and hypertension in different populations, though probably not within a given population. Spontaneous hypertension is rarely observed in free-living animals; however, hypertension is readily produced in a variety of experimental animals (monkey, chicken, and rat) by the feeding of sodium chloride. Meneely and Ball [41] summarized their observations of blood pressure and of other responses in rats to the dietary manipulation of sodium, chloride, and potassium. There is no difference in growth, longevity, or blood pressure among rats fed between 0.15 and 2 percent salt in their dry rations. Those fed 2.8 or 5.6 percent salt (10 or 20 meq sodium per 100 kcal) developed moderate hypertension, grew slightly less, and had a shorter life span; when fed 7 percent salt or more, more severe hypertension and growth retardation resulted and they had a much shorter life span. Resulting damage to organs included cardiac and renal enlargement, glomerulosclerosis, and renal failure. Increased intake of potassium chloride lessened but did not eliminate the effects of salt feeding on blood pressure and life span. Dahl [42] demonstrated that feeding 8 percent salt or more in dry rations to rats resulted in irreversible hypertension, but with considerable variation in blood pressure response within the general population. He then developed, by selective breeding, strains of salt-sensitive and salt-resistant rats. Salt-sensitive rats developed hypertension on a high sodium intake but remained normotensive on a low-sodium diet. A salt intake in the salt-sensitive rats of 0.4 to 11 percent of the diet correlated with progressive elevation of blood pressure [43]. When rats of the sensitive strain were fed 8 percent salt from weaning to the age of six weeks, they developed hypertension by the age of 1 year and their life span was shortened [44]. The effect, both on blood pressure and life span, was less when extra salt intake was provided between the ages of 3 and 6 months.

In summary, these results indicate the following:

1 High intake (10 to 30 meq sodium per 100 kcal per day) is necessary to induce hypertension in nonselected laboratory rats.

2 Lesser amounts of sodium induce hypertension in genetically selected rats.

3 Early feeding of salt to sensitive rats predisposes them to hypertension later.

4 Adding potassium to the diet to maintain the ratio Na:K < 2 protects against the induction of hypertension.

5 Resistant rats tolerate high sodium intake.

One might assume that in order to develop sodium-induced hypertension, some initial accumulation of sodium in the body occurs, which in turn brings about a rise in pressure. The salt-sensitive Dahl rats do not have excessive body sodium levels, either on high- or low-sodium diets. Moreover, when rats with established hypertension are challenged with a sodium load, they excrete sodium as expeditiously as do normotensive controls. However, the hypertensive kidney is perfused at an elevated pressure, while the normotensive kidney is perfused at a normal pressure. Selkurt [45] showed that high perfusion pressure in the renal artery greatly facilitates the urinary excretion of sodium and increases urine volume. Therefore, in order to compare the ability of kidneys to excrete sodium, the same inflow pressure should be applied. Tobian et al. [46] used isolated perfused kidneys from the salt-sensitive and salt-resistant Dahl rats which had been eating a low-sodium diet and hence had blood pressures within the normal range. Figure 9-3 shows the urinary sodium excretion per 100 g of isolated kidney per minute at various inflow pressures. When compared at the same pressure, the salt-sensitive kidneys seem to have a pronounced natriuretic handicap at each inflow pressure. However, raising the inflow pressure can overcome the natriuretic handicap. For instance, the sensitive kidneys, perfused at 160 mmHg, excrete about 50 percent more sodium per minute than the normotensive, salt-resistant kidneys, perfused at a normal 130 mmHg. Thus it is apparent that the pressure-natriuresis curve of the salt-sensitive rat has been shifted to the right. In either strain, on a very low sodium intake, there is virtually no tendency for sodium retention and thereby little stimulus for a rise in blood pressure. However, when the salt-sensitive rats eat a high-sodium diet, the resetting of the pressure-natriuresis curve could be important. If the relative rates of natriuresis of isolated salt-sensitive and salt-resistant kidneys occurred also in the intact rat during high sodium intake, the salt-sensitive rat would tend to retain more sodium than the sodium-resistant rat and would tend to reach a sodium balance characterized by elevated body sodium and extracellular volume. High body sodium and high extracellular volume frequently produce a rise in blood pressure. If the arterial blood pressure were to rise into the hypertensive range, the salt-sensitive kidney would then increase its rate of

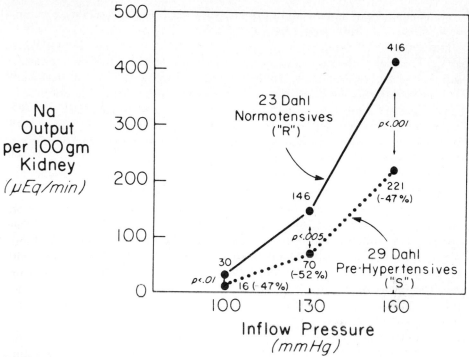

FIGURE 9-3
Sodium excretion of isolated kidneys from salt-sensitive and salt-resistant rats, at varying inflow pressures. The distance between the large black dot (the mean value) and the tip of the arrowhead represents the SEM. (*From L. Tobian, Am. J. Clin. Nutr., 32:2739, 1979.*)

sodium excretion through the mechanism of pressure natriuresis and its natriuretic handicap would be overcome.

PATHOGENESIS

High blood pressure is a physical finding associated with an increased incidence of vascular pathology, such as coronary artery and cerebrovascular disease [47]. A variety of pathophysiological processes may result in elevated blood pressure. Hypertensive patients are classified as (1) those in whom the underlying pathophysiology is understood, i.e., patients with "secondary" forms of hypertension, and (2) those in whom the pathophysiology of elevated blood pressure is not presently understood, i.e., patients with "essential" hypertension [48]. Secondary forms of hypertension occur in diseases such as pheochromocytoma, primary hyperaldosteronism, coarctation of the aorta, and renovascular disease. However, secondary hypertension is found only in a small percentage of patients with elevated blood pressure. The pathophysiology of primary hypertension is unknown, and it is not even known whether the patients suffer from a single disease or from many diseases of different etiologies.

The dynamics of hypertension are essentially those of normal blood pressure per se. The blood pressure in determined by the rate of blood flow, or cardiac output, and the resistance to blood flow offered by vessels of the peripheral vascular bed, particularly the arterioles. Blood pressure is simply determined by the product of cardiac output and peripheral vascular resistance (BP = CO × PVR). An elevation in either of these two factors can increase blood pressure. Most individuals with essential hypertension have normal cardiac output and increased peripheral vascular resistance.

The primary factors determining cardiac output are blood volume and inotropism, or the pumping action of the heart. Blood volume is determined by the balance of salt and water intake, retention, and excretion. Blood volume and body fluid balance are carefully regulated by a complex network of mechanisms involving renal filtration pressures, variable permeability of membranes to fluid and changing electrolyte transport in renal tubules, and a system of hormones including, among others, renin, angiotensin, aldosterone, antidiuretic hormone, and prostaglandins [49,50]. A complex system of sensor mechanisms for blood volume, osmolarity, and pressure are located in the heart, large blood vessels, kidneys, and brain. They connect with the nervous system, which in turn provides feedback pathways for the control of hormones and smooth muscle tone of vessels, influencing blood volume and blood pressure. The pumping action of the heart is controlled by the sympathetic nervous system through neural pathways and catecholamine hormone release.

Peripheral vascular resistance, the other main determinant of blood pressure, is largely controlled by the sympathetic nervous system, but humoral systems, including those that secrete norepinephrine, epinephrine, antidiuretic hormone (ADH), adrenocorticotropic hormone (ACTH), renin-angiotensin, and aldosterone, are also involved. Thus a number of mechanisms normally operate to regulate heart performance and systemic blood pressure. In essential hypertension, apparently some component of this regulatory system fails to function satisfactorily.

In this complex regulatory network, changes in any one variable of the system usually result in subsequent changes in several of the other variables. Hence it is difficult to interpret isolated measurements of a variable in experiments relating to hypertension. Observed changes in any specific parameter can be either primary or simply due to reflex responses to change in some other component of the system.

Systolic and diastolic blood pressure are affected similarly by many of these physiological factors. Generally, when factors increase diastolic blood pressure, systolic pressure also rises. However, systolic pressure can be elevated alone by some inotropic states or by decreased distensibility of the normally elastic aorta and greater vessels.

Many theories have been proposed to explain the etiology of essential hypertension. Both Swales [51] and Page [52] have recently reviewed the major current hypotheses. Among the mechanisms suggested are (1) neural mechanisms, (2) "inappropriate" renin-angiotensin activity, (3) sodium retention, (4) vascular hypertrophy, and (5) renal dysfunction.

CLINICAL MANIFESTATIONS

Hypertension is a silent disease. In the early stages there may be no symptoms that cause the patient to seek medical attention. In most cases the hypertensive patient will be identified in the course of a physical examination. Though popularly considered a symptom of elevated blood pressure, headache is characteristic only of severe hypertension. Most frequently the headache is frontal or occipital in distribution and is present in early morning when the patient awakens. Other possibly related complaints include fatigue, tinnitus, dizziness, and epistaxis.

DIAGNOSIS

HISTORY

In approaching the hypertensive patient, an accurate history will provide valuable information for evaluating the possible causes of hypertension. Hypertension is familial, and so the family history is important in determining the approach to treatment. If the parents of a patient with hypertension died at relatively young ages (under 60) from cerebral vascular accident, myocardial infarction, or renal failure or if siblings have hypertension, the physician may elect to treat the patient more aggressively. A strong family history of hypertension, along with the reported findings of intermittent pressure elevation in the past, favors the diagnosis of essential hypertension. A history of muscle weakness, muscle cramps, and polyuria suggests further screening for hyperaldosteronism. A history of headaches, palpitations, or excessive sweating suggests further study for pheochromocytoma. Both are rare. Several drugs, including steroids, carbenoxolone, nonsteroidal anti-inflammatory drugs (e.g., phenylbutazone, indomethacin, birth control pills, and other estrogens), and excess use of nephrotoxic analgesics such as phenacetin may cause hypertension. Licorice overingestion should be considered when hypokalemia is present. In some of these situations, discontinuing the chemical agent is often the only treatment necessary. A dietary history should be obtained, including salt (sodium) and potassium intake. Concomitant drug usage should be established, because this may affect the success of the therapeutic dietary regimen. Many prescription, patent, and over-the-counter medications have a high sodium content (see Table 9-2). Associated disorders such as hyperlipemia, gout, diabetes, polycythemia vera, and obesity may contribute to increased risk of cardiovascular complications or may make pharmacological management of the hypertension more complex. Other risk factors that may be elicited include cigarette smoking and use of alcohol.

TABLE 9-2
SELECTED MEDICATIONS AND THEIR SODIUM CONTENT

Drug	Average dose	Sodium content,* mg
Alka-Seltzer (blue)	2 tablets	1064
Bisodol power	1 packet	1540
Bromo Seltzer	1.25 g	717
Basaljel suspension	15 ml	27
Creamalin tablets	2 tablets	50
Effergel powder	1 tsp (rounded)	200
Fizrin	1 packet	763
Gelusil liquid	15 ml	21
Kolantyl tablets	2 tablets	20
Kaopectate concentrate	15 ml	135
Maalox suspension	15 ml	18
Metamucil instant mix	1 packet	250
Milk of Magnesia	30 ml	36
Mylanta II liquid	10 ml	20
Phosphaljel suspension	15 ml	39
Rolaids	2 tablets	100
Sal Hepatica	1 tsp (rounded)	1000
Sodium bicarbonate tablets, 325 mg	2 tablets	178
Titralac liquid	15 ml	37.5
Tums	2 tablets	40

*The milliequivalent content of sodium may be obtained by dividing the amount in milligrams by 23.
Sources: A. G. Lipman, Mod. Med., 45:59, 1977; Sodium and Medicinals, Tables of Sodium Values, San Francisco Heart Association, San Francisco, 1966.

Physical Examination

Blood pressure should be measured on both arms. Measurements in the supine position should be compared with measurements taken erect. A rise in diastolic pressure when the patient rises from the supine to the standing position is most compatible with essential hypertension; a fall, in the absense of antihypertensive medication, suggests some form of secondary hypertension. Bilateral funduscopic examination for hemorrhages, exudates, and papilledema is mandatory, since these provide some of the best indications of the duration of hypertension and of prognosis. Such an examination is especially important in persons with diastolic blood pressure of 110 mmHg or higher [53].

All peripheral pulses should be palpated, and auscultation for bruits over the carotid, brachial, femoral, and radial arteries should be performed. Narrowing of a carotid artery may be a manifestation of hypertensive vascular disease, while bruits due to renal arterial narrowing may be the result of arteriosclerosis or fibrous dysplasia. The heart responds to hypertension by enlargement of the left ventricle. Cardiac assessment through palpation and auscultation may detect increased rate, precordial heave, murmurs, arrhythmias, and gallops.

Laboratory Tests

There is controversy about what laboratory studies should be done in patients presenting with hypertension. Most of the disagreement pertains to the vigor with which the patient is evaluated for secondary forms of hypertension. The initial laboratory evaluation is intended (1) to help the physician assess vascular disease in the target organs, (2) to assess coexisting factors for atherosclerotic vascular disease, and (3) to determine the likelihood that there is underlying curable cause of the hypertension. Moser [54] suggested that a workup should involve only five simple laboratory tests—urinalysis, serum potassium, blood urea nitrogen, and cholesterol and glucose determinations—and an electrocardiogram. A 24-hour urinary sodium measurement can help confirm the dietary history, since 90 percent of the sodium intake is excreted in the urine. Stool and sweat losses are less than 10 meq per day for adults.

Blood urea nitrogen (BUN) is an indicator of glomerular filtration rate (GFR) and is available as part of a standard battery of chemical tests. Measurement of serum potassium concentration is made to rule out hyperaldosteronism. It is unusual for a patient with primary hyperaldosteronism to have a normal serum potassium concentration. Hypokalemia and hypertension secondary to ingestion of large amounts of licorice (with the mineralocorticoid effects of its glycyrrhizinic acid) can be excluded by a careful dietary history. An initial estimation of serum potassium concentration is also useful as a base line for subsequent diuretic therapy.

Urinalysis includes measurement of osmolarity to assess concentrating ability, which is impaired in chronic renal failure, hypokalemia, and hypercalcemia. Some degree of proteinuria is present in nearly half of all untreated hypertensives. It is only of diagnostic significance when protein is present in amounts greater than 1+. The presence of red blood cell casts is indicative of active glomerulonephritis. Proteinuria, nonspecific casts, and microscopic hematuria may be the first clues to the presence of polycystic renal disease. Plasma glucose concentrations may reveal coexisting diabetes mellitus in the hypertensive patient, while serum cholesterol may serve as a means to evaluate the risk of atherosclerotic vascular disease.

Physiological Tests

Electrocardiographic evidence of cardiac hypertrophy may be found in as many as 60 percent of untreated hypertensive individuals. The electrocardiogram can be used as a base line and should be evaluated for evidence of conduction disturbance and ischemic heart disease.

Management

The initial therapeutic approach to the patient with primary hypertension is the establishment of a reasonable nutritional program. Most hypertensive patients are adequately nourished, and a majority are more than 15 percent above mean normal weight for height, age, and sex. For information about calorie-restricted diets, the reader is referred to Chapter 7, Table 7-3.

Hypertensive patients frequently know that salt should be restricted as part of their antihypertensive therapy, but a "salt-free diet" to most means that the saltshaker should not be used at the table. Few hypertensive patients (and few physicians!) realize that the preponderance of sodium intake comes through nondiscretional use. The average daily consumption of table salt in the American home is estimated at 3.4 g per person, corresponding to approximately 1.4 g sodium (60 meq). Thus a substantial portion of the estimated average daily 10- to 15-g sodium chloride intake comes from the addition of salt in the processing of food [55].

Hunt et al. [56] report that it is rare to find a patient with a daily dietary sodium intake of less than 100 meq, even though he or she may believe that the diet followed is "salt-free." When sodium intake is controlled to 75 meq or less, short-term studies [57] indicate that most patients with mild hypertension (diastolic blood pressure from 90 to 104 mmHg) will become normotensive without supplemental therapy (Table 9-3). Patients with moderate hypertension (diastolic blood pressure of 105 to 114 mmHg) respond in a less predictable fashion; however, a majority will become normotensive without additional therapy. When dietary sodium ranges from 75 to 149 meq, the percentage of patients who become normotensive as the result of dietary therapy in the absence of additional antihypertensive agents decreases markedly. When sodium excretion in a 24-hour urine sample exceeds 150 meq, it is uncommon for patients with mild or moderate hypertension to achieve a normotensive state unless pharmacological therapy is initiated; however, the effectiveness of supplemental diuretic antihypertensive therapy is nullified unless dietary sodium is also decreased below 150 meq per day.

For help in planning a sodium-restricted diet Table 9-4 lists the sodium content of selected foods. In planning diets, it should be remembered that certain ethnic diets may have a particularly high salt content (e.g., kosher,

TABLE 9-3
RESULTS OF NUTRITIONAL THERAPY IN 300 PATIENTS WITH ESSENTIAL HYPERTENSION
[Percentage of Subjects Becoming Normotensive (90 mmHg diastolic)]

24-h urinary sodium, meq	Pretreatment diastolic blood pressure, mmHg		
	90–104	105–114	≥ 115
< 75	84	64	49
75–149	37	16	2
≥ 150	11	3	0

Source: J. C. Hunt, in Hypertension, J. Genest, E. Koiw, and O. Kuchel (eds.), McGraw-Hill, New York, 1977.

TABLE 9-4
SODIUM CONTENT OF SELECTED FOODS

Food	Serving size	Sodium content,* mg
Kentucky Fried Chicken, original recipe dinner	3-piece dinner	2285
McDonald's Big Mac	1 (7 $\frac{1}{2}$ oz)	1510
Soy sauce	1 tbsp	1319
Pizza Hut pizza supreme	$\frac{1}{2}$ of 10-in pizza (3 slices)	1281
Swanson's chicken TV dinner	1	1152
Dill pickle	1 large	1137
Bouillon	1 cube	960
Olives, green	10 large	926
Baked ham	3 oz	770
Frankfurter	2 oz	627
Jack-in-the-Box taco	1	463
American cheese, processed	1 oz	406
Tomato juice, canned	6 oz	364
Salad dressing, Italian	1 tbsp	314
Corn flakes	1 oz	260
Peas, canned	$\frac{1}{2}$ cup	200
Potato chips	1 oz	191
Cheddar cheese	1 oz	176
Bacon, cooked	3 slices	156
Bread, white, enriched	1 slice	134
Milk, whole	1 cup	120
Egg, whole	1 large	69
Celery	1 stalk	50
Hamburger, 21% fat, cooked	3 oz	49
Butter, salted	1 tsp	41
Carrots, cooked	$\frac{1}{2}$ cup	26
Orange	1 medium	2
Peas, fresh, cooked	$\frac{1}{2}$ cup	1

*The milliequivalent content of sodium may be obtained by dividing the amount in milligrams by 23.

Sources: C. F. Adams, Nutritive Value of American Foods in Common Units, U.S. Department of Agriculture Handbook no. 456, U.S. Government Printing Office, Washington, 1975; Consumer Reports, 44:147 (March 1979), 44:508 (September 1979).

Chinese, and American black diets), so that expectations for sodium restriction must be realistic. Salt substitutes (Table 9-5) may help to make diets more appetizing, and various herbs and spices can be used in food preparation. Even when prepared by knowledgeable sources, like the American Heart Association, these diets may appear so complex that they discourage all but the most persistent patient. Most patients are unaware of the naturally high sodium content of cow's milk, the added salt in cheese, and the added salt in most processed foods. To overcome these impediments to the widespread adoption of a moderately

TABLE 9-5
SODIUM AND POTASSIUM CONTENT OF SALT SUBSTITUTES

Name	Potassium per gram		Sodium per gram	
	mg	meq	mg	meq
Co-salt	476	12.18	1	0.06
Adolph's salt substitute	333	8.51	2	0.09
Morton's salt substitute	493	12.62	1	0.06
Morton's lite salt	240	6.15	195	8.47
Regular salt (NaC1)	0	0.00	393	17.00

Source: M. J. Oexmann-Wannamaker, Am. J. Clin. Nutr., 29:599, 1976.

restricted sodium diet, Dahl [58] suggested these simple rules:

1 Never add salt to food during preparation or at the table.
2 Avoid milk and milk products.
3 Avoid all processed foods except fruits and juices, and read the labels of the latter.

Like all rules of thumb, these are not foolproof, but most people can remember them and will achieve a far lower sodium intake than if they use a regimen which they may abandon because of its complexity.

Additional problems may make sodium restriction difficult to achieve. The amount of sodium in drinking water varies considerably. In Galveston, Texas, the municipal water supply contains 34 mg sodium per deciliter (1.5 meq), and in Crandal, Texas, it contains 170 mg/dl (7.4 meq). The latter water is rarely drunk, but it is used for cooking (27). Water treated in most water-softening equipment is often much higher in sodium because two atoms of sodium replace each atom of calcium or magnesium exchanged.

There are many medications which contain considerable amounts of sodium, including many antacids and laxatives (see Table 9-2). These should be avoided by subjects on sodium-restricted diets. Riopan (2 mg sodium per 15 ml or per 3 tablets) is the drug of choice for sodium-restricted patients who use antacids frequently or in large doses [59].

Many high-sodium compounds are used in food manufacturing and in food preservation, including baking powder, sodium bicarbonate, sodium propionate, sodium alginate (found in chocolate milk drinks and ice cream), sodium nitrate, and monosodium glutamate.

Table 9-6 gives the approximate sodium content of the exchange lists when foods are produced, processed, or prepared without the addition of any sodium compound. Table 9-6 also gives adjusted meal patterns for diets containing 22, 44, and 88 meq sodium. Foods that are comparatively high in sodium content and must be restricted in low-sodium diets are listed in Table 9-7.

Not all hypertensive patients respond to diet, and supplemental therapy will

TABLE 9-6
SODIUM IN EXCHANGE LISTS AND SUGGESTED MEAL PATTERNS FOR SODIUM-CONTROLLED DIETS

Food exchange	Amount	Sodium content meq	Sodium content mg	22 meq (500 mg)	44 meq (1000 mg)	88 meq (2000 mg)
Milk, regular	1 cup	5.2	120	2 cups	2 cups	2 cups
Meat	1 oz	1.0	25	5 oz	6 oz	6 oz
Egg	1	3.0	70	1	1	1
Vegetables	½ cup	0.4	9	ad lib.	ad lib.	ad lib.
Fruit	1 serving	0.1	2	5 servings	ad lib.	ad lib.
Bread, unsalted	1 serving	0.2	5	4 servings	1 serving	ad lib.
Bread, salted	1 serving	8.5	200	0	3 servings	6 servings
Fat, unsalted	1 tsp	0.0	0	ad lib.	ad lib.	ad lib.

then be needed. Oral diuretic drugs are usually employed first. The three main classes of diuretics, shown in Table 9-8, are (1) thiazides (2) "loop" diuretics, and (3) potassium-sparing agents. Both the thiazides and loop diuretics produce saluresis (salt loss) and diuresis (water loss), resulting in a reduction of extracellular fluid volume, plasma volume, and total exchangeable sodium and the desired fall in blood pressure.

Side effects of these diuretics include hypokalemia, hyperuricemia, and hyperglycemia. Hypokalemia is especially common and can be treated with dietary therapy or with potassium supplements. Dietary sources of potassium are usually preferred because of the unpleasant taste of most potassium supplements. Table 9-9 lists some common sources of potassium. If potassium depletion becomes a problem, a potassium-sparing diuretic can be used. Also, various salt substitutes (Table 9-5) substitute potassium for sodium, but the patient should be told to check labels thoroughly, as many available substitutes are not completely sodium-free. The use of these may be contraindicated or restricted if there is associated renal disease. Serum potassium concentration should be measured.

If the therapeutic goal is not achieved with the diuretic alone, additional drugs should be added as a second step. This stepped-care approach is recommended by the Joint National Committee of the recently completed Hypertension Detection and Follow-up Program (HDFP) [53]. They suggest using an adrenergic blocker, such as Reserpine (0.1 to 0.25 mg per day) or methyldopa (500 to 2000 mg per day). Reserpine blocks the transport of norepinephrine into its storage granules, so that less of the neurotransmitter is available when the adrenergic nerves are stimulated. The resultant decrease in sympathetic tone results in a decrease in peripheral vascular resistance. Methyldopa also decreases peripheral vascular resistance. Methyldopa is closely related to the natural precursor of norepinephrine, dihydroxyphenylalanine (dopa), and enters into the biosynthetic pathway within nerve endings. The

TABLE 9-7
FOODS WITH RELATIVELY HIGH SODIUM CONTENT

Exchange group	Food high in sodium
Milk	Buttermilk
	Malted milk
	Cocoa mix
Meat	Canned, salted, or smoked meats and fish
	Ham, bacon, sausage, bologna, salami, and cold cuts
	Corned beef
	Frankfurters
	Cheese
	Tuna, oil-packed
	Peanut butter
Vegetable	Regular canned vegetables
	Brine-cured vegetables, sauerkraut, pickles
	Olives
	Tomato paste
	Chili sauce
	Potato chips
	Frozen green peas and lima beans
	Regular vegetable juices
Bread	Salted crackers
	Yeast breads prepared with salt
	Muffins, biscuits, cornbread, etc., prepared with salt and baking powder
	Cakes and cookies prepared with salt, soda, or baking powder
	Ready-to-eat cereal
	Precooked dehydrated cereal
	Pretzels and snack chips
	Pastry made with salt
Fat	Commercial salad dressings
	Salted nuts
	Salt pork
Miscellaneous	Catsup
	Prepared mustard
	Worcestershire sauce
	Soy sauce
	Monosodium glutamate (MSG)
	Bouillon cubes
	Canned, frozen, or dried soup
	Garlic salt
	Meat sauces
	Meat tenderizer

TABLE 9-8
ORAL DIURETICS

	Daily dosage, mg	Duration of action, h
Sulfonamide-derived diuretics		
Thiazides and thiazide derivatives		
Chlorothiazide (Diuril)	500–1000	6–12
Hydrochlorothiazide (Esidrix, HydroDiuril, Oretic)	25–200	12–18
Benzthiazide (Aquatag, Exna)	25–200	12–18
Hydroflumethiazide (Saluron)	50–100	12–24
Bendroflumethiazide (Naturetin)	5–20	18–24
Methyclothiazide (Enduron)	2.5–10	24
Trichlormethiazide (Metahydrin, Naqua)	2–4	24
Polythiazide (Renese)	1–4	24–48
Cyclothiazide (Anhydron)	1–2	18–24
Quinethazone (Hydromox)	50–200	18–24
Metolazone (Zaroxolyn)	1–10	12–24
Loop diuretics		
Furosemide (Lasix)	40–120	4–6
Ethacrynic acid (Edecrin)	50–400	12
Potassium-sparing diuretics		
Spironolactone (Aldactone)	25–100	8–12
Triamterene (Dyrenium)	100–300	12

Sources: Joint National Committee on Detection, Evaluation, and Treatment of High Blood Pressure, J. Am. Med. Assoc., 237:255, 1977; N. Kaplan, Clinical Hypertension, 2d ed., Williams & Wilkins, Baltimore, 1978.

TABLE 9-9
GOOD SOURCES OF POTASSIUM

Food	Amount	Potassium,* mg
Apricots, canned	4 apricots, 4 tbsp liquid	422
Orange juice	½ cup	248
Banana	1 small	350
Potato	1 medium	555
Raisins	½ cup	553
Beans, red kidney, cooked	1 cup	629
Prunes, dried, uncooked, pitted	10 prunes	708
Peanuts, roasted, unsalted	1 ounce	196

*The milliequivalent content of potassium may be obtained by dividing the amount in milligrams by 39.
Source: C. F. Adams, Nutritive Value of American Foods, U.S. Department of Agriculture Handbook no. 456, November 1975.

methylnorepinephrine (a "false" neurotransmitter) that is produced displaces norepinephrine from the stores in the adrenergic nerves and central nervous system.

When a third step is needed, hydralazine hydrochloride (30 to 200 mg per day) can be added to the regimen. Hydralazine causes direct relaxation of vascular smooth muscle, but since it increases cardiac work, it should be used cautiously in patients with angina. If the first three steps of the drug regimen are ineffective, addition of the antiadrenergic drug guanethidine sulfate (10 to 200 mg per day), with or without continuation of the medication used in the second and third steps, is then suggested. Guanethidine is taken into adrenergic nerves by an active transport mechanism and blocks the exit of norepinephrine from storage granules, thereby depleting the reserve pool of the neurotransmitter and decreasing the amount released when the nerve is stimulated. The interference with norepinephrine release causes a decrease in arteriolar constriction and a modest reduction in peripheral resistance.

While the recommendations outlined above are satisfactory for most patients, it is important to use a flexible approach, since individual patients may respond differently to each combination of drugs. Additional information on treatment regimens and potential drug side effects is available in Kaplan [4].

Additional measures that can be employed are relief of stress and regular exercise. Relief of emotional and environmental stress is one of the reasons for the improvement in hypertension that occurs when the patient is hospitalized. Though it is usually impossible to extricate hypertensive patients from all their internal and external stresses, they should be advised to avoid unnecessary tension. Regular exercise is indicated within the limits of the patient's cardiovascular status. Not only is exercise helpful in maintaining and controlling weight, but in addition there is evidence that physical conditioning itself may lower arterial pressure. Isotonic exercises (jogging and swimming) are better than isometric exercises (weight lifting).

Management of hypertension must be considered a lifelong endeavor. Patients must be periodically monitored to ensure blood pressure control and to overcome problems in treatment, especially poor patient adherence to both dietary and drug therapy. After control has been demonstrated and the patient's blood pressure has stabilized, most patients should be monitored every 3 to 6 months. It may be possible to reduce drug therapy after normal blood pressure levels are achieved. However, it is rarely possible to discontinue treatment. This point should be emphasized to the patient.

PREVENTION

Primary prevention involves monitoring those factors which, when present in a normotensive individual, may eventually lead to elevated blood pressure, for example, obesity, excessive salt ingestion, and a family history indicating a predisposition to hypertension. Those factors that can be modified, should be changed. Since genetic factors cannot be changed, we need to know whether their operation is direct or whether they simply determine a susceptibility to some necessary environmental agent or agents, as in inbred rat strains whose blood pressure is highly sensitive to salt loading [43].

Although the evidence is not complete, a large body of evidence links hypertension to dietary sodium intake in humans. The evidence suggests some general conclusions.

1 Only a fraction of the human population is genetically susceptible to developing essential hypertension. This fraction varies from 9 to 20 percent in the American population [60]. The remainder of the population (80 to 91 percent) can be considered genetically resistant to developing essential hypertension. Apparently the genetically resistant individual can eat the usual American sodium intake of 150 to 200 meq without developing elevated blood pressure.

However, for genetically susceptible individuals, a lifelong modest salt restriction will probably prevent the onset of hypertension indefinitely and will also prevent all subsequent hypertensive complications. For absolute prevention of hypertension, the epidemiological evidence suggests a daily intake of 230 mg (10 meq) or less of sodium [61]. However, there are examples of tribes with a daily sodium intake of 230 to 1610 mg (10 to 70 meq) in which the prevalence of hypertension is very low. The current average daily intake in the United States is about 3450 to 4600 mg (150 to 200 meq) of sodium. Thus, a moderate restriction to one-third of current levels, i.e., 60 meq, ought to be an effective preventive measure. Unfortunately, there are no certain techniques that will identify individuals who are hypertension-prone, but we do know that individuals at increased risk include (*a*) individuals with a family history of hypertension, (*b*) people of the black race of both sexes, (*c*) individuals with a blood pressure in the upper 20th percentile of the population (*d*) individuals whose resting heart rate is considerably more rapid than would be expected from their state of physical conditioning, and (*e*) individuals who are more than 15 percent above optimal body weight.

2 Control of body weight and correction of obesity are beneficial both in the prevention of hypertension for persons at risk and in the reduction of blood pressure in persons with established hypertension. Weight control, therefore, is a prudent recommendation for all segments of society.

3 The risks of a low-sodium diet appear negligible. It is estimated that our primarily herbivorous ancestors consumed at most 10 meq of sodium per day and a strictly carnivorous man consuming 4000 kcal might have consumed 60 meq of sodium on successful hunting days [62]. The minimum sodium requirement of a healthy adult living in a moderate climate is estimated to be 22 meq (500 mg) or less [62]; the dietary standards for Canada [63] recommend an intake for adults of 15 meq (345 mg).

Since a 60-meq sodium diet has not been applied to wide segments of the American population, there may be subsets of the population, such as the elderly and pregnant women, who may need higher levels of dietary sodium. In addition, occasional severe exertion or heavy physical effort in hot environments may cause an acute loss of sodium in sweat, and additional sodium intake may be required.

To facilitate consumption of a low-sodium diet, considerable assistance is needed from the American food industry. Salt-free convenience foods, food snacks, and restaurant meals should be available. The food industry to date has failed to recognize the considerable needs of hypertensives and their families, as well as other health-conscious consumers who need and/or prefer to limit their salt intake. The Food and Drug Administration is moving to ensure that the labeling of all packaged foods will list sodium and potassium content.

REFERENCES

1 The Pooling Project Research Group, Relationship of blood pressure, serum cholesterol, smoking habit, relative weight, ECG abnormalities to incidence of major coronary events: final report of the Pooling Project, J. Chronic Dis, 31:201, 1978.

2 Williams, G. H., J. I. Jagger, and E. Braunwald: Hypertensive vascular disease, in *Harrison's Principles of Internal Medicine*, 9th ed., K. J. Isselbacher et al. (eds.), McGraw-Hill, New York, 1980.

3 *Blood Pressure Levels of Persons 6–74 Years, United States 1971–1974*, National Health Survey, ser. 11, no. 203, 1977.

4 Kaplan, N. M.: *Clinical Hypertension*, 2d ed., Williams & Wilkins, Baltimore, 1978.

5 Havlik, R. J., and M. Feinleib (eds.), *Proceedings for the Conference on the Decline in Coronary Heart Disease Mortality*, U.S. Department of Health, Education, and Welfare Publication no. (NIH) 79–1610, 1979.

6 Stamler, J., R. Stamler, and T. N. Pullman (eds.), *The Epidemiology of Hypertension*, Grune & Stratton, New York, 1967.

7 Fregly, M. J., and M. S. Fregly: *Oral Contraceptives and High Blood Pressure*, Dolphin Press, Gainesville, Fla. 1974.

8 Paul, O. (ed.): *Epidemiology and Control of Hypertension*, Stratton Intercontinental Medical Book, New York, 1975.

9 Klatsky, A. L., G. D. Friedman, A. B. Siegelaub, and M. J. Gerard: Alcohol consumption and blood pressure, N. Engl. J. Med., 296:1194, 1977.

10 Feinleib, M.: The contribution of family studies to the partitioning of population variation of blood pressure, in *Genetic Analysis of Common Diseases: Applications to Predictive Factors in Coronary Disease*, C. F. Sing and M. Skolnick (eds.), Alan R. Liss, New York, 1979.

11 Feinleib, M., R. Garrison, N. Borhani, R. Rosenman, and J. Christian, Studies of hypertension in twins, in *Epidemiology and Control of Hypertension*, O. Paul (ed.), Symposia Specialists, Miami, 1975.

12 Biron, P.: Pediatric aspects of hypertension, in *Genetic Analysis of Common Diseases: Applications to Predictive Factors in Coronary Disease*, C. F. Sing and M. Skolnick (eds.), Alan R. Liss, New York, 1979.

13 MacLean, C. J., M. S. Adams, W. C. Leyshon, P. L. Worksman, T. E. Reed, H. Gershowitz, and L. R. Weitkamp: Genetic studies on hybrid populations. III. Blood pressure in an American black community, Am. J. Hum. Genet., 26:614, 1974.

14 Veith, I.: *The Yellow Emperor's Classic of Internal Medicine*, University of California Press, Berkeley, 1972.

15 Isaacson, L. C., M. Modlin, and W. P. U. Jackson: Sodium intake and hypertension, Lancet, 1:946, 1963.

16 Meneely, G. R. and L. K. Dahl: Electrolytes in hypertension: the effects of sodium chloride. The evidence from animals and human studies. Hypertension and its treatment, Med. Clin. North Am., 45:271, 1961.

17 Prior, I. A. M., J. G. Evans, H. P. B. Harvey, F. Davidson, and M. Lindsey: Sodium intake and blood pressure in two Polynesian populations, N. Engl. J. Med., 279:515, 1968.

18 Prior, I. A. M., and J. G. Evans: Sodium intake and blood pressure in Pacific populations, Isr. J. Med. Sci., 5:608, 1969.

19 Shaper, A. D.: Cardiovascular disease in the tropics. III. Blood pressure and hypertension, Br. Med. J., 3:805, 1972.

20 Dahl, L. K., and R. A. Love: Etiological role of sodium chloride intake and essential hypertension in humans, J. Am. Med. Assoc., 164:397, 1957.

21 Joosens, J. V., J. Willems, J. Claessens, J. Claes, and W. Lissens: Sodium and hypertension, in *Nutrition and Cardiovascular Diseases,* F. Fidaza et al. (eds.), Morgagni Edizioni Scientifiche, Rome, 1971.

22 Dawber, T. R., W. B. Kannel, A. Kagan, R. K. Donabedian, P. M. McNamara, and G. Pearson: Environmental factors in hypertension, in *The Epidemiology of Hypertension,* J. Stamler, R. Stamler, and T. N. Pullman (eds.), Grune & Stratton, New York, 1967.

23 Langford, H. G., and R. L. Watson: Electrolytes and hypertension, in *Epidemiology and Control of Hypertension,* O. Paul (ed.), Stratton Intercontinental Medical Book, New York, 1975.

24 Pickering, G. W.: *High Blood Pressure,* Churchill, London, 1968.

25 Platt, R.: Heredity in hypertension, O. J. Med., 16:111, 1947.

26 Tobian, L.: Dietary salt (sodium) and hypertension, Am. J. Clin. Nutr., 32:2659, 1979.

27 Mcneely, G. R.: Toxic effects of dietary sodium chloride and the protective effect of potassium, in *Toxicants Occurring Naturally in Foods,* National Academy of Sciences, National Research Council, Food and Nutrition Board, Committee on Food Protection, Washington, 1973.

28 Kempner, W.: Treatment of hypertensive vascular disease with rice diet, Am. J. Med., 4:545, 1948.

29 Medical Research Council: The rice diet in the treatment of hypertension, Lancet, 2:509, 1950.

30 Grollman, A., T. R. Harrison, M. F. Mason, J. Baxter, J. Crampton, and F. Reichsman: Sodium restriction in the diet for hypertension, J. Am. Med., Assoc., 129:533, 1945.

31 Dahl, L. K.: The role of salt in the fall of blood pressure accompanying reduction in obesity, N. Engl. J. Med., 258:1186, 1958.

32 Reisen, E., R. Abel, M. Modan, D. S. Silverberg, H. E. Eliahou, and B. Modan: Effect of weight loss without salt restriction on the reduction of blood pressure in overweight hypertensive patients, N. Engl. J. Med., 298:1, 1978.

33 Morgan, T., N. Adam, A. Gillies, M. Wilson, G. Morgan, and S. Carney: Hypertension treated by salt restriction, Lancet, 1:227, 1978.

34 Murray, R. H., F. C. Luft, R. Block, and A. E. Weyman: Blood pressure responses to extremes of sodium intake in normal man, Proc. Soc. Exp. Biol. Med., 159:432, 1978.

35 McDonough, J., and C. M. Wilhelmj: The effect of excessive salt intake on human blood pressure, Am. J. Dig. Dis., 21:180, 1954.

36 McQuarrie, I., W. H. Thompson, and J. Anderson: Effects of excessive ingestion of sodium and potassium salts on carbohydrate metabolism and blood pressure in diabetic children, J. Nutr., 11:77, 1936.

37 Mark, A. L., W. J. Dawton, F. M. Aboud, A. E. Fitz, and W. E. Connor: Effects of high and low sodium intake on blood pressure and vascular reactivity in borderline hypertensive subjects, Circulation, 50(suppl. 3):107, 1974.

38 Dustan, H. P., G. R. Cumming, A. C. Corcoran, and I. H. Page: A mechanism of chlorothiazide enhanced effectiveness of antihypertensive ganglioplegic drugs, Circulation, 19:360, 1959.

39 Wilson, I. M., and E. D. Fried: Relationship between plasma and extracellular fluid volume depletion and the antihypertensive effect of chlorothiazide, Circulation, 20:1028, 1959.

40 Parijs, J., J. V. Joosens, L. Van de Linden, G. Verstreken, and A. Amery: Moderate sodium restriction and diuretics in the treatment of hypertension, Am. Heart J., 85:22, 1973.

41 Meneely, G. R., and C. O. Ball: Experimental epidemiology of chronic sodium chloride toxicity and the protective effect of potassium chloride, Am. J. Med., 25:713, 1958.

42 Dahl, L. K.: Effects of chronic excess salt feeding: induction of self-sustaining hypertension in rats, J. Exp. Med., 114:231, 1961.

43 Dahl, L. K., M. Heine, and L. Tassinari: Effects of chronic excess salt ingestion. Evidence that genetic factors play an important role in susceptibility to experimental hypertension, J. Exp. Med., 115:1173, 1962.

44 Dahl, L. K., K. D. Knudsen, M. A. Heine, and G. J. Leitl: Effects of chronic excess salt ingestion. Modification of experimental hypertension in the rat by variations in the diet, Cir. Res., 22:11, 1968.

45 Selkurt, E. E.: Effect of pulse pressure and mean arterial pressure modification on renal hemodynamics and electrolyte and water excretion, Circulation, 4:541, 1951.

46 Tobian, L., J. Lange, S. Azar, J. Iwai, D. Koop, K. Coffee, and M. A. Johnson: Reduction in natriuretic capacity and renin release in isolated, blood-perfused kidneys of Dahl hypertension-prone rats, Cir. Res., 43(Part II):I–92, 1978.

47 Pickering, G. W.: Hypertension: definitions, natural history and consequences, Am. J. Med., 52:570, 1972.

48 Sambhi, M. P., M. G. Crane, and J. Genest: Essential hypertension: new concepts about mechanism, Ann. Intern. Med., 79:411, 1973.

49 Gottschak, C. W., and W. E. Lassiter: Mechanism of urine formation, in *Medical Physiology,* V. B. Mountcastle (ed.), Mosby, St. Louis, 1974.

50 Slottkoff, L. M.: Prostaglandins and hypertension, Angiology, 29:320, 1978.

51 Swales, J. D.: *Clinical Hypertension,* University Press, Cambridge, England, 1979.

52 Page, I. H.: Arterial hypertension in retrospect, Cir. Res., 34:133, 1974.

53 Joint National Committee on Detection, Evaluation and Treatment of High Blood Pressure: Report of the Joint National Committee on Detection, Evaluation, and Treatment of High Blood Pressure, J. Am. Med. Assoc., 237:255, 1977.

54 Moser, M.: Management of hypertension, J. Am. Med. Assoc., 235:2297, 1976.

55 Mertz, W.: Effect of dietary components on lipids and lipoproteins: mineral elements, in *Nutrition, Lipids and Coronary Heart Disease,* R. Levy et al. (eds.), Raven, New York, 1979.

56 Hunt, J. C., C. G. Strong, E. G. Harrison, W. L. Furlow, and F. J. Leary: Management of hypertension of renal origin, Am. J. Cardiol., 26:280, 1970.

57 Hunt, J. C.: Management and treatment of essential hypertension, in *Hypertension,* J. Genest, E. Koiw, and O. Kuchel (eds.), McGraw-Hill, New York, 1977.

58 Dahl, L. K.: Salt and hypertension, Am. J. Clin. Nutr., 25:231, 1972.

59 Lipman, A. G.: Sodium content of frequently used analgesics and gastrointestinal drugs, Mod. Med., 45:59, 1977.

60 Tobian, L.: The relationship of salt to hypertension, Am. J. Clin. Nutr., 32:2739, 1979.

61 Freis, E. D.: Salt, volume and the prevention of hypertension, Circulation, 3:589, 1976.

62 Meneely, G. R., and H. D. Battarbee: Sodium and potassium, in *Present Knowledge of Nutrition,* 4th ed., The Nutrition Foundation, New York, 1976.

63 Committee for Revision of the Canadian Dietary Standard: *Dietary Standard for Canada,* Information Canada, Ottawa, 1975.

CHAPTER 10

NUTRITIONAL ASPECTS
OF HEMATOPOIESIS

CONTENTS

INTRODUCTION

The deficiency anemias most commonly encountered in clinical practice are due to lack of iron, folacin, or cobalamin, either independently or in various combinations. So far as we know, the other deficiencies listed in Table 10-1

TABLE 10-1
NUTRIENTS INVOLVED IN HEMATOPOIESIS: EFFECTS OF DEFICIENCY

Nutrient	Type of anemia	Other hematological changes

Iron	Microcytic
	Hypochromic
		Poikilocytosis
		Normal white cells
		Normal platelets
		Erythroid hyperplasia of
		  marrow
		Absence of stainable iron in
		  marrow

Folic acid and
  cobalamin
	Macrocytic	Poikilocytosis
		Neutropenia
		Hypersegmentation of neutrophil
		  nucleus
		Thrombocytopenia
		Megaloblastic marrow
		Giant myelocytes and mega-
		  karyocytes in marrow

Pyridoxine	Microcytic Hypochromic	Poikilocytosis Leukopenia Sideroblasts in marrow
α-Tocopherol	Hemolytic	
Protein	Normocytic, partly dilutional	

rarely occur in the United States. However, prolonged total parenteral feeding has revealed hitherto unsuspected hematopoietic effects of deficiencies. Table 10-2 provides an approach to the diagnosis of the cause of anemia. The purpose of Table 10-3 is to present in an accessible way the categories of subjects in whom each type of deficiency anemia may be expected, relevant dietary or other information to be sought in taking a history, and symptomatology and physical findings. Further information is available in the sections which follow. Current concepts of the ways in which all the nutrients listed in Table 10-1 are involved in red blood cell formation can be found in Figure 10-1.

It must be emphasized that recognition of the possibility of a nutritional anemia in a patient is a major step in the direction of effective therapy. Thoughtful and logical diagnostic steps should establish the cause or likely cause of the anemia and lead to appropriate, specific therapy, without risk of aggravating the effects of the deficiency.

Nutritional anemias may be due to lack of a single nutrient or of more than one nutrient. For instance, most anemia in young women is due to iron deficiency alone. However, in anemia associated with disease of the small bowel, changes in the blood which are consistent with deficiency of both iron and folacin may occur. In pernicious anemia in middle-aged women, deficiency of both cobalamin and iron may be found.

TABLE 10-2

DIAGNOSTIC APPROACH TO CHRONIC ANEMIA*

Lack of hematinics due to:	Consider:
Dietary deficiency:	
Iron	Dietary history
Folacin (rare)	Dietary idiosyncracy
Cobalamin (rare)	Dietary idiosyncracy
Malabsorption:	
Iron	Gastric surgery, celiac-sprue
Folacin	Celiac-sprue
Cobalamin	Inflammatory small-bowel disease
	Resection of distal small bowel
Increased need:	
Iron	Pregnancy: rapid growth
Folacin	Pregnancy
Recurrent or chronic blood loss:	
Iron	Menorrhagia
	Gastrointestinal bleeding
Repeated hemolysis:	
Folacin	Paroxysmal nocturnal hemoglobinuria

*Anemia in women is indicated by a hemoglobin concentration < 12.3 g/dl, and in men by a hemoglobin concentration < 12.9 g/dl (both lower limits of normal).

TABLE 10-3

NUTRITIONAL ANEMIAS

Deficiency	Relevant information	Symptomatology and findings
	Infants	
α-Tocopherol	Prematurity:	
	Occurs weeks or months after birth	Hemolytic anemia
	Low birth weight	Pallor
		Other stigmata rare
		Noted after infection
Iron	Milk-based iron-deficient diets	
	Milk allergy	Abnormal stools
		Blood in stools
	Possibility of celiac disease	Abnormal stools
		Other deficiencies
Iron and folacin	Strong possibility of celiac disease	Abnormal stools
		Other deficiencies

TABLE 10-3 (Continued)

Deficiency	Relevant information	Symptomatology and findings
	Adolescents	
Iron	Females:	
	Menstrual loss	Fatigue
		Pallor
	Both sexes:	
	Rapid growth and inadequate intake of iron	
	Adults	
Iron	Females of childbearing age:	
	Menstrual loss	Fatigue
	Pregnancy	Glossitis
	Low calorie intake	Koilonychia
	Idiosyncrasies of diet	Dysphagia
	Pica	
	Middle age, both sexes:	
	Bleeding peptic ulcers	Symptoms of ulcer disease
	and other sites of gastro-	Rectal bleeding
	intestinal tract	Melena
	Malabsorption due to small	Abnormal stools
	bowel disease, post	Other deficiencies
	gastrectomy	
	Old age, both sexes:	
	Low calorie intake	Weight loss
	Low iron content of diet	Glossitis
		Angular stomatitis
Folacin	Females of childbearing age:	
	Pregnancy	
	Any age, both sexes:	
	Alcoholism	Other deficiencies
Iron and	Malabsorption due to small	Abnormal stools
folacin	bowel disease	Other deficiencies
Cobalamin	Pernicious anemia	Glossitis
	Postgastrectomy	Neurological changes
	Resection or disease of	
	terminal small bowel	
	Vegetarian diet	

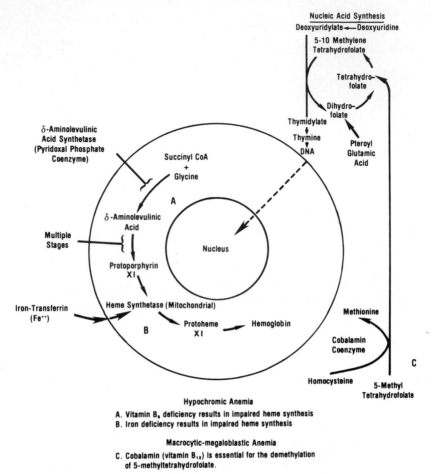

FIGURE 10-1
Metabolic pathways involving nutrients essential for red blood cell formation.

The effects of either folacin or cobalamin depletion are indistinguishable in the hematopoietic system. Treatment of the cobalamin-deficient subject with folic acid alone may result in severe damage to the central nervous system, since folacin can substitute to some extent for cobalamin in hematopoiesis, but it cannot do so in those processes which maintain myelin integrity in the nervous system.

In the United States, anemia due to iron deficiency is the most common type of anemia, affecting particularly infants, adolescent girls, and young women. Anemia due to deficiency of folacin is the next most common anemia; those individuals who are most commonly affected are chronic alcoholics. Clinical manifestations of cobalamin deficiency are rather uncommon and are confined to subjects with pernicious anemia, to those who have had extensive gastric resections, to a small proportion of those with inflammatory bowel disease, and to those who have had resection of the second half of the small bowel. Cobalamin deficiency may also occur in a small number of total vegetarians.

IRON IN NUTRITION

Distribution in the Body

Iron is an integral component of oxygen-transporting proteins and of enzymes essential to tissue respiration, the major ones of which are hemoglobin, myoglobin, the cytochrome system, peroxidase, and catalase. In these compounds iron is incorporated in a porphyrin to form heme. Some iron is also present as ferritin and hemosiderin, which are iron-storage protein complexes present mainly in the liver, spleen, and bone marrow. The total amount of iron in the body varies according to size and sex. In a 70-kg adult it is about 4 g, the amount present in a medium-sized carpenter's nail; of this, 75 percent is found in the red blood cells as hemoglobin, 5 percent as myoglobin, less than 0.5 percent as heme-containing enzymes, and less than 0.1 percent in circulation, bound to a specific β-globulin called *transferrin*. Ferritin and hemosiderin together constitute about 20 percent of the total load of iron in the body (Figure 10-2).

Dietary Requirements

Iron requirements vary greatly between groups of healthy individuals because of differential rates of growth, losses of iron due to menstruation, and the increased needs of pregnancy. Lactation is responsible for a daily loss of less than 1 mg, or approximately the daily loss due to menstruation, which is usually suppressed during lactation.

Until recently, stated daily requirements in terms of iron intake were based on the crude assumption that 10 percent of dietary iron was absorbed. For adult males the Recommended Daily Allowance is 10 mg [1], which provides 1 mg of

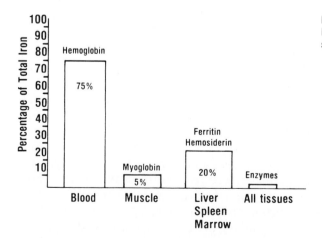

FIGURE 10-2
Distribution of iron in the replete subject.

absorbable iron, and for women of childbearing age the RDA is 18 mg, which provides 1.8 mg of absorbable iron. The RDA for infants during the first year of life is 1.5 mg dietary iron per kilogram of body weight. The RDA for male adolescents, who are still growing, is also 18 mg.

Iron Deficiency

The development of iron deficiency involves different tissue compartments sequentially. When losses exceed absorption, reduction in iron stores in liver, spleen, and bone marrow occurs first, then increasing desaturation of transferrin. It is sometimes stated that the number of red blood cells then falls, but this is not the case. What happens is that an increasing number become smaller than normal, and finally there is a fall in red cell hemoglobin concentration. Fully developed iron-deficiency anemia is thus microcytic and hypochromic. Although not a sensitive indicator of iron depletion, the appearance of microcytes occurs quite early and studies suggest that it is still useful as an indicator of iron depletion [2]. Alternatively, direct or indirect measurements of iron stores can be made, the former by staining bone marrow for iron and the latter by estimating serum ferritin by radioimmunoassay.

Epidemiology   Iron deficiency is one of the commonest forms of malnutrition worldwide. Low intake of dietary iron, often in a poorly absorbed form or in association with other dietary constituents which inhibit absorption, is common and in many areas of the world is aggravated by parasitic infestation, which causes chronic blood loss from the intestinal or urinary tract. The commonest such infestations are hookworm disease (ancylostomiasis) and flukes (schistosomiasis). This low intake of dietary iron results in morbidity due to severe anemia and impaired physical performance. When pregnancy complicates existing iron-deficiency anemia under these conditions, the anemia may become profound and may even precipitate heart failure. Rates of miscarriage, prematurity, and perinatal morbidity and mortality are all significantly raised. In North America, available data from surveys suggest that those at risk of iron deficiency are young children, young women and, particularly, pregnant women. A Canadian study reported by Valberg et al. [3] showed that only 2 percent of subjects had abnormally low hemoglobin concentrations. However, by measuring serum ferritin concentration, which is a valid indicator of bone marrow stores in populations, though not necessarily for individuals, it was shown that 19 percent of subjects, mainly children and nonpregnant young women, and 60 percent of pregnant women had depleted iron stores. The results of the Ten-State Nutrition Survey conducted in the United States in 1968 to 1969 suggested that significantly low hemoglobin values and iron intake were present in up to 20 percent of subjects sampled in states such as Texas and Louisiana [4]. All age groups and both sexes were affected. In some areas blacks were more affected than whites, and there was a positive correlation between levels of hemoglobin and educational achievement of homemakers. Inadequate iron intakes were found most commonly in infants, but were not rare in other groups. One survey in the inner city of Baltimore revealed that 30 percent of 15-year-old males had hemoglobin values below 12 g/dl and a daily mean iron intake of 9.5 ± 4.2 mg, compared to the calculated daily need of 16 mg for the male adolescent [5]. Surveys have shown significantly low levels of iron-dependent indexes in older age groups and both sexes. Others have established that 5 to 20 percent of a population 65 years old or older are anemic, usually from iron deficiency. However, mean iron stores tend to rise in elderly populations, and currently there is agreement that in the United States iron-deficiency anemia in the elderly is almost always due, in part, to gastrointestinal bleeding, which is sometimes compounded by poor dietary intake of iron or by malabsorption. However, iron deficiency in the elderly due to low iron intake may occur, particularly when the total daily intake from a conventional diet is less than 1400 kcal.

In clinical practice in the United States the common causes of iron deficiency in adults are, in order of frequency, chronic occult bleeding into the gastrointestinal tract; menstruation, both heavy and normal; and pregnancy. Inadequate intake of iron without excessive loss of blood is a cause of deficiency in women of menstrual age (see Figure 10-3), which group constituted about 25 percent of all

FIGURE 10-3
Mean iron intakes of persons aged 1 to 74 years, by age, race, and sex: United States, 1971 to 1974. (*Adapted from U.S. Department of Health, Education, and Welfare Publication no. (PHS) 79–1657, June 1979.*)

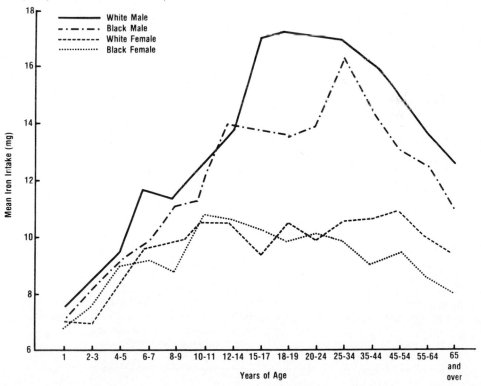

cases of iron-deficiency anemia in a survey made in Oxford 15 years ago [6]. Malabsorption of iron occurs less frequently. However, after gastric surgery there may be failure to absorb iron from food and failure of the mechanism which is responsible for increasing the percentage of absorption of iron from the small bowel when the iron stores of the body are depleted.

In children under 2 years of age, low birth weight and inadequate dietary iron are the usual causes of iron deficiency. A survey by Sturgeon [7] of apparently healthy children in lower-income groups in California revealed mean hemoglobin concentrations of 10.8, 9.9, and 10.7 g/dl at the ages of 6, 12, and 18 months, respectively. The 12-month figure is 2 g/dl lower than the mean figure at this age obtained by the Health and Nutrition Examination Survey (HANES) of the National Center for Health Statistics [8].

Table 10-4 lists the diagnoses which should be considered when iron-deficiency anemia is found to be present.

Etiology and Pathogenesis   In simplest terms iron deficiency occurs because of inadequate intake, inadequate absorption, excessive loss of iron, or any combination of these three factors.

The normal regulatory mechanisms for maintaining iron homeostasis reside in the epithelial cells of the small intestine, where absorption of iron occurs.

TABLE 10–4
POSSIBLE DIAGNOSES BASED UPON PRESENCE OF HYPOCHROMIC MICROCYTIC (IRON-DEFICIENCY) ANEMIA

Infants

Low birth weight	Celiac disease
Inadequate dietary iron	Pica
(breast- or bottle-fed)	Intestinal infestations (in tropics)
Allergic enteritis	

Women of menstrual age

Menstruation and inadequate	Pregnancy
iron intake	Intestinal infestations (in tropics)
Menorrhagia	

Men of all ages and postmenopausal women

Peptic ulcer and erosions	Esophageal varices
Aspirin and other anti-	Celiac-sprue
inflammatory drugs	Esophagitis and hiatus hernia
Polyps: colon	Inflammatory bowel disease
Cancer: colon, stomach, ampulla	Hemorrhoids
of Vater	Postmenopausal uterine bleeding
Gastric surgery	Intestinal infestations (in tropics)
Diverticulosis	

Absorption of Iron   Iron is currently considered to be present in food in only two forms: heme and nonheme iron. That this is all we can say about the composition of iron in food is a reflection of our ignorance of some of the complexities of iron absorption; nevertheless, it represents a considerable advance over what we knew 10 years ago. The amounts of heme and nonheme iron available for absorption in a single meal can now be estimated by taking into account the influence of other dietary constituents on the absorption of both iron components [9]. Nonheme iron is absorbed by an active process into the epithelial cells (enterocytes) in the upper part of the small intestine, mainly in the duodenum and proximal jejunum. Heme iron is absorbed into the enterocytes by a different process and possibly over a more extensive length of small bowel. Whether the difference in the site of absorption is due to the influence of intraluminal factors operating differently on these two forms of iron or whether it is due to specificity of type and distribution of enterocyte receptors is not known. On the basis of available data the former seems more likely.

The proportion of total iron as heme iron in animal, fish, poultry, and mammalian tissues, though variable, averages 40 percent. The remainder is classed as nonheme, as is all the iron in vegetable sources. Heme iron is far more efficiently absorbed than nonheme iron, and its absorption appears to be little influenced by intraluminal factors. Monsen et al. [9] estimate that the mean absorption of the total iron content of heme iron is 23 percent. Absorption of the nonheme iron is much more affected by intraluminal factors. Phosphate, phytate, and antacids, even tannin in tea, inhibit its absorption. Ascorbic acid in oral doses of up to 1 g enhances absorption in a linear manner. The presence of animal tissues enhances nonheme iron absorption.

Monsen et al. suggest that iron absorption from a single meal can be predicted by computing the following:

1 Total iron in the meal from food composition tables. Forty percent of the iron in animal tissues will be heme iron, and the rest will be nonheme. All of the iron in vegetable sources is nonheme iron.
2 The amount of ascorbic acid in the meal.
3 The amount of animal tissue.

The values given in Table 10-5, which are derived from Monsen et al. [9], allow estimation of absorbable iron.

The amount of either category of iron absorbed beyond the enterocyte and transported to stores for subsequent utilization depends on the iron stores of the body and rates of hemoglobin synthesis. The iron-depleted subject absorbs more than the replete subject. The mechanisms involved have still not been satisfactorily elucidated. Inorganic iron given orally as ferrous sulfate, labeled with radioiron, enters by a different mechanism from heme iron, which passes into the enterocyte as the intact heme molecule after proteolytic cleavage of globin and is subsequently degraded, probably by the enzyme heme oxygenase in the enterocyte.

TABLE 10-5

AVAILABILITY OF FOOD IRON

	Percentage of absorption of iron	
	Nonheme iron	Heme iron
Low availability meal < 30 g meat, poultry, or fish < 25 mg ascorbic acid	3	23

Medium availability meal
  30–90 g meat, poultry, or fish
  or 25–75 mg ascorbic acid
	5	23

High availability meal
  > 90 g meat, poultry, or fish
  or > 75 mg ascorbic acid
  or 30–90 g meat, poultry, or fish
   plus 25–75 mg ascorbic acid
	8	23

Source: E. R. Monsen, L. Hállberg, M. Layrisse, D. M. Hegstead, J. D. Cook, W. Mertz, and C. A. Finch, Am. J. Clin. Nutr., 31:143, 1978.

The current view of regulation of absorption is that some iron is transferred from plasma transferrin into the enterocyte as it differentiates in the crypts of Lieberkühn; the amount transferred is an expression of transferrin saturation and thus of iron stores. The amount of nonheme iron, which is moved from the lumen into the enterocyte by an active process, against a concentration gradient, is not influenced by the amount of iron already present in the enterocyte. But the amount which is transported out of the enterocyte and bound to transferrin is a function of the primary load of iron in the enterocyte. If this is high, the major part of absorbed nonheme iron gets no further; it is incorporated with apoferritin to form ferritin and is lost as the enterocyte is shed into the lumen of the gut.

This mechanism appears to fail sometimes. In the evolution of hemochromatosis the absorption of iron is enhanced in spite of adequate body stores. It is only in the late iron-overloaded state that the inhibitory mechanism appears to exert its effect.

Iron absorbed beyond the enterocyte, from heme or nonheme sources, is bound to a specific plasma β-globulin, transferrin, for transport through the body. A contribution to plasma iron also comes from the breakdown of hemoglobin from red blood corpuscles, which are destroyed at the end of their life span in the reticuloendothelial system. The total daily turnover of iron through the plasma is about 25 to 45 mg in the adult. The major components of iron metabolism are summarized in Figure 10-4.

Malabsorption of iron occurs in a number of gastrointestinal diseases. The most important is a consequence of gastric surgery, particularly when the

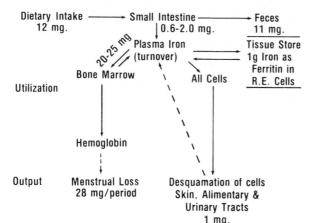

FIGURE 10-4
Summary of daily iron metabolism in humans.

duodenum has been bypassed as in a Billroth II partial gastrectomy. Studies have shown that after any of the surgical procedures used for peptic ulcer disease, absorption of dietary iron is impaired and that the percentage of absorption of heme iron and nonheme iron given with food is more affected than is the absorption of tracer doses of inorganic iron. There is also some evidence that the mechanism which increases absorption when the subject is iron-deficient is impaired, but the evidence is not conclusive. Since many subjects are iron-depleted before surgery and may continue to bleed chronically, either continuously or intermittently, from gastric erosions or stomach ulcers after surgery, there may be increasingly severe iron deficiency following gastric surgery unless iron stores are repleted.

Another cause of malabsorption of iron is mucosal disease of the small intestine such as gliadin-induced enteropathy, tropical sprue, and regional enteritis. Malabsorption of iron may also be a sequela to small bowel bypass for gross obesity.

The complexity of interplay of different factors which affect iron absorption from a diet consisting of many constituents is well-illustrated by concern about vegetarian diets. If eggs are excluded, the iron in such diets is present almost exclusively in nonheme forms, and, in addition, vegetarian diets contain inhibitors of iron absorption such as phytate. Cow's milk itself may inhibit iron absorption. The best practical advice for the vegetarian is to undergo annual checks of hemoglobin and serum iron levels and not to rely on calculations of intake and absorption.

The effect of alcohol (ethanol) has not been adequately examined. Experiments with healthy volunteers have shown that acute ingestion of alcohol enhances absorption of ferric chloride but not absorption of heme iron or inorganic iron given with ascorbic acid [10]. Studies of iron absorption in chronic alcoholics have not been reported.

Some substances impair the absorption of nonheme iron. Among these are medications such as tetracylines and antacids. Phytate (in cereals), tannin (in tea), oxalate (in green leafy vegetables), and nondigestible fibers are examples of naturally occurring factors which inhibit iron absorption. Inquiry into iron deficiency should include questions about intake of such foods.

Of importance both in the United States and in other countries is the phenomenon of pica, which is a perversion of the appetite causing individuals to consume clay, laundry starch, chalk, and other substances, often in surprisingly large quantities. Young children and pregnant women, especially in black communities, seem especially prone to the condition. Some of these substances inhibit iron absorption. Inquiry about consumption of unusual substances should always be made of patients suffering from iron deficiency.

Loss of Iron   There is no mechanism for regulating the excretion of iron. In the adult, after growth has ceased, daily loss is of the order of 0.5 mg in cells shed from internal and external body surfaces.

In addition, according to a study in Sweden, daily loss due to menstruation when averaged over 1 month amounts to a mean of 0.6 mg per day, but in half the women in this study the loss was more than 1.1 mg per day, in one-fourth it was more than 1.5 mg per day, and in 10 percent it exceeded 2 mg per day [11]. If these figures are fairly typical, daily iron loss in one-third of women of menstrual age is four times that of an adult male. However, a recent study by Hallberg et al. [12] reveals a striking fall in prevalence of iron-deficiency anemia in the same general female population, from 25 to 30 percent to 6 to 7 percent. How much of this has been due to better control of menstrual loss by the use of oral contraceptives, how much to increasing fortification of flour with iron, how much to use of iron tablets, and how much to consumption of ascorbic acid is derived by factorial analysis (Figure 10-5).

In pregnancy, a single fetus accumulates about 300 mg of iron and the placenta 70 mg; the increased maternal red blood corpuscular mass requires an average 290 mg, and loss of blood at delivery may represent 100 to 250 mg. Fifteen months of associated amenorrhea conserves 250 to 500 mg, so that the overall deficit is approximately 0.5 g or more if the infant is breast-fed for 6 months. Human milk contains 0.5 mg of highly absorbable iron per liter, and lactation is responsible for a loss of 0.5 to 1.5 mg iron daily.

The other principal source of loss is the gastrointestinal tract. The main causes of abnormal loss have been tabulated (Table 10-4). There are rare ones, such as a bleeding Meckel's diverticulum, multiple telangiectasia, and pseudo-xanthoma elasticum, which are outside the scope of this book.

In temperate regions occult fecal blood loss may be detected in some infants with iron-deficiency anemia who are being fed cow's milk formula diets. It appears they are allergic to β-lactoglobulin. The lesions are not unlike those of inflammatory bowel disease [13]. A different type of small intestinal lesion with some shortening and clubbing of the villi and occult blood loss and malabsorption of fat and vitamin A has been described [14]. This lesion is said to respond to treatment with iron. We have found no similar lesions in rats maintained in a markedly iron-deficient state for some months [15].

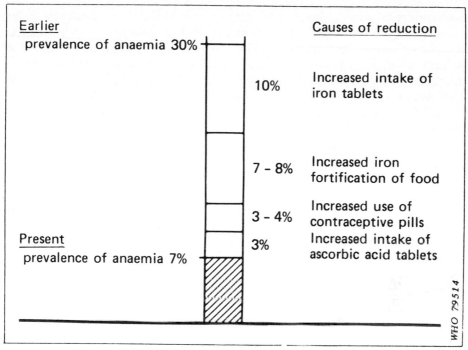

FIGURE 10-5
Factorial analysis of causes of reduction in prevalence of anemia in Swedish women of fertile age. (*From L. Hallberg, C. Bengttsson, L. Garby, J. Lennartsson, L. Rossander, and E. Tibblin, Bull. WHO, 57:947, 1979.*)

One cause of excessive loss which is now attracting attention are conditions of the skin such as psoriasis and exfoliative dermatitis, in which cell turnover is much increased. In these conditions, if a sufficient area of body surface is involved, daily losses of iron may be considerably increased [16].

A final consideration which illustrates the efficiency of the mechanisms responsible for maintaining an appropriate iron balance is their capacity to meet the needs of the growing child through puberty. The fetus at term contains some 250 mg iron, or less if underweight. By 18 years of age a male must accumulate an additional 5000 mg, or approximately 2 mg daily, in addition to the daily loss during this period. After menarche, the daily requirements of a female, until growth has ceased, may be 3 mg. It is remarkable that most young men do not become anemic, though some instances were documented after the Second World War in the United Kingdom [17] and recently some instances have been observed in the United States [5]. It is small wonder that young women show a significant prevalence of iron-deficiency anemia.

Clinical Findings   The onset of symptoms of iron-deficiency anemia is insidious. Although weakness, easy fatigability, palpitations, breathlessness, pallor, and headaches are usually present, some patients with low circulating hemoglobin concentrations do not complain at all. When the condition is very severe, the pulse is rapid, cardiac output is much increased, and there is a precordial systolic murmur and ankle edema. Glossitis occurs in about 40 percent of patients (Color Figure 8). The tongue is reddened and papillae disappear, leaving the surface, and particularly the edge, denuded and smooth. The patient complains of a burning tongue, which is probably responsible for the craving for ice sucking, or pagophagia, which some iron-deficient young women display. Angular stomatitis also occurs, particularly in the edentulous or those with too shallow a "bite" due to poorly fitting dentures (Color Figure 7).

Concave spooning of the fingernails, or koilonychia, has been described in 18 percent of iron-deficient subjects in the United Kingdom, but it appears to be uncommon in the United States. Some patients complain of a dry throat and difficulty in swallowing. In about 10 percent of subjects with chronic iron deficiency, predominantly women, there is significant dysphagia, and a post-cricoid web, a midline backward-projecting fold of mucosa in the uppermost part of the esophagus, may occur. There is usually some degree of stenosis in the upper esophagus. The associated findings of hypochromic anemia, glossitis, and dysphagia have been termed the Plummer-Vinson, or Paterson-Kelly, syndrome. Whether depression of gastric secretory function and chronic atrophic gastritis occur as a consequence of continuing iron deficiency in humans is unresolved, but there is no doubt that there is a significant association, and the bulk of evidence favors the possibility that iron deficiency damages the gastric mucosa. However, recovery of the mucosa does not occur after iron therapy.

Surprisingly, in the iron-deficient infant none of the buccal or nail changes are found, but gastric achlorhydria is common, which responds to iron repletion. The spleen is palpable in about 10 percent of iron-deficient adults.

Iron is an essential part of a number of vital electron-transporting enzyme systems in the body, and it is surprising that depletion of iron, which is known to precede the development of the typical microcytic, hypochromic anemia, is not associated with the symptoms and signs which occur before the onset of anemia. In fact symptoms of iron deficiency without anemia have not been shown conclusively to occur, and the clinical picture as described is rarely if ever seen unless the hemoglobin level is below 10 g/dl. Significant functional impairment of the nonanemic iron-deficient subject has yet to be demonstrated. Although some investigators have found reductions in cytochrome oxidase activity and reductions of other iron-containing enzymes in buccal mucosal tissue in iron deficiency, these results have not been confirmed.

There is much speculation about the role of iron in the immune response and in modifying infections, but no conclusive data are available.

Laboratory Diagnosis   The degree of anemia in iron deficiency in the United States is usually moderate and quite unlike that seen in those parts of the world where infestation is rife, dietary intake of iron low, and multiple pregnancies common. In Table 10-6 the values of various hematological indexes found in iron-deficient anemia are compared with the normal observed ranges.

Examination of the blood film reveals small red blood cells (microcytosis) of

TABLE 10-6

COMPARISON OF HEMATOLOGICAL INDEXES FOUND IN NORMAL SUBJECTS AND IN
SUBJECTS WITH IRON-DEFICIENCY ANEMIA*

Index	Iron-deficient	Normal range (sea level)
Hemoglobin, g/dl	< 12.0	14.7 ± 1.8 (M)
		13.5 ± 1.2 (F)
Red blood corpuscles, $10^6/\mu l$	< 4.67 ± 0.86	5.0 ± 0.6 (M)
		4.6 ± 0.5 (F)
Mean cell volume, fl	< 80	85.52 ± 4.8 (M)
		85.8 ± 3.9 (F)
Packed cell volume, %	< 37.9 (M)	42.8 ± 4.9 (M)
	< 35.8 (F)	39.5 ± 3.7 (F)
Mean cell diameter, μm	< 6.7	7.2 ± 2.6
Mean cell hemoglobin concentration, %	< 31	34.4 ± 1.3 (M)
		34.0 ± 1.3 (F)
Red cell free protoporphyrin, $\mu g/dl$	60-600	39 (16-67)
Plasma		
Iron, $\mu g/dl$	15-50	71-201 (M)
		62-173 (F)
Iron binding capacity, $\mu g/dl$	350-400[†]	253-435
Serum ferritin, $\mu g/dl$	< 1.0	6.9 (M)[‡]
		3.6 (F)[‡]

* Some normochromic, normocytic cells are always present. The indexes may mask the presence of a population of markedly abnormal cells.
[†] Iron saturation may be as low as 5 percent.
[‡] Mean value.

variable size (anisocytosis) and shape (poikilocytosis). There is always a
population of apparently normal cells as well. The microcytic, hypochromic cells
appear as rings of hemoglobin. Occasional nucleated red cells are seen in a blood
smear of peripheral blood. The unavailability of iron is manifested by the
abnormally high concentration of free protoporphyrin in the red cells and the
reduction in circulating ferritin and transferrin-bound iron. Reticulocyte,
platelet, and white cell numbers are usually within the normal range. If either of
the last two is deficient, an additional deficiency of folacin or cobalamin is to be
suspected.

The bone marrow has a notable excess of red cell precursor cells, which are
smaller than normal, and absence of iron stores, which are normally present
mainly as hemosiderin granules in reticuloendothelial cells.

Treatment   Chronic blood loss from the gastrointestinal tract is the commonest cause of iron deficiency, and its detection and management lie outside the
scope of this text. Most of the sites of bleeding must be treated by specific
medical or surgical means, and the iron stores subsequently restored—an

important matter that is sometimes overlooked. In patients, usually old and frail, in whom the rate of blood loss is such that the bone marrow can compensate if adequate amounts of iron are present and in whom surgery is contraindicated because of inoperability or extragastrointestinal disease that is liable to make abdominal surgery unjustifiably life-threatening, the aim is to maintain adequate iron intake. In many patients with chronic inflammatory bowel disease, particularly Crohn's disease of the small bowel, intermittent blood loss occurs in spite of medical treatment. It may be compounded by a degree of malabsorption, and surgery may be contraindicated. Iron therapy is essential in such cases. Judicious blood transfusion may help to keep the patient active. Women with menorrhagia who do not wish to have a hysterectomy should be treated as skillfully as possible with hormones to reduce menstrual loss and should receive adequate iron therapy. In pregnancy, iron supplementation is strongly advocated by all but a small minority who argue that there is no advantage to attempting to correct an anemia which is largely physiological and due to hemodilution.

The route of administration of iron is determined by clinical expediency. Oral, intravenous, and intramuscular preparations of iron are available. Convenience, cost and, to a lesser extent, safety favor the oral route. However, a significant number of patients without gastrointestinal disease complain of nausea, vomiting, diarrhea, constipation, colic, or any combination of these when taking a therapeutic course of ferrous iron.

Some of the preparations available and their iron content are listed in Table 10-7. Of these, ferrous sulfate elicits intolerance about three times as frequently as the others. A daily intake of 100 to 200 mg of elemental iron is the maximum tolerated dose, and from this some 10 to 15 percent will be absorbed. If larger

TABLE 10-7
PREPARATIONS OF IRON

Compound	Iron, %	Dose
Oral		
Ferrous sulfate (hydrated)	20	300 mg t.i.d.
Ferrous fumarate	33	200 mg t.i.d.
Ferrous gluconate	12	300 mg t.i.d.
Ferrous lactate	19	300 mg t.i.d.
Parenteral (intramuscular and intravenous)		
Iron-dextran complex (Imferon)	5	25 mg* (infants) 100 mg* (adults < 50 kg) 250 mg* (adults > 50 kg)

*Daily maximum.

intakes are encouraged, side effects will increase and compliance fall. This daily intake should be continued until the hemoglobin level is restored to within the normal range except in pregnancy in which the dilutional factor usually makes it impossible to achieve this end-point.

It has been observed that large numbers of iron tablets are not taken and lie in medicine cupboards or drawers, constituting a hazard to young children, since they are brightly colored, are usually sugarcoated, and have an elemental iron content which is sufficient to cause death if 20 tablets or more are ingested by a toddler. Relapse of iron-deficiency anemia in young women is common. These two observations clearly suggest poor compliance, and when a history is taken, poor compliance is found in many patients to be due to minor intolerance of the treatment. Continuing follow-up and supervision of patients will mitigate the problem. Another approach is to switch to an elemental iron preparation in which the dose is halved but ascorbic acid is added, which markedly enhances the percentage of the dose of iron absorbed. Young women should always be encouraged to select a diet of higher iron content (Table 10-8).

Parenteral administration of iron may be necessary in patients with malabsorption syndromes, before response to gliadin-exclusion in celiac-sprue, and in those who are bleeding chronically or episodically from inflammatory bowel disease or multiple hereditary telangiectasia. Subjects with Crohn's disease or nonspecific ulcerative colitis tolerate oral iron poorly and commonly lose abnormal amounts of blood from the GI tract. Before surgery for chronic bleeding from ulcer disease, it is recommended that iron stores be repleted parenterally.

A major advantage of parenteral iron therapy is that repletion of depleted iron stores can be achieved by using the following simple calculation:

$$\text{mg iron to be injected} = \left[\left(\frac{\text{normal Hb (g/dl)} - \text{patient's Hb (g/dl)}}{100} \right) \times 3.4 \right] \times 4000 + 500 \text{ mg}$$

where 4000 is the average blood volume in milliliters, 3.4 is a conversion factor

TABLE 10-8
DIETARY SOURCES OF HEMATINICS

Iron	Folacin	Cobalamin
Liver	Liver	Liver
Red meat	Green vegetables	Red meat
Shellfish	Nuts	Fish
Nuts	Yeasts	Milk and cheese
Beans and peas		
Apricots		
Raisins		
Enriched bread		

(grams of hemoglobin to milligrams of iron), and 500 mg is added to replenish iron stores. In the pregnant woman in the third trimester, add 1 g instead of 500 mg. Normal hemoglobin values are listed in Table 10-6.

Another formula that can be used is the following:

$$\text{mg iron to be injected} = [15 - \text{patient's Hb (g/dl)}] \times \text{body weight (kg)} \times 3$$

Preparations of iron-dextran complex are given either intramuscularly or intravenously. Reluctance to administer iron intramuscularly is due to fear of subsequent skin discoloration. This can be avoided by using a Z injection track and injecting not more than 5 ml at any one site.

If given intravenously, it is best to infuse the calculated dose in 500 ml sterile normal saline over the course of 30 to 180 minutes. Should dizziness, flushing, headache, or nausea become too severe or should vomiting occur, the infusion is stopped until the symptoms clear and is then begun again at a much slower rate. Severe reactions are rare (less than 0.5 percent in the case of intramuscular iron), but are more likely to occur in patients with asthma or chronic infection and possibly in patients with allergies.

In all cases, a small test dose of the iron preparation, given by the route to be used, should precede the full treatment.

Reticulocyte response follows parenteral administration of iron, reaching a peak in 1 to 2 weeks. With oral administration of iron, the response may start as early but is usually not of the same magnitude and the peak has a much broader base.

Hemoglobin concentration should be restored to within the normal range in 9 to 10 weeks. If this does not occur, continuing blood loss from multiple hematinic deficiencies may be responsible. Folic acid deficiency is common with pregnancy, alcoholism, and small bowel malabsorption.

Prevention   This may be achieved in two ways. One consists of ensuring iron supplementation of groups of subjects recognized as being at risk. Thus infant formulas should be supplemented, breast-fed infants should be given iron supplements, especially if of low birth weight, and adolescent girls and young women should be encouraged to take a daily supplement of iron containing 18 mg of elemental iron (the RDA). Pregnant women should double or triple this iron intake as soon as pregnancy is confirmed.

In theory, an alternative method of preventing iron deficiency would be to encourage subjects at risk to eat foods which contain iron (Table 10-8). In practice, many of these foods, such as calf's liver, are not universally popular with subjects most at risk. For women, it is very difficult to achieve a dietary intake of 18 mg (the RDA). Because of this, fortification with iron of a food which is universally consumed has been advocated and tested. The food widely used for this purpose is wheat flour. Proponents of this practice argue that there may be as many as 5 million women with iron-deficiency anemia in the United States and another 25 million with deficient iron stores [18]. The proposed level of fortification is calculated so that the daily diet will on the average provide 18 mg of iron daily for women. Since calorie consumption is the major determinant of iron intake, the average consumption by men would be 30 mg daily. Opponents of iron fortification in the United States question its value and its effectiveness on the one hand and express fears that it may significantly increase the expression of hemochromatosis in those who have the unrecognized disease [19]. In Sweden, a program of increasing the iron content of flour incrementally has been in operation for about 15 years; the initial supplement of 30 mg/kg was increased first to 50 mg/kg and then, in 1970, to 75 mg/kg. During this time there has been a marked decline in iron-deficiency anemia in women. There has been no evidence of an increase in overt hemochromatosis, but there is wide variation in the estimates of frequency of homozygous idiopathic hemochromatosis [20] and, therefore, in the likelihood of iron overload in different populations.

If the rate of heterozygosity proves to be 3 percent in most populations and if a carrier is at risk of iron overload, as seems possible from transferrin percentage saturation data, then the argument against iron fortification is hard to resist. Nor is there good evidence that minor degrees of iron-deficiency anemia have functional importance. Thus, Elwood [21] has argued that significant reduction in sense of well-being and performance occurs only when hemoglobin concentrations fall below 10 g/dl. The problem is unresolved.

In summary, if hemoglobin estimations were done routinely in the following populations:

1 In infants at the age of one
2 In children and adolescents at annual intervals during rapid growth phases
3 In pregnant women at their first clinic visit and at regular intervals throughout their pregnancy
4 In all subjects after gastric surgery and at yearly intervals thereafter, or more frequently
5 In women of menstrual age as part of an annual physical checkup
6 In patients presenting with gastrointestinal symptoms or disease
7 In any subject in whom anemia or iron deficiency is suspected on the basis of medical history or findings of glossitis, koilonychia, or occult blood in the stool

and if iron therapy were to be started when indicated, a major part of iron-deficiency anemia in the United States would be eradicated.

Iron Overload: Hemochromatosis

Abnormally high tissue iron concentrations are toxic and cause damage to tissues, possibly as a result of free radical formation. The result is fibrotic change in the liver, heart, pancreas, and other organs so that liver failure, heart failure, diabetes mellitus, or other endocrine disorders may ensue. The most important recognized causes are hemochromatosis and heavy consumption of alcoholic beverages containing large amounts of iron. The most quoted example is that of the African Bantu, who use iron pots for fermentation and cooking.

Hemochromatosis is a genetic disease, transmitted as an autosomal recessive allele. The carrier state is now believed to have a frequency of 3 percent and may itself confer the capacity for abnormally high absorption of dietary iron, which is the basic defect. The benefits in terms of natural selection in an environment without iron fortification are obvious.

Why the enterocyte in hemochromatosis transports excess iron until iron stores are grossly and toxically overloaded is still unclear.

Since the body has no means of increasing iron excretion, the standard treatment is phlebotomy (removal of blood), repeated over several years. Iron-chelating agents, such as deferoxamine, infused subcutaneously on a daily basis will mobilize iron from stores and are excreted by the kidneys together with the bound iron. This treatment is currently under trial; it may prove to be superior to phlebotomy.

FOLACIN IN NUTRITION

Folacin is the name now used to describe a group of related compounds which have nutritional properties and chemical structures similar to folic acid. Folic acid is a water-soluble vitamin that is found, together with other folacins, in green foliage (hence the name) and also in yeasts, liver, and meat. The molecule of folic acid consists of two cyclical structures, a pteridine ring and p-aminobenzoic acid, and one or more glutamic acid residues. The pteroylgluta-mates therefore constitute a group. Mammals are incapable of synthesizing pteroylglutamates, but some microorganisms have this capability, including some of the intestinal flora. Their contribution to folacin requirements in humans is uncertain.

The pteridine ring acts as a hydrogen acceptor, and in the naturally occurring folate there are four extra hydrogens on this ring, forming tetrahydrofolic acid. Folacins participate in metabolic pathways involving transfer of single-carbon units, such as formyl (—CHO) and methyl (—CH_3), from one molecule to another. Thus, folic acid deficiency expresses itself in disturbed nucleic acid and amino acid synthesis, and the results of deficiency are seen in cells of rapid turnover, such as those of the bone marrow and the intestinal epithelium.

Distribution in the Body

The liver is the main site of storage of folacins. When depletion of folacin occurs, this is first reflected in a fall in serum folacin below the lower limit of normal (3 ng/ml) and later by a fall in red blood cell folacin levels.

Dietary Requirements

Adults The amount of folacin absorbed is currently believed to be 25 to 50 percent of the total available in one's diet. Evidence suggests that 100 to 200 μg of pteroylglutamate is needed daily to maintain tissue concentrations, so the

RDA has been set at 400 μg of total folacin activity for nonpregnant, nonlactating healthy adults. There is considerable variation in the assayable folacin content of mixed diets.

Infants and Children The daily folacin requirement is estimated to be 5 μg per kilogram of body weight. Fresh milk (human and bovine) contains 2 to 3 μg folacin per deciliter, but some of this is heat-labile; if heated milk is the only source of folacin, the diet should be supplemented. For children eating a mixed diet the RDA is increased and a calculated 8 to 10 μg per kilogram of body weight should be consumed daily. This allows for variations in the dietary folacin available.

Pregnancy and Lactation Megaloblastic anemia of pregnancy remains a concern even in developed countries. However, in areas where there is good prenatal care, this previously serious complication of pregnancy has virtually disappeared, as a consequence possibly of better diet and the introduction of folacin supplementation. The RDA for folacin in pregnancy is 800 μg per day. In lactation, it is calculated that the maternal folacin reserves are depleted at the rate of 20 μg per day. Because of the large number of variables, the recommended supplement above the basic 400 μg of folacin is purposely set high to ensure complete safety; the total RDA is 500 μg/kg.

Folacin Deficiency

Epidemiology Folacins are ubiquitous in most diets. Yet the commonest cause of folacin deficiency in the United States is inadequate dietary intake due to poor diet, which is sometimes aggravated by overcooking green vegetables, which destroys heat labile folacins. Folacin deficiency is seen in chronic alcoholics, in pregnant women, in subjects with gastrointestinal disease, and rather rarely in subjects intolerant of liver and green vegetables. Inadequate intake cannot be precisely defined and quantified. Many alcoholics eat a poor diet, and, in addition, alcohol inhibits intestinal absorption of a number of dietary factors, including folacin. In some gastrointestinal conditions, such as Crohn's disease, intestinal malabsorption and suppression of appetite and dietary exclusions occur together. There is the added complication that folacin deficiency, like cobalamin deficiency, may itself induce a malabsorptive state because of abnormalities in the enterocytes. The causes of folacin deficiency which are likely to be encountered are listed in Table 10-9.

Folacins have a shorter biological half-life than iron or cobalamin (vitamin B_{12}). Thus deficiency may be precipitated by a period of dietary exclusion or malabsorption of months rather than of years. Increased requirements for folacin occur in pregnancy and to a lesser extent during lactation. In the United States and other developed countries there is a significant incidence, of the order of 2.5 to 5.0 percent, of megaloblastic anemia due almost exclusively to folacin deficiency in pregnant women attending prenatal clinics. It is estimated that

TABLE 10-9
CAUSES OF FOLACIN DEFICIENCY

Cause	As a consequence of:
Deficient ingestion	Alcoholism
	Crohn's disease
	Small bowel bypass
	Aging
	Dietary idiosyncrasy
	Overcooked food
	Partial gastrectomy
Malabsorption	Gliadin-induced enteropathy
	Tropical sprue
	Crohn's disease
	Alcohol abuse
	Small bowel bypass
	Short bowel syndrome
	Anticonvulsants
	Partial gastrectomy
Increased requirements	Pregnancy
	Hemolytic anemia
	Some tumors

megaloblastic changes occur in the marrow of about 25 percent of all pregnant women, and abnormally low serum folate concentrations occur in about 50 percent. In some developing countries the figure for megaloblastic anemia in pregnancy is as high as 20 percent, and marrow changes due to folacin deficiency are found in more than 50 percent. There is considerable variation between different countries, and in some areas the picture is complicated by cobalamin deficiency.

When infants and children in the developed countries present with megaloblastic anemia due to folacin deficiency, the only likely cause is gliadin-sensitive enteropathy or celiac disease (see Chapter 15). In some developing countries folacin deficiency occurs in association with protein-calorie malnutrition, especially in children fed on goat's milk. Folacin deficiency is an almost invariable finding in tropical sprue (see Chapter 15). In areas where malaria is endemic, hemolytic processes and use of some antimalarial drugs, which have an antifolate effect, may result in both low tissue folacin levels and megaloblastic anemia or marrow changes. In continuing or intermittent hemolytic diseases such as paroxysmal nocturnal hemoglobinuria, in which increased hematopoiesis results in increased demand, severe folacin deficiency may occur. A similar deficiency may occur in patients with prosthetic cardiac valves, in whom chronic hemolytic anemia due to mechanical injury to red cells is an invariable finding.

In nonpregnant adults in the United States folacin deficiency is usually the result of excessive alcohol consumption, the use of drugs such as anticonvulsants (see Chapter 6), or some small intestinal malabsorption.

In the elderly, dietary deficiency of folacin may occur as a consequence of much reduced caloric intake or overcooking of vegetables. Megaloblastic anemia due to folacin deficiency has been noted in 2 to 3 percent of patients admitted to geriatric wards, suggesting that preanemic folacin deficiency must be quite common in older people.

Etiology and Pathogenesis   The metabolic pathways in which folacins are involved are described in Figure 10-1. Folacin deficiency results in abnormal nucleic acid synthesis, amino acid metabolism, and protein synthesis.

Absorption of Folacin   The absorption of folacins from ingested food is complex and not fully quantified. Folacins vary very much in stability, availability, and nutritional effectiveness. Some are heat-labile, others heat-stable. The major part (75 percent) of folacin in an American diet is in the form of polyglutamates [22], which are available neither for microbiological assay nor for absorption across the human enterocyte until the number of L-glutamyl molecules on the side chain has been reduced, possibly to three or fewer. Pteroylpolyglutamyl hydrolases are present in the enterocyte brush border and probably within the cell. Activity in the small intestinal lumen is low. Deconjugation of heptaglutamates downward probably occurs mainly at the enterocyte surface [23,24]. The complexity of factors determining availability is increased by the demonstrated presence of conjugase (γ-L-glutamyl carboxypeptidase) inhibitors of varying activity in foodstuffs. The folacin which enters the portal system as free pteroylmonoglutamate and the metabolically important endogenous 5-methyltetrahydrofolate circulate either free or loosely bound to a protein carrier.

Pteroylpolyglutamates are synthesized from monoglutamate derived from the plasma mainly in the liver, but probably in all other cells which retain folates. It has been shown that the polyglutamate forms function as more efficient cofactors than the monoglutamate forms. Not surprisingly, the overall bioavailability of folacin is further complicated by differential intracellular binding, either loosely or tightly, to high-molecular-weight complexes.

Malabsorption of folacins occurs in inflammatory small bowel disease, of which Crohn's disease, untreated gliadin-induced enteropathy, and tropical sprue are the important examples. In all of these, depression of appetite may be a significant contributory factor.

Clinical Findings   Normal human subjects maintained on diets of very low folacin content develop frank macrocytic anemia after approximately 20 weeks from the outset. This is preceded, in order, by a low serum folacin (at 2 weeks), neutrophilic nuclear hypersegmentation (at 10 weeks), low red cell folacin levels (at 16 to 20 weeks), and megaloblastic changes in the marrow a few days before the appearance of macrocytosis. This clinical picture is not characteristic of the preanemic phase. Fatigue, irritability, and listlessness are subjective and in the clinical, in contrast to the experimental, setting have no diagnostic value.

When chronic folacin deficiency has advanced to the stage of a macrocytic-megaloblastic anemia, glossitis is often present. The tongue is sore, inflamed, and depapillated (Color Figure 9). Sometimes a peripheral neuritis occurs, characterized by paresthesia, when the anemia is advanced. These changes disappear upon treatment with folic acid.

Laboratory Diagnosis   Examination of peripheral blood and of the bone marrow and estimation of folacin concentrations in red blood cells or serum are the standard diagnostic tests used by physicians.

Peripheral blood in mild or early folacin deficiency may show only some nuclear hypersegmentation of neutrophils (Color Figure 19).

Low folacin levels in red blood cells are not observed for 4 to 5 months. The red cell folacin level is a good index of tissue folacin stores; the serum level is not. The ranges of normal and abnormal values are shown in Table 10-10. Megaloblastic changes in the marrow precede the onset of anemia by several weeks (Color Figure 19). The number of circulating neutrophils and platelets may become significantly low as the anemia develops. The red cells become macrocytic, and there is marked anisocytosis and poikilocytosis.

All of these changes also occur in association with deficiency of cobalamin, and there are no distinguishing features in the *hematopoietic* system or in the cells of mucosal surfaces. In both folacin and cobalamin deficiency the mucosal epithelial cells of mouth, stomach, and small bowel display megaloid changes; i.e., the cells are rather large, with immature, large nuclei. In both folacin and cobalamin deficiency an intermediary metabolite, formiminoglutamic acid, appears in the urine in abnormally large amounts after an oral loading dose of histidine.

It must be pointed out that in alcoholics and in patients after partial gastrectomy, serum and sometimes red cell folacin levels may fall below the lower limit of normal without megaloblastic changes in the marrow.

Treatment and Prevention   The first approach to treatment should be to recognize the subgroups of subjects who are at risk of developing folacin deficiency and to supplement their diets with folacin before frank deficiency occurs.

TABLE 10-10
TISSUE FOLACIN AND COBALAMIN LEVELS

	Normal range	Deficiency
Folacin, ng/ml:		
Red blood cells	⩾ 160	< 140
Serum	⩾ 6.0	< 3.0
Cobalamin, pg/ml:		
Serum	⩾ 200	< 100

In pregnancy and lactation there has been considerable success in preventing folacin deficiency as a part of better pre- and postnatal care. In subjects with gastrointestinal disease who are receiving continuing care, folacin deficiency can also be anticipated and supplementation given when appropriate, from the time of first diagnosis. In tropical sprue and gliadin-induced enteropathy, sufficient folacin is absorbed from an oral dose of 5 mg tid of folic acid to restore body folacin stores, but it is wise, after making certain that there is no coexistent deficiency of cobalamin, to give 1 mg of folic acid parenterally for 10 days before changing to the oral route. Other supplements of water-soluble and fat-soluble vitamins and minerals are usually indicated while awaiting response to the major therapeutic factors (namely, tetracycline in tropical sprue and gliadin exclusion in celiac-sprue). In tropical sprue the usual recommendation is to continue 5 mg folic acid daily for 1 to 2 years to ensure complete restoration of the small intestinal mucosa.

The need to educate the elderly and those who prepare food for them about the importance of preserving nutrients in the cooking process cannot be overemphasized and is discussed elsewhere in the book (Chapter 4). Good sources of folacin are listed in Table 10-8. If there are insurmountable problems preventing improved dietary intake, folacin and other supplements can be given.

The alcoholic will always be at risk nutritionally if he or she cannot comply with sound nutritional recommendations. Presently, we have no estimate of how important varying degrees of nutrient deficiency may be in perpetuating alcohol addiction and jeopardizing the treatment of alcoholism.

Patients receiving anticonvulsants should receive an oral dose of 1 mg folic acid daily as prophylaxis against developing folacin deficiency. This is absorbed without need of deconjugation; it will maintain serum folacin activity within the normal range and ensure that deficiency, from whatever cause does not occur. Similar maintenance should be given to patients with hemolytic anemia, including those with prosthetic cardiac valves.

COBALAMIN (VITAMIN B$_{12}$) IN NUTRITION

Cobalamin is an essential nutrient, lack of which results in megaloblastic anemia in humans and other primates. Sometimes severe damage to the peripheral and central components of the nervous system may occur. Cobalamin is a rather large molecule, in which four pyrrole groups are bonded together to form a corrin ring and by their nitrogen atoms are bonded with one atom of cobalt. The full structural details and metabolic implications may be found in Appendix 6.

Cobalamin can be synthesized only by certain microorganisms, including some molds. Major sources of cobalamin for all animals in which it is an essential food factor are the rumen of herbivors and the cecum and colon of some other mammals. Microorganisms in these structures synthesize cobalamin. Cobalamin produced in the rumen is absorbed from the small intestine and stored in liver and other organs, including muscle. Animals in which colonic synthesis occurs almost certainly lack the mechanisms for colonic absorption. The rabbit obtains its cobalamin, therefore, by coprophagy, and it is likely that many other species do likewise.

Dietary Requirements

Humans obtain cobalamin by eating cobalamin-containing foods (see Table 10-11), all of which are of animal origin. In some parts of the world fermented fish and vegetable products are eaten as condiments, and some contain large amounts of cobalamins due to synthesis by molds. In other parts of the world, especially in underdeveloped areas where people subsist on diets lacking any animal protein, fecal contamination is thought to provide sufficient cobalamin to support life. The daily requirement for an adult is extremely small.

Adults The RDA is set at 3 μg daily for adults on the assumption that at least one-third will be absorbed from the diet. The considerations from which this figure was derived are of some interest and should be consulted [1]. Unfortunately, the total body content of cobalamin for an adult is not easy to determine. Tissue assays and isotope dilution techniques have been applied, and the range is believed currently to be 2.2 to 3.0 mg. In general, daily intake in the United states is usually greatly in excess of the RDA, and deficiency is unlikely to occur unless there is malabsorption.

Infants and Children The RDA for the suckling infant is set at 0.5 μg per day. The cobalamin content of human milk is dependent on the serum cobalamin concentration of the donor. Daily output during lactation has been shown to be of the order of 0.2 to 0.8 μg. Children on cow's milk-based foods

TABLE 10-11
COBALAMIN CONTENT IN VARIOUS FOODS

	Cobalamin content, μg/100 g
Eggs	1.5
Cow's milk	0.36
Cow's milk cheeses	0.6–3.0
Yogurt	0.5
Beef	1–3
Beef liver	50–100
Chicken	0.35
Chicken liver	22.0
Shellfish	0.5–3.0
Human milk	0.045

Source: Composition of Foods, U.S. Department of Agriculture Handbooks, 1976–1979.

should receive 1.5 µg per 1000 kcal, and this is the figure applied to preadolescents. In pregnancy and during lactation 4 µg per day is recommended. There is need for more data in order to derive more confident estimates.

Cobalamin Deficiency

Epidemiology   The causes of cobalamin deficiency are listed in Table 10-12. Inadequate dietary intake is rare in the United States. A pure vegetarian, such as a so-called vegan, can become deficient in cobalamin. Fortunately, many who do eat an exclusively vegetarian diet are aware of the potential danger and take an oral cobalamin supplement. Commercially available cobalamin is synthesized by a mold, *Streptomyces griseus,* and is not of animal origin, so that vegans need have no scruples about taking it.

In India, studies of Hindu lacto-vegetarian students [25] have revealed abnormally low serum cobalamin levels and body stores despite their being in apparently good health. Daily consumption of milk ranged from 150 to 300 ml. Some Hindu women consuming lacto-vegetarian diets do show evidence of pathology due to deficiency of the vitamin, for reasons which are unclear. Megaloblastic anemia is more common than in a population eating a mixed diet, and it may be severe. Neurological damage is rare. In women deficiency is associated with infertility.

There are now quite large numbers of subjects living on lacto-vegetarian diets

TABLE 10-12
CAUSES OF COBALAMIN DEFICIENCY

Cause	As a consequence of:
Dietary lack	Pure vegetarian diet
	Lacto-vegetarian diet (inadequate milk)
Failure of absorption	Lack of gastric intrinsic factor, due to:
	Pernicious anemia
	Total gastrectomy
	Partial gastrectomy
	Disease of small bowel:
	Crohn's disease
	Celiac-sprue
	Tropical sprue
	Radiation enteritis
	Strictures: Diverticula
	Absence of ileal receptors
Failure of transport	Transcobalamin II deficiency

in the United States. Women consuming such diets should be monitored for evidence of progressive cobalamin deficiency.

Pernicious anemia is one of the better-known examples of disease due to a deficiency of a specific nutrient. The underlying defect is in the gastric mucosa, the parietal cells of which normally produce a glycoprotein of 55,000 molecular weight called *intrinsic factor*. Intrinsic factor mediates the absorption of cobalamin at specific receptor sites in the second half of the small intestine. In pernicious anemia there is an absence of, or a marked reduction in, parietal cells. The disease very rarely presents until adult life. Its prevalence in the United States is not known. In the United Kingdom it is 127 per 100,000 of the population.

Total gastrectomy results inevitably in cobalamin deficiency, which may also follow years after a partial gastrectomy. The biological half-life of cobalamin has been estimated to be between 1.5 and 4 years. Body stores may be adequate to meet demands for the vitamin for 1 to 5 years from the time any significant absorption ceases, as is the case after total gastrectomy. In pernicious anemia and after partial gastrectomy, the secretion of intrinsic factor usually decreases gradually, so that the absorption of dietary cobalamin and the reabsorption of the endogenous cobalamin present in bile, which is normally recycled in an efficient enterohepatic circulation, decreases over the course of months or years, and cobalamin deficiency develops slowly.

Cobalamin deficiency also occurs in about 50 percent of patients with Crohn's disease of the small bowel, presumably depending on the extent of involvement of the receptor sites. In gliadin-induced enteropathy and tropical sprue, impaired absorption of cobalamin occurs less commonly than does impaired absorption of iron or folacin but may lead to significant depletion of cobalamin stores. Resection or bypass of the terminal 30 percent of the ileum will almost always result in cobalamin deficiency occurring 1 year or more subsequently.

Etiology and Pathogenesis   Cobalamin deficiency occurs because of inadequate dietary intake or lack of absorption. There are no known mechanisms which vary the amount excreted.

Dietary deficiency has been discussed. It is essentially due to exclusion of all animal products. Cobalamin is relatively heat-stable, and only a small percentage is destroyed by cooking. When cow's milk is the sole source of cobalamin, there is the possibility of deficiency, since milk contains rather less than 1 μg/dl. The percentage of cobalamin absorbed from a meal has not been satisfactorily estimated, but it likely varies between 10 and 60 percent. Inferences from data on the percentage of absorption from oral doses of labeled cobalamin given alone and consideration of the data of Mehta et al. [25] support the recommendation that the lacto-vegetarian should consume 1 liter of milk daily.

Failure of cobalamin absorption occurs for many reasons. Lack of gastric intrinsic factor, as in pernicious anemia or following gastrectomy, is a major cause. In pernicious anemia the gastric mucosa is atrophic and the normal glandular structure and specialized cells are destroyed. Acid, pepsinogen, and intrinsic factor secretions are lost. The disease is familial and possibly, but not certainly, genetically transmitted.

There are rare variants that usually become manifest in childhood, in which the capacity of the parietal cell to elaborate intrinsic factor, or biologically active intrinsic factor, is lost.

The other principal cause of malabsorption of cobalamin is disease of the surface of the ileum, which may be due to tropical sprue, ionizing radiation enteritis, inadequate blood supply, or inflammatory changes of unknown cause, as in Crohn's disease. Rare causes are chronic pancreatitis, infestation with the fish tapeworm, and bacterial overgrowth in the upper small intestine, which may occur as a result of strictures, surgical intervention, or jejunal diverticulosis. Malabsorption due to bacterial overgrowth responds, at least temporarily, to treatment with oral antibiotics.

There is a rare condition occurring in children in which the transport of cobalamin across the ileal enterocyte is impaired (Gräsbeck-Imerslund syndrome). The defect is associated with proteinuria and appears to be in the enterocyte, but it has not yet been elucidated.

Clinical Findings In pernicious anemia the clinical findings are seen in a form least complicated by other deficiencies. The onset is insidious. Loss of appetite, some tongue soreness, and tiredness are very common. There is frequently loss of weight, but this rarely exceeds 2 to 3 kg. There is often paresthesia of a tingling, pins-and-needles type in the extremities, and minor personality changes occur. Epigastric pain is rare, but mild discomfort quite common.

The descriptions of blue-eyed, silver-haired patients are colorful but these associations do not quite reach statistical significance. Patchy depigmentation (vitiligo) is less colorful but is a significant association (Color Figure 6). The forehead, wrists, and neck are often affected.

Nowadays extremely sick patients with heart failure, dyspnea, and severe neurological damage, including loss of position sense, long-tract motor-neuron involvement, and loss of sphincteric control are rare. Screening of in-patients for cobalamin deficiency in hospitals for the chronic mentally sick has frequently disclosed patients whose mental illness responds to parenteral treatment with cobalamin and who have pernicious anemia.

Laboratory Findings These are essentially the same as those for folacin deficiency. However, there are additional features. The most valuable, since it provides a direct estimate of cobalamin status and thus reduces the real risks of treating cobalamin deficiency with large doses of folic acid, is measurement of serum cobalamin activity by various techniques. Further, tests of cobalamin absorption are routine. The urinary excretion test is the one usually applied. It is possible to use two tracer doses of 0.5 μg cobalamin labeled with two different cobalt radioisotopes (usually ^{57}Co and ^{58}Co), one of which is complexed with intrinsic factor. In this way it is possible to estimate simultaneously the percentage absorption of each preparation, one without and the other with intrinsic factor. This test avoids to some extent the problems of complete 24-hour urine collections, since a ratio of concentration of one cobalt isotope to the other can provide information as to whether intrinsic factor enhances absorption. A full 24-hour urine collection is still desirable. In pernicious anemia, the gastric mucosa is incapable of secreting any hydrochloric acid in response to even a maximal dose of gastrin or betazole (Histalog), but gastric analyses are rarely done today. In addition, in pernicious anemia circulating antibodies to two gastric parietal-cell antigens are found. One antigen is intrinsic factor, and the sera of about 70 percent of pernicious anemia patients are positive for antibodies to this antigen. The other antigen is intimately associated with acid-secretory activity of the parietal cell, and about 90 percent of sera from pernicious anemia patients are positive for antibodies to this antigen.

In about 70 percent of pernicious anemia subjects, circulating gastrin activity is abnormally high (plasma levels > 400 pg/ml).

Treatment   When the cause of deficiency is dietary and there is no reason to suspect malabsorption, cobalamin may be given orally. Frequently the most appropriate preparation is a tablet or capsule containing 5 μg of cobalamin and the whole array of water-soluble vitamins, including vitamin C, since this will ensure adequate intake in what are often ill-defined dietary situations.

Therapy with cobalamin is indicated in pernicious anemia and, to a lesser degree, in other states of malabsorption. Cobalamin is given by subcutaneous injection. Initially, various regimens are used. We give 100 μg daily for 10 days and then 100 μg monthly or, occasionally, every 3 weeks if patients complain of having felt fatigued after a previous injection, although this may express more of a psychological than organic reaction. Cobalamin is an inexpensive drug and injections can be given by the patient, so there need be no call on professional time.

The early days of response to cobalamin in severe pernicious anemia are not without hazard, owing to the dramatic change to effective red cell production which sometimes occurs. This may be associated with a significant fall in extracellular potassium concentration. Some deaths can be attributed to this. The appropriate place for treatment of the very anemic is the hospital, where serum electrolytes can be monitored. The peripheral neuropathy of cobalamin deficiency usually responds to therapy with cobalamin. The long-tract damage, which consists of patchy demyelination and punctate hemorrhages, may be partly and sometimes wholly irreversible. The same is true of mental changes.

In many patients suffering from a deficiency of cobalamin, radiological or endoscopic examination of the gastrointestinal tract is indicated because of increased incidence of gastric cancer and because in patients who do not have pernicious anemia, small bowel abnormalities should be looked for. It is well worth delaying such examinations until patients have responded to cobalamin therapy. They are able to cooperate better, and more definitive studies can be done.

In conclusion it cannot be emphasized enough that the earlier treatment is instituted, the better, and this requires above all that the practitioner should entertain the diagnostic possibility of cobalamin deficiency.

Prevention   Deficiency of cobalamin occurs classically in pernicious anemia. It also may occur years after partial gastric resections and resection of the terminal part of the ileum. Cobalamin levels in the sera of siblings and other close relatives of subjects known to have pernicious anemia should be measured annually. The same monitoring should be done following gastric and ileal surgery. Any trend downward below 200 pg/ml is an indication for monthly intramuscular injections of 100 to 1000 μg cobalamin.

The only other subjects at risk are pure vegetarians. They should take a daily oral vitamin preparation containing 4 to 5 μg of cobalamin.

OTHER DEFICIENCY ANEMIAS

Pyridoxine Deficiency

Hereditary sideroblastic anemia is a rare condition, believed to be inherited as an X-linked recessive trait. It is therefore almost exclusively a disease of males. The anemia may first be apparent in infancy, but more usually, it is first noted in the young adult. It is of the hypochromic, microcytic type. Iron overload is almost invariably present. The liver and spleen are enlarged, the liver from containing excessive iron. There is variable parenchymal damage and scarring, but liver function is usually not severely affected. Diabetes mellitus may occur, as in hemochromatosis. The bone marrow contains excess hemosiderin, and almost half of the nucleated red cell precursors are ring sideroblasts, with punctate dots of hemosiderin in their cytoplasm.

Treatment is with large doses of pyridoxine (50 to 200 mg daily) on a continuing basis. Response ranges from complete, through partial, to no response. The anemia is corrected, iron stores are mobilized, and tissue damage is minimized in the good responders, but in others the course progresses from cardiac arrhythmias, liver failure, or infection to death.

Pyridoxine-responsive sideroblastic anemia is rarely seen in chronic alcoholism [26].

α-Tocopherol Deficiency

In the premature, underweight newborn infant, a deficiency of vitamin E is associated with hemolytic anemia. The role of the vitamin is in some way to protect the lipids of the red cell membrane. The red blood cells of α-tocopherol-deficient infants are more easily damaged by hydrogen peroxide than the cells of normal infants.

It is now recommended that premature infants should receive supplements of α-tocopherol in formula feeds of the order of 0.7 IU per 100 kcal, or as a separate oral supplement of 5.0 IU of water-soluble α-tocopherol daily.

Protein Deficiency

Since an uncomplicated deficiency of protein in humans is exceptional, the type of anemia seen in this condition has not been much studied. The fall in hemoglobin levels seen in kwashiorkor is due in part to hemodilution, and the red cells are usually normal in appearance and contain normal levels of hemoglobin.

Iron or folate deficiency is frequently superadded.

REFERENCES

1 *Recommended Dietary Allowances,* 9th ed., National Academy of Sciences, National Research Council, Washington, 1980.

2 England, J. M., S. M. Ward, and M. C. Down: Microcytosis, anisocytosis and the red cell indices, Br. J. Haematol., 34:389, 1976.

3 Valberg, L. S., J. Sorbil, J. Ludwig, and O. Pelletiero: Serum ferritin and the iron status of Canadians, Can. Med. J., 114:417, 1976.

4 *Highlights, Ten-State Nutrition Survey 1968-1970,* U.S. Department of Health, Education, and Welfare Publication no. 72-8134, 1972.

5 Hepner, R: General Discussion, in *Nutrient Requirements in Adolescence,* J. I. McKigney and H. N. Munro (eds.), MIT, Cambridge, Mass., 1976.

6 Witts, L. J.: *Hypochromic Anaemia,* Heinemann Medical, London, 1969.

7 Sturgeon, P.: Iron requirements in infants and children, in *Iron in Clinical Medicine,* R. O. Wallerstein and S. R. Mettier (eds.), University of California Press, Berkeley, 1958.

8 *HANES, Health and Nutritional Examination Survey,* National Center for Health Statistics, Advance Data no. 46, 1979.

9 Monsen, E. R., L. Hallberg, M. Layrisse, D. M. Hegsted, J. D. Cook, W. Mertz, and C. A. Finch: Estimation of available dietary iron, Am. J. Clin. Nutr., 31:134, 1978.

10 Charlton, R. W., P. Jacobs, H. Seftel, and T. H. Bothwell: Effect of alcohol on iron absorption, Br. Med. J., 5422:1427, 1964.

11 Hallberg, L., A. M. Hogdahl, L. Nilsson, and G. Rybo: Variation of iron loss in women, in *Occurrence, Causes and Prevention of Nutritional Anaemias, Symposia of the Swedish Nutrition Foundation,* G. Blix (ed.), Almquist & Wiksells, Uppsala, 1968.

12 Hallberg, L., C. Bengtsson, L. Garby, J. Lennartsson, L. Rossander, and E. Tibblin: An analysis of factors leading to a reduction in iron deficiency in Swedish women, Bull. WHO, 57:947, 1979.

13 Wilson, J. F., D. C. Heiner, and M. E. Lahey: Milk induced gastrointestinal bleeding in infants with hypochromic microcytic anemia, J. Am. Med. Assoc., 189:568, 1964.

14 Kimber, C., and L. R. Weintraub: Malabsorption of iron secondary to iron deficiency, N. Engl. J. Med., 279:453, 1968.

15 Bannerman, R. M., B. Creamer, and K. B. Taylor: Gastrointestinal cell turnover and morphology in experimental iron deficiency (unpublished).

16 Marks, J., and S. Shuster: Iron metabolism in skin disease, Arch. Dermatol., 98:469, 1968.

17 Leonard, B. J.: Hypochromic anaemia in R.A.F. recruits, Lancet, 1:899, 1954.

18 Finch, C. A., and E. R. Monsen: Iron nutrition and the fortification of food with iron, J. Am. Med. Assoc., 219:1462, 1972.

19 Crosby, W. H.: Improving iron nutrition, West. J. Med., 122:499, 1975.

20 Motulsky, A.: Genetics of hemochromatosis, N. Engl. J. Med., 301:1291, 1979.

21 Elwood, P. C.: Evaluation of the clinical importance of anemia, Am. J. Clin. Nutr., 26:958, 1973.

22 Butterworth, C. E., Jr., R. Santini, Jr., and W. B. Frommeyer, Jr.: The pteroylglutamate composition of American diets as determined by chromatographic fractionation, J. Clin. Invest., 42:1929, 1963.

23 Halsted, C. H., C. M. Baugh, and C. E. Butterworth, Jr.: Jejunal perfusion of simple and conjugated folates in man, Gastroenterology, 68:261, 1975.

24 Baugh, C. M., C. L. Krumdieck, H. J. Baker, and C. E. Butterworth, Jr.: Absorption of folic acid poly-γ-glutamates in dogs, J. Nutr., 105:80, 1975.

25 Mehta, B. M., D. V. Rege, and R. S. Satoskar: Serum vitamin B_{12} and folic acid activity in lactovegetarian and non-vegetarian healthy adult Indians, Am. J. Clin. Nutr., 15:77, 1964.

26 Hines, J. D., and D. H. Cowan: Studies on the pathogenesis of alcohol-induced sideroblastic bone-marrow abnormalities, N. Engl. J. Med., 283:441, 1970.

For an excellent account of current views of iron deficiency without anemia see P. R. Dallman, E. Beutler, and C. A. Finch, Effects of iron deficiency exclusive of anaemia, Br. J. Haematol., 40:179, 1978.

Excellent accounts of anemias due to folacin and cobalamin deficiencies are found in I. Chanarin, *The Megaloblastic Anaemias*, 2d ed., Blackwell, Oxford, 1969.

CHAPTER 11

NUTRITIONAL ASPECTS OF DIABETES MELLITUS

CONTENTS

INTRODUCTION

Diabetes mellitus (DM) can be counted among the world's major public health problems on the basis of its prevalence, its morbidity and mortality rates, and its socioeconomic impact on the world's populations. According to the National Institutes of Health (NIH), 10.2 million Americans have diabetes, although the disease has been diagnosed in only 5.2 million [1]. The number of diabetics in the United States is increasing at a rate of 5 to 6 percent a year. One reason for this growth is that DM affects mainly older people, whose numbers are on the rise. Another is that because of better medical care, more diabetics than previously are able to have children, some of whom grow up to become diabetics themselves.

Diabetologists are not agreed on a definition of diabetes. West [2] has simply defined diabetes as "too much glucose in the blood" (hyperglycemia). Frequently, there are other metabolic aberrations involved, including qualitative and quantitative abnormalities of carbohydrate and lipid metabolism, characteristic pathological changes in small blood vessels and nerves, and intensification of atherosclerosis. Among the many complications of diabetes are kidney disease and gangrene. Heart disease and stroke are twice as common among diabetics as among nondiabetics. The life expectancy of the average diabetic in the United States is about a third less than that of the general population. Among the serious but nonlethal complications of diabetes are cataracts, retinal damage, and eventual blindness.

A report published in 1979 by the National Diabetes Data Group [3] of the National Institutes of Health provides a working classification of diabetes and appropriate diagnostic criteria. The classification (Table 11-1) includes the clinical classes characterized by either fasting hyperglycemia or abnormality of glucose tolerance (as described in Table 11-2) and two statistical risk classes with normal glucose tolerance, which may be stages in the natural history of diabetes.

In this chapter we will focus on the two major clinical patterns of the diabetic syndrome—insulin-dependent diabetes mellitus (type I) and non-insulin-dependent diabetes mellitus (type II). Although it is recognized that this is not a new categorization, the Data Group classification calls attention to the fact that these two types of diabetes are distinct in terms of etiology, pathogenesis, clinical presentation, and requisite treatment strategies. Insulin-dependent and non-insulin-dependent forms of diabetes are compared in Table 11-3.

Insulin-dependent diabetes mellitus (IDDM), or type I diabetes, is characterized by severe and pathognomonic changes in the pancreatic islets, by an

TABLE 11-1

CLASSIFICATION OF DIABETES MELLITUS AND OTHER CATEGORIES OF GLUCOSE INTOLERANCE

Clinical class	Former terminology
Diabetes mellitus (DM)	
Type I: Insulin-dependent (IDDM)	Juvenile diabetes
	Juvenile-onset diabetes
	Juvenile-onset type diabetes (JOD)
	Ketosis-prone diabetes
	Unstable or brittle diabetes
Type II: Noninsulin-dependent (NIDDM)	Adult-onset diabetes
	Maturity-onset diabetes
	Maturity-onset type diabetes (MOD)
	Ketosis-resistant diabetes
	Maturity-onset type diabetes of the young (MODY)
	Stable diabetes
Other types including diabetes mellitus associated with certain conditions and syndromes:	Secondary diabetes
Pancreatic disease	
Hormonal	
Drug or chemical induced	
Certain genetic syndromes	
Insulin receptor abnormalities	
Other types	
Impaired glucose tolerance (IGT)	
Nonobese IGT	Asymptomatic diabetes
Obese IGT	Chemical diabetes
IGT associated with certain conditions and syndromes	Latent diabetes
	Borderline diabetes
Pancreatic disease	Subclinical diabetes
Hormonal	
Drug or chemical-induced	
Insulin receptor abnormalities	
Certain genetic syndromes	
Gestational diabetes (GDM)	Gestational diabetes

Statistical risk classes	Former terminology
Previous abnormality of glucose tolerance (previous AGT)	Prediabetes
	Latent diabetes
Potential abnormality of glucose tolerance (potential AGT)	Prediabetes
	Potential diabetes

Source: National Diabetes Data Group, Diabetes 28:1039, 1979.

TABLE 11-2

VENOUS PLASMA GLUCOSE CONCENTRATIONS DIAGNOSTIC FOR VARIOUS
CONDITIONS IN NONPREGNANT ADULTS*

Condition	Fasting level, mg/dl	Level on oral glucose tolerance test,[†] mg/dl	
		$\frac{1}{2}$-, 1-, and $1\frac{1}{2}$-h samples	2-h sample
Normal	< 115	< 200	< 140
Diabetes mellitus	⩾ 140[‡]	At least one value ⩾ 200	⩾ 200
Impaired glucose tolerance	< 140	At least one value ⩾ 200	140–199

*Full report of National Diabetes Data Group (Diabetes, 28:1039, 1979) should be consulted for details, including conditions for performance of glucose tolerance tests, diagnostic levels of venous whole blood and capillary whole blood glucose, and diagnosis of diabetes mellitus in children.

[†]Glucose, 75 g, or equivalent commercially prepared carbohydrate administered in morning after 10- to 16-h overnight fast, with blood samples taken before carbohydrate administration and at $\frac{1}{2}$-h intervals for following 2 h.

[‡]Either (1) classic symptoms of diabetes with gross and unequivocal elevation of plasma glucose or (2) a fasting venous plasma glucose concentration ⩾ 140 mg/dl on more than one occasion is diagnostic of diabetes mellitus, and a glucose tolerance test is not required.

eventual absolute deficiency of endogenous pancreatic insulin secretion, by insulinopenia, by proneness to ketosis, and by a dependence on daily insulin administration for the maintenance of life. Genetic factors are thought to be of importance in the majority of patients.

The failure of pancreatic beta cells to produce sufficient hormone may be due to a variety of causes including genetic, viral, autoimmune, and toxic factors or a combination of these [4,5]. Classically, this type of disease occurs in juveniles; however, it can be recognized and may become symptomatic for the first time at any age.

However, the majority of DM cases encountered in clinical practice are of the non-insulin-dependent type, and this form of the disease accounts for over 80 percent of the diabetes cases in the United States. Onset is usually in later adulthood (after the age of 40), and obesity is very common in these patients. Non-insulin-dependent diabetes mellitus (NIDDM), or type II diabetes, also has a genetic basis, which is commonly expressed by a more frequent familial pattern of occurrence than is seen in IDDM. It also includes the category maturity-onset diabetes of the young (MODY), in which autosomal dominant inheritance has been established [6]. It is usually characterized by retention of endogenous pancreatic secretion (although with altered secretory dynamics), by the absence of ketosis, and by insulin resistance due to diminished target-cell response to insulin. Insulin therapy, although often used to normalize glycemia, is not required for the maintenance of life.

TABLE 11-3
COMPARISON OF TYPE I AND TYPE II DIABETES MELLITUS

	I. Insulin-dependent	II. Non-insulin-dependent
Age of onset	Most often in childhood, but may occur in adulthood	Frequently after 40 years of age, but may occur in children
Body habitus	Normal to wasted	Usually obese
Symptoms	Polydipsia, polyphagia, polyuria	May be asymptomatic or symptomatic
HLA type association	Yes	No
Etiology	Genetic Viral Autoimmune	Obesity Genetic Insulin receptors
Plasma insulin	Low to absent	Normal to high
Plasma glucagon	High, suppressible	High, resistant
Acute complication	Ketoacidosis	Hyperosmolar coma
Insulin therapy	Essential	Required by some
Diet therapy	Maintain ideal weight for height Prevent hypoglycemia Maintain good glycemic control Prevent hyperlipidemia	Reduce weight Maintain good glycemic control Prevent hyperlipidemia
Exercise	Important in daily management	Needed for weight reduction

EPIDEMIOLOGY

Controversy persists regarding the relative importance of hereditary and environmental factors in the diabetic state. It is the consensus that both factors are relevant and that in certain populations one factor or the other may predominate. We will briefly review some of the factors that are suggested to influence the appearance of the diabetic state (Table 11-4).

TABLE 11-4
FACTORS ASSOCIATED WITH OCCURRENCE OF DIABETES MELLITUS

Genetics	Viral infections
Obesity	Dietary factors
Aging	Dietary energy
Sex	Dietary carbohydrate
Exercise	and fiber

Genetics

It has been recognized only recently that IDDM and NIDDM have different genetic roots. Moreover, family and twin studies have provided evidence that there is genetic heterogeneity within each of these two types of DM. The nearly complete concordance in twin pairs for NIDDM suggests that genetic factors are predominant in the etiology of this disease. However, family studies have not clearly delineated a single pattern of inheritance. Pedigree analysis studies in families with maturity-onset diabetes of the young (MODY) [7] showed that MODY was vertically transmitted from generation to generation, with approximately half the offspring of each affected person being affected. This finding is consistent with autosomal dominant inheritance.

There appears to be an association between certain histocompatibility antigens and IDDM and no association with NIDDM. Human leukocyte (HLA) antigens HLA-B8, HLA-Bw15, HLA-Dw3, and HLA-Dw4 appear to represent the primary association sites. Population studies in Caucasians in western Europe have revealed positive associations on the order of twofold increased risk for IDDM with HLA-B8, HLA-B15, and HLA-B18 antigens. Even stronger associations on the order of a fivefold increase were found with HLA-Dw3 and HLA-Dw4 [8]. These observations suggest that either (1) the disease predisposition is due to the HLA antigen itself or (2) the predisposition results from the presence of another gene or genes carried in the same haplotype as the associated HLA allele.

Obesity

It has long been known, and it is now quite generally accepted, that obesity is an important risk factor for DM. West and Kalbfleisch [9] found a correlation coefficient of 0.89 for diabetes prevalence and percentage of standard weight in 10 populations in different countries. Recently the National Commission on Diabetes pointed to the twofold risk of developing DM with every 20 percent addition of excess body weight [10].

In general, diabetes has been looked upon as a hereditary disorder in which obesity often plays a "precipitating" role. More recently the view that obesity per se is diabetogenic has evolved. This view is based on the fact that in simple obesity there is insulin resistance in muscle [11] and hyperinsulinism [12], which is reversed by weight reduction [13].

Aging

Figure 11-1 shows the age of discovery of diabetes in a large group of diabetics in London who were cared for at King's College Hospital. A similar distribution is also observed in data from U.S. National Health Surveys [14]. To what extent the increasing appearance of diabetes with age is an effect of aging itself is not clear. It seems likely that other factors such as obesity and decreasing exercise account to some extent for the rise of incidence with age.

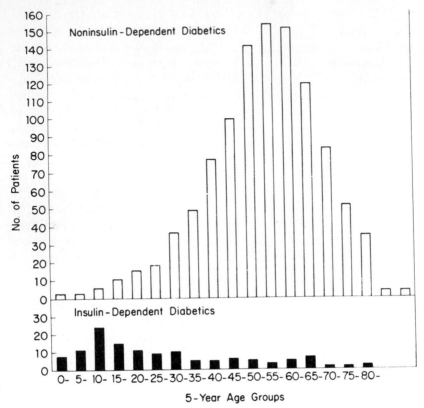

FIGURE 11-1
Frequency distribution of age of diagnosis of diabetes, in clinic of King's College
Hospital, London. (*From D. R. Gamble, and K. W. Taylor, Br. Med. J., 3:631,
1969.*)

Sex

It is widely believed that females are more susceptible to IDDM, and in most
affluent societies there is female dominance of varying degree. The World
Health Organization, in its 1964 report [15], calculated an average of mortality
rates for males and females in the 45 countries from which it received reports.
The mean male-female ratio was 1:1.5. There is much to suggest that the female
preponderance in the prevalence of diabetes observed in many societies is
mainly the result of the greater fatness of women in these populations. West and
Kalbfleisch [9] did not find any differences between the sexes in their
international studies in 11 countries which could not be explained by differences
in adiposity.

Exercise

West [14] has stated that exercise is "probably a potent protective factor" in
DM. Unfortunately, there are little quantitative data addressing this issue, and

furthermore, the short- and long-term effects of exercise on carbohydrate metabolism are incompletely understood. There are two mechanisms by which inactivity could lead to diabetes: (1) inactivity favors obesity or (2) inactivity per se impairs glucose tolerance. It has been shown that inactivity impairs glucose tolerance [16] and that physical conditioning improves glucose tolerance [17].

Viral Infections

The less constant genetic pattern in IDDM than in NIDDM suggests that environmental factors may exert a greater impact. Mounting evidence implicates viruses as an environmental etiologic factor in IDDM. Association of diabetes with infections of mumps, rubella (German measles), influenza, hepatitis, and Coxsackie infections has been reported [18]. Some of the best evidence of the role of viruses in diabetes has come from laboratory animals. Craighead and coworkers reported that a variant of encephalomyocarditis (EMC) virus (which attacks the central nervous system and heart muscle as well as the pancreas) can produce diabetes in susceptible strains of mice [18]. The virus causes diabetes in these animals by infecting and destroying the beta cells of the pancreas. In 1978 the first direct evidence was obtained that viruses can cause diabetes in humans. A 10-year-old boy who died after developing a viral illness resembling influenza had very high levels of blood glucose and suffered from diabetic ketoacidosis [19]. Studies showed that the pancreas contained a virus with properties similar to those of Coxsackie B4 virus. When cultured virus was injected into susceptible mice, many developed diabetes within a week. This work does not establish Coxsackie virus as a cause of all cases of IDDM. However, it may be one of the several different causes, and many different viruses may be diabetogenic under favorable circumstances.

Dietary Factors

A number of workers have studied the extent to which dietary factors may influence the incidence of clinical DM. Regrettably few studies distinguish patients with IDDM from those with NIDDM. Excess energy consumption has emerged as the most consistent finding in all these studies.   adiposity

Dietary Energy Precise measurement of energy consumption is difficult both in populations and in individuals except under very carefully controlled circumstances. In addition, it is seldom possible to control such conditions over long periods of time. These difficulties have limited the epidemiological approach to the study of energy consumption as a risk factor. There are, however, some observations which suggest the influence of energy consumption. Diabetes rates appear to have increased markedly in the last generation in Japan at a time when food consumption per capita was rising sharply [20]. In Taiwan there has been a sharp increase in the prevalence of diabetes, coinciding with an increase in daily food consumption from 1217 kcal per person per day in 1948 to 2509 kcal per person per day in 1968 [21]. In privileged societies where diabetes is more common, consumption averages 3000 kcal daily. In the developing world where diabetes is uncommon, consumption in adults averages 2150 kcal [22].

Dietary Carbohydrate and Fiber   Cleave and Campbell [23] and Yudkin [24] have argued forcibly in favor of the hypothesis that excessive consumption of sugar and other refined carbohydrates has an important role in determining the prevalence of diabetes in a population. Cleave and Campbell believe that the consumption of concentrated carbohydrates is harmful to beta cells because it overtaxes them and also tends to induce obesity, thereby further increasing the risk of diabetes. Cleave and Campbell's conclusions may be better explained by the work of West and Kalbfleisch, who carefully studied the interrelationship between nutritional factors and diabetes in 12 age-matched populations in different countries [9]. A positive correlation was found between diabetes prevalence and sugar consumption, but a very similar association was also present between fat intake and prevalence of the disease. Keys has pointed out that intake of sugar and fat in different population groups is closely related [25]. The most striking correlation in the investigation carried out by West and Kalbfleisch was between prevalence of diabetes and prevalence of obesity ($r = 0.89$).

Yudkin [26] examined for each of 22 countries the diabetes mortality rate for either 1955 or 1956 and the levels of sugar consumption about 20 years earlier in these countries. He found a positive correlation coefficient of 0.73. West [14] reexamined the original sources of data that Yudkin used and found that when all available data (on 37 populations) were used, the correlation coefficient was considerably less (0.52) than with the 22 pairs selected by Yudkin. Strong evidence against the sugar hypothesis emerged from the prospective study of 10,000 Israeli civil servants [27]. Those destined to develop diabetes during the observation period actually consumed less sugar during the prediabetic period than those who remained nondiabetic.

During the past 10 years, substantial interest has developed regarding the etiological role of dietary fiber in the development of human disease and the potential therapeutic role for fiber. Trowell has suggested that fiber-depleted diets may lead to the development of diabetes and that fiber-rich starchy foods are a protective factor [28]. This hypothesis is based on epidemiological studies of societies in rural Africa where diets contain large quantities of unrefined carbohydrates, as compared to diets of societies in more-developed countries, which have a low incidence of diabetes. Although provocative, such data do *not* establish causation, since many other factors, especially obesity, also varied fundamentally in prevalence in rural Africa as opposed to western cultures. On the other hand, the improvement in glucose tolerance and the decreased insulin secretion in response to glucose in fiber-treated patients [29] suggest that the addition of fiber to the diabetic diet might be of therapeutic importance.

METABOLIC CHANGES ASSOCIATED WITH DIET

There are a limited number of studies examining the effect of varying carbohydrate and/or fat intakes on diabetic control. Most are short-term studies, and many have used extreme dietary measures which would be unpalatable or monotonous for long-term maintenance. Weinsier and colleagues [30] observed that increasing dietary carbohydrates from 40 to 60 percent did not lead to deterioration of diabetic control in adult diabetics treated with diet and, in some cases, with oral hypoglycemic agents. Serum cholesterol and triglycerides were unchanged. The role of carbohydrate intake in the control of the plasma lipid levels was noted by Stone and Connor [31]. They increased the carbohydrate intake from 40 to 64 percent and manipulated other aspects of the diet, and they noted improvement in hyperglycemia, hypertriglyceridemia, and hypercholesterolemia in their patients. Kiehm et al. [32] increased dietary carbohydrate from 43 to 75 percent in 13 diabetic patients treated with either insulin or sulfonylurea agents. In 10 patients the high-carbohydrate diet led to a fall in fasting plasma glucose, cholesterol, and triglyceride concentrations, as well as a reduction or cessation of treatment with insulin or sulfonylurea agents. When Brunzell et al. [33] fed a diet containing 85 percent carbohydrate and no fat to insulin- or sulfonylurea-treated diabetics, fasting plasma glucose significantly decreased and glycosuria did not change. The high-carbohydrate diet used by Kiehm and associates [32] featured natural food and was high in fiber, in contrast to the liquid formula diet of Brunzell et al. [33].

Dietary fiber appears to modify plasma glucose and insulin responses in patients with diabetes. Jenkins et al. [34] indicated that both plasma glucose and insulin levels were lowered when insulin-independent diabetics ate a meal containing pectin and guar gum. In a randomized crossover study, 18 NIDDM and 9 IDDM diabetics ate a 60 percent carbohydrate-containing leguminous fiber diet for 6 weeks and also a conventional 40 percent carbohydrate diet. Preprandial and postprandial blood glucoses were significantly lower on the high-carbohydrate, high-fiber diet for both groups of diabetics. Total serum cholesterol was also reduced in both groups and the HDL cholesterol–LDL cholesterol ratio increased significantly in the NIDDM group [35]. Anderson believes high-carbohydrate, high-fiber diets (70 percent carbohydrate, 19 percent protein, and 11 percent fat, with 35 to 40 g plant fiber per 1000 kcal) are most effective for reducing insulin needs in IDDM [36]. When 20 lean insulin-treated diabetic men were fed weight-maintaining, high-carbohydrate, high-fiber diets for 16 days, a 58 percent reduction in insulin requirements was observed [37]. However, patient acceptance may be a problem with a diet that restricts meat intake to 5 oz or less per day and requires eating 8 to 10 slices of whole wheat bread (see Table 11-5). Crapo and coworkers [38] measured serum glucose, insulin, and glucagon levels as well as urinary glucose excretion in 20 subjects with nonketotic, non-insulin-requiring DM after the ingestion of 50-g amounts of four different kinds of dietary starch (potato, rice, corn, and wheat) or dextrose. The data suggest that rice and corn were less glycemia-inducing than wheat or potato. The differences in metabolic response did not correlate with plant fiber content of the starch sources. Since these are ordinary foods, diets enriched in them are feasible and could be incorporated in the dietary management of patients. However, since these studies involved short-term testing of single foods, long-term feeding studies incorporating these starches into otherwise normal diets are necessary.

TABLE 11-5
1800-CALORIE HIGH-FIBER MAINTENANCE DIET

Breakfast:	Dinner:
1 cup skim milk (240 g)	$\frac{2}{3}$ cup mushrooms (50 g)
1 small peach (85 g)	1 thin slice chicken (40 g)
1 large whole wheat muffin (50 g)	$\frac{1}{2}$ cup brown rice (100 g)
$\frac{1}{3}$ cup bran buds (30 g)	Salad
2 pats margarine (10 g)	1 cup shredded lettuce (50 g)
1 multivitamin	$\frac{1}{2}$ small tomato (20 g)
Lunch:	$\frac{1}{2}$ stalk celery (20 g)
1 thin slice roast pork (30 g)	3 slices whole wheat bread (75 g)
2 slices whole wheat bread (50 g)	3 pats margarine (15 g)
1 tsp mayonnaise (5 g)	$\frac{1}{2}$ cup cooked brown beans (30 g dry)
1 cup white potatoes (150 g raw)	$\frac{3}{4}$ cup cooked green beans (100 g)
$\frac{2}{3}$ cup cooked lima beans (40 g dry)	Evening snack:
$\frac{1}{2}$ cup summer squash (100 g cooked)	1 small apple (150 g)
3 pats margarine (15 g)	7 rye wafers (45 g)
$\frac{3}{4}$ cup blackberries (110 g)	

Source: J. W. Anderson, K. Ward, and B. Sieling, HCF Diets: A Professional Guide, University of Kentucky Diabetes Fund, Lexington, 1979.

PATHOGENESIS

Current data suggest that a deficiency in insulin secretion by the pancreatic beta cell is the predominant or primary lesion in IDDM. This secretory abnormality may vary from complete failure to a partial defect. However, endogenous insulin secretion is generally not detectable in juvenile-onset diabetics who have received insulin therapy for more than 5 years [39]. The islets are reduced in number, and most are small. The islets are composed of small cells, which in the past have been regarded as atrophic and inactive but which are now known, by the use of immunocytochemical techniques, to be glucagon- and somatostatin-secreting cells [40]. Insulin-secreting cells are present at clinical onset, but their number is reduced to less than 10 percent of normal [41]. There is also a profound distortion of islet organization, and many endocrine cells are scattered as single cells in the exocrine tissue. The cause of the destruction of beta cells in juvenile-onset diabetes is not known. Lymphocytic infiltration or insulitis has been reported [42], but the actual frequency of insulitis is controversial. The etiology of insulitis is still unknown. A viral infection or an autoimmune reaction to beta cells, either primary or triggered by a viral infection, on a background of a genetic predisposition, is an attractive hypothesis.

Paradoxical hyperglucagonemia is a well-established characteristic of juvenile diabetes. The source of the high levels of circulating glucagon is not certain. Gepts and De Mey have reported that alpha cells, or glucagon-secreting cells, persist in large numbers throughout the course of the disease [43] and provide a reasonable explanation for the preserved glucagon secretion.

In NIDDM the insulin secretory failure is less severe or insulin secretion may be intact. Basal insulin levels are generally normal or increased, whereas glucose-stimulated insulin secretion is generally diminished. The pancreatic pathology is variable and not pathognomonic. A numeric reduction in beta cells can be demonstrated in many maturity-onset diabetic patients, but this reduction is much more moderate than in IDDM patients. The same amount of beta-cell reduction can be found in some elderly subjects without clinical evidence of diabetes. Cahill has suggested that NIDDM may be a kind of premature senescence of the beta cells [44].

It is still not clear what is the primary derangement in the development of NIDDM. Some have advocated that it is impairment in the insulin response of the beta cell to glucose stimulation [45]. Other authors, mainly Reaven and coworkers, hold the view that the primary defect is a decreased sensitivity of target tissues to insulin [46,47]. Olefsky and Reaven described a decrease in insulin binding to mononuclear cells in insulin-independent diabetes and suggested that a decrease in insulin receptors was part of the diabetic syndrome [48]. Savage et al. have published data in which the insulin binding to mononuclear cells was no different between obese controls and diabetic subjects [49]. Thus it is unclear whether insulin resistance in diabetic subjects is due to decreased insulin receptors, impaired postreceptor insulin action, or a combination of the two. Very recently, Luft and coworkers [50] presented a working hypothesis for the development of NIDDM that incorporates both mechanisms. The earliest phase of the disease would be characterized by low insulin response to glucose. The next state, characterized by borderline or decreased oral glucose tolerance, would be precipitated by the appearance of decreased insulin sensitivity. The latter derangement is, at least partially, compensated for by enhancement of the ability of glucose to potentiate insulin release. The interaction of these two processes—decreased insulin sensitivity and increased potentiation—is reflected by the enhancement of the late phase of insulin release, at least in absolute terms. Progression of the impairment of insulin release and/or of decreased insulin sensitivity results in manifest diabetes.

Fuel Homeostasis and Diabetes

Insulin is the primary factor that controls the storage and metabolism of the body's metabolic fuels—carbohydrate, fat, and protein—in three principal tissues—liver, muscle, and adipose tissue. When insulin is deficient, there is decreased uptake and oxidation of glucose in muscle tissue and there is loss of muscle glycogen and failure to synthesize more. There is also release of amino acids by muscle, particularly alanine [51], to supply the liver with substrate for gluconeogenesis. In adipose tissue there is decreased fatty acid uptake and increased lipolysis. Decreased glucose uptake by adipose tissue causes a lack of α-glycerophosphate and fatty acid for triglyceride synthesis. The liver receives much of the fatty acids released by adipose tissue and metabolizes part of them to produce ketone bodies (β-hydroxybutyric acid and acetoacetic acid). The liver responds to persistent insulin lack with increased gluconeogenesis, using amino acids from muscle as substrate. Glycogenolysis is enhanced, glucose phosphorylation is decreased, and little or no new glycogen is synthesized in the liver. There is an excess of glucose in the system, resulting from both underutilization by tissues and overproduction by the liver. In the severe manifestations of diabetes (diabetic ketoacidosis), there is overproduction of glucose and marked acceleration of all catabolic processes (lipolysis and proteolysis).

CLINICAL MANIFESTATIONS

IDDM usually begins before the age of 40, often in childhood or adolescence. Onset of symptoms may be abrupt, with polyphagia, polyuria, polydipsia, weight loss, lassitude, and irritability. In some cases the disease is heralded by the appearance of ketoacidosis during an intercurrent illness or after surgery. If the condition remains undiagnosed, nausea, vomiting, dehydration, acidosis, stupor, coma, and finally death will result. This progression may be rapid, or it may continue over a period of weeks to months. Females with glycosuria are particularly susceptible to bacterial and fungal infections of the vulva and vagina.

In NIDDM the patient is usually 40 years old or older. Classically the patient is overweight. The patient may be asymptomatic, and the diagnosis may be made by finding elevated plasma glucose on routine laboratory examination. In contrast to IDDM, plasma insulin levels are normal to high in absolute terms, although they are probably lower than predicted for the level of plasma glucose.

Patients may also present with symptoms due to one of the complications of diabetes: e.g., failing vision; paraesthesia in the limbs or pain in the legs due to diabetic neuropathy or peripheral vascular disease, or a combination of the two; impotence; and infection of the skin, lungs, or urinary tract. Many of these patients also admit to symptoms attributable to glycosuria.

DIAGNOSIS

The recent National Diabetes Data Group report [3] clarified criteria for the diagnosis of diabetes and advocated use of the label "impaired glucose tolerance" for patients in whom glucose tolerance is a degree between normal and diabetic. In nonpregnant adults, the criteria for diagnosis of diabetes are (1) classic symptoms of diabetes with unequivocal hyperglycemia (venous plasma glucose > 200 mg/dl), (2) fasting venous plasma glucose ≥ 140 mg/dl on more than one occasion, or (3) sustained venous plasma glucose ≥ 200 mg/dl during an oral glucose tolerance test (demonstrated both at 2 hours after glucose ingestion and at some other time between the glucose ingestion and 2 hours later). Persons with gross hyperglycemia usually have glycosuria and symptoms of diabetes such as polyuria. These persons do *not* need a glucose tolerance test. In these cases, the diagnosis can be confirmed by the fasting blood glucose determination.

History

There are no standard conventions with respect to the form or type of questions intended to elicit information about the symptoms of DM. West [14] has suggested the following line of questioning for determining presence and degree of symptoms relating to diabetes.

In the past two months:
- Have you been unusually thirsty?
- Have you been passing more urine than usual?
- Have you been unusually hungry?
- Have you lost weight?
- Have you been unusually tired?
- Have you been unusually weak?
- Have you had blurred vision?

Physical Examination

In the mild and even moderately severe diabetic there may be no abnormal physical signs. On the other hand, the severe untreated diabetic may look ill and wasted, with loss of weight due to a combination of dehydration and loss of subcutaneous fat. Heavy glycosuria and hyperglycemia often produce vulvitis or, less commonly, balanitis; extension of monilial infection from the vulva to the perianal region can cause pruritus ani. Many subjects with NIDDM are overweight. Other findings that sometimes suggest the diagnosis of diabetes are carbuncles, gangrene, retinopathy, and xanthomata, but none of these has a high degree of sensitivity or specificity for diabetes.

Laboratory Tests

Blood Glucose Methods Several methods are available for determining the concentration of glucose in the blood: the Autoanalyzer ferricyanide and neocuprine methods, the glucose oxidase and hexokinase methods, and the o-toluidine and Somogyi-Nelson methods. For clinical purposes results with these six methods are interchangeable.

Urine Tests Most persons with occult fasting hyperglycemia have glycosuria in specimens obtained 2 hours after a large meal, and most people with fasting glycosuria have diabetes. Glycosuria is usually detected by the reduction of copper sulfate using a Clinitest tablet with 5 drops of urine and 10 drops of water. Reduction tests may give false-positive results if a reducing substance such as lactose or aspirin is present in the urine. Proteinuria delays the development of results with Clinitest tablets and may give falsely low readings. Enzyme tests are preferred in the presence of proteinuria. Specific tests for glucose in the urine are based upon the release of hydrogen peroxide by the enzyme glucose oxidase and are easily performed with Clinistix, Diastix, or Tes-

Tape reagent strips. Lactose gives a positive result with Clinitest tablets but a negative result with an enzyme test. Because of the occasional presence of interfering substances in the urine (ascorbic acid) and the possible deterioration of the enzyme glucose oxidase, a negative test must be accepted with caution. The high sensitivity of the glucose oxidase method may lead to detection of glucosuria in concentrations that are too low to be of clinical significance.

Oral Glucose Tolerance Test (OGTT)   When an OGTT is administered, it should be performed in the morning after at least 3 days of unrestricted diet (>150 g carbohydrate) and physical activity. The subject should have fasted for at least 10 hours but no more than 16 hours; water is permitted during this period. The Diabetes Data Group of the NIH recommends a glucose dose for nonpregnant adults of 75 g (1.75 g per kilogram of ideal body weight for children, up to a maximum of 75 g). A commercially prepared carbohydrate load equivalent to this glucose dose is also acceptable. A fasting blood sample should be collected after which the glucose dose in a concentration no greater than 25 g per deciliter of flavored water should be drunk in about 5 minutes. Zero time is the beginning of the drink, and blood samples should be collected at 30-minute intervals for 2 hours. If possible, venous blood samples should be collected, and plasma glucose is the preferred measurement. The recommended diagnostic concentrations are 140 mg/dl or more for the initial, or fasting, measurement and/or 200 mg/dl or more at 2 hours. A new category, "impaired glucose tolerance," has been introduced for values between normal and diabetic. The diagnostic values for this category are below 140 mg/dl for the initial, or fasting, measurement and between 140 and 200 mg/dl at 2 hours.

Differential Diagnosis of Hyperglycemia

Secondary forms of hyperglycemia also occur and are important to recognize in order that the underlying disorder may be treated. The differential diagnosis includes chronic pancreatitis, Cushing's syndrome, acromegaly, hemochromatosis, pheochromocytoma, glucagonoma, somatostatinoma, and certain rare insulin resistance syndromes such as acanthosis nigricans and Werner's syndrome. Hyperglycemia can also appear in the context of acute stress, such as burns. If glucose appears in the urine when the blood glucose level is less than 180 mg/dl, the individual has a low renal threshold for glucose or renal glycosuria. This is a benign condition and may occur temporarily in pregnancy.

MANAGEMENT

Dietary

Treatment of all diabetics involves some type of dietary modification. Depending on the severity of the disorder, any one of three regimens may be selected: (1) diet alone (2) diet and oral hypoglycemic drugs, or (3) diet and insulin. The nature of the diet has been and continues to be controversial. Until recently, most "diabetic diets" in western industrial countries prescribed 40 to 45 percent of energy as carbohydrate. In 1979, the Committee on Food and Nutrition of the American Diabetes Association published a report [52] which stated that the dietary carbohydrate intake for *insulin-dependent diabetics* "should usually account for 50–60% of total energy intake." No comments were made concerning the amount of dietary carbohydrate to be included in the diet of insulin-independent diabetics. However, the chairman of the committee subsequently stated in an editorial that "for most persons the diet should contain 50–60% carbohydrate" [53]. Furthermore, Arky, in the fifth volume of *Diabetes Mellitus,* published under the sponsorship of the American Diabetes Association [54], states that carbohydrate should comprise 55 to 60 percent of total calories in the diet. This stance has been challenged by Reaven [55] on the basis that (1) sound experimental data are lacking, (2) high-carbohydrate diets may cause elevations in plasma triglycerides, and (3) high-carbohydrate diets may have undesirable effects on untreated or poorly controlled diabetics.

It is the authors' view that although more research is still required, the following recommendations can be made:

1 The main objective of dietary management is to achieve and maintain body weight.

2 Carbohydrate restriction is unnecessary.

3 Consuming large amounts of sucrose and glucose should be avoided.

4 Though the optimal carbohydrate intake has yet to be determined, increasing complex carbohydrate and "fiber" in the diet is at the least benign and is probably beneficial.

5 Circumstantial evidence seems good enough to recommend that fat constitute 30 percent of dietary caloric intake and polyunsaturated fat comprise 50 percent of total fat.

Few measures are more important than proper instruction in diet at the onset of diabetes mellitus. Since most physicians do not have the time necessary for adequate dietary counseling, referral to a dietitian for instruction is strongly recommended.

Insulin-Dependent Diabetes Mellitus (IDDM) The cornerstone of dietary therapy in insulin-treated patients is to provide a consistent schedule of energy intake to match exogenous insulin action, particularly with the intent to prevent hypoglycemic episodes. This requires consistency of dietary composition from day to day as well as consistency in meal timing during the day. To facilitate meal planning, daily energy intake may be divided into tenths, so that two-tenths to four-tenths of calories are taken at meal time and one-tenth at snack time. The exchange diet is one of the available tools which can facilitate meal planning (see Chapter 2). Dietary patterns must be tailored to fit the individual's activity and exercise schedule. Extra energy is required before strenuous exercise. Quickly absorbed monosaccharide- and disaccharide-containing foods are to be avoided or consumed in moderation, since they aggravate hyperglycemia and cause wide fluctuations in blood glucose.

Non-Insulin-Dependent Diabetes Mellitus (NIDDM)   For patients who do not require insulin, the main objective of dietary management is to achieve and maintain ideal body weight. The method of weight reduction in obese patients is much less important than the maintenance of weight loss once it has been achieved (see Chapter 7). Other dietary adjustments, including additional snacks (not mandatory for patients not receiving insulin) and altered dietary composition (e.g., fat reduction), should assume a strictly secondary role to calorie intake control. A stable maturity-onset diabetic who is non-insulin-dependent may distribute his or her energy intake approximately in thirds.

Special Considerations

Energy   In constructing the individual diet, it is essential to estimate the energy requirements of each patient. These are dependent upon age, sex, vocation, physical activity, and deviation from "ideal" body weight. In the very young or adolescent insulin-dependent patient, additional calories should be included to provide for growth. Methods are outlined in Appendix 2 to calculate an energy prescription.

Protein   The amount of protein required by the average diabetic is similar to that required by the normal person. Daily protein intake should be 0.8 g per kilogram of desirable body weight for adults (see Appendix 3); additional allowance should be made for growing children. Fifteen to twenty percent of total calories are often derived from protein in a diabetic diet, although the usual intake of protein for nondiabetics in the United States is 10 to 15 percent [56]. The necessity to control fat intake and limit sugar tends to raise the level of protein in the diet.

Carbohydrate   Within the framework of the total caloric intake for weight maintenance, it is not necessary to restrict carbohydrate. Depending on individual preference, 50 to 60 percent of the daily caloric intake should consist of carbohydrate. Research suggesting that a liberal intake of carbohydrate is advantageous for a diabetic is reviewed earlier in this chapter. Increasing the level of carbohydrate in the diet allows a corresponding decrease in fat.

In general, complex carbohydrates commonly found in cereal grains, legumes (peas or beans), and tubers (potato) cause less dramatic excursions of blood glucose than simple carbohydrates such as sucrose, glucose, or lactose. These simple carbohydrates (monosaccharides and disaccharides) are found in corn syrups, soft drinks and many bakery goods, ice creams, and canned goods.

Fat   Liberalized proportions of carbohydrate automatically necessitate reduced fat intake. Fat intake should supply no more than 35 percent of the total calories ingested by the diabetic. Since saturated fat consumption is linked to atherosclerosis, it seems prudent to reduce the consumption of saturated fat (e.g., animal fats and coconut oil) and to increase the proportion of fat derived from polyunsaturated fats (e.g., vegetable oils and special margarines) and from monounsaturated fats (e.g., nuts, poultry fat, and olive oil). Limitation of saturated fat also tends to limit cholesterol consumption. For many patients saturated-fat intake can be reduced considerably by limiting fried foods or by frying in polyunsaturated oil.

Fiber Dietary fibers are the skeletal remains of plant cells that resist digestion by human enzymes. Most dietary fibers are indigestible polysaccharides (cellulose, pectin, and guar) which are found in fibrous plants such as bran cereals, while lignins are phenylpropane polymers [57]. Ingestion of plant fibers improves carbohydrate tolerance. The fibers may act by slowing gastric and intestinal transit time or by interfering with glucose transport across the intestinal wall [58]. A potential concern is the possibility of decreased absorption of calcium and other minerals [59].

Alcohol Alcohol, which is frequently disallowed for diabetics, can be safely included in the diet provided that certain guidelines are observed—among them, that alcohol be consumed with food or at least shortly before or after a meal.

Alcohol does not require insulin for its metabolism but can affect carbohydrate metabolism in several ways. In fasting insulin-dependent patients, alcohol in large amounts may precipitate hypoglycemia by abetting insulin in reducing liver glucose output, and this hypoglycemia may be confused with symptoms of intoxication. In the nonfasting state, blood glucose levels tend to rise after alcohol administration, partly because of glycogenolysis in the liver [60]. Alcohol is a concentrated source of energy, and it is devoid of nutritional value, except as a source of calories. The energy in alcohol is used by the body or stored as fat. Hence, any alcohol consumed must be included in considering the total energy intake if weight gain is to be avoided. Beer and most mixed drinks also contain sugar, or carbohydrate. Hence these drinks contain "insulin-dependent" calories in addition to the calories derived from alcohol. The average alcohol, carbohydrate, and caloric content of various alcoholic beverages is summarized in Table 11-6. Liqueurs (or cordials) are omitted, since they are not recommended for diabetics. Nearly all liqueurs are sweet, with sugar content as high as 50 percent. Distilled spirits, such as whiskey, gin, vodka, and rum contain no carbohydrate and are preferable. Drink mixers, if used, should be low in carbohydrate or carbohydrate-free. As a rule of thumb, a jigger (1½ oz) of most standard liquors is equivalent to about 125 kcal and is therefore equivalent to about three fat exchanges. Other exchange substitutions are given in Table 2-7.

There are several other considerations for the diabetic who drinks. Alcohol ultimately acts as a depressant to the brain and clouds thinking. The diabetic individual may not differentiate the effects of alcohol from the early symptoms of hypoglycemia. Another effect of drinking is appetite stimulation. Because hors d'oeuvres and other delectables may be abundant at social occasions at which people are drinking, the diabetic individual may overindulge. If a diabetic individual chooses to drink, it has been suggested that alcohol contribute not more than 6 percent of the total calories per day [61]. Furthermore, a diabetic person would be well-advised to develop a taste for liquor itself or to limit

TABLE 11-6
AVERAGE ALCOHOL, CARBOHYDRATE, AND CALORIC CONTENT OF ALCOHOLIC
BEVERAGES

Beverage	Average serving, oz	Alcohol, g per serving	Carbo-hydrate, g per serving	Calories per serving*
Beer	12.0	13.0	13.7	151
Beer, light†	12.0	10.1	5.5	97
Distilled spirits, 86 proof	1.5	15.3	trace	107
Table wines				
Red	4.0	11.6	0.2	83
Rosé	4.0	11.6	1.3	88
White, dry	4.0	11.3	0.4	80
White, sweet	4.0	11.8	4.9	102
Champagne	4.0	11.9	3.6	98
Kosher wine, sweet	4.0	11.9	12.0	132
Sherry wine, dry	2.0	9.5	1.2	72
Vermouth				
French type	3.0	12.6	4.2	105
Italian type	3.0	12.2	13.9	141

*Calculated by multiplying grams of alcohol, carbohydrate, and protein by 7, 4, and 4, respectively.

†Anheuser-Busch Natural Light contains 1.0 g protein per 12-oz serving.
Source: Adapted from J. McDonald, Diabetes Care, 3:629, 1980.

himself or herself to drinks mixed with water, club soda, or diet soda. *Dry* table wines are well-suited for the diabetic diet because of their low carbohydrate content (less than 2 percent reducing sugars).

Sweeteners The nutritive sweeteners fructose, xylitol, and sorbitol have the same caloric density as glucose and sucrose but produce a lessened postprandial hyperglycemia in the absence of severe insulin deficiency when given as pure substances [62]. However, their safety and effectiveness in diabetics when ingested in substantial quantities in mixed meals have not been established.

Saccharin and its salts are the most extensively used artificial nonnutritive sweeteners in the United States. The American Diabetes Association has concluded that there is insufficient evidence to warrant a ban on saccharin use because of its alleged relationship to urinary bladder cancer. However, the American Diabetes Association does recommend that it be used in prudent amounts by pregnant women and by children [63].

Calculation of Diet Patterns Using Exchange Lists The system of exchanges discussed in Chapter 2 was originally developed in 1950 by a joint committee of the American Dietetic Association, the American Diabetes Association, and the Diabetes Branch of the U.S. Public Health Service; it was updated in 1976. The exchange system allows the amount of food that can be eaten to be accurately estimated.

Before developing a diet plan, information on what, when, and how much the patient would eat if he or she did not have diabetes must be gathered. Knowledge of the individual's economic status, usual food preparation procedures, personal food likes and dislikes, patterns of physical exercise, meals eaten away from home, and type of insulin or oral hypoglycemic agent prescribed is necessary in the development of an appropriate diet pattern.

In assigning specific amounts from each exchange list one should begin with milk, vegetables, and fruits (see Table 11-7). A patient should be encouraged to include 2 cups of milk in the diet pattern each day unless there is a particular reason why milk should be avoided. If milk fat is inappropriate in a diet, skim milk or buttermilk may be used. Choices from the vegetable list should be encouraged in liberal amounts. Desserts for the diabetic patient will usually be fruit, and since most listed servings of fruits are limited to 10-g quantities of carbohydrate, several daily fruit exchanges are appropriate.

After an estimated number of milk, vegetable, and fruit exchanges have been determined, a subtotal of carbohydrates included in them should be made. The only remaining exchange list that contains carbohydrates is the bread group. The remainder of the carbohydrate in the diet prescription may be divided by 15 to determine the number of bread exchanges to be included. The bread exchange supplies complex carbohydrate (starch).

The next step is to subtotal the amount of protein included thus far. All the remaining protein will come from meat exchanges; therefore this figure can be divided by 7 to determine the number of meat choices to be included. The

TABLE 11-7
DAILY DIET PATTERN FOR 1800-kcal DIET
(90 g Protein, 60 g Fat, and 225 g Carbohydrate)

Exchange List	No. of exchanges	Pro- tein, g	Fat, g	Carbo- hydrate, g	Energy, kcal
Milk, skim	2	16	0	24	160
Vegetables	2	4	0	10	56
Fruit	7	0	0	70	280
Subtotal				104	
Bread	8	16	0	120	544
Subtotal		36			
Meat, lean	6	42	18	0	330
Meat, medium fat	2	14	11	0	155
Subtotal			29		
Fat	6	0	30	0	270
Total		92	59	224	1795

amount of fat in the pattern may then be subtotaled, and the remaining grams of fat divided by 5 to determine the number of fat exchanges. This completes the diet pattern on a daily basis (see Table 11-7).

The daily total diet pattern must then be divided into meals and snacks, with the carbohydrate distributed as indicated in the prescription. Division into meals is illustrated in Table 11-8 for an 1800-kcal diet (50 percent carbohydrate, 30 percent fat, and 20 percent protein), and illustrative menus are shown in Table 11-9.

Physical Activity

The fall in blood glucose levels reported in diabetics after vigorous exercise has been the basis for recommending exercise to diabetic patients. This acute glucose-lowering action of exercise is most pronounced in insulin-treated diabetics and occurs only if therapy is sufficient to prevent ketosis [64]. On the other hand, poorly controlled diabetics may experience increases in plasma glucose, free fatty acids, and ketone bodies during exercise [65]. The mechanism for the fall in blood glucose with exercise is not clear. Dandona et al. [66] and Koivisto and Felig [67] have reported that leg exercise (bicycling) increases the absorption of insulin from injection sites on the leg. Vranic and his colleagues [68,69] suggest that when the insulin level is sufficiently high, hepatic glucose

TABLE 11-8
DIET PATTERN OF MEALS FOR 1800-kcal DIET

| Meal | Exchanges | |
	Type	No.
Morning	Milk	1
	Fruit	2
	Bread	2
	Fat	2
	Meat, medium-fat	1
Noon	Meat, lean	2
	Meat, medium-fat	1
	Vegetable	1
	Bread	2
	Fat	2
	Fruit	2
Evening	Meat	4
	Vegetable	1
	Bread	3
	Fat	2
	Fruit	2
Bedtime	Milk	1
	Bread	1
	Fruit	1

TABLE 11-9
SAMPLE MENU FOR 1800-kcal DIET

| Meal | Exchanges | | Food | Amount |
	Type	No.		
Breakfast	Milk	1	Skim milk	1 cup
	Fruit	2	Oranges	2 small
	Bread	1	Cornflakes	$^{3}/_{4}$ cup
	Bread	1	Whole wheat toast	1 slice
	Fat	2	Margarine	2 tsp
	Meat, medium-fat	1	Soft-cooked egg	1
Lunch			Sandwich:	
	Meat, medium-fat	1	Mozzarella cheese	1 oz
	Meat, lean	2	Sliced turkey	2 oz
	Bread	2	Whole wheat bread	2 slices
	Fat	2	Mayonnaise	2 tsp
	Vegetable	1	Celery and carrot sticks	$^{1}/_{2}$ cup
	Fruit	2	Banana	1 small
Dinner	Meat	4	Baked halibut	4 oz
	Vegetable	1	Green beans	$^{1}/_{2}$ cup
	Bread	2	Baked potato	1 large
	Bread	1	French bread	1 slice
	Fat	2	Margarine	2 tsp
	Fruit	2	Cantaloupe	$^{1}/_{2}$ small
Bedtime	Milk	1	Skim milk	1 cup
	Bread	1	Graham crackers	2 squares
	Fruit	1	Fresh grapes	12

production induced by exercise is suppressed. Exercise also lowers the blood glucose concentration in patients with NIDDM. Because this patient population tends to be obese and sedentary, an increase in physical activity is indicated as a way of helping them to combat this lifestyle. Regular physical exercise can be an important adjunct to diet and can facilitate weight reduction.

Exercise-induced hypoglycemia is a well-recognized complication in insulin-treated diabetics. Flood [70] recently suggested the following guidelines for physicians in establishing a safe exercise program for diabetics:

1 Evaluate the overall health status of patients, especially with regard to their cardiovascular system.

2 Encourage proper physical training and conditioning.

3 Consider the type of diabetes. Insulin-dependent diabetics tend to be younger and to have fewer general health problems, but they may need more day-to-day adjustment in their management. Non-insulin-dependent diabetics usually are older and may have more health problems, but their diabetes may be simpler to manage.

4 Be sure the current level of diabetic management is adequate. Exercise should be used as an adjunct to, not a replacement for, management of diabetes by diet and hypoglycemic agents.

5 Work with the patient to establish a solid basic program. The simple addition of exercise without proper attention to diet, oral agents or insulin, and urine and blood tests for diabetic control may lead to hypoglycemia or deterioration of diabetic control.

6 Encourage detailed record keeping for the insulin-treated diabetic. As the exercise program progresses, adjustments to diet or insulin dosage must be based on data, not guesswork.

7 Be prepared to revise the diet. For some patients, the addition of regular physical exercise will usually mean that daily caloric intake can be increased. For other patients, carbohydrate supplementation prior to or subsequent to exercise will be necessary to ward off episodes of hypoglycemia.

8 Be prepared to revise the insulin dosage. Some insulin-treated diabetics decrease their daily insulin requirements after they initiate an exercise program.

9 Guard against hypoglycemia. The vast majority of patients who are willing to observe urine or blood tests and to be alert for early signs of hypoglycemia can successfully participate in an exercise program with minimal risk.

10 Encourage regularity. Most studies of diabetic athletes have shown that changes in diet and insulin dosage, which are necessary to maintain a proper balance, should generally be made early in an exercise program.

Hypoglycemic Agents

Oral Agents   Maturity-onset diabetes (type II) that cannot be controlled by careful dietary management usually responds to sulfonylurea drugs. These drugs have a common core component, $-SO_2-NH-CO-NH-$, which is responsible for their pharmacological actions. Differences in the molecular structure alter their hypoglycemic potency, duration of action, and metabolism. Pharmacological data concerning the four oral agents currently marketed in the United States are shown in Table 11-10.

Stimulation of pancreatic insulin secretion is presumed to be the major mode of action of sulfonylureas. Several extrahepatic actions have also been ascribed to these agents. Increased insulin receptor binding capacity was reported by Olefsky and Reaven [71], who observed a doubling of insulin binding to receptors after 3 months of chlorpropamide therapy. The suppression of hepatic gluconeogenesis during sulfonylurea administration has been described by Blumenthal [72].

Insulin   Insulin is required for treatment of all juvenile (type I) diabetic patients and many patients with maturity-onset (type II) disease. The symptoms of diabetes can be controlled with insulin, but it is very difficult to normalize blood glucose levels throughout the day. A variety of forms of insulin are available, but crystalline (regular) and NPH or lente preparations are most

TABLE 11-10
ORAL SULFONYLUREA DRUGS SOLD IN UNITED STATES

Generic name (trade name)	Structural formula a	U.S. supplier	Tablet size, mg	Dosage, mg Usual	Dosage, mg Range	Daily Dose	Duration of action, h
Tolbutamide (Orinase)	H_3C—⬡—$SO_2NHCNHCH_2CH_2CH_2CH_3$	Upjohn	500	1500	500–2000	2–3	6–10
Chlorpropamide (Diabinese)	Cl—⬡—$SO_2NHCNHCH_2CH_2CH_2CH_3$	Pfizer	100 250	250	50–500	1	36–60
Acetohexamide (Dymelor)	CH_3C—⬡—SO_2NH—NH	Lilly	250 500	750	250–1500	1–2	10–20
Tolazamide (Tolinase)	H_3C—⬡—SO_2NHC—N	Upjohn	100 250 500	500	100–1000	1–2	12–24

commonly used. The three major characteristics distinguishing insulin preparations are time course of action, species of origin, and degree of purity. These characteristics of insulin currently marketed in the United States are summarized in Table 11-11. Insulin preparations are generally available in concentrations of 40, 80, and 100 units per milliliter. In the future only U-100 (100 units per milliliter) will be used. Regular insulin given subcutaneously will ordinarily have an onset of action within a period of minutes and its effect will last for 4 to 6 hours. Plasma insulin concentrations following injection of lente or NPH insulin rise at slightly slower rates, and the biological effects persist for 12 to 24 hours.

Therapy in each patient has to be determined by trial and error, since individual diabetics exhibit wide differences in their response to a given form of insulin. Foster [73] has suggested the following guidelines regarding insulin use:

1 In emergencies such as diabetic ketoacidosis or hyperosmolar coma always use regular insulin.

2 For initiation of therapy (in the absence of an emergency) try a single injection of intermittent-acting insulin (lente or NPH).

3 Start treatment with small amounts and increase gradually.

4 Allow several days to a week between changes in dose.

5 If control is difficult, give intermediate insulin twice daily with or without the addition of regular insulin.

6 Avoid hypoglycemia.

DIABETIC CONTROL

Good control of blood glucose levels is difficult, at best, in stable diabetics and may not be possible in unstable diabetics. Considerable controversy continues regarding the relationship of blood glucose control to the development of the "chronic" complications of diabetes (retinopathy, neuropathy, and arteriosclerosis). Whether hyperglycemia causes or accelerates the development of these long-term complications is not certain.

At the same time, there are compelling reasons to try to keep the diabetic patient's blood glucose level as close to normal as possible, without inducing severe hypoglycemia. A major aim of therapy is to keep the patient symptom-free. The prevention of diabetic ketoacidosis and hyperosmolar nonketotic coma are important reasons to strive for control of diabetes. Good control also appears to decrease the incidence of infections, to promote normal growth and development of the diabetic, and to decrease perinatal morbidity and mortality and possibly to inhibit the development of congenital defects in the infants of pregnant diabetic mothers [74].

Monitoring Diabetic Control

The assessment of long-term blood glucose regulation in the diabetic relies on (1) urine testing, (2) blood glucose estimations, and (3) glycosylated hemoglobin

TABLE 11-11

INSULINS AVAILABLE IN THE UNITED STATES
(Listed by Manufacturer)

Species, purity, and type of action	Lilly products	Novo products	Nordisk products	Squibb products
Purified pork (<10 ppm):				
Rapid-acting	Regular	Actrapic (regular) Semitard (semilente)	Velosulin Quick (regular) Mixtard (30% regular: 70% NPH)	
Intermediate-acting	NPH Lente	Monotard (lente)	Insulatard (NPH)	
Long-acting	PZI			
Purified beef (<10 ppm):				
Rapid-acting	Regular			
Intermediate-acting	NPH Lente			
Long-acting	PZI	Ultratard (ultralente)		
Purified beef-pork (<10 ppm):				
Intermediate-acting		Lentard (lente)		
Improved single peak (USP beef-pork, < 50 ppm):				
Rapid-acting	Regular Semilente			
Intermediate-acting	NPH Lente			
Long-acting	PZI Ultralente			
USP beef-pork (conventional, <10,000 ppm):				
Rapid-acting				Regular
Intermediate-acting				NPH Globin PZI
Long-acting				
USP beef (conventional, <10,000 ppm):				
Rapid-acting				
Intermediate-acting				Semilente Lente
Long-acting				Ultralente

Source: J. A. Galloway, Diabetes Care, 3:615, 1980.

measurements. None of these measurements permits the determination with certainty of the chemical state of patients during their day-to-day life and activity.

Urine testing for glucose and ketones before breakfast and 2 to 4 hours after meals helps the physician and/or the experienced patient to decide whether the dose of insulin or hypoglycemic drug should be adjusted or whether the carbohydrate content of the diet or the time when it is taken should be altered. While the patient is being stabilized, tests have to be carried out three to four times daily; when control is established, the frequency is greatly reduced.

Fasting or postprandial blood glucose determinations are a routine part of diabetes care, although their value is doubtful. Variation in glucose in most insulin-treated diabetic patients is so great that isolated observations on one day, or at the same time on successive days, are likely to give an incomplete and often misleading impression [75].

Measurement of glycosylated hemoglobin (Hb A_{1c}) provides a means to assess objectively long-term blood glucose regulation in the diabetic patient. Measurement of hemoglobin A_{1c} is more useful to the physician than to the patient, who cannot use the results to modify his or her therapy.

Hemoglobin A_{1c} is a minor red cell component that comprises 3 to 6 percent of the total hemoglobin in normal individuals but up to 15 percent in patients with DM [76]. Formation of Hb A_{1c} has been considered a slow, nonenzymatic, posttranslational, irreversible process occurring within the erythrocyte at a rate dependent on the blood glucose concentration. These measurements correlate with mean serum glucose determination over time and may be a better marker of diabetic control over a sustained time (4 to 12 weeks) than of hyperglycemia per se. Elevated concentration of Hb A_{1c} in diabetics can be reversed by adequate insulin treatment.

The advantages of this test are that it is objective, independent of the patient's cooperation, and reduces diabetic control to a single number. As a clinical tool this measurement is most useful in labile diabetes, i.e., IDDM and diabetes in pregnancy [77]. Furthermore, objective results may have a positive motivating influence on the patient by providing a target number for average blood glucose control. Recent reviews of this subject have been published by Jovanovic and Peterson [77] and by Gabbay and Fluckiger [78].

PREVENTION

Non-insulin-dependent diabetes mellitus is a disease of the prosperous and well-nourished and is much more common among overweight individuals. Joslin, in an article written in 1921, stated: "Obese patients should be frankly told they are candidates for diabetes. The physician should consider it as important to prevent his patient acquiring diabetes as he feels it incumbent on himself to vaccinate them against smallpox" [79]. The importance for health of sufficient exercise and of avoiding dietary excess has been stated repeatedly. Diabetes, like obesity and atherosclerosis, is likely to occur in predisposed individuals who eat too much and exercise too little.

CASE STUDY

A 46-year-old woman was referred for an endocrine consultation after an ophthalmologist diagnosed myopia and found a casual plasma glucose of 260 mg/dl. Her history revealed no other problems; her mother is a type II diabetic who is managed with diet alone. She, herself, had one child 24 years ago, with a birth weight of 7½ lb. Physical examination of the patient was negative. Her height was 5 feet 5 inches and her weight was 156 lb.

Study Questions

1 What laboratory studies would be needed to make the diagnosis of diabetes?

2 What treatment would you recommend?

3 What calorie level would you recommend in the diet?

REFERENCES

1 National Center for Health Statistics: *Diabetes Data,* U.S. Department of Health, Education, and Welfare Publication no. (NIH) 78-1468, 1978.

2 West, K. M.: Epidemiology of diabetes mellitus and its cardiovascular manifestations, in *Genetic Analysis of Common Diseases: Application to Predictive Factors in Coronary Disease,* C. F. Sing and M. Skolnick (eds.), Alan R. Liss, New York, 1979.

3 National Diabetes Data Group: classification and diagnosis of diabetes mellitus and other categories of glucose intolerance, Diabetes, 28:1039, 1979.

4 Ganda, O. P., and S. S. Soeldner: Genetic, acquired and related factors in the etiology of diabetes mellitus, Arch. Intern. Med., 137:461, 1977.

5 Prosser, P. R., and J. H. Karam: Diabetes mellitus following rodenticide ingestion in man, J. Am. Med. Assoc., 239:1148, 1978.

6 Fajans, S. S., M. C. Cloutier, and R. L. Crowther: Clinical and etiologic heterogeneity of idiopathic diabetes mellitus, Diabetes, 27:1112, 1978.

7 Fajans, S. S., J. C. Floyd, R. B. Tattersall, J. R. Williamson, S. Peh, and C. I. Taylor: The various faces of diabetes in the young, Arch. Intern. Med., 136:194, 1976.

8 Christy, M., A. Green, B. Christau, H. Kromann, J. Nerup, P. Platz, M. Thomsen, L. P. Ryder, and A. Sregaard: Studies of the HLA system and insulin-dependent diabetes mellitus, Diabetes Care, 2:209, 1979.

9 West, K. M., and J. M. Kalbfleisch: Influence of nutritional factors on prevalence of diabetes, Diabetes, 20:99, 1971.

10 *Report of the National Commission on Diabetes to the Congress of the United States,* vol. 1, U.S. Department of Health, Education, and Welfare Publication no. (NIH) 76-1018, 1975.

11 Butterfield, W. J. H., and M. Whichelow: Effect of diet, sulfonylureas and phenformin on peripheral glucose uptake in diabetes and obesity, Lancet, 2:785, 1968.

12 Karam, J. H., G. M. Grodsky, and P. H. Forsham: Excessive insulin response to glucose in obese subjects as measured by immunochemical assay, Diabetes, 12:197, 1963.

13 Butterfield, W. J. H., T. Hanely, and M. J. Whichelow: Peripheral metabolism of glucose and free fatty acids during oral glucose tolerance test, Metabolism, 14:851, 1965.

14 West, K. M.: *Epidemiology of Diabetes and Its Vascular Lesions,* Elsevier, New York, 1978.

15 World Health Organization: Statistical Yearbook, Epidemiol. Vital Statist. Rep., 17:47, 51, 307–330, 1964.

16 Altman, D. E., S. D. Baker, M. McCally, and T. E. Piemme: Carbohydrate and lipid metabolism in man during prolonged bed rest, Clin. Res., 17:543, 1969.

17 Bjorntorp, P., G. Holm, B. Jacobsson, K. Schiller-de Jounge, P. A. Lundberg, L. Sjostrom, U. Smith, and L. Sullivan: Physical training in human hyperplastic obesity. 4. Effects of hormonal status, Metabolism, 26:319, 1977.

18 Sanders, H. J.: Diabetes: rapid advances, lingering mysteries, Chem. Eng. News, 59:30, 1981.

19 Yoon, J. W., M. Austin, T. Onodera, and A. L. Notkins: Virus-induced diabetes mellitus. Isolation of a virus from the pancreas of a child with diabetic ketoacidosis, N. Engl. J. Med., 300:1173, 1979.

20 Oiso, T.: Recent changes in nutrition in Japan, in *Diabetes Mellitus in Asia,* Proc. Symp. Kobe, S. Tsuji, and M. Wada (eds.), Excerpta Medica, Amsterdam, 1970.

21 Tsai, S.: Epidemiology of diabetes mellitus in Taiwan, J. Jpn. Diabet. Soc., 14:33, 1971.

22 Sukhatme, P. V.: On the trend of obesity in advanced countries, in *Diabetes: Proceedings of the 6th Congress of the International Diabetes Federation,* J. Oestman and R. D. G. Milner (eds.), Excerpta Medica, Amsterdam, 1967.

23 Cleave, T. L., and G. D. Campbell: *Diabetes, Coronary Thrombosis and the Saccharine Disease,* John Wright and Sons, Bristol, 1969.

24 Yudkin, J.: *Sweet and Dangerous,* Bantam, New York, 1972.

25 Keys, A.: Sucrose in the diet in coronary heart disease (letter to the editors), Atherosclerosis, 18:352, 1973.

26 Yudkin, J.: Dietary fat and dietary sugar in relation to ischemic heart disease and diabetes, Lancet, 2:4, 1964.

27 Kahn, H. A., J. B. Herman, J. H. Medalie, H. N. Neufeld, E. Riss, and U. Goldbourt: Factors related to diabetes incidence: a multivariate analysis of two years observation on 10,000 men, J. Chronic Dis., 23:617, 1971.

28 Trowell, H. C.: Dietary fiber hypothesis of the etiology of diabetes mellitus, Diabetes, 24:762, 1975.

29 Jenkins, D. J. A., A. R. Leeds, M. A. Gassull, B. Cochet, and K. G. M. M. Alberti: Decrease in postprandial insulin and glucose concentrations by guar and pectin, Ann. Intern. Med., 86:20, 1977.

30 Weinsier, R. L., A. Seeman, M. G. Herrera, J. P. Assal, J. S. Soeldner, and R. E. Gleason: High- and low-carbohydrate diets in diabetes mellitus, Ann. Intern. Med., 80:332, 1974.

31 Stone, D. B., and W. E. Conner: The prolonged effects of a low cholesterol, high carbohydrate diet upon the serum lipids in diabetic patients, Diabetes, 12:127, 1963.

32 Kiehm, T. G., J. W. Anderson, and K. Ward: Beneficial effects of a high carbohydrate, high fiber diet on hyperglycemic men, Am. J. Clin. Nutr., 29:895, 1976.

33 Brunzell, J. D., R. L. Lerner, D. J. Porte, and E. L. Bierman: Effect of a fat-free, high carbohydrate diet on diabetic subjects with fasting hyperglycemia, Diabetes, 23:138, 1974.

34 Jenkins, D. J. A., A. R. Leeds, R. M. S. Wolever, D. V. Goff, K. G. M. M. Alberti, M. A. Gassull, and T. D. R. Hockaday: Unabsorbable carbohydrates in diabetes: decreased post-prandial hyperglycaemia, Lancet, 2:172, 1976.

35 Simpson, H. C. R., S. Lousley, M. Geekie, R. W. Simpson, R. D. Carter, T. D. R. Hockaday, and J. I. Mann: A high carbohydrate leguminous fiber diet improves all aspects of diabetic control, Lancet, 1:1, 1981.

36 Anderson, J. W.: New approaches to diabetes diets, Med. Times, 108:41, 1980.

37 Anderson, J. W., and K. Ward: High carbohydrate, high fiber diets for insulin-treated men with diabetes mellitus, Am. J. Clin. Nutr., 32:2312, 1979.

38 Crapo, P. A., J. Insel, M. Sperling, and O. G. Kolterman: Comparison of serum glucose, insulin and glucagon responses to different types of complex carbohydrate in noninsulin-dependent diabetic patients, Am. J. Clin. Nutr., 34:184, 1981.

39 Steiner, D. F. and P. E. Oyer: The biosynthesis of insulin and a probable precursor of insulin by a human islet cell tumor, Proc. Natl. Acad. Sci. U.S.A., 57:473, 1967.

40 Gepts, W., and P. M. Lecompte: The pancreatic islets in diabetes, Am. J. Med., 70:105, 1981.

41 Doniach, I., and A. G. Morgan: Islets of Langerhans in juvenile diabetes mellitus, Clin. Endocrinol., 2:233, 1973.

42 Gepts, W.: Pathological anatomy of the pancreas in juvenile diabetes mellitus, Diabetes, 14:619, 1965.

43 Gepts, W., and J. De Mey: Islet cell survival determined by morphology. An immunochemical study of the islet of Langerhans in juvenile diabetes mellitus, Diabetes, 27(suppl. 1):251, 1978.

44 Cahill, G. F.: Diabetes mellitus: a brief overview, John Hopkins Med. J., 143:155, 1978.

45 Cerasi, E., and R. Luft: The plasma insulin response to glucose infusion in healthy subjects and in diabetes mellitus, Acta Endocrinol., 55:278, 1967.

46 Reaven, G. M., R. Bernstein, B. Davis, and J. M. Olefsky: Non-ketotic diabetes mellitus: insulin deficiency or insulin resistance? Am. J. Med., 60:80, 1976.

47 Reaven, G. M., and J. M. Olefsky: The role of insulin resistance in the pathogenesis of diabetes mellitus, in *Advances in Metabolic Disorders*, Vol. 9, R. Levine and R Luft (eds.), Academic, New York, 1978.

48 Olefsky, J. M., and G. M. Reaven: Effect of sulfonylurea therapy on insulin binding to mononuclear leukocytes of diabetic patients, Am. J. Med., 60:89, 1976.

49 Savage, P. J., L. J. Bennion, E. V. Flock, M. Nagulesparam, D. Mott, J. Roth, R. H. Unger, and P. H. Bennett: Diet-induced improvement of abnormalities in insulin and glucagon secretion and in insulin-receptor binding in diabetes mellitus, J. Clin. Endocrinol. Metab., 48:999, 1979.

50 Luft, R., A. Wajngot, and S. Efendic: On the pathogenesis of maturity-onset diabetes, Diabetes Care, 4:58, 1981.

51 Felig, P., E. Pozefsky, E. Marliss, and G. F. Cahill, Jr.: Alanine: key role in gluconeogenesis, Science, 167:1003, 1970.

52 Committee of the American Diabetes Association on Food and Nutrition: Special report—principles of nutrition and dietary recommendations for individuals with diabetes mellitus, Diabetes, 28:1028, 1979.

53 Nuttall, F. Q.: Dietary recommendations for individuals with diabetes mellitus, 1979: summary of report from the Foods and Nutrition Committee of the American Diabetes Association, Am. J. Clin. Nutr., 33:1311, 1980.

54 Arky, R. A.: Diet and diabetes, in *Diabetes Mellitus,* vol. V, H. Rifkind and P. Raskin (eds.), Robert J. Brady, Bowie, Md., 1981.

55 Reaven, G. M.: How high the carbohydrate? Diabetologia, 19:409, 1980.

56 Bennion, M.: *Clinical Nutrition,* Harper & Row, New York, 1979.

57 Kritchevsky, D.: Dietary fiber: what it is and what it does, Ann. N.Y. Acad. Sci., 300:283, 1977.

58 Einsinck, J. W., and E. L. Bierman: Dietary management of diabetes mellitus, Annu. Rev. Med., 30:155, 1979.

59 Reinhold, J. G., K. Nasr, A. Lahimgarzadeh, and H. Hedayati: Effects of purified phytate and phytate-rich bread upon metabolism of zinc, calcium, phosphorus and nitrogen in man, Lancet, 1:283, 1973.

60 Wallgren, H., and H. Barry: *Actions of Alcohol,* vol. 1, Elsevier, Amsterdam, 1970.

61 West, K. M.: Diabetes mellitus, in *Nutritional Support of Medical Practice,* H. A. Schneider, C. E. Anderson, and D. B. Coursin (eds.), Harper & Row, Hagerstown, Md., 1977.

62 Olefsky, J. M., and P. Crapo: Fructose, xylitol and sorbitol, Diabetes Care, 3:390, 1980.

63 American Diabetes Association: Saccharin, Diabetes Care, 2:380, 1979.

64 Wahren, J., L. Hagenfeldt, and P. Felig: Splanchnic and leg exchange of glucose, amino acids, and free fatty acids during exercise in diabetes mellitus, J. Clin. Invest., 55:1303, 1975.

65 Richter, E. A., N. B. Ruderman, and S. H. Schneider: Diabetes and exercise, Am. J. Med., 70:201, 1981.

66 Dandona P., P. Hook, and J. Bell: Exercise and insulin absorption from subcutaneous tissue, Br. Med. J., 1:479, 1978.

67 Koivisto, V. A., and P. Felig: Effect of leg exercise on insulin absorption in diabetic patients, N. Engl. J. Med., 298:77, 1978.

68 Vranic, M., and M. Berger: Exercise and diabetes mellitus, Diabetes, 28:147, 1979.

69 Zinman, B., M. Vranic, A. M. Albisser, B. S. Leibel, and E. B. Marliss: The role of insulin in the metabolic response to exercise in diabetic man, Diabetes, 28(suppl. 1):76, 1979.

70 Flood, T. M.: Ten steps to a successful exercise program, Med. Times, 108:19, 1980.

71 Olefsky, J. M., and G. M. Reaven: Effects of sulfonylurea therapy on insulin binding to mononuclear leukocytes of diabetic patients, Am. J. Med., 60:89, 1976.

72 Blumenthal, S. A.: Potentiation of the hepatic action of insulin by chlorpropamide, Diabetes, 26:485, 1977.

73 Foster, D. W.: Diabetes mellitus, in *Harrison's Principles of Internal Medicine,* 9th ed., K. J. Isselbacher et al. (eds.), McGraw-Hill, New York, 1980.

74 Rifkin, H., and H. Ross: Control of diabetes and long-term complications, in *Diabetes Mellitus,* vol. V, H. Rifkin and P. Raskin (eds.), Robert J. Brady, Bowie, Md., 1981.

75 Molnar, G. D.: Clinical evaluation of metabolic control in diabetes, Diabetes, 27(suppl. 1):216, 1978.

76 Trivelli, L. A., H. M. Ranney, and H. T. Lai: Hemoglobin component in patients with diabetes mellitus, N. Engl. J. Med., 284:353, 1971.

77 Jovanovic, L., and C. M. Peterson: The clinical utility of glycosylated hemoglobin, Am. J. Med., 70:331, 1981.

78 Gabbay, K. H., and R. Fluckiger: Clinical significance of glycosylated hemoglobin, in *Diabetes Mellitus,* vol. V, H. Rifkind and P. Raskin (eds.), Robert J. Brady, Bowie, Md., 1981.

79 Joslin, E. P.: The prevention of diabetes mellitus, J. Am. Med. Assoc., 76:79, 1921.

CHAPTER 12

NUTRITIONAL ASPECTS OF RENAL DISEASES

CONTENTS

INTRODUCTION

Both acute and chronic progressive failure of kidney function were recognized long before the introduction of various techniques of dialysis and artificial kidneys. The contributions that manipulation of nutrient intake can make in either situation were poorly worked out at that time, largely because of the grave prognosis and short survival of the bulk of patients with severe renal disease, which supportive treatment, including some attention to nutrition, influenced very little. However, effective hemodialysis, and the success of renal transplantation, which requires that a patient be kept alive until a suitable kidney donor is found, have stimulated efforts to prolong survival by dietary management. Manipulation of the diet in a number of different ways and improvement of the general nutritional status of the patient have contributed significantly to survival and to the quality of life of survivors. There is some cause for optimism that rigorous dietary control may significantly reduce or postpone the need for use of hemodialysis or renal transplantation.

Acute renal failure due to acute tubular necrosis (ATN) is a self-limiting disease in a substantial number of patients. During the period of acute failure it is usually impossible, because of nausea and vomiting, for the patient to ingest sufficient glucose and lipids to reduce significantly the mobilization of tissue nitrogen. The development of materials and techniques for intravenous infusion of adequate amounts of calories as glucose and fat, together with hemodialysis, has been a major advance, permitting a degree of nutritional adequacy consonant with tissue repair and healing, until recovery of tubular function occurs and the patient can eat again.

Useful lessons in nutritional biochemistry have also been learned from earlier experiences. It is evident that the quality of life of the subject with progressive renal failure or terminal end-stage renal disease can be significantly enhanced by improving the quality of the nutritional support provided.

The kidney is primarily an excretory organ. By virtue of variations in its selective excretory functions it maintains the balance between the volumes of extra- and intracellular fluids and thus the blood pressure and the pH of the internal milieu. It also serves as an endocrine organ, being the source of (1) renin, which is involved in maintenance of blood pressure; (2) 1,25-dihydroxycholecalciferol, which is derived from 25-hydroxycholecalciferol and controls calcium absorption by the small intestine; and (3) erythropoietin, which stimulates hematopoiesis. In consequence, instability of blood pressure, calcium deficiency, and a normochromic, normocytic (aregenerative) anemia commonly occur in patients with both acute and chronic renal disease. The kidney is also a source of other hormones, such as prostaglandins, but their roles both in health and in chronic and acute renal failure in humans are uncertain.

The kidney is also a major site of destruction or excretion of gastrin and some other hormones. Increased gastric secretion and peptic ulceration may occur in the patient with chronic renal failure, and decreased insulin requirements may occur in the insulin-dependent diabetic who develops chronic renal damage. These effects are most marked in the anephric patient.

EFFECTS OF NUTRITIONAL DEFICIENCY ON RENAL FUNCTION

Little is known about the response of the kidney to the degrees of malnutrition likely to be encountered in clinical practice. The exception to this is the effect of chronic deficiency of potassium, which most commonly results from excessive use of potassium-wasting diuretics without proper monitoring. It may also occur in diseases associated with intestinal malabsorption and chronic diarrhea, such as celiac-sprue, Crohn's disease and, occasionally, ulcerative colitis.

Chronic abuse of purgatives may also result in potassium depletion, a cause which is frequently unsuspected and which sometimes gives rise to a false diagnosis of primary or secondary hyperaldosteronism. Occasionally long-term treatment with corticosteroids results in hypokalemia.

Potassium wasting may be an expression of chronic renal failure itself or of a specific renal tubular dysfunction and may thus aggravate the disturbances of kidney function.

Potassium deficiency affects the proximal and distal convoluted tubules of the kidney. The endothelial cells become vacuolated. Later, interstitial fibrosis occurs, and the lesions may then be irreversible.

Patients develop polydipsia and polyuria with nocturnal frequency of urination, as a consequence of failure of renal tubular concentration. The osmotic pressure of the urine declines, approximating that of the plasma. Treatment consists of treating the cause of potassium loss or providing potassium supplements, either in the form of increased consumption of orange or prune juices, bananas, dried apricots, tomatoes, and other foods of high potassium content (see Table 9-9) or as a potassium chloride–potassium carbonate salt.

Severe protein-calorie malnutrition in children may result in disturbance of renal function. Reduced creatinine clearance has been observed in some severely malnourished Guatemalan Indian children [1].

In adults it appears that starvation may or may not affect renal function significantly. Thus of four subjects from the concentration camp at Belsen, two displayed normal renal clearance and two reduced clearance. The latter were suffering from famine edema; the former were not [2]. In another study reduced inulin clearance was found in only one of eleven undernourished subjects [3].

There is some evidence that urea clearance falls much more than inulin clearance in protein-deficient subjects [4], and it has been postulated that increased urea absorption by the renal tubule occurs as a compensatory device to conserve nitrogen. This postulation has been well reviewed by Klahr and Alleyne [4].

NUTRITIONAL MANAGEMENT OF SPECIFIC RENAL DISEASE

Acute Renal Failure

Epidemiology Acute renal failure is defined as a degree of functional disturbance of the kidneys sufficient to cause substantial alteration in the plasma biochemistry, which develops over days or, at most, weeks. It may be associated, but not invariably, with significant reduction of urinary volume below 500 ml per day (oliguria) or with absence of urine production (anuria).

It is estimated that in the United States more than 12,000 patients per year require dialysis for transient renal failure. The causes are very numerous. Acute tubular necrosis (ATN) is the most common cause and constitutes about three-quarters of all cases. Some patients with this condition recover spontaneously and are never dialyzed; others, in whom there may be severe impairment of other systems, are too sick to be benefited by dialysis. But the majority are treated by dialysis. Other causes of acute renal failure are acute glomerulonephritis, urinary obstruction by stones or tumor, occlusion of renal blood vessels, and drug-induced papillary necrosis. Analgesics such as phenacetin are the most common culprits in drug-induced renal failure.

Etiology   There are several recognized causes of ATN. The most common is posttraumatic or surgical shock, which causes transient ischemic anoxia of the kidneys due to failure of renal perfusion. The usual antecedents are a fall of blood pressure of considerable magnitude sustained for 5 minutes or more during or after major surgery or as a result of severe trauma, burns, or hemorrhage (e.g., during obstetric delivery or from a bleeding peptic ulcer), and septicemia. The most common associations in pregnancy are early septic abortion or preeclampsia.

Despite observations in humans and in animal experiments, which emphasize that the hypotensive episode must be a severe one, a number of patients, especially after surgery, develop ATN without recorded antecedent cardiovascular failure. Other important causes are the toxic effects of some metals, such as gold used therapeutically or mercury or chromium salts ingested by accident or by murderous design; of organic compounds such as methanol and carbon tetrachloride and other halogenated hydrocarbons, some of which are used as anesthetic agents; of sulfonamides; rarely of some antibiotics such as neomycin, polymyxin, and methicillin; and of radiographic contrast media. Surgery, trauma, and pregnancy make up three-quarters of all cases of ATN.

Acute renal failure may complicate many forms of acute or progressive glomerulonephritis. The most common are acute, poststreptococcal glomerulonephritis, the type associated with subacute bacterial endocarditis, disseminated lupus erythematosus, and polyarteritis nodosa.

Pathology   During the acute phase of ATN the endothelial cells of the kidney tubules are swollen and edematous, with vacuolated cytoplasm. Damaged renal tubules usually recover in days or weeks.

Symptoms   In the early stages of ATN the patient may be asymptomatic, but symptoms of the after effects of major surgery, trauma, or another cause will of course be present. Since severe surgical trauma or other trauma or illness is a common association, the patient may be in a markedly catabolic state, with increased gluconeogenesis making demands on tissue protein and reactive insulin resistance reducing entry of glucose into cells. Even when oliguria is present, thirst may persist, and unless intake of fluid has been restricted from the time of onset (which may not be recognized unless the possibility is entertained and appropriate laboratory monitoring is begun), there is real danger of overexpansion of the extracellular space with resulting hyponatremia and consequent cellular overhydration, leading to convulsions and vomiting early in the course of renal failure. Vomiting that occurs without warning sometimes results in inhalation of gastric contents, which can be catastrophic. However, if the cause of shutdown of renal function is associated with severe burns or heavy metal or other toxic agents, symptoms may be minimal until other profound metabolic effects of failure of renal function begin to produce toxic effects. Anorexia, nausea, or intestinal ileus (paralysis) may occur later, in consequence.

A major danger to survival is elevation of extracellular potassium concentrations (hyperkalemia), which can cause cardiac arrhythmias or arrest. This rise may occur and reach fatal levels within hours of onset. It occurs as a complication of acidosis, a hypercatabolic state, or blood transfusions, each acting alone or all acting in concert. The acidosis reflects the inability of the kidneys to synthesize ammonium ions.

Another complication is gastrointestinal bleeding, which may be due to acute erosions and may be compounded by disturbance of normal function of the blood platelets [5]. It is possible that increased blood gastrin activity may be responsible in part for the upper gastrointestinal erosions, as a consequence of hypersecretion of gastric acid.

A significant reduction in urinary output or, less commonly, anuria occurs in 90 percent of subjects. The change may be noted within hours, or it may be delayed by as much as 24 to 48 hours from the onset of renal failure. In the remaining 10 percent of patients there may be no reduction of urine volume, only increased retention of electrolytes and nonelectrolytes. This is especially true after severe burns.

If the patient survives, recovery of function occurs in a few days to 3 weeks or more. The first indication of recovery of function in the oliguric patient is an increase in urinary volume. The urine is initially of low specific gravity and in osmolarity approximates plasma (hyposthenuria). Subsequently there may be partial or complete return of renal function to normal. The average length of the oliguric or anuric phase is 11 days.

Increased susceptibility to infection is well-recognized in both acute and chronic renal failure. This is due possibly to impaired immune responsiveness. Monilial infection is common and may result in large, shallow, painful ulcers on the tongue and buccal mucosa and sometimes in the esophagus; any of these lesions may produce severe dysphagia and make eating difficult or impossible.

Laboratory Findings. Examination of the urine in acute renal failure is essential to distinguish between ATN and glomerulonephritis. In the former, microscopic findings are usually normal, but, more importantly, in the latter the urine invariably contains red cells or protein, or both, and red cell casts.

Monitoring of serum electrolytes is essential in order to recognize early hyponatremia, with its dangers of cellular overhydration and edema of the central nervous system, and to follow the concentration of serum potassium. Hyperkalemia may be asymptomatic until severe disturbances of the electrocardiogram or cardiac arrest occurs. Early dialysis has markedly reduced this risk, but serial serum estimations are still mandatory. Serum calcium concentrations almost always fall in acute renal failure, and serum phosphate rises. The cause is unclear, since circulating parathyroid hormone concentrations measured immunologically tend to rise. The hypocalcemia is rarely symptomatic. Plasma urea concentrations may rise at the rate of 5 to 10 mmol per liter per day or, in the markedly hypercatabolic posttraumatic or infected patient, at more than double that rate (greater than 25 mmol per liter per day).

Standard measurements of hemoglobin and packed cell volume and red cell morphology reveal progressive aregenerative anemia due to marrow shutdown, and a varying degree of hemolysis can be demonstrated by red cell survival studies. In about one-fifth of patients, gastrointestinal hemorrhage occurs, usually as the result of bleeding gastroduodenal erosions. The stools should therefore be examined serially for overt and occult blood.

Treatment   A problem in managing ATN is that there is no reliable indicator of how long the functional disturbance will last. The important factor in management is to monitor changes in serum bicarbonate and potassium, in order to assess whether the patient is becoming acidotic, and to monitor changes in serum sodium as an index of water intake. Daily hemodialysis is now widely used for acute renal failure so as to avoid the risks of cardiac arrest and other complications. There is no simple, controlled trial showing that dialysis improves survival or hastens recovery, but it is clear that it permits a less restrictive diet and fluid intake and may reduce the incidence of gastrointestinal bleeding [6].

Current practice is to control uremia at a much lower level than in the past; a predialysis figure below 30 mmol per liter can be attained easily with daily dialysis during the severe hypercatabolic phase, if present. When this phase is controlled, dialysis on alternate days is sufficient. In the mildly hypercatabolic patient dialysis every 3 days may be sufficient to permit free access to water and protein.

Oral intake of food is impossible in patients who have undergone abdominal surgery and is seldom adequate to meet metabolic needs during the first week in the sick patient with acute renal failure, because of anorexia, nausea, or even disturbed consciousness. Attempts to give high-protein, oral feeds such as Sustacal or Precision and sufficient extra calories as fat and carbohydrate are usually successful only in the less severely sick patient.

In the early stage total parenteral feeding is the method of choice, using subclavian or other deep-vein catheterization. Standard amino acid solutions are used. There are two types of solution, each appropriate to a different approach to the problem. Both recognize the need to meet calorie requirements in order to reduce gluconeogenesis from tissue proteins to a minimum. This is done by infusing dextrose, and Intralipid may be given in addition by peripheral vein two or three times in the first week.

The first approach is now more widely used. Both essential and nonessential amino acids are given at a daily rate of 1 to 1.5 g per kilogram of body weight, which is equivalent to 70 to 100 g protein for an adult. Two widely used preparations are FreAmine II and Aminosyn 10%. Each is made up with 70 percent dextrose in water so that each liter contains 400 g dextrose and the equivalent of 40 g protein, a kilocalorie-protein ratio of approximately 40:1. Infusion initially at 20 ml per hour is gradually increased over 2 to 4 days to 70 to 100 ml per hour, depending on the patient's size. Electrolytes, including trace minerals, and all vitamins are added. In addition, insulin must be given, since relative insulin resistance is likely to be present; the dose should be adjusted to maintain blood glucose concentrations below 300 mg/dl. This requires monitoring on at least a 6-hourly basis during the first 3 days.

This regimen is not directed to keeping nitrogen intake to a minimum. It is confidently assumed that dialysis and supplementation can take care of the uremia and other metabolic problems and, of course, remove surplus fluid. Dialysis is performed by using a forearm Scribner-Quinton shunt which has a siliconized rubber segment.

The second approach has few advocates for use in *acute* renal failure. The goal is to keep nitrogen intake to a minimum, to maintain a supply of essential amino acids only, and to encourage reutilization of urea produced by breakdown of endogenous tissue proteins in building new protein. However, only a small fraction of the total nitrogen used for albumin synthesis is derived from urea (about 6 percent), which is approximately only 2 to 2.5 percent of all the urea available [7]. The amino acid preparation used is Nephramine, which is made up so that a liter of infusion fluid contains approximately 17 g essential amino acids and 470 g dextrose. The initial rate of infusion is 20 ml per hour, increased fourfold gradually over 2 to 4 days. Two liters daily supply 34 g essential amino acids and over 3000 kcal. Electrolytes and vitamins are added and insulin also in an amount which will allow peripheral utilization of glucose and will maintain a blood level below 300 mg/dl. However, there is some evidence that mixtures of essential and nonessential amino acids are metabolically handled more efficiently by the hypercatabolic patient. Since repeated dialysis is now widely utilized and is able to handle both problems of nitrogen retention and other important and potentially life-threatening disturbances such as hyperkalemia and, to some extent, intestinal bleeding, the first approach, which uses both essential and nonessential amino acids, is much more favored.

If the patient's condition warrants it, increased mobility can be achieved by removing the deep venous line as soon as it is indicated. Supplements of calories and essential amino acids can be given during dialysis, and glucose can be used in the dialysate; blood glucose concentrations should be monitored, and insulin used if necessary. As improvement continues and renal function is restored, the patient will be able to take increasing amounts of food by mouth and the need for dialysis and intravenous feeding will disappear.

In some patients, especially children, peritoneal dialysis is preferable to hemodialysis. It is, in general, not so efficient in removing metabolic products, and serum protein losses are significantly higher, but when considered on a 24-hourly basis, the results are comparable.

Patients who have attempted suicide by taking overdoses of nephrotoxic drugs should not receive arteriovenous shunts, which can be taken apart by the patient with lethal consequences. In such patients, peritoneal dialysis or hemodialysis by catheterization of the femoral vein should be used.

Supportive Treatment   Adequate protein and calories, protection from infection, and early mobilization are important components of successful treatment of acute renal failure. Precautions should be taken against cross infection in intensive care units, hourly mouth hygiene should be performed, nystatin lozenges or mouthwashes should be used if a thrush infection develops, and indwelling catheters should be removed as soon as patients are able to void urine. All drug prescription orders must be constantly reviewed. There is still a great deal of ignorance about the effect of hemodialysis on the concentrations of various drugs in the circulation, due in part to differential effects of protein binding and binding affinities. Aminoglycoside antibiotics, which are nephrotoxic, should be used only when there is no substitute.

Regular doses of oral antacid or cimetidine, an inhibitor of gastric acid secretion, are given in the hope of reducing the chances of upper gastrointestinal bleeding. There is no evidence, however, of significant prophylaxis.

Chronic Renal Failure

Chronic renal failure is a life-threatening condition for which there are many causes, the most common of which are chronic glomerulonephritis (48 percent), pyelonephritis (20 percent), cystic kidney disease (8 percent), renal vascular disease (5 percent), and drug-induced renal damage (3 percent). The introduction of renal dialysis and renal transplantation has revolutionized the treatment and prognosis of chronic renal failure.

Epidemiology   In the United States approximately 40,000 to 45,000 people develop chronic uremia annually, and of these some 20 percent are selected for dialysis; the rest are not dialyzed, by reason of old age or other severe disease, and consequently die.

Approximately 95 people per million in the United States, a total of 25,000 to 30,000 people, are currently supported by chronic dialysis. The cost is now well over a half-billion dollars annually. Further, 32 or more people per million, or about 8000 to 9000 total, have received renal transplants.

The mortality rate in the first year of chronic dialysis is 10 to 15 percent and thereafter about 10 percent per annum. The life expectancy is determined largely by the nature of the primary disease. Thus patients with disseminated lupus erythematosus or diabetes mellitus do far less well than those with polycystic kidney disease. The survival rates appear to be better when dialysis is performed in large centers.

Causes of death include degenerative vascular disease, infection, hyperkalemia, and suicidal depression, in that order of importance.

Etiology   Detailed discussion is outside the scope of this chapter. The major causes of chronic renal failure are the result of infections with microorganisms, both bacteria and viruses. In the case of glomerulonephritis the classification according to the renal micropathology and immunological studies offers a large variety of causes, in most of which antibodies to both exogenous and endogenous antigens or components of humoral mediating systems, such as complement, play a primary or essential secondary role.

In pyelonephritis the etiology is currently debatable. Infection of the urinary tract with various single-serotype *Escherichia coli* organisms in early childhood seems to be a major cause in females. As a cause of chronic renal disease and failure, pyelonephritis is twice as common in females as in males. Cystic kidney, another cause of renal failure, is a congenital defect.

Pathology   In this text it is more appropriate to address the disturbances of the internal environment of the body associated with chronic renal failure than the range of pathological lesions which may impair renal function. In brief, progressive structural changes in the renal glomeruli and gradual reduction in their number are the hallmarks of chronic glomerulonephritis, but damage to the tubules occurs also to a varying degree. The histological classification is a highly specialized field. In pyelonephritis, the kidneys become scarred and shrunken as a consequence, it is believed, of direct damage by coliform bacteria, for instance, and subsequent healing by fibrosis, without intervention of immune mechanisms. The functional pathology in all cases is impairment of renal clearance with retention of nitrogenous waste products, abnormalities in electrolyte balance, and inability to secrete an acid urine, which results in acidosis.

Clinical Manifestations   Some patients with chronic renal failure remain relatively well until late in the course of the illness and present for the first time in near-stage failure with salt and water retention. Elevated blood pressure may cause heart failure, visual disturbances, or headache. They may have anorexia and nausea or hiccups. Others complain much earlier of tiredness or of tiring easily and of muscle weakness. They may have to get up at night to urinate.

Gastrointestinal bleeding may occur. Persistent thirst and an unpleasant metallic taste are moderately common complaints. The skin may itch, locally or all over (pruritus), and patients may produce widespread excoriation of the skin by scratching. Pericarditis and pericardial pain are common.

Salt and water depletion rarely occur instead of retention. In these cases, persistent vomiting and diarrhea are contributory factors.

Terminally, irritability, drowsiness, and confusion may occur.

Symmetrical peripheral neuropathy may develop, usually insidiously, the legs being affected earlier than the arms. The dysfunction is both motor and sensory. The skin may show purpuric lesions, and when the plasma urea rises to high concentrations, a fine bloom of urea may appear on the skin.

The cause of all these changes except the last is not well-established. Uremia represents far more than an accumulation of urea and other nitrogenous compounds derived from proteins. Although serum concentrations of urea, creatinine, phosphate, sulfate, uric acid, and potassium are elevated in uremia, none of these appears to be responsible for the toxic effects observed [8]. Various candidates have been considered for the toxic role, without confirmation, and uremia must currently be considered a clinical entity without a known chemical basis. This uncertainty must be borne by those treating patients by both dialysis and dietary means, but the problem seems to be solved in patients who receive a successful transplant.

Laboratory and Special Findings   Elevations of plasma urea and creatinine occur rapidly after 50 to 75 percent of renal function (as glomerular filtration) has been lost. With advancing disease the rate of creatinine production may fall, so that the plasma level may underestimate the degree of renal failure.

Serum potassium concentration rises later than creatinine concentration, unless potassium-retaining diuretics are given or the patient receives blood transfusions. Both phosphate and bicarbonate levels remain unchanged until the glomerular filtration rate falls below 20 to 25 ml per minute; below this rate acidosis begins to develop. Rises in uric acid also tend to appear late. Serum calcium concentrations fall as phosphate rises. Magnesium concentrations tend to remain within the normal range, but a sudden oral load of magnesium may precipitate hypermagnesemia. Magnesium-containing antacids should therefore be used cautiously in subjects with chronic renal failure. The urinary concentrating power of the kidney is lost to a greater degree than diluting power in a majority of patients with chronic renal failure. The loss in concentrating power is due to an increased solute load and glomerular filtration rate per nephron, which occur in uremia.

Blood findings reveal normochromic, normocytic anemia with depression of marrow function, believed to be due to reduced production of the hormone erythropoietin. In addition, red cell survival is shortened, because of a serum factor or factors, or there may be increased blood loss from the gastrointestinal tract and iron reutilization in hemoglobin synthesis may be disturbed. Increases in red cell 2,3-diphosphoglycerate, a consequence of elevated plasma phosphate, alter the oxygen dissociation curve, shifting it to the right, so that the affinity between hemoglobin and oxygen is reduced and better tissue oxygenation occurs at a given arterial oxygen saturation. This may be a compensatory mechanism contributing to tolerance of severe anemia [9]. When acidosis supervenes, the compensation breaks down, since at lower pH red cell 2,3-diphosphoglycerate concentration is reduced.

The plasma alkaline phosphatase activity is increased when osteomalacia is present in a degree causing clinical symptoms. However, the significance of bone disease in chronic renal failure remains uncertain because of the difficulties of comparison with patients with other debilitating diseases. Assessments of prevalence of demineralization of bone range from 40 to over 90 percent [10].

The theory of causation is that elevated phosphate concentrations depress ionized plasma calcium concentration, which stimulates parathyroid secretion. This produces extra loss of phosphate from the kidney (depressed renal tubular resorption) and increased mobilization of calcium from bone [11]. Other contributory factors are acidosis and reduced ingestion of calcium. Poor calcium absorption by the gut may occur because of depressed levels of 1,25-dihydroxycholecalciferol, which is synthesized by the kidney [12].

Arterial degenerative disease constitutes the most common cause of death in patients with chronic renal failure. The incidences of ischemic heart disease and strokes are both significantly raised, compared with age- and sex-matched nonrenal controls [13]. The reason is unclear. Hypertension is a common association, and abnormal patterns of plasma lipids occur and are not altered by dialysis [14]. The common pattern is that of so-called type IV hyperlipidemia, that is, elevated triglycerides and pre-β-lipoproteins (very low density lipoproteins).

Disturbances of carbohydrate metabolism occur in the majority of patients with chronic renal failure. There may be impaired degradation and excretion of insulin as the kidneys fail [15]; this phenomenon is frequently observed in patients with diabetic nephropathy (Kimmelstiel-Wilson kidney). A more important factor, operating antagonistically, is increased insulin resistance, the causes of which are undetermined [16]. Increased circulating glucagon and growth hormone concentrations do not appear to be responsible. The likely explanation is that peripheral handling of insulin and, thus, of carbohydrate is deranged in the presence of uremia, since dialysis temporarily improves the abnormality. Hypoglycemic attacks may occur in fasting nondiabetic subjects with chronic renal failure. Impaired gluconeogenesis from amino acids may be responsible [17].

Treatment   Attempts to treat chronic renal failure without dialysis have been disappointing. Survival and reversibility are quite unpredictable, although the time of death or of commencing dialysis as a lifesaving measure seemed to occur, in one series of subjects studied, within 51 to 68 days from time of diagnosis [18]. However, these patients were in a stage of advanced renal failure at the time of entering the study.

Early recognition of hypertension may lead to effective hypotensive treatment, and in severe hypertension, this may help to preserve or to improve renal function [19]. Whether treatment of moderate hypertension is beneficial in improving prognosis and, in the current context particularly, in preserving good renal function will not be shown until current trials are completed.

Satisfactory dietary management of chronic renal failure is still far from being achieved. The pioneer approach of Borst applied more to acute failure than chronic failure. The principles are, of course, similar, but there are major practical differences. Long-term management must include an adequate intake of essential amino acids and of essential nutrients, both vitamins and trace elements. Borst utilized replacement of measured and calculated fluid and electrolyte loss and provision of energy in the form of carbohydrate and fat only, with no added nitrogenous sources. An early attempt to provide nitrogenous sources was that of Giordano [20]. Giovanetti and Maggiore subsequently [21] devised diets in which food proteins of high biological value or amino acids were provided together with high levels of fat and carbohydrate.

The problem of feeding patients with chronic renal disease is that many have intermittent or continuous anorexia and nausea and they are often depressed, sometimes to the point of suicide. The depression is both endogenous and exogenous and may be due to the monotonous, unappetizing low-protein diet, sexual impotence in males, premature cessation of menstruation in women, or the recurrent stresses of hemodialysis. Medications for recurrent infections or other illnesses may add to anorexia and depression.

Nutritional support is considered here in two parts: first, for the nondialysed patient and, second, for the patient who receives regular hemodialysis.

Management of the Nondialyzed Patient Feeding the nondialyzed patient requires experience and careful adjustment to individual needs in order to steer an optimal course between undernutrition, particularly of protein, and toxic uremia. A useful principle is to use the patient's condition and symptomatology as a guide rather than the blood urea concentration. Many patients live in a state of chronic malnutrition because this has not been appreciated.

The approach we have adopted at Stanford consists of a series of guidelines which can be partly tabulated (Table 12-1). The dietary regimen outlined is designed to maintain patients with chronic renal failure as long as possible without dialysis. The current practice is to introduce dietary control at the time of diagnosis of chronic renal failure or shortly thereafter. Few patients accept the monotonous, restricted diet. Many attempts have been made to relieve the monotony. One novel way has been to permit a lower daily intake of protein (15 to 20 g) but in any form and supplement the protein with essential amino acids [23]. Good compliance was achieved. Histidine must be added, since it is not adequately synthesized in uremic subjects [24].

Many patients prefer a high fat intake at the expense of carbohydrate, but this may contribute to the development of degenerative vascular disease, which is associated with chronic renal failure.

Management of the Dialyzed Patient An increase in the capability for dialysis over the past decade has resulted in the current emphasis on curtailing dietary management alone and applying modified dietary control to patients, together with regular dialysis. The advantages are that dietary protein need not be rigorously restricted, fluid intake can be more flexible, and an overall diet can be devised in keeping with the current concepts of a prudent diet, in which intake of saturated fats and intake of total fat are reduced in order to reduce the incidence of stroke and ischemic heart disease [25]. The three modifications employed in the study of Gokal et al. were (1) a change of the polyunsaturated-saturated ratio to 1.0 from 0.25, (2) an increase of total carbohydrate calories, and (3) a reduction of oral cholesterol intake.

The problems of recurrent hemodialysis are the time involved, the added risks of infection to a patient already at risk, and the removal by the dialytic procedure of unknown amounts of trace elements and other essential nutrients. In terms of quality of life it is hard to argue against the apparent advantages of

TABLE 12-1
MANAGEMENT OF NONDIALYZED PATIENT

Problem	Process	Outcome
1 Potential imbalance of caloric intake	**a** Obtain height and weight.	Maintenance of or trend toward desired weight.
	b Calculate ideal weight from age, sex, and height.	
	c Calculate caloric requirement from Harris-Benedict equation:	
	Male:	
	66 + [13.7 × weight (kg)]	
	+ [5 × height (cm)] − [6.8 × age (years)]	
	× activity factor × stress factor	
	Female	
	655 + [9.6 × weight (kg)]	
	+ [1.7 × height (cm)] − [4.7 × age (years)]	
	× activity factor × stress factor	
	Activity factors:	
	Bed rest	1.2
	Ambulatory, light	1.3
	Ambulatory, moderate	1.4
	Stress factors:	
	Skeletal trauma	1.3
	Sepsis	1.8
	Ventilation	1.8
	Minor surgery	1.2
	Cancer	1.2
	Growth	1.4
	Pregnancy	1.1
	Lactation	1.4
	d Adjust energy input if need to change patient's weight, by adding or subtracting calories.	

371

TABLE 12-1 (Continued)

Problem	Process	Outcome
	e Use sunflower and other vegetable oils and low-protein wheat or rice, starch, Hycal (flavored glucose solution), or similar preparation.	
	Note: A ratio of % fat calories–% carbohydrate calories between approximately 0.5 and 1.0 appears not to affect nitrogen balance [22]. However the number of patients studied was small. In general the fat-carbohydrate mixture should be palatable, non-flatulent, high in complex carbohydrate, and low in fat to reduce hyperlipidemia to a minimum, and it should not delay gastric emptying.	
2 Protein depletion or nitrogen retention	**a** Restrict daily protein intake below 0.7 g per kilogram of body weight in patient without uremic symptoms.	**a** Patient asymptomatic. **b** Serum albumin in accepted range($>$ 3.2 g/dl). **c** Delay of onset of dialysis. **d** Delay development of hyperparathyroidism as consequence of transient elevations of serum phosphorus.
	b Restrict daily protein intake below 0.55–0.6 g per kilogram of body weight when uremic symptoms appear (usually GFR = 10–15 ml/min, creatinine clearance = 20 ml/min).	
	c Two thirds of daily protein allowance should be of high biological value (egg white, chicken, lamb). For most men, protein intake should not be less than 40 g/day; for women and small men, not less than 35 g/day.	

d If serum albumin falls below 3.2 g/dl, use amino acid supplements (Amin-Aid or Travesorb), but introduce gradually and diluted to avoid osmotic

3 Potassium imbalance

Recommend level of intake based on 24-h urine output of potassium, serum potassium concentration, and body size. Usually 38–78 mmol/day. Potassium content of food protein precludes restriction below 30 mmol/day.

Maintenance of safe serum potassium concentration.

4 Sodium and water imbalance

a Recommend intake based on 24-h urine output, fecal output if diarrhea, insensible fluid loss, presence of dependent edema, stability of blood pressure, absence of pulmonary edema.

b Sodium intake usually ranges from 43 to 130 mmol/day.

c Water intake ranges from 2.0 to 2.5 liters daily in adult.

d Patients should be advised to increase water intake if fever or diarrhea present.

Control of blood pressure.

5 Hyperphosphatemia

If serum phosphorus concentration is rising although calculated intake is less than 1200 mg/day, do not further restrict diet but use liquid phosphate-binding agent such as Amphojel (320–960 mg aluminum hydroxide) three times or more daily. This also serves as an antacid.

Serum phosphorus concentration remains within accepted range for renal disease.

TABLE 12-1 (Continued)

Problem	Process	Outcome
6 Vitamin and mineral deficiencies	Analyze intake in diet using food composition tables. Ensure total daily intake by supplementation if necessary in following amounts (adult consuming 2500 kcal daily):	Avoidance of nutrient deficiency.
	Thiamine 1.5 mg	
	Riboflavin 1.8 mg	
	Pantothenic acid 5.0 mg	
	Niacin 20.0 mg	
	Cobalamin 3.0 μg	
	Pyridoxine 5.0 mg	
	Ascorbic acid 50.0 mg	
	Folacin 1.0 mg	
	Tocopherols 15.0 IU	
	Vitamin D 10,000–100,000 IU*	
	Calcium 1000–2000 mg	
7 Poor dietary intake due to anorexia	Review diet with care and discuss with patient. Evaluate need for oral supplementation or tube feeding.	Improvement of intake.
8 Faulty intake due to noncompliance	Review diet with patient. Reinforce prescribed diet; attempt appropriate modifications to make diet more acceptable.	Improved compliance.

*Higher doses if osteomalacia is present.

renal transplantation, the only disadvantages of which are the need for continuing immunosuppression and the acceptable but nonetheless increased risk of developing malignant lymphoid tumors. Rehabilitation rates are significantly higher in patients who have had transplants. The dietary management of patients treated by regular hemodialysis, two or three times weekly, is addressed in a way similar to that used for patients with chronic renal failure treated with diet alone.

Caloric needs are assessed according to the Harris-Benedict equations (Table 12-1; Appendix 2). Adjustments to achieve reduction in obesity can be made with greater confidence because optimal depression of nitrogen turnover is not as critical as it is in the nondialyzed patient. Complex carbohydrate is preferred to simple sugars and to fat. Protein is given in daily amounts on the order of 1 to 1.2 g per kilogram of body weight. Two-thirds of the total protein is of high biological value. When dietary intake is insufficient to maintain satisfactory serum albumin concentrations, supplements of essential amino acids alone or mixtures of essential and nonessential amino acids are given orally, diluted and gradually increased in quantity to minimize diarrhea. If the patient is receiving peritoneal dialysis, protein losses are much greater and protein intake may need to be doubled. Hemodialysis removes about 15 to 20 g amino acids in 4 to 6 hours, which is as much as the supplements given daily. This should be borne in mind.

Recommended daily intake of potassium ranges from 38 to 78 meq daily. If predialysis serum potassium concentrations exceed 6.0 meq per liter when dialysis is performed three times weekly, dietary compliance should be scrutinized.

Sodium and water intake are controlled so that gain in weight between dialyses is not more than 2 kg. However, if there are significant predialytic elevations of blood pressure, reduced intake of sodium is advisable. The concentration of serum inorganic phosphorus should likewise present no problem, but in noncompliant patients an oral aluminum gel may need to be used to reduce phosphorus absorption.

Because of the possible removal of some essential nutrients during the dialytic procedure, larger daily amounts are recommended. These include 10 mg pyridoxine and 100 mg ascorbic acid.

Recently zinc depletion, associated with reduction in or loss of sensation of taste (ageusia), has attracted concern [26], and daily oral zinc supplements (220 mg zinc sulfate) together with oral iron (300 mg tid of ferrous sulfate) should be given. This should ensure that iron deficiency plays no part in the anemia almost invariably present. Some advocate giving parenteral iron. There is, however, a risk of toxic overload by this route, and, in addition, untoward reactions may occur after multiple infusions.

A major advantage of hemodialysis is that calcium may be used in the dialysis fluid at an optimal concentration of 3.5 meq per liter to suppress parathyroid stimulation and to maintain normal skeletal mineralization [27].

In recent years much interest has been directed to techniques for encouraging reutilization of urea nitrogen in amino acid and protein synthesis. All amino acids except threonine and lysine can be synthesized in vivo from their corresponding α-keto acid analogues [28]. The use of infusions of α-keto acid analogues has been encouraging. It appears that amino groups from amino acids derived from endogenous protein breakdown may be incorporated into new amino acids when the appropriate α-keto acids are available [29], instead of nitrogen being recirculated via urea, which is an inefficient mechanism.

There would seem to be potential for significant advances in the dietary management of chronic renal failure toward an ultimate goal of the nitrogen-free diet. However two problems would still remain to be solved: the possible unpalatability of a protein-free diet and the true cause of the toxic nature of uremia.

In children with chronic renal failure the same principles in management apply, but maintenance of satisfactory growth poses a special problem and control of water and electrolyte homeostasis is more difficult, since the small child constitutes a smaller pool size and damage to the kidney seems to cause disturbance of distal tubular function and sodium balance more than in the adult. Sodium wasting is therefore common. Systemic acidosis is also likely to occur early in renal failure because of a low level of circulating base (bicarbonate). Dietary compliance, especially at puberty and in the adolescent, is a major problem, requiring perseverance, understanding, and great ingenuity.

Formerly childhood was a contraindication to hemodialysis; today some centers specialize in pediatric renal failure. However, hemodialysis is probably best regarded as a temporizing step toward renal transplantation. Strict protein restriction is clearly contraindicated, and the lowest daily limit is 1 g per kilogram of body weight. Essential amino acid supplements are given. Low growth rates result from low energy intake, and energy intake should be encouraged at levels even higher than those calculated from the Harris-Benedict equation with a growth factor of 1.5 included. Drinks, ice cream, and mousses made of fat and carbohydrate without other nutrients are good sources of energy and are well tolerated by children.

What are not so well tolerated are nonnutritious soft drink beverages of high phosphate content; these drinks must be rigorously excluded.

Acute Glomerulonephritis

There are numerous types of nephritis included under this heading, distinguished by histopathology and clinicopathological outcome.

From the standpoint of nutrition the important points are to provide a good diet during the acute illness and to anticipate a period of acute renal failure and of sodium and potassium retention. There is no immediate or long-term benefit to be gained from severe protein restriction, which characterized the management of acute nephritis 30 years ago or more, unless renal failure with uremic symptoms supervenes. If this occurs, the patient is treated for acute renal failure. Edema is a common association of acute glomerulonephritis, as is hypertension. The latter may cause encephalopathy with seizures or strokes and congestive heart failure with pulmonary edema. Sodium intake should be restricted to less than 40 meq daily from the outset (see Table 9-6). This can be achieved by adding no salt while cooking food or after it is served at the table. If, despite this, significant hypertension occurs, a salt-free regimen (<22 meq daily) must be commenced.

Foods high in potassium, such as apricot and citrus juices and bananas, should be excluded until renal function improves (see Table 9-9).

The prognosis, in terms of full recovery of renal function, is good in infants and children, not as good in young adults, and poor in older adults.

Nephrotic Syndrome

This is a condition in which excessive amounts of plasma proteins leak into the urine because of disease of the kidneys. This proteinuria results in reduced levels of plasma albumin if the rate of loss exceeds the synthetic capability of the liver. Peripheral edema due to reduced plasma oncotic pressure may then ensue. The degree of edema is variable and is affected by age, by intake of sodium and, to some extent, dietary protein, by the protein-synthesizing capacity of the liver, and by the use of diuretics.

Epidemiology Protein-losing nephropathy may occur at any age and in either sex. It is not possible to produce meaningful figures for incidence or prevalence. Many subjects with mild changes are almost certainly not diagnosed, and others are misdiagnosed as having postural albuminuria.

Etiology In some patients the causes are known: diabetes mellitus, disseminated lupus erythematosus, myelomatosis, or poisoning with heavy metals. In other patients the cause is unknown, and the syndrome is classified according to the nature of the lesions involved, as in minimal lesion, membranous, and proliferative glomerulonephritis. Deposition of immunoglobulins and complement in the basement membrane of the glomeruli is a well-recognized phenomenon in the latter two forms of the syndrome.

Pathology The integrity of the renal glomerular basement membrane is at fault, although this is not always clear from light- or even electron-microscopic appearances. Deposition of immunoglobulin in the basement membrane is a feature of some types of glomerulonephritis. Functionally, leakage of protein is the predominant abnormality.

Treatment Even when daily urinary losses of protein are as high as 20 to 25 g, adequate protein intake, careful use of diuretics, and sodium restriction to 40 meq daily (see Table 9-6) will usually control edema, but some protein components of the diet may have to be low in salt. Sodium intake may be further reduced by using low-sodium milk products (Lonolac) or peptide supplements (Vital).

Daily intake of protein or protein equivalents should be approximately 2 g per kilogram of body weight in adults to allow for urinary loss and 50 percent higher in children to allow for growth.

Calorie supplements, such as Hycal, Polycose, or Controlyte, can be used to reduce diversion of amino acids for energy production. However, Controlyte contains fat. Hyperlipidemia is found in many nephrotic patients, in whom an abnormally high prevalence of ischemic heart disease occurs, and although the benefits are unproven, it is probably best to keep fat intake below 30 percent of total calories.

Corticosteroids produce impressive improvement in children with minimal lesion glomerulonephritis, but their value in other types of nephrotic syndrome is uncertain.

Hepatorenal Syndrome

The term *hepatorenal syndrome* describes a progressive form of impairment of renal function that occurs in cirrhosis and severe viral hepatitis [30].

Epidemiology   There is no known association with age or sex. The most common presentation is in the chronic alcoholic, usually a middle-aged male, who has cirrhosis and superadded acute alcoholic hepatitis.

Etiopathogenesis   Marked renal vasoconstriction occurs in the kidneys. Currently, the likeliest cause is thought to be endotoxemia [31,32], in which the damaged liver fails to filter out endotoxins absorbed from the gut wall, but this is still speculative.

Clinical Picture   The disturbance in renal function is prerenal uremia. The urine is hyperosmolar and of remarkably low sodium content (some set an arbitrary ceiling of 10 meq per liter). Expansion of the intravascular volume, however, with infusions of salt-free albumin rarely if ever corrects the renal failure, although it is usual to give any patient who appears to be suffering from hepatorenal syndrome at least one infusion in case plasma volume is reduced. Despite these infusions, the glomerular filtration rate falls, approaching 2 ml per minute [33]. This reduction persists to death, which may occur in days or sometimes after weeks or months. Occasionally, spontaneous recovery occurs.

Treatment   There is no specific dietary or nutritional therapy. However, survival has occasionally followed hemodialysis and the nutritional management used in support of dialysis.

URINARY CALCULI (STONES)

Kidney stones are of different types, classified according to their chemical composition. At least 90 percent contain calcium in the form of phosphate or phosphate and oxalate. The remainder contain calcium oxalate, uric acid, or magnesium ammonium phosphate. In the rare inborn metabolic disease cystinuria, calculi of pure cystine may occur.

Epidemiology   Kidney stones may form or be found in any part of the urinary tract. Since 1900, stones in the pelvis of the kidney have become increasingly common and bladder stones have shown a marked reduction in prevalence.

Overall, hospitalization figures would set the chances of developing symptomatic renal stones during a lifetime within a range of 0.16 to 3.4 percent, with an average of approximately 2 percent. The incidence is significantly higher in hotter climates.

Approximately 40 percent of urinary calculi are bilateral. The recurrence rate is high; in some series, as high as 75 percent. Calculi consist of calcium oxalate, calcium phosphate, a mixture of the two, magnesium ammonium phosphate, cystine, or uric acid. Approximately 80 percent of all renal calculi consist of calcium phosphate, calcium oxalate, or both, 1 to 2 percent consist of cystine, and 5 to 15 percent consist of uric acid. The last are much commoner in males than females, whereas calcium calculi are commoner in females.

Etiology   Formation of the majority of calculi requires that the urine be supersaturated with the material composing the stone. Other factors, however, play a role in a complex interplay: some encourage crystallization; some inhibit it. Hypercalciuria may occur in males and females as a consequence of ingestion of large amounts of calcium in milk, hard water, or calcium antacids; increased intestinal absorption of calcium due to excessive consumption of vitamin D; and hyperparathyroidism. Daily excretion of more than 15 meq (300 mg) calcium by females and 17.5 meq (350 mg) by males is the usual definition of hypercalciuria. Alkaline urine, which is found in renal tubular acidosis and which is sometimes associated with a vegetarian diet, encourages precipitation of calcium.

Oxalate stones form as a result of a rare inborn error of metabolism called *oxalosis*, in which endogenous oxalate production is increased. Oxalate stones also occur in conditions associated with increased absorption of oxalate from the large intestine, such as inflammatory disease or resection of the small bowel, in which steatorrhea is present and calcium in the lumen forms insoluble soaps instead of binding oxalate to prevent its absorption.

Magnesium ammonium phosphate calculi are associated with chronic infections of the urinary tract with urea-splitting organisms such as *Proteus*, which make the urine alkaline and increase ammonium concentration. In the past 50 years these calculi have become much less frequent.

Cystine calculi occur in a rare, genetically determined disease, cystinuria, in which the mode of inheritance is autosomal dominant; the gene frequency is 1:20,000 or thereabouts. Uric acid calculi occur in gout, if the urine is acidic and has a high uric acid content, and sometimes for the same reason in patients being treated with cytotoxic agents for malignant disease.

Pathology   Calculi in the urinary tract may occur as a consequence of some extrarenal metabolic defect, or as a result of chronically inadequate intake of water; or they may be the result of pathology of the tract, such as medullary sponge kidney, or of chronic or recurrent infections, such as pyelitis or pyelonephritis.

Once calculi have formed, they may cause damage to the kidney or urinary tract. They may obstruct the outflow of urine, and renal failure or dilatation of the renal pelvis or ureters may ensue. There is always the risk of superadded infection when the free flow of urine is impeded.

The very marked reduction in magnesium ammonium phosphate calculi, which were the most common at the turn of the century, is probably due to control of infection and earlier surgery. These calculi were sometimes of great size, lying in the grossly dilated renal pelvis and conforming to the structure of the renal calyces, so that they were known as staghorn calculi.

Symptoms and Clinical Features   Renal calculi may be asymptomatic. However, they are associated with recurrent urinary infection; with intermittent or continuous hematuria, either microscopic or macroscopic; with attacks of severe pain (renal colic), particularly when a stone in the renal pelvis passes into the ureter and stretches the smooth muscle of the ureteric wall during its passage down to the bladder; and, finally, with renal failure.

Treatment   Increased ingestion of water has an important therapeutic role. The water should have a low calcium content. Primary calcium calculi are best treated with low calcium intake of no more than 300 to 600 mg daily. Omission of milk from the diet or the use of low-calcium milk, as well as the use of softened water, will achieve this. When calcium calculi are secondary to hypoparathyroidism, sarcoidosis, or overdoses of vitamin D, treatment of the primary condition is indicated.

Cellulose phosphate (5 g tid) may be ingested to inhibit calcium absorption by the small intestine, or sodium and potassium pyrophosphate (500 mg tid) will lower the urinary calcium and inhibit stone formation.

Persistent treatment has been shown clearly to reduce the need for surgical removal of calcium calculi [34]. Many calcium calculi contain oxalate, and if the urinary oxalate concentration is high, small intestinal function should be checked in case the patient has steatorrhea. In any event the oxalate content of the diet should be reduced by avoiding oxalate-containing foods (see Table 15-10), such as spinach, rhubarb, strong teas, stone fruit, chocolate, and nuts, and vitamin C (an oxalate precursor).

Some studies have suggested that the treatment of oxalosis by continued administration of oral magnesium salts, which serve to solubilize calcium oxalate in the renal pelvis, significantly slows the rate of renal stone formation [35].

Cystine calculi are treated by encouraging the patient to consume at least 3 liters of water per day and by alkalinizing the urine with a high-vegetable diet and sodium citrate to raise the urinary pH above 7.5.

Penicillamine and low-methionine diets have also been used [36]. Magnesium ammonium phosphate calculi are usually treated surgically. Efforts to delay or to prevent recurrence include increasing water intake, acidifying the urine with high-protein diets and ascorbic acid (500 qid), and initiating appropriate antibiotic therapy. Irreversible damage to the kidney or ureter tends to encourage reinfection, and recurrence is common.

Uric acid stones are treated by similar encouragement to increase daily water intake, by urinary alkalinization, and with the drug allopurinol, a hypoxanthine oxidase inhibitor that depresses uric acid production in the gouty subject. Although low-purine diets are still recommended (excluding sweetbreads, oysters, and other high-purine foods), they probably have little value now that allopurinol is available.

REFERENCES

1 Arroyave, G., D. Wilson, M. Behar, and N. S. Scrimshaw: Serum and urinary creatinine in children with severe protein malnutrition, Am. J. Clin. Nutr., 9:176, 1961.

2 Mollison, P. L.: Observations on cases of starvation, Br. Med. J., 1:4, 1946.

3 McCance, R. A.: Aspects of renal function and water metabolism in studies of undernutrition, Wuppertal 1946–49, Medical Research Council Special Report Series 272–276, 1950–1951, pp. 1–192.

4 Klahr, S., and G. A. O. Alleyne: Effects of chronic protein-calorie malnutrition on the kidney, Kidney Int., 3:129, 1973.

5 Stewart, J. H., and P. A. Castaldi: Uraemic bleeding. A reversible platelet defect corrected by dialysis, Q. J. Med., 36:409, 1967.

6 Kleinknecht, D., P. Jungers, J. Chanard, C. Barbanel, and D. Gavenal: Uremic and non-uremic complications in acute renal failure. Evaluation of early and frequent dialysis on prognosis, Kidney Int., 1:190, 1972.

7 Varcoe, R., D. Halliday, E. R. Carson, P. Richards, and A. S. Tavill: Efficiency of utilization of urea nitrogen for albumin synthesis by chronically uraemic and normal man, Clin. Sci. Mol. Med., 48:3, 1975.

8 Herkin, R. I., N. D. Levine, H. H. Sussman, and M. M. Maxwell: Evidence for the presence of substances toxic for HeLa cells in the serum and in the dialysis fluid of patients with glomerulonephritis, J. Lab. Clin. Med., 64:79, 1964.

9 Blumberg, A., and H. A. Marti: Adaptation to anorexia by decreased oxygen affinity of haemoglobin in patients on dialysis, Kidney Int., 1:263, 1972.

10 Ledingham, J. G. G.: Chronic renal failure, in *Renal Disease*, 4th ed., D. Black and N. F. Jones (eds.), Blackwell, Oxford, 1979.

11 Slatopolsky, E., and N. S. Bricker: The role of phosphorus restriction in the prevention of secondary hyperparathyroidism in chronic renal disease, Kidney Int., 4:141, 1973.

12 Fraser, D. R., and E. Kodicek: Unique biosynthesis by the kidney of a biologically active vitamin D metabolite, Nature, 228:764, 1970.

13 Lindner, A., B. Charra, D. J. Sherrard, and B. H. Scribner: Accelerated atherosclerosis in prolonged maintenance hemodialysis, N. Engl. J. Med., 290:697, 1974.

14 Ibels, L. S., L. A. Simons, J. O. King, P. F. Williams, F. C. Neale, and J. H. Stewart: Studies of the nature and causes of hyperlipidaemia in uraemia, maintenance dialysis and renal transplantation, Q. J. Med., 44:601, 1975.

15 Navalesi, R., A. Pilo, S. Lenzi, and L. Donato: Insulin metabolism in chronic uremia and in the anephric: effect of dialytic treatment, J. Clin. Endocrinol. Metab., 40:70, 1975.

16 De Fronzo, R. A., R. Andres, P. Edgar, and W. G. Walker: Carbohydrate metabolism in uremia: a review, Medicine, 52:469, 1973.

17 Garber, A. J., D. M. Bier, P. E. Cryer, and A. S. Pagliera: Hypoglycemia in compensated chronic renal insufficiency. Substrate limitation of gluconeogenesis, Diabetes, 23:982, 1974.

18 Maher, J. F., K. D. Nolph, and G. W. Bryan: Prognosis of advanced chronic renal failure. 1. Unpredictability of survival and reversibility, Ann. Intern. Med., 81:43, 1974.

19 Pohl, J. E. F., H. Thurston, and J. D. Sivales: Hypertension with renal impairment: influence of intensive therapy, Q. J. Med., 43:569, 1974.

20 Giordano, C.: Use of exogenous and endogenous urea for protein synthesis in normal and uremic subjects, J. Lab. Clin. Med., 62:231, 1963.

21 Giovanetti, S., and Q. Maggiore: A low nitrogen diet with proteins of high biological value for severe chronic uraemia, Lancet, 1:1000, 1964.

22 Fowell, E., J. W. T. Dickerson, J. M. Duckham, and H. A. Lee: The influence of energy source and intake on nitrogen metabolism in chronic renal failure: relevance to hyperlipoproteinaemia, J. Hum. Nutr., 32:87, 1978.

23 Noree, L. O., and J. Bergstrom: Treatment of chronic uremic patients with protein-poor diets and oral supplements of essential amino acids. II. Clinical results of long-term treatment, Clin. Nephrol., 3:195, 1975.

24 Furst, P.: ^{15}N-Studies in severe renal failure. II. Evidence for the essentiality of histidine, Scand. J. Clin. Lab. Med., 30:307, 1972.

25 Gokal, R., J. I. Mann, D. O. Oliver, and J. G. G. Ledingham: Dietary treatment of hyperlipidemia in chronic hemodialysis patients, Am. J. Clin. Nutr., 31:1915, 1978.

26 Goddard, B. W., J. O'Nion, R. L. Stephen, and W. J. Kolff: Hypogeusia and zinc depletion in chronic dialysis patients, Am. J. Clin. Nutr., 31:1948, 1978.

27 Johnson, W. J.: Optimum dialysate calcium concentration during maintenance hemodialysis, Nephron, 17: 241, 1976.

28 Walser, M., A. W. Coulton, A. Dighe, and F. R. Crantz: The effect of keto-analogues of essential amino acids in severe chronic uremia, J. Clin. Invest., 52:678, 1973.

29 Kopple, J. D., and M. E. Swendseid: Amino acid and keto acid diets for therapy in renal failure, Nephron, 18:1, 1977.

30 Bartoli, E., and L. Chiandushi: *Hepato-Renal Syndrome*, Piccin Medical Books, Padua, Italy, 1979.

31 Liehr, H., M. Grun, D. Brunswig, and T. H. Sautter: Endotoxinaemie bei Leberzirrhose, Gastroenterology, 14:14, 1976.

32 Clemente, C., J. Bosch, J. Rodes, U. Arroyo, A. Mas, and S. Maragall: Functional renal failure and haemorrhagic gastritis associated with endotoxaemia in cirrhosis, Gut, 18:556, 1977.

33 Wilkinson, S. P., D. Hirst, D. W. Day, and R. Williams: The spectrum of renal tubular damage in renal failure secondary to cirrhosis and fulminant hepatic faiure, J. Clin. Pathol., 31:101, 1978.

34 Pak, C. Y. C., C. S. Delea, and F. C. Bartter: Successful treatment of recurrent

nephrolithiasis (calcium stones) with cellulose phosphate, N. Engl. J. Med., 290:175, 1974.

35 Dent, C. E., and T. C. B. Stamp: Treatment of primary hyperoxaluria, Arch. Dis. Child., 45:735, 1970.

36 Lee, H. A.: The nutritional management of renal diseases, in *Nutrition in the Clinical Management of Disease,* J. W. T. Dickerson and H. A. Lee (eds.), Arnold, London, 1978.

CHAPTER 13

NUTRITIONAL ASPECTS
OF OSTEOPOROSIS

CONTENTS

INTRODUCTION

The term *osteoporosis* refers to a group of diseases of many causes, characterized anatomically by a reduction in bone mass. The chemical composition of the bone, or the ratio of mineral to organic matrix, remains normal; this characteristic distinguishes osteoporosis from osteomalacia, a bone disorder in which this ratio is decreased. Osteoporosis is said to be present when bone mass is reduced to such an extent that the skeleton becomes vulnerable to fractures arising from mild trauma or from the physical stress of daily activities. Typically, the fracture affects the neck of the femur, the vertebrae, or the distal radius and ulna. "Dowager's hump," which is caused by compression and wedging of the vertebrae, typifies the disease in elderly women.

Osteoporosis is probably the most common and yet most poorly understood bone disorder which confronts the average clinician. It can occur at any age, but it is most common in older persons, especially postmenopausal women. It has been estimated that one in three postmenopausal women has osteoporosis; one in five suffers a hip or vertebral crush fracture. The occurrence of osteoporosis is lower in black women than in white women, and the incidence of senile osteoporosis (including postmenopausal osteoporosis) appears to be four times greater in women than in men.

Demographic data indicate that the over-50 age group is the fastest-growing minority in the world, particularly in the United States. The estimated increases in the population that is 64 and over can be expected to lead to a greater incidence of fractures. In short, bone health is fast becoming a major health problem which deserves, if not demands, the early establishment of preventive measures. Unfortunately, health care programs designed to detect early osteoporosis and to prevent its progression are hindered by apathetic public health efforts and controversy over the efficacy of preventive measures. As a result, the diagnosis is usually made only after the patient has lost a significant portion of total body calcium and many years after skeletal calcium loss first began.

Osteoporosis has been divided into primary (idiopathic) and secondary forms. The etiology of primary osteoporosis is multifaceted and is still unclearly defined, although inactivity and prolonged periods of immobilization, estrogen deficiency, and diet are among the possible etiological factors. In contrast, the causes of secondary osteoporosis are known, and the bone disorder is usually named after the etiological agent (Table 13-1). This chapter focuses on primary osteoporosis, which occurs in middle-aged and older women and men.

EPIDEMIOLOGY

On the basis of the age of onset, primary osteoporosis is labeled juvenile, adult, postmenopausal, or senile. *Juvenile osteoporosis* is very uncommon. *Adult osteoporosis*, which affects the 20 to 40 age group, is also rare. Between the ages

TABLE 13-1
CLASSIFICATION OF OSTEOPOROSIS ACCORDING TO CAUSE

Primary (idiopathic) disease (suspected causes)	Secondary disease
Estrogen deficiency	Hypogonadism
Inactivity	Hypercortisolism
High phosphate intake	Hyperthyroidism
Decreased calcium intake	Heparin therapy
Vitamin D deficiency	Malabsorption
Impaired calcium absorption	Immobilization
Decreased dietary Ca:P ratio	Hyperparathyroidism
	Homocystinuria
	Osteogenesis imperfecta

of 40 and 60, osteoporosis becomes a more common disease, especially in women. Since menopause also occurs around this time, this osteoporosis has been called *postmenopausal osteoporosis*. The over-60 age group provides most of the osteoporotic patients seen, and this type of osteoporosis is often referred to as *senile osteoporosis*. Up to the age of 80, women are affected four times more often than men; after the age of 80 the sex incidence is the same. Caucasians and northern Europeans are particularly susceptible.

Bone loss has been found to occur with aging in all contemporary human societies examined [1], and there is archeological evidence for its occurrence over the past 2000 years [2]. Moreover, it occurs in experimental animals at an analogous physiological age, even when they are fed a diet that is apparently optimal in nutrient content [3]. These observations have prompted some investigators to regard bone loss as an inevitable accompaniment of aging which has no adverse implications except for certain individuals who are susceptible by reason of race, sex, heredity, or small mature skeletal size. Although bone loss evidently occurs with aging in all populations, regardless of socioeconomic status, food culture and life style, there are, nevertheless, unexplained differences in the rate of bone loss among individuals within as well as between populations. Additionally, there are systematic differences attributable to heredity, race, and sex, and in a minority of both sexes, aging is not associated with significant bone loss [4].

PATHOGENESIS

Our present state of knowledge does not certify a single variable as the specific cause of osteoporosis. Osteoporosis seems to have a multifactorial genesis, but in individual patients a single etiological factor may dominate. Morphometric analyses of biopsied specimens reveal that bone resorption is increased, whereas bone formation is in general (but not invariably) reduced [5]. There are data to suggest that the following factors may all play important roles in the genesis of osteoporosis.

Genetics

There is a distinct racial difference in vulnerability to osteoporosis between blacks and whites, the order of increasing susceptibility being black males, black females, white males, and white females. This difference is attributable in part to a greater mature bone mass in blacks [6] and possibly to a slower rate of bone loss. The reduced rate of bone loss, which appears to be due to decreased resorption, has been related to a reportedly higher concentration of serum calcium and a lower concentration of parathyroid hormone (PTH) in black postmenopausal women [7].

In addition to differences in susceptibility to osteoporosis between black and white races, which appear to be genetic in origin, there are clear familial differences among individuals of the same sex in both races. Bone mass at the time of early adulthood is a major risk factor in the development of osteoporotic bone disease in later life, especially in women. The most likely prospective osteoporotic patient is a white postmenopausal female of small bone structure.

Physical Activity

It has long been known that bone loss will occur in both sexes at any age if physical activity is markedly reduced. Astronauts [8] and almost completely immobilized, bedridden humans [9] have shown negative calcium balance and rapid bone loss. The mechanism is not understood, but the decline in physical activity associated with senescence and the sedentary lifestyle of affluent societies may be a factor in osteoporosis. This bone atrophy is prevented only by weight-bearing ambulation [10].

While reduced physical activity may be a contributing factor in the etiology of osteoporosis, it is unlikely that it is a primary cause of the condition. In a cross-sectional study of women aged 50 to 96, Smith et al. [11] demonstrated that the rate of bone mineral loss was significantly greater in the postmenopausal years and then decreased with age. Since physical activity declined with advancing age, this decrease in activity may have been less important than other factors in determining rates of bone loss in postmenopausal osteoporosis.

There is little direct experimental evidence on the effectiveness of exercise in preventing bone loss in human subjects. Cross-sectional comparisons indicate that bone density is greater in persons with occupations requiring physical exertion than in those involved in sedentary work. Furthermore, athletes have greater bone density than nonathletes [12].

Age

It has been well documented that bone density increases from childhood throughout adolescence to maturity, remains approximately constant through the second and third decades, and falls thereafter at varying rates. The rate of bone loss does not increase with age and appears to be linear at a rate of 8 percent per decade in women and 3 percent per decade in men. Age-related bone loss proceeds at different rates in different parts of the body. There is a greater proportional loss of trabecular bone (20 percent of the skeleton by weight), which forms the axial skeleton, than of cortical bone (80 percent of the skeleton by weight), which is found in the peripheral skeleton. These observations, indicating that bone loss is an aging phenomenon, are based on cross-sectional studies of individuals of different ages. However, carefully controlled longitudinal studies, over an 11-year period, of persons initially 55 to 64 years old have demonstrated that a significant number did not lose bone mass [13].

It seems probable that osteoporosis will become clinically manifest in individuals who have a relatively small bone mass at maturity and in whom the same percentage of bone loss occurs as they become older as in nonosteoporotic individuals. However, fractures occur in osteoporotic individuals because they reach a state of greatly reduced bone mass earlier in life. The cause of age-related calcium loss is unknown. Diminished physical activity, reduced dietary calcium intake, impaired intestinal calcium absorption, increased renal calcium loss, and reduced endogenous secretion of anticatabolic hormones such as estrogens may all play a role.

Estrogen Deficiency

The work of the last 40 years has confirmed the original observation of Albright and coworkers that an association exists between osteoporosis and the postmenopausal state [14]. Women lose bone faster than men after the age of 35 [15], and this decline in bone mass is more strongly related to time after menopause than to age [16]. Heaney et al. [17,18] recently used observations of calcium kinetics to show that bone remodeling increases after menopause and bone resorption increases to a greater extent than bone formation. Estrogen treatment was found to reduce skeletal calcium resorption and to improve calcium balance. The principal estrogen formed in both physiological and postcastration menopause is estrone [19], which is derived from circulating androstenedione made by the adrenal cortex. Plasma androstenedione is reported to be significantly lower in osteoporotic women than in age-matched controls, below the age of 65 [20].

Increased Parathyroid Hormone (PTH) Secretion

The role of PTH in osteoporosis is controversial. Since bone loss occurs progressively in osteoporosis and since osteoclastic bone must form in order for bone resorption to occur, some investigators suggest that the hormone that governs osteoclastic activity must be associated with the pathogenesis of the disorder. Wiske and coworkers [21] demonstrated that PTH increased with advancing age after the age of 40 and that this increase was associated with a significant decrease in serum ionized calcium and inorganic phosphate. Furthermore, elderly women had higher serum PTH levels than elderly men. Riggs et al. [22] showed that 10 to 15 percent of patients with primary osteoporosis have increased levels of PTH despite normocalcemia. Proponents of the theory that PTH action causes primary osteoporosis disagree as to the exciting stimulus. Berlyne and his associates [23] claim that elderly patients tend to acquire secondary hyperparathyroidism and "age-related bone atrophy" as a consequence of waning renal function, and some of them then develop osteoporosis. In contrast, Nordin and associates [24] have provided controversial evidence that patients doomed to acquire primary osteoporosis fail to conserve calcium adequately by means of renal tubular reabsorption. Hence, a tendency to become hypocalcemic follows, which is corrected for by the development of a subtle degree of secondary hyperparathyroidism, leading to the development of osteoporosis. These theories, however, do not address the contradiction that hypoparathyroidism does not protect against the development of bone loss [25,26].

Dietary Calcium Deficiency and Malabsorption

While there is definite evidence that calcium deficiency causes osteoporosis in a variety of experimental animals [27,28], dietary evidence is less convincing in humans, possibly because of the difficulty in obtaining reliable dietary information spanning many years of an individual's life. Cross-sectional studies on bone loss in different countries indicate that there is no simple relationship between the prevalence of bone loss and the calcium content of the national food supplies [1]. However, epidemiological studies and dietary surveys may prove misleading until more specific emphasis is placed on other factors which influence calcium balance, i.e., dietary habits, the degree of mobilization, the daily intake of minerals other than calcium, the dietary intake of protein and vitamin D, and the degree of exposure to sunlight. For example, a wide variety of food constituents are known to affect the utilization of calcium. Absorption is decreased by phosphates, oxalates (found in green vegetables), and phytates (found in unleavened wheat bread) and by high fat intake. Vitamin D, either from the diet or from exposure to sunlight, increases calcium absorption.

In cross-cultural studies on the relationship between osteoporosis and calcium intake, it is generally assumed that the calcium requirement of different populations is the same; for example, if 400 mg per day is adequate in a cereal-based diet, it is also adequate in the mixed diet of western industrial countries. This assumption fails to take into account the higher protein and phosphorus content of western diets. Animal studies clearly show that the dietary calcium-phosphorus ratio has a major impact on bone mass. The optimal dietary ratio for calcium and phosphorus appears to be 1:1. In animals, if phosphorus intake is supplemented to create a low calcium-phosphorus ratio, bone loss is observed in rats [29], dogs [30], and horses [31]. In humans, phosphorus supplementation may stimulate secondary hyperparathyroidism [32]. However, even on a relatively low calcium intake, if it is greater than the phosphorus intake, bone will not be lost. It appears that the ingested phosphorus transiently reduces the ionized calcium level in the serum, thereby promoting increased PTH secretion and mobilizing calcium from bone to restore the serum calcium concentration.

In humans, adherence to the Recommended Dietary Allowances (RDA) would theoretically achieve a calcium-phosphorus ratio of 1:1 (800 mg calcium, 800 mg phosphorus). However, for many Americans, widespread consumption of soft drinks, meat, snack foods, and processed cheese (all high-phosphorus foods) may substantially reduce this ratio. Another factor that results in increased phosphorus ingestion is the addition to food of additives such as orthophosphates (for acidifying food), diphosphonates, and "polyphosphates." Furthermore, almost all estimates of average daily calcium intake in the United States, especially among females, fall far short of the RDAs (Figure 13-1). The

FIGURE 13-1
Mean calcium intake of persons aged 1 to 74, by age, race, and sex: United States, 1971 to 1974. (Adapted from *U.S. Department of Health, Education, and Welfare Publication no. (PHS) 79-1657, June 1979.*)

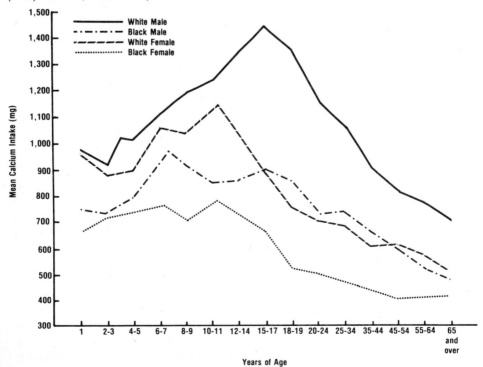

National Health Survey reported in 1977 that postmenopausal women in the United States typically ingest less than 500 mg calcium per day [33].

The calcium requirement for normal adults is a debatable issue, although it is generally set between 600 and 1000 mg per day [34]. Most young and middle-aged adults are capable of maintaining a positive calcium balance with this intake, but higher intakes may be necessary to maintain calcium balance in older individuals [35,36]. Heaney et al. showed that the calcium intake necessary to produce calcium balance in normal perimenopausal women aged 35 to 50 is 1.241 g per day [37]. The age-related need for additional dietary calcium may result from the calcium malabsorption which has been observed in older individuals [38].

The strongest evidence for dietary calcium deficiency is experimental work showing that treatment of osteoporosis with oral calcium supplements decreases bone loss [39,40]. In a prospective study Riggs and associates [41] showed by bone biopsy that a high calcium intake reduced bone-resorbing activity; they attributed the favorable response to suppression of endogenous PTH secretion.

The evidence for a prophylactic effect of calcium on bone loss is stronger than the evidence for its therapeutic value. Recker et al. [40] concluded from radiographic and photon absorptiometric measurements that supplementing the diet of postmenopausal women with 1 g calcium per day for a 2-year period significantly inhibited bone loss. Supplementing the diet of elderly women having a history of low calcium intake with 750 mg calcium and 375 IU of vitamin D prevented bone loss during the subsequent 3 years [36]. Avioli [5] has recommended that females from the fifth decade onward consume 1 to 1.5 g calcium per day at the calcium-phosphorus ratio of 1:1 or higher.

Dietary Phosphorus Excess

The possibility that excess dietary phosphorus may have an adverse effect on human calcium metabolism, as it is known to have in domestic animals, is an idea that only recently has been considered. Excess dietary phosphate has been shown to induce osteoporosis in several laboratory animal species [29,42]. Krook's [43] proposal that excess dietary phosphate induces secondary parathyroidism has been substantiated by experimental observation in several laboratories [30,32,44]. Under conditions of mild hyperphosphatemia, calcium in the serum forms an isoluble complex with phosphate [45]. The resulting depression in serum calcium stimulates PTH secretion and the resorption of bone [46].

The enhancement of bone loss produced by phosphate is frequently attributed to an adverse ratio of calcium to phosphorus in the diet. In studies in rabbits, the absolute amount of dietary phosphorus varied by a factor of 10, but only when the ratio of calcium to phosphorus was low did holes appear in bone (Table 13-2). Draper and Bell [46], however, caution that characterizing the nutritional relationship of calcium and phosphorus by their ratio in the diet may be simplistic. When the dietary concentrations of these elements are increased at a fixed ratio (even at the most favorable ratio of 2:1), a point is reached beyond

TABLE 13-2
BONE CHANGES IN RELATION TO DIETARY CALCIUM-PHOSPHORUS RATIO IN ADULT
RABBITS

Diet	Calcium, mg/kg/day	Phos-phorus, mg/kg/day	Ca : P ratio	Bone findings
8-week study				
Control	385	221	1.7	Normal
High-phosphate	385	682	0.6	Increased porosity
6-month study				
Control	30	28	1.1	Normal
High-phosphate	29	67	0.4	Increased porosity

Source: J. Jowsey, Osteoporosis: its nature and the role of diet, Postgrad. Med., 60:27, 1976.

which bone resorption is increased. This is explained by the fact that inorganic phosphate is efficiently absorbed even at very high intakes, whereas the efficiency of calcium absorption at high intakes decreases sharply. Therefore, as the intake of both elements is increased proportionately, the ratio of absorbed calcium to absorbed phosphorus shifts in favor of the latter. This indicates that the absolute intake of phosphorus, as well as the calcium-phosphorus ratio must be considered in relation to the influence of phosphate on bone loss.

In the diet of most Americans, phosphorus intake is much higher than calcium intake because phosphorus is naturally more abundant than calcium in most of our major food sources (Table 13-3). In general, meats, poultry, and fish furnish 15 to 20 times as much phosphorus as calcium, while organ meats such as liver provide 25 to 50 times as much. Eggs, grains, nuts, dried beans, peas, and lentils provide lesser amounts of phosphorus. Milk, most natural cheeses, and a large number of green leafy vegetables contain more calcium than phosphorus (Table 13-3). Although cow's milk provides only slightly more calcium than phosphorus, some natural cheeses contain almost twice as much. In light of these natural variations, it is easy to understand why a calcium-phosphorus ratio as high as 1:1 is rarely achieved, especially in diets which are as high in meat as the usual American diet. Very few foods contain calcium and no phosphorus (sesame seeds, seaweed, and molasses).

In adults, the dietary intake of phosphorus is likely to be several times that of calcium. For instance, an individual who does not drink milk ingests 300 to 500 mg of calcium and 700 to 1500 mg phosphorus daily, whereas a milk drinker ingests 900 mg of calcium and 2000 mg of phosphorus [42]. Furthermore, various phosphate additives (orthophosphate, pyrophosphate, and polyphosphates) are being used increasingly in many areas of food processing, especially in processed meats and cheeses, soft drinks, and modified food starches. The magnitude of their contribution to dietary phosphorus is not well documented, but Bell et al. [47] showed that maximum substitution of phosphate-containing food items for

TABLE 13-3
CALCIUM AND PHOSPHORUS CONTENT OF SELECTED FOOD ITEMS AND THEIR
CALCIUM-PHOSPHORUS RATIO

Food	Serving size	Calcium, mg	Phosphorus, mg	Ca : P ratio
Yogurt, fruit-flavored, low-fat + milk solids	8 oz	345	271	1 : 0.8
Milk, skim	1 cup	302	247	1 : 0.8
Milk, whole	1 cup	291	228	1 : 0.8
Cheddar cheese	1 oz	204	145	1 : 0.7
American cheese, pasteurized, processed	1 oz	174	211	1 : 1.2
Collard greens, cooked	½ cup	110	50	1 : 0.5
Spinach, cooked	½ cup	100	34	1 : 0.3
Ice cream, 10% fat	½ cup	88	67	1 : 0.8
Orange	1 medium	54	33	1 : 0.6
Egg	1 large	28	90	1 : 3.2
Bread, white, enriched	1 slice	21	28	1 : 1.3
Liver, calf, cooked	3 oz	11	405	1 : 37
Hamburger, 21% fat, cooked	3 oz	9	159	1 : 18
Peanut butter	1 tbsp	9	61	1 : 6.7
Gator-Ade	10 oz	0.6	21	1 : 35
Bologna	3 oz	32	581	1 : 18
Coca-Cola	10 oz	9	48	1 : 5.3

Source: C. F. Adams, Nutritive Value of American Foods in Common Units, U.S. Department of Agriculture Handbook 456, U.S. Government Printing Office, Washington, 1975.

similar items free of phosphate additives (processed meat for fresh meat, refrigerator rolls for yeast bread, processed cheese for natural cheese, etc.) resulted in an increase in phosphorus intake of 1.1 g per day. These changes were associated with a rise in serum phosphate, a decrease in serum calcium (Figure 13-2), and indications of parathyroid stimulation.

Although the effects of a high-phosphorus diet on serum calcium and PTH secretion are similar to those produced by a low-calcium diet, there is an important distinction in the metabolic response. In calcium deficiency, activation of vitamin D–dependent adaptation mechanisms leads to a stimulation of dietary calcium absorption [48]. In animals consuming a high-phosphorus diet, the phosphaturic action of PTH appears to be inadequate to cause a decrease in phosphate ion concentration in the renal cells sufficient to increase 25-hydroxycholecalciferol-l-hydroxylase activity [46]. Such animals may be unable to restore normocalcemia by increasing calcium absorption.

Whether the high phosphorus content of the modern processed diet has some influence on bone mineral loss is not known. Studies on animals and humans suggest, however, that the addition in recent years of substantial amounts of

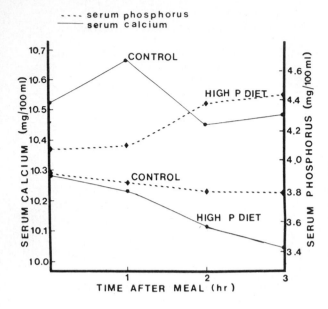

- - - - serum phosphorus
——— serum calcium

FIGURE 13-2
Effect of a meal high in foods containing phosphate additives, on serum calcium and phosphate levels in human adults. [*From H. H. Draper and R. R. Bell, in Advances in Nutritional Research, vol. 2, H. H. Draper (ed.), Plenum, New York, 1977.*]

phosphorus to the diet has increased the intake of calcium required to suppress bone loss. In light of these recent observations it is interesting to note once again that Avioli has suggested that postmenopausal women consume 1 to 1.5 g calcium per day with a calcium-phosphorus ratio of 1:1 or higher [5].

Protein Intake

A few studies have shown that when adult human subjects are introduced to a high-protein diet composed of purified proteins such as lactalbumin, they exhibit calciuria and a negative calcium balance [49,50]. On the basis of these observations, the high protein content of the western diet has been implicated as a factor in osteoporosis. However, Spencer et al. [51] recently showed that in subjects who were fed a diet high in protein (2 g/kg per day) in the form of meat for 70 days, there was no change in fecal calcium excretion, calcium balance, or intestinal calcium absorption.

Since phosphorus intake also was allowed to rise with protein, as it normally does in a high-meat diet, it appears that the hypercalciuric effect of protein was offset by the hypocalciuric effect of phosphorus. Recently, Linkswiler et al. [52] proposed that the hypercalciuria of high-protein feeding is due to an increase in the metabolic production of acid as sulfate arising from the oxidation of excess methionine and cystine. Dietary sulfate is acutely calciuric in animals, and methionine loading results in an increase in acid excretion in the amount of 2 equivalents of hydrogen ion per mole of sulfur oxidized [53]. Additionally, a decrease in the fractional renal tubular reabsorption of calcium and an increase in glomerular filtration rate are seen in adults fed high levels of protein [54]. The clinical significance of these studies and the net effect of the interaction of protein, calcium, and phosphorus intake on bone homeostasis under practical conditions await resolution.

CLINICAL MANIFESTATIONS

In the majority of patients with osteoporosis there are no presenting symptoms—there may only be localized pain when actual fracture or progressive bony collapse occurs. The major clinical manifestations of osteoporosis usually involve the axial skeleton, most commonly the thoracic and lumbar spine, where anterior wedge compression fractures occur. Manifestations may include severe midline, low-back pain that is worsened by bending over or pain of segmental distribution. These are the events that usually bring the patient to a physician. However, such compression fractures may be silent and may only be discovered by x-ray examination for some unrelated problem. When a patient does not have vertebral crush fractures, osteoporosis may be discovered after a fall results in a Colles' fracture of the forearm or in a fracture of the neck of the femur, often called a *hip fracture*. The compression fractures of the vertebral body contribute to the loss in height. These are particularly common in the upper dorsal region, where collapse may be unassociated with pain but may result in a dorsal kyphosis and exaggerated cervical lordosis described as *dowager's* or *widow's hump*.

DIAGNOSIS

According to Skillman [55] the following are three major considerations in making a timely diagnosis of osteoporosis:

1 To select young women who have an increased risk of the disorder
2 To diagnose the disorder prior to the development of fractures
3 To exclude causes of reduced bone density other than osteoporosis

The concentration of calcium and inorganic phosphorus in the blood is usually normal in patients with osteoporosis; slight hyperphosphatemia may be present in women who are past the menopause. Serum alkaline phosphatase is usually normal, although slight increases may be seen after fractures. Urinary calcium is usually normal in elderly patients. However, in some cases with functional kidney defects, hypercalciuria is observed [5]. Urinary hydroxyproline, an indirect measure of bone collagen turnover, is also generally normal, but care in the interpretation of values is essential. Excretion normally decreases with age, so that "normal urinary hydroxyproline" may reflect accelerated bone resorption in individuals with reduced skeletal mass.

Recognition of osteoporosis is based on roentgenological evidence of bone rarefaction. Typically, changes involve all bones but are often most prominent in the axial skeleton. Conventional x-ray films of the vertebrae, ribs, and femoral neck are only grossly quantitative. Increased radiolucency in these bony regions is probably not detectable until about 35 percent of the bone mass has been lost.

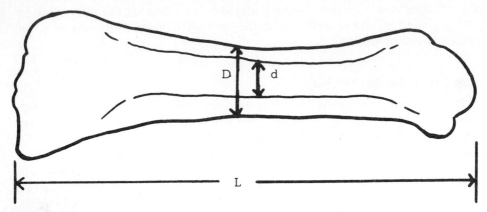

FIGURE 13-3
Metacarpal index, (D-d)/D. (*From E. Barnett and B. E. C. Nordin, Clin. Radiol., 11:166, 1961.*)

If osteoporosis is to be diagnosed before there is a risk of fracture, special radiological or densitometric technology must be employed.

Although accelerated calcium turnover is expressed earliest in trabecular bone, quantification of bone mass may be made fairly early by a study of cortical bone. If one examines a carefully made x-ray film of the hand, the area of cortical bone in the second metacarpal may be expressed as a percentage of the cross-sectional area of the outer dimension of the tubular structure. (The area of the medullary cavity is subtracted.) A ratio (cortical area/total area) then gives a value that decreases from about 0.85 in women aged 50 to near 0.7 in women aged 70 (see Figure 13-3). While this method cannot measure cortical resorption, it is inexpensive and can be easily adapted to clinical practice.

The mineral content of bone can be more accurately measured by using low-energy photons emitted from a radioactive source. Such photon absorption has proved quite reproducible. This method employs the ability of gamma rays from radioiodine 125 to be absorbed by selected bony landmarks of the radius or to be transmitted to a gamma detector. If this technique is applied sequentially every 2 years, it can identify people who will in the future have an increased risk of fracture [55].

MANAGEMENT

Since the cause(s) of postmenopausal or senile osteoporosis is still unknown, the therapy is largely empirical and frequently controversial and unsatisfactory. Reexpansion of collapsed vertebrae cannot be expected on any therapy, but there are several treatments which will delay or prevent further bone loss. Treatments which have been tried include estrogens, fluoride, calcium and vitamin D (alone or in combination), PTH, and calcitonin. Treatment is aimed at reducing bone resorption, and it appears that calcium supplementation, vitamin D therapy, or estrogen therapy (each by itself or in combination) is the most effective treatment [56].

Estrogen

Oral estrogen administration has proved most effective in reducing negative calcium balance and stimulating positive calcium balance. Estrogens are best used to *prevent* osteoporosis in high-risk individuals rather than "cure" patients with the disorder. A commonly used dosage regimen is 25 μg of ethinyl estradiol daily for three weeks out of four [56]. But postmenopausal estrogen treatment increases the incidence of endometrial carcinoma [57]. A recent report suggests an increased risk of breast cancer in postmenopausal women taking 1.25 mg of conjugated estrogens daily for about 3 years [58]. Estrogen therapy produces lithogenic bile and more than doubles the risk of gallbladder disease. Whether estrogens increase the risk of thromboembolic phenomena, stroke, or heart disease in postmenopausal women remains to be determined.

Calcium

The hallmark of osteoporosis is gross deficiency of calcium. Intestinal calcium absorption apparently decreases with age and osteoporotic patients generally absorb less calcium than age-matched controls. Dietary calcium supplements can retard bone loss in some patients with postmenopausal osteoporosis, although less effectively than estrogens [39,40]. Despite some of the uncertainty about its effectiveness, use of oral calcium supplements is gaining wide acceptance [59,60]. Large doses of 1 to 1.5 g of elemental calcium per day are generally recommended.

Vitamin D

Vitamin D supplements may also be recommended, particularly for patients who do not have adequate exposure to sunlight or who have peculiar dietary habits. Vitamin D stimulates the production of calcium-binding protein by intestinal epithelial cells and increases the absorption of calcium that reaches the gut. However, oral vitamin D supplementation should be strictly limited to 10,000 IU per day or less to avoid hypercalcemia, hypercalciuria, and renal stone formation, and it should be avoided altogether in patients with impaired renal function.

Fluoride

Treatment of osteoporosis with combined fluoride, calcium, and vitamin D is still experimental [61] and controversial. Sodium fluoride, in large doses of 40 to 65 mg per day, can increase bone mass, but it has not been established that the new bone is of normal strength or that the incidence of fracture is reduced. If fluoride is used, it is given as capsules of sodium fluoride with meals to avoid gastrointestinal side effects.

Exercise

Weight-bearing movement is important in maintaining mineralization of bone, so that programmed exercise to improve muscle tone is useful.

PREVENTION

The universality of bone loss with aging has fostered an attitude on the part of some that skeletal infirmities are inevitable among that fraction of the population that is predisposed to osteoporosis because of race, sex, genetics, or environmental factors. While some of these factors cannot be changed, others are under individual control, particularly level of physical activity and choice of foods. Lifestyles for the prevention of osteoporosis must be designed to result in a state of positive calcium balance. An approach to achieve this end would include the following:

1 An adequate amount of calcium in the diet. Amounts greater than the present RDA of 800 mg have been suggested as optimum intakes for the prevention of bone disease in humans [36,37].

2 Adequate amounts of nutrients other than calcium, such as protein, vitamin C, and vitamin D, since osteoporosis involves loss of bone matrix as well as bone mineral.

3 Adequate dietary supply of vitamin D and of lactose, which promotes calcium absorption.

4 Distribution of total calcium allowance in several portions, since it is documented that the rate of calcium absorption is inversely related to the amount of calcium ingested at any one time.

5 Adequate physical exercise. Draper and Bell [46] have suggested that osteoporosis may be another manifestation of the limit of human adaptability to a lack of exercise.

The main dietary sources of calcium in most western diets are milk and milk products [62]. In 1976 milk and milk products contributed 75 percent of the total calcium available to the American civilian population [63]. It is a challenge to meet the calcium RDA with the exclusion of dairy products from the diet.

There have been many retrospective studies showing that bone status is better in estrogen-treated women than in untreated controls, but these have been superseded by four prospective studies all showing that postmenopausal bone loss is prevented by estrogens in ordinary replacement doses [39,40,64,65]. Two of these studies [39,40] also showed that large calcium supplements (about 1 g daily of extra calcium) effectively delay postmenopausal bone loss, though this therapy may not be quite as effective as estrogens. Since estrogen replacement therapy, if initiated more than 6 years following cessation of ovarian function, has proved incapable of reversing the progressive fall in bone mass [16] and since long-term therapy with estrogen may be hazardous, it would appear inappropriate to subject women to this form of therapy. On the other hand, on the basis of present evidence it would appear prudent for white females and white males of small bone structure to consume liberal amounts of calcium and to avoid excess dietary phosphorus.

REFERENCES

1 Garn, S. M., C. G. Robmann, B. Wagner, H. G. Dairla, and W. Ascioli: Population similarities in the onset and rate of adult endosteal bone loss, Clin. Orthop. Relat. Res., 65:51, 1969.

2 Dewey, J. R., C. J. Armelagos, and M. H. Bartley: Femoral cortical involution in three Nubian archeological populations, Hum. Biol., 41:13, 1969.

3 Krishnarao, G. V. G., and H. H. Draper: Age-related bone changes in the bones of adult mice, J. Gerontol., 24:149, 1969.

4 Singh, M., B. L. Riggs, J. W. Beaubout, and J. Jowsey: Femoral trabecular-pattern index for evaluation of spinal osteoporosis, Ann. Intern. Med., 77:63, 1972.

5 Avioli, L. V.: Osteoporosis: pathogenesis and therapy, in *Metabolic Bone Disease,* vol. I., L. V. Avioli and S. M. Krane (eds.), Academic, New York, 1977.

6 Trotter, M., G. E. Broman, and R. R. Peterson: Densities of bone of white and Negro skeletons, J. Bone Jt. Surg., 42A:50, 1969.

7 Roof, B. S., C. F. Piel, J. Hansen, and H. H. Fredenberg: Serum parathyroid hormone levels and serum calcium levels from birth to senescence, Mech. Ageing Dev., 5:289, 1976.

8 Mack, P. B., and P. L. LaChance: Effects of recumbence in space flight on bone density, Am. J. Clin. Nutr., 20:1194, 1967.

9 Donaldson, C. L., S. B. Hulley, J. M. Vogel, R. S. Hattner, J. H. Bayers, and D. E. McMillan: Effect of prolonged bed rest on bone mineral, Metab. Clin Exp., 19:1071, 1970.

10 Hulley, S. B., J. M. Vogel, C. L. Donaldson, J. H. Bayers, R. J. Friedman, and S. N. Rosen: The effect of supplemental oral phosphate on the bone mineral changes during prolonged bed rest, J. Clin. Invest., 50:2506, 1971.

11 Smith, B. M., M. R. A. Khairi, J. Norton, and C. C. Johnston, Jr.: Age and activity effects on rate of bone mineral loss, J. Clin. Invest., 58:716, 1976.

12 Nilsson, B. E., and N. E. Westlin: Bone density in athletes, Clin. Orthop., 77:179, 1971.

13 Adams, P., G. T. Davies, and P. Sweetnam: Osteoporosis and the effects of aging on bone mass in elderly men and women, Q. J. Med., 39:601, 1970.

14 Albright, F., P. H. Smith, and A. M. Richardson: Postmenopausal osteoporosis: its clinical features, J. Am. Med. Assoc., 116:2465, 1941.

15 Garn, S. M.: The earlier gain and later loss of cortical bone, in *Nutritional Prospective,* Charles C Thomas, Springfield, Ill., 1970.

16 Aitken, J. M., D. M. Hart, and R. Lindsay: Oestrogen replacement therapy for prevention of osteoporosis after oophorectomy, Br. Med. J., 3:515, 1973.

17 Heaney, R. P., R. R. Recker, and P. D. Saville: Menopausal changes in bone remodeling, J. Lab. Clin. Med., 92:964, 1978.

18 Heaney, R. P., R. R. Recker, and P. D. Saville: Menopausal changes in calcium balance performance, J. Lab. Clin. Med., 92:953, 1978.

19 Radar, M. D., G. L. Flickinger, G. O. DeVilla, Jr., J. J. Mikuta, and G. Mikhail: Plasma estrogens in postmenopausal women, Am. J. Obstet. Gynecol., 116:1069, 1973.

20 Nordin, B. E. C., M. Peacock, J. Aaron, R. G. Crilly, P. J. Hegburn, A. Horsman, and D. Marshall: Osteoporosis and osteomalacia, Clin. Endrocrinol. Metab., 9:177, 1980.

21 Wiske, P. S., S. Epstein, N. H. Bell, S. F. Queener, J. Edmondson, and C. C. Johnston: Increases in immunoreactive parathyroid hormone with age, N. Engl. J. Med., 300:1419, 1979.

22 Riggs, B. L., C. D. Arnaud, J. Jowsey, R. S. Goldsmith, and P. J. Kelly: Parathyroid function in primary osteoporosis, J. Clin. Invest., 52:181, 1973.

23 Berlyne, G. M., J. Ben-Ari, A. Kushelevsky, A. Idelman, D. Galinsky, M. Hirsch, R. Shainken, R. Yagil, and M. Zlontnick: The etiology of senile osteoporosis: secondary hyperparathyroidism due to renal failure, Q. J. Med., 44:505, 1975.

24 Marshall, D. A., A. Horsman, and B. E. C. Nordin: The prevention and management of postmenopausal osteoporosis, Acta Obstet. Gynecol. Scand., 65(suppl):49, 1977.

25 Parfitt, A. M.: the state of bones in uremic hyperparathyroidism—the mechanisms of skeletal resistance to PTH in renal failure and pseudohypoparathyroidism and the role of PTH in osteoporosis, osteopetrosis and osteofluorosis, Metabolism, 25:1157, 1976.

26 Dimich, A., P. B. Bedrossian, and S. Wallach: Hypoparathyroidism—clinical observations in 34 patients, Arch. Intern. Med., 120:449, 1967.

27 Jowsey, J., and J. Gershon-Cohen: Effect of dietary calcium levels on production and reversal of experimental osteoporosis in cats, Proc. Soc. Exp. Biol. Med., 116:437, 1964.

28 Shah, B. G., G. V. G. Krishnarao, and H. H. Draper: The relationship of Ca and P nutrition during adult life and osteoporosis in aged mice, J. Nutr., 92:30, 1967.

29 Draper, H. H., T. L. Sie, and J. G. Bergan: Osteoporosis in aging rats induced by high phosphorus diets, J. Nutr., 102:1133, 1972.

30 LaFlamme, G. H., and J. Jowsey: Bone and soft tissue changes with oral phosphate supplements, J. Clin. Invest., 51:2834, 1972.

31 Argenzio, R. A., J. E. Lowe, H. F. Hintz, and H. F. Schryver: Calcium and phosphorus homeostasis in horses, J. Nutr., 104:18, 1974.

32 Reiss, E., J. M. Canterbury, M. A. Bercovitz, and E. L. Kaplan: The role of phosphate in the secretion of parathyroid hormone in man, J. Clin. Invest., 49:2146, 1970.

33 Marx, J.: Osteoporosis: new help for thinning bones, Science, 207:628, 1980.

34 Irwin, M. I., and E. W. Kienholz: A conspectus of research on calcium requirements of man, J. Nutr., 103:1019, 1973.

35 Heaney, R. P., R. R. Recker, and P. D. Saville: Calcium balance and calcium requirements in middle-aged women, Clin. Res., 22:649A, 1974.

36 Albanese, A. A., A. H. Edelson, E. J. Lorenze, Jr., M. L. Woodhull, and E. H. Wein: Problems of bone health in elderly, N.Y. State Med. J., 75:326, 1975.

37 Heaney, R. P., R. R. Recker, and P. D. Saville: Calcium balance and calcium requirements in middle-aged women, Am. J. Clin. Nutr., 30:1603, 1977.

38 Ireland, P., and J. S. Fordtran: Effect of dietary calcium and age on jejunal calcium absorption in humans studied by intestinal perfusion, J. Clin. Invest., 52:2672, 1973.

39 Horsman, A., J. L. Gallagher, M. Simpson, and B. E. C. Nordin: Prospective trial of oestrogen and calcium in postmenopausal women, Br. Med. J., 2:789, 1977.

40 Recker, R. R., P. D. Saville, and R. P. Heaney: The effect of estrogens and calcium carbonate on bone loss in postmenopausal women, Ann. Intern. Med., 87:649, 1977.

41 Riggs, B. L., J. Jowsey, P. J. Kelly, D. L. Hoffman, and C. D. Arnaud: Effects of oral therapy with calcium and vitamin D in primary osteoporosis, J. Clin. Endocrinol. Metab., 42:1139, 1976.

42 Jowsey, J.: Osteoporosis: its nature and the role of diet, Postgrad. Med., 60:75, 1976.

43 Krook, L.: Dietary calcium-phosphorus and lameness in the horse, Cornell Vet., 58(suppl. 1):59, 1968.

44 Sie, T. L., H. H. Draper, and R. R. Bell: Hypocalcemia, hyperparathyroidism, and bone resorption induced by dietary phosphate, J. Nutr., 104:1195, 1974.

45 Herbert, L. A., J. Lemann, Jr., J. R. Petersen, and E. J. Lennon: Studies on the mechanism by which phosphate infusion lowers serum calcium concentration, J. Clin. Invest., 45:1886, 1966.

46 Draper, H. H., and R. R. Bell: Nutrition and Osteoporosis, in *Advances in Nutritional Research,* vol. 2, H. H. Draper (ed.), Plenum, New York, 1977.

47 Bell, R. R., H. H. Draper, D. Y. M. Tzeng, H. K. Shin, and G. R. Schmidt: Physiological responses to human adult foods containing phosphorus additives, J. Nutr., 107:42, 1977.

48 DeLuca, H. F., and H. K. Schnoes: Metabolism and mechanism of vitamin D, Annu. Rev. Biochem., 45:631, 1976.

49 Johnson, N. E., E. N. Alcantara, and H. Linkswiler: Effect of level of protein intake on urinary and fecal calcium retention in young adult males, J. Nutr., 100:1425, 1970.

50 Margen, S., J.-Y. Chu, N. A. Kaufman, and D. H. Calloway: Studies in calcium metabolism. I. The calciuric effect of dietary protein, Am. J. Clin. Nutr., 27:584, 1974.

51 Spencer, H., L. Kramer, D. Osis, and C. Norris: Effect of high protein (meat) intake on calcium metabolism in man, Am. J. Clin. Nutr., 31:2167, 1978.

52 Schuette, S. A., M. B. Zemel, and H. M. Linkswiler: Studies on the mechanism of protein-induced hypercalciuria in older men and women, J. Nutr, 110:305, 1980.

53 Lemann, J., Jr., and A. S. Relman: The relation of sulfur metabolism in acid-base balance and electrolyte excretion: the effects of DL-methionine in normal man, J. Clin. Invest., 38:2215, 1959.

54 Allen, L. H., R. S. Bartlett, and G. D. Block: Reduction of renal calcium reabsorption in man by consumption of dietary protein, J. Nutr., 109:1345, 1979.

55 Skillman, T. G.: Can osteoporosis be prevented? Geriatrics, 35:95, 1980.

56 Nordin, B. E. C., A. Horsman, R. G. Crilly, D. H. Marshall, and M. Simpson: Treatment of spinal osteoporosis in postmenopausal women, Br. Med. J., 1:451, 1980.

57 Autune, C. M. F., P. D. Stolley, N. B. Rosenshein, J. L. Davies, J. A. Tonascia, C. Brown, L. Burnett, A. Ruledge, M. Pokempher, and R. Garcia: Endometrial cancer and estrogen use, N. Engl. J. Med., 300:9, 1979.

58 Ross, R. K., A. Pagganini-Hill, V. R. Gerkins, T. M. Mack, R. Pfeffer, M. Arthur, and B. E. Henderson: A case-control study of menopausal estrogen therapy and breast cancer, J. Am. Med. Assoc., 243:1635, 1980.

59 Treatment of osteoporosis (editorial), Br. Med. J., 1:1303, 1978.

60 Avioli, L. B.: What to do with postmenopausal osteoporosis? Am. J. Med., 65:881, 1978.

61 Riggs, B. L., S. F. Hodgson, D. L. Hoffman, P. J. Kelly, K. A. Johnson, and D. Taves: Treatment of primary osteoporosis with fluoride and calcium, J. Am. Med. Assoc., 243:446, 1980.

62 National Survey Committee: *Domestic Food Consumption and Expenditure 1961,* H. M. Stationery Office, London, 1963.

63 Marston, R., and B. Friend: *National Food Situation,* U.S. Department of Agriculture, Economic Research Service, Publication NFS-158, November 1976.

64 Lindsay, R., D. M. Hart, J. M. Aitken, E. B. McDonald, J. B. Anderson, and A. C. Clarke: Long-term prevention of postmenopausal osteoporosis by oestrogen, Lancet, 1:1038, 1976.

65 Nachtigall, L. E., R. H. Nachtigall, R. D. Nachtigall, and E. M. Beckman: Estrogen replacement therapy. I. A 10-year prospective study in the relationship to osteoporosis, Obstet. Gynecol., 53:277, 1979.

CHAPTER 14

NUTRITIONAL ASPECTS
OF RICKETS
AND OSTEOMALACIA

CONTENTS

INTRODUCTION

During the industrial revolution, the prevalence of rickets, particularly in winter and among children confined to sunless sweat shops and smog-ridden cities implicated insufficient exposure to sunlight in its etiology. Despite the discovery of the antirachitic action of cod-liver oil more than 200 years ago, rickets remained a serious health problem until the early part of the twentieth century, when the identification, isolation, and addition of vitamin D to the food supply and more exposure to the ultraviolet rays of the sun rendered conventional rickets a disorder of mere academic interest in developed countries. Today in developing countries where children and women are customarily shielded from the sun, where vitamin D enrichment of food is not practiced, and where vitamin D supplementation is not given, rickets remains a substantial public health problem.

Over the past 30 years the increased recognition of rickets in developed countries in new, more subtle forms necessitates that the physician be able to recognize the clinical manifestations of the disease and the clinical settings under which it most often occurs. Rickets has been reported in children (1) who have a variety of inborn or acquired derangements of vitamin D, (2) who have renal and nonrenal disturbances of the handling of phosphate, (3) who have been breast-fed for a prolonged period without supplementation of their diet with other foods or vitamins, and (4) who are fed a vegan diet [1]. Rickets has also been reported among Asian immigrants in Britain [2].

The term *osteomalacia,* meaning literally "softening of the bone," refers to a generalized bone disease of various etiologies characterized by a greatly increased amount of osteoid (unmineralized bone) in the skeleton, which is due to inadequate concentrations of calcium or phosphate ions in body fluids. In *rickets* the growing skeleton is involved; defective mineralization occurs not only in bone but also in the cartilaginous matrix of the growth plate. The term *osteomalacia* is usually reserved for the disorders of mineralization of the adult skeleton in which the epiphyseal growth plates are closed. Rickets and osteomalacia were for decades synonymous with vitamin D deficiency, and from a global perspective it is still their commonest cause. However, the definition of rickets has been broadened to include all of the disturbances of growing bone in which there is a lag in the mineralization of the matrix. The failure in bone mineralization may occur as a result of a rare disorder, such as Fanconi syndrome, but the varieties most frequently encountered are due to vitamin D deficiency, abnormal vitamin D metabolism, or hypophosphatemia, and these are the ones to be considered in this chapter (Table 14-1). In renal tubular disorders, rickets and osteomalacia develop in the presence of normal intestinal function and are not cured by treatment with doses of vitamin D that are adequate to cure rickets due to vitamin D deficiency. Thus, the term *vitamin D–resistant* is sometimes applied to these cases.

Since at least some of the clinical aspects and causes of rickets can be explained in terms of vitamin D metabolism, we will briefly summarize the metabolic steps leading to the formation of biologically active vitamin D and the physiological effects of this activated form. Further information can be obtained in Appendix 5 or in the review article by Haussler and McCain [3].

Vitamin D is a collective term identifying a group of compounds that have antirachitic activities; it is present in animals (as cholecalciferol, or vitamin D_3) and plants (as ergocalciferol, or vitamin D_2). In humans, vitamin D is either ingested or synthesized by photochemical activation of 7-dehydrocholesterol in the skin by ultraviolet light. The metabolism of vitamins D_2 and D_3 in the body is very similar, and that of vitamin D_3 will be further described. Cholecalciferol

TABLE 14-1
CLASSIFICATION OF MAIN CAUSES OF RICKETS AND OSTEOMALACIA

Main etiological defect	Causes	Main clinical forms
Vitamin D deficiency	Dietary deficiency Malabsorption Lack of sunlight	Asian Elderly Unusual dietary practices Hepatic biliary cirrhosis Pancreatic insufficiency
25-OH vitamin D_3 deficiency	25-Hydroxylase abnormalities	Liver disease Anticonvulsants
1,25-$(OH)_2$ vitamin D_3 deficiency	1α-Hydroxylase failure 1α-Hydroxylase deficiency	Renal failure Vitamin D–dependent rickets
Hypophosphatemia	Decreased renal tubular phosphate reabsorption	Sporadic Tumor-associated Fanconi syndrome Familial (vitamin D-resistant)
	Phosphate depletion	Use of oral phosphate binders
	Low phosphate intake	Premature infants
Bicarbonate deficit	Impaired renal tubular excretion of H^+	Renal tubular acidosis

(vitamin D_3) is carried in the blood to the liver, where it is converted into 25-hydroxycholecalciferol [25-$(OH)D_3$]. This in turn is carried to the kidney, where it undergoes a second hydroxylation to form 1,25-dihydroxycholecalciferol [1,25-$(OH)_2D_3$], the most active metabolite in the series. Renal 1-hydroxylation is stimulated by many agents, of which the most important are parathyroid hormone (PTH) and hypophosphatemia. Because the synthesis of 1,25-$(OH)_2D_3$ in the body is regulated in response to homeostatic demands, 1,25-$(OH)_2D_3$ is more properly regarded as a hormone than as a vitamin. Increased formation of 1,25-$(OH)_2D_3$ is usually accompanied by decreased formation of another dihydroxy metabolite, 24,25-$(OH)_2D_3$. Although this compound is thought by some to be the first stage in the inactivation of vitamin D [4], there is evidence that it is an independent metabolite with its own biological effects [5].

Once vitamin D is activated, its primary effect is on the epithelial cells of the small intestine (enterocytes), where it induces the formation of a transport protein which enhances the absorption of dietary calcium and phosphate. The active metabolites of vitamin D also directly increase the rate of bone resorption. This effect, while not requiring the presence of PTH, is less marked in its absence. Whether the active metabolites of vitamin D alter renal tubular transport of calcium or phosphate is not known.

Phosphate concentration also plays an important role in the regulation of 1,25-$(OH)_2D_3$ synthesis. Hypophosphatemia stimulates production of active vitamin D and thus increases intestinal absorption of calcium and phosphate. In addition, low blood phosphate levels induce the kidney tubule to reabsorb this ion maximally. The net result of these processes is an elevation in blood phosphate and a decrease in $1,25\text{-}(OH)_2D_3$ production.

EPIDEMIOLOGY

In the United States, nutritional deprivation of vitamin D has not been considered an important cause of osteomalacia. However, in elderly persons who eat sparingly and have little or no exposure to sunlight and in infants and children (especially blacks) whose diets do not include animal-derived products, it may be more common than is generally appreciated [6,7]. During a 4½-year period, 24 cases of rickets due to vitamin D deficiency were reported in Philadelphia in black breast-fed infants who were otherwise healthy and had no underlying malabsorptive or renal diseases. Most of these children were members of families who belonged to one of the Black Muslim sects which subscribe to various dietary restrictions and to clothing habits that minimize their exposure to sunlight. Cases have also been reported in white children in San Francisco [8] and Boston [9] who adhere to macrobiotic vegetarian diets that provide very little or no animal food and often no milk after weaning. Most dietary vitamin D is obtained in this country through the ingestion of fortified foods, especially dairy products (Table 14-2). Deficiency then can be due to poverty, but ignorance, apathy, and food faddism are also important considerations. Vitamin D deficiency also occurs in patients as a complication of vitamin D malabsorption due to the effect of gastrectomy, small intestinal disease, pancreatic insufficiency, chronic obstructive jaundice, or long-term administration of a bile salt chelator such as cholestyramine. Poor intake of vitamin D and calcium and antacid-induced phosphate depletion are additional causes of osteomalacia after gastric surgery.

Osteomalacia is an infrequent complication of liver disease, but serum $25\text{-}(OH)D_3$ concentrations are low in some patients with parenchymal and cholestatic disease. Rickets and hypocalcemia can occur in premature infants apparently because of delayed production of the 25-hydroxylase enzyme in liver and the consequent impairment of $25\text{-}(OH)D_3$ synthesis. Rickets has also been reported in epileptic populations treated with anticonvulsants, especially individuals on combinations of phenobarbital and phenytoin (Dilantin). It is thought that the plasma level of $25\text{-}(OH)D_3$ in these individuals is low, possibly as a result of the induction of hepatic microsomal enzymes that catalyze the formation of inactive polar metabolites of both vitamin D_3 and $25\text{-}(OH)D_3$, which are then excreted in the bile.

Patients with many forms of renal disease, especially those in whom tubular reabsorption of phosphorus is impaired, are candidates for osteomalacia. The failure of bone mineralization is a consequence of low serum phosphate rather than low serum calcium levels. Secondary hyperparathyroidism is not usually present in these patients. The three most common disorders of this type are (1) primary renal hypophosphatemic rickets (familial vitamin D–resistant rickets

TABLE 14-2
VITAMIN D CONTENT OF SELECTED FOODS

Food	Serving size	Vitamin D content*, IU/serving
Sardines	$3\frac{1}{2}$ oz	1150–1570
Cod-liver oil	1 tbsp	1275
Salmon, canned	$3\frac{1}{2}$ oz	220–440
Herring, canned	$3\frac{1}{2}$ oz	330
Tuna, canned in water	$3\frac{1}{2}$ oz	250
Milk, whole or skim, fortified	1 cup	100
Liver, chicken, raw	$3\frac{1}{2}$ oz	50–67
Liver, beef, raw	$3\frac{1}{2}$ oz	9–42
Egg, whole	1 large	25
Cheese, cottage	$\frac{1}{2}$ cup	10
Milk, cow, unfortified	1 cup	0.7–10
Cheese, cheddar	1 oz	3–8
Cream, heavy	1 tbsp	5
Butter	1 pat	2

*Ranges are given for food items in which a significant variability in vitamin D content can occur.
   Source: C. F. Church and H. N. Church, Food Values of Portions Commonly Used, 12th ed., Lippincott, Philadelphia, 1975.

and osteomalacia), (?) renal tubular acidosis, and (3) Fanconi syndrome. Renal hypophosphatemia rickets is a familial disorder usually transmitted as an X linked dominant trait, thus rendering the hemizygous-X male the more severely affected. Absorption of phosphorus from the gut also appears diminished. Phosphorus malabsorption is manifested early in life by hypophosphatemia and growth failure.

In patients with renal tubular acidosis the tubular mechanism that is responsible for maintaining a H^+ ion gradient between the tubular lumen and the cell does not function properly. These patients also usually have a vasopressin-resistant polyuria, indicating another abnormality in distal tubular function. The mechanism of this renal hypophosphatemia secondary to bicarbonate deficit is unknown. In the untreated state there is impairment of renal tubular reabsorption of phosphate. This type of hypophosphatemia is readily correctable; administration of sodium bicarbonate or a bicarbonate precursor such as sodium lactate or sodium citrate can return serum phosphate levels to normal.

Fanconi syndrome is manifested by disturbed function of the proximal tubule, i.e., by renal glycosuria, aminoaciduria, and hypophosphatemia. Aside from the well-known causes of this syndrome, such as cystinosis, tyrosinosis, heavy metal poisoning (particularly cadmium and lead), glycogen storage disease, multiple myeloma, and toxic organic compounds such as degraded tetracycline, there are so-called idiopathic cases, those without known cause. Clinical presentation of Fanconi syndrome is similar to that of renal tubular acidosis.

Finally among the types of rickets associated with vitamin D deficiency is so-called vitamin D–dependent rickets (pseudovitamin D deficiency, or increased requirement for vitamin D), a disorder caused by a functional reduction in the concentration of the kidney 1α-hydroxylase enzyme. This syndrome is often mistakenly confused with vitamin D–resistant rickets. It is characterized by signs and symptoms which usually appear in the first year of life and which mimic those seen in simple nutritional vitamin D deficiency. The syndrome, transmitted as an autosomal recessive trait, is due to incomplete conversion of 25-$(OH)D_3$ to $1,25\text{-}(OH)_2D_3$ [10]. Use of the word *dependent* is a result of the observation that the skeletal and biochemical derangements in this syndrome respond dramatically to vitamin D in doses 100 times the normal daily recommendation of 400 IU per day.

PATHOGENESIS

Clinically, rickets develops in otherwise normal bone matrix when the concentrations of calcium and inorganic phosphate in the plasma (and extracellular fluid) are too low for normal bone mineralization. The bone matrix or osteoid continues to be produced at its usual rate, and its accumulation becomes disproportionate to the amount of calcification. Once the epiphyses have closed, this process is called osteomalacia.

As shown in Table 14-3, the various forms of rickets can be divided into two types according to their pathogenesis: (1) those in which an abnormality of vitamin D metabolism leads to a deficiency of $1,25\text{-}(OH)_2D_3$; and (2) those due to a target-tissue abnormality, specifically the renal tubular disorders characterized by defective renal tubular reabsorption of phosphate.

It is not known whether vitamin D, through one of its metabolites, has a major effect on mineralization. Its primary role after conversion to 25-$(OH)D_3$ and $1,25\text{-}(OH)_2D_3$ is to enhance absorption of calcium and phosphate ions from the intestinal lumen. The pathogenesis of inadequate skeletal mineralization when there is insufficient vitamin D present, from whatever cause, is likely to be as follows. Insufficient concentrations of the active vitamin D metabolites lead to decreased intestinal calcium absorption and decreased mobilization of calcium from bone, resulting in hypocalcemia. Hypocalcemia stimulates increased parathyroid hormone (PTH) secretion, which tends to raise plasma calcium concentration but also stimulates increased renal phosphate clearance, which, in turn, produces hypophosphatemia. When the concentration of phosphorus in the extracellular fluid falls below a critical level, mineralization cannot proceed normally. In severe vitamin D deficiency, normocalcemia cannot be maintained and the impetus for mineralization is further decreased.

TABLE 14-3
CLASSIFICATION, DIAGNOSIS, AND TREATMENT OF RICKETS AND OSTEOMALACIA

	Classification	
	Type I	Type 2
Cause	Abnormality of vitamin D metabolism causing deficiency of biologically active vitamin D	Renal tubular disorders leading to defective reabsorption of phosphate
Diagnosis		
Clinical	Enlarged, distorted bones	
	Muscle weakness	
	Chest deformities	
	Kyphoscoliosis	
	Growth failure	
	Tetany	
	Craniotabes	
	Delayed fontanelle and suture closing	
	Frontal thickening and bossing	
Biochemical		
Parathyroid hormone	↑↑	N or ↑
Alkaline phosphatase	↑↑	↑
Aminoaciduria	↑↑	N or ↑
Serium calcium	N or ↓	N
Serum phosphate	↓	↓↓
Treatment	Vitamin D, DHT, or 1,25-$(OH)_2D_3$ in appropriate doses to normalize serum alkaline phosphatase, calcium, and phosphate Monitor healing with serial radiographs	Phosphate in an amount sufficient to maintain serum levels greater than 4 mg/dl Vitamin D, DHT, or 1,25-$(OH)_2D_3$ in an amount sufficient to prevent hypocalcemia Other electrolytes if appropriate

Phosphate depletion alone can cause osteomalacia, as is seen in patients who consume large amounts of nonabsorbable antacids. Excessive renal loss of phosphate due to decreased tubular reabsorption may also result in the hypophosphatemia that is responsible for osteomalacia in some renal tubular disorders.

CLINICAL MANIFESTATIONS

It is convenient to consider the clinical aspects of rickets and osteomalacia separately, since although they share the same abnormality, the manifestations differ considerably. In infants and young children the features of rickets include listlessness, irritability, and often profound hypotonia and muscular weakness. The failure of adequate calcification affects mostly those parts of the skeleton in which bone growth is most rapid. At birth the skull grows faster than any other bone, and craniotabes is, therefore, the main manifestation of congenital rickets. The membrane bones of the vault of the skull may be reversibly depressed by minor pressure, which to the uninitiated may cause considerable alarm. Suture and fontanelle closure are delayed, and frontal thickening (bossing) becomes evident. In the first year, the upper limbs and ribs grow quickly, leading to signs at the wrist and costochondral junctions (rachitic rosary) (Color Figure 14). Indentation of the lower rib at the site of attachment of the diaphragm is known as *Harrison's groove* or *sulcus*. Later the legs grow faster, with most signs manifesting around the growing ends at the knees. Weight bearing and normal muscle tension cause twisting, bending, rotation, and eventually distortion of many bones. A waddling gait secondary to grotesque femoral bowing and tibial torsion is common (Color Figure 15). Dental eruption is often delayed, and enamel defects are common. Pelvic bone deformation from rickets is an important cause of dystocia in adult women. Deformity of the birth canal is a major cause of difficult labor and stillbirth in certain parts of the world. General muscle weakness may result in a "potbellied" appearance.

In contrast to rickets in children, presentation of osteomalacia in adults is not as dramatic and is often difficult to diagnose clinically. Vague, poorly localized skeletal pains and bony tenderness are the first manifestations of osteomalacia. The dorsolumbar and pelvic regions are usually first affected. The pain is made worse by muscle strain, weight bearing, or pressure. Bone tenderness can be elicited by pressure on the tibiae, the pubic rami, or the rib cage. If the disease has been present for a long time, the vertebral bodies begin to collapse and measurable loss of trunk height ensues; gross deformity such as kyphosis or scoliosis is usually a late sign. Proximal muscle weakness in the lower extremities may lead to a waddling gait similar to that seen in muscular dystrophy. Many patients with long-standing osteomalacia have had previous incorrect diagnoses of muscular rheumatism, arthritis, and herniated lumbar disks. When the diagnosis is overlooked for many years, a diagnosis of psychoneurosis or malingering may be mistakenly entertained.

RADIOLOGICAL FEATURES

Radiological changes in the skeleton in rickets and osteomalacia reflect the pathological changes. Again, it is convenient to deal with rickets and osteomalacia separately. Radiographic confirmation of rachitic bone changes is helpful, except in the newborn period, when it has little diagnostic value. The cardinal signs of rickets are widening of the growth plate and an irregular appearance at the end of the metaphysis. The metaphysis is widened and cupped and has a ragged edge. The trabecular pattern of the metaphyses is abnormal, cortices of the diaphyses may be thin, and bowing of the shaft may be present.

The radiological signs of osteomalacia are not at all precise. Because longitudinal growth has stopped, only the shaft of the long bones and the flat bones, such as the pelvis, are affected. However, the most distinctive feature is the occurrence of Looser zones (pseudofractures, or Milkman fractures) or symmetric radiolucent bands adjacent and usually perpendicular to the periosteal surface in ribs, pubic rami, and outer borders of the scapulae and near the ends of long bones [11]. Their origin is almost certainly a consequence of trauma, since the localization of these zones usually follows the well-known distribution of various forms of stress fractures occurring in the normal skeleton [12].

LABORATORY DIAGNOSIS

Biochemical findings depend upon the stage of the disease and its etiology (Table 14-1). Changes in serum concentrations of calcium, inorganic phosphorus, alkaline phosphatase, 25-$(OH)D_3$, and 1,25-$(OH)_2D_3$ vary depending on the cause of the disease. In states of vitamin D deficiency caused by dietary lack, malabsorption, or inadequate sunlight exposure, serum calcium levels are normal or low, phosphorus and 25-$(OH)D_3$ levels are characteristically low, and alkaline phosphatase levels are increased (Table 14-3). In adults phosphorus concentrations less than 2.8 mg/dl are abnormal; in children the lower limit of normal is closer to 4.0 to 4.5 mg/dl. In *severe* states of vitamin D deficiency, hypocalcemia may also be seen, occasionally sufficient to produce tetany.

Generally, patients with renal tubular disorders maintain normal serum calcium levels, while hypophosphatemia is characteristic. Other laboratory findings such as glycosuria, aminoaciduria, acidosis, and hypouricemia reflect variable degrees of renal proximal tubular function disturbance. In chronic renal failure, hyperphosphatemia and some degree of hypocalcemia are usually seen, accompanied by normal 25-$(OH)D_3$ and low 1,25-$(OH)_2D_3$ levels. Circulating alkaline phosphatase may be normal or slightly elevated. Because the method of analysis and the expression of results differ in various laboratories, numerical values have not been given.

MANAGEMENT

Vitamin D is the cornerstone of the medical treatment of rickets and osteomalacia, and the form of vitamin D used and the dose are of great importance. Since vitamin D accumulates and vitamin D toxicity can be produced, it is important to use the correct dose. The recent explosion of knowledge concerning the metabolism of vitamin D has led to the synthesis of several potent substances with vitamin D action.

The generic term, vitamin D, includes ergocalciferol (vitamin D_2), cholecalciferol (vitamin D_3), and dihydrotachysterol (DHT or AT 10) together with their biologically active metabolites and a variety of synthetic analogues. Because D_2 and DHT were synthesized first, they have been mainly used in treatment. It is traditional to express quantities of vitamin D in units of antirachitic activity in the rat, but for the pure substances used in treatment it is preferable to use either units of weight or molar units. For vitamins D_2 and D_3, 40,000 IU = 1 mg and 1 IU = 0.025 µg. Dihydrotachysterol, a sterol with steric similarity to the biologically active form of vitamin D [$1,25\text{-}(OH)_2D_3$], does not require renal hydroxylation for activation. This substance has a 3-hydroxyl group that is sterically positioned so that it mimics the position of the 1-hydroxyl group of $1,25\text{-}(OH)_2D_3$. Its advantage lies in its short half-life (50 hours versus 20 days for vitamin D) and its rapid onset of action; 1 mg of DHT has at least the equivalent effect of 3 mg of vitamin D in humans. The vitamin D metabolite $1,25\text{-}(OH)_2D_3$ is now available as calcitriol (Rocaltrol, Roche Laboratories); its onset of action is rapid, and its half-life is short (less than 24 hours). The metabolite $25\text{-}(OH)D_3$ (Calderol, UpJohn) is also available, but less is known about optimal dose regimens. The synthetic sterol $1\alpha\text{-}(OH)D_3$, which requires hepatic hydroxylation before it is active, is available in Europe but can be obtained in the United States only with an Investigational New Drug (IND) number.

The therapeutic approach to each of the disorders associated with rickets and osteomalacia is somewhat different. In rickets and osteomalacia due to dietary lack of vitamin D or inadequate exposure to sunlight, vitamin D_2 or vitamin D_3 is given orally in doses of 2000 to 4000 IU (0.05 to 0.1 mg) daily for 6 to 12 weeks, followed by daily supplements of 200 to 400 IU, which are adequate to prevent development of the disorder in otherwise normal subjects. Calcium supplements and larger initial doses of vitamin D may be necessary in infants and children with tetany.

Patients with osteomalacia due to intestinal malabsorption do not respond to the relatively small doses of vitamin D that can cure osteomalacia due to vitamin D deficiency. In the presence of active steatorrhea, oral doses of vitamin D of 40,000 to 100,000 IU daily may be required in addition to large doses of calcium (e.g., 15 to 20 g calcium lactate per day, administered orally). Small doses of $1\alpha\text{-}(OH)D_3$ (2.5 to 5.0 µg daily) or $1,25\text{-}(OH)_2D_3$ (0.5 to 1.0 µg daily) are also effective in treating this form of osteomalacia [13]. In all patients receiving large doses of vitamin D, monitoring the plasma calcium level is essential.

In patients who have been using anticonvulsants, it is often necessary to continue the drugs while adding supplemental vitamin D and monitoring levels of serum calcium biweekly until a therapeutic response is obtained. Doses varying from 4000 to 40,000 IU daily have been recommended.

The treatment for vitamin D–dependent rickets is the administration of large doses of vitamin D; the exact amount must be determined individually. As much as 50,000 IU per day has been needed by some patients. The required dose is determined by serial measurements of serum calcium concentration and urine calcium excretion and should be sufficient to raise serum calcium into the normal range without producing hypercalciuria. Treatment with $1,25\text{-}(OH)_2D_3$ would be the most specific therapy, but it is currently approved only for treatment of patients with renal insufficiency [14].

Treatment of rickets and osteomalacia in the presence of renal tubular disorders is more difficult, and there is no uniform agreement as to the regimen to be followed. The basic treatment for X-linked hypophosphatemic vitamin D–resistant rickets is oral phosphate in sufficient amount to raise serum phosphate to levels at which mineralization of bone generally occurs (> 4 mg/dl). Elemental phosphorus, 1.5 to 2 g per day, is also required. Because high phosphate intake lowers calcium absorption, it is also necessary to administer vitamin D, 25,000 to 100,000 IU daily, or dihydrotachysterol, 0.2 to 1 mg per day. The appropriate dose of sterol is one which maintains normal serum calcium levels and normal urinary excretion of calcium (50 to 150 mg per day). Rickets associated with renal tubular acidosis may be healed with correction of the acidosis by administration of excess cation. A solution of sodium and potassium citrates (Polycitar) is administered in divided doses of 20 to 60 ml per day; monitoring is by determination of serum bicarbonate concentrations [15].

In chronic renal failure high doses of vitamin D are administered. Dihydrotachysterol, at doses of 0.2 to 1.0 mg daily, is effective in treating hypocalcemia and osteodystrophy resulting from chronic renal failure. $1,25$-$(OH)_2D_3$ and 1α-$(OH)D_3$ in small doses are also effective. $1,25$-$(OH)_2D_3$ is approved for use in the United States in the treatment of hypocalcemic patients using hemodialysis; the recommended initial dose is 0.25 µg per day. If after 2 to 4 weeks biochemical parameters are unaltered, the dose is increased by 0.25 µg per day every 2 to 4 weeks until a satisfactory biochemical response (elevation of serum calcium levels and a decrease in PTH levels) is obtained. The usual dose is 0.5 to 1.0 µg per day. Because there are no physiological feedback regulatory mechanisms to control the biological responses to 1α-$(OH)D_3$, hypercalcemia can occur, especially during initial treatment. Frequent serum calcium determinations are encouraged during the initial months of therapy. Hypercalcemia can be reversed by discontinuing or decreasing the dose of 1α-$(OH)D_3$ [13].

PREVENTION

Dietary vitamin D deficiency rickets can be prevented by adequate exposure of the infant to sunlight or by vitamin D supplementation. The latter is less subject to the vagaries of climate and season and thus is more dependable. The Recommended Dietary Allowance (RDA) is 400 IU (10 µg) of vitamin D per day for infants and children. This can be provided by 1 quart of fortified cow's milk or by an equivalent amount of prepared infant formula or evaporated milk.

It is clear that if breast milk is to be used as the sole food, the mother must be well nourished. Jackson [16] claims that human milk from well-nourished mothers meets all the nutritional needs of full-term babies for 4 to 6 months of postnatal life. Human milk has been called a poor source of vitamin D [17]. Earlier assays of human milk for vitamin D concentration were done on the lipid fraction of milk, and the aqueous phase was discarded. It is now clear that most of the vitamin D in human milk is present as a water-soluble conjugate of vitamin D with sulfate [18], so that the intake of the breast-fed infant may be appreciably higher than has previously been believed.

Small or premature infants may not ingest adequate amounts of vitamin D and should receive supplements of vitamin D for a total intake of 400 IU per day. Older children may obtain 400 IU of the vitamin daily by exposure to sunlight and by ingestion of foods such as tuna, salmon, sardines, liver, eggs, and vitamin D–fortified milk (Table 14-2). There is no need for other supplemental vitamin D unless there is a defect of absorption or of hepatic or renal function. It is especially important to encourage parents who adhere to macrobiotic and other vegetarian patterns of eating to supplement the diet of their infants and young children with a source of vitamin D and to expose their infants to the sun.

Patients with renal, liver, or bowel absorption disease may require 2000 to 5000 IU per day. For patients on anticonvulsant medications or with cystic fibrosis, especially those with minimal exposure to sunlight, a dose of up to 2000 IU per day may be necessary.

CASE STUDY

A 14-month-old black girl was brought to the pediatric clinic; the chief complaint was a swollen right leg that followed mild trauma to the leg. Her prenatal history was unremarkable. The mother was a strict vegetarian and also wore copious garments which covered all of her body except her face and hands. The child had been entirely breast-fed since birth, without supplemental vitamins, until 2 months prior to admission. The family, which was Muslim, had been receiving dietary advice from a neighborhood health food store.

On physical examination, the patient was irritable, potbellied, and pale. She had a widely patent anterior fontanelle, a rachitic rosary, widened metaphyses at the elbows, wrists, knees, and ankles, and a palpable liver edge. She had only two lower central incisors. A skeletal survey showed a fracture of the mid-shaft right fibula. Her length was 73.5 cm, and her weight was 6.95 kg.

Laboratory data:

Serum calcium	9.3 mg/dl
Serum phosphorus	3.4 mg/dl
Alkaline phosphatase	408 units
Serum PTH	385 pg/ml
	(normal = 163–347 pg/ml)

Study Questions

1 What features did this patient have which are commonly seen in nutritional rickets?

2 What acute treatment would you begin for this child?

3 What dietary recommendations would you make for this child?

REFERENCES

1 Bachrach, S., J. Fisher, and J. S. Parks: An outbreak of vitamin D deficiency rickets in a susceptible population, Pediatrics, 64:871, 1979.

2 Rickets in Asian immigrants (editorial), Br. Med. J., 1:1744, 1979.

3 Haussler, M. R., and T. A. McCain: Basic and clinical concepts related to vitamin D metabolism and action, N. Engl. J. Med., 297:974, 1041, 1977.

4 DeLuca, H. F.: Vitamin D endocrinology, Ann. Intern. Med., 85:367, 1976.

5 Kanis, J. A., G. Heynen, G. G. Russell, R. Smith, R. J. Walton, and G. T. Warner: Biological effects of 24,25-dihydroxycholecalciferol in man, in *Proceedings of the Third Workshop on Vitamin D,* A. W. Norman et al. (eds.), Walter de Gruyter, Berlin, 1977.

6 Zmora, E., and R. Goridscher: Multiple nutritional deficiencies in infants from a strict vegetarian community, Am. J. Dis. Child., 133:141, 1979.

7 Edidin, D. V., L. L. Levitsky, W. Schey, N. V. Dumbovic, and A. Campos: Resurgence of nutritional rickets associated with breast-feeding and special dietary practices, Pediatrics, 65:232, 1980.

8 Erhard, D.: The new vegetarians, part 2, Nutr. Today, 9:20, January-February 1974.

9 Dwyer, J. T., W. H. Dietz, G. Hass, and R. Suskind: Risk of nutritional rickets among vegetarian children, Am. J. Dis. Child., 133:134, 1979.

10 Fraser, D., S. W. Kooh, H. P. King, M. F. Holick, Y. Tanaka, and H. F. DeLuca: Pathogenesis of hereditary vitamin D metabolism involving defective conversion of 25-hydroxyvitamin D to 1,25-dihyroxyvitamin D, N. Engl. J. Med., 289:817, 1973.

11 Parfitt, A. M., and H. Duncan: Metabolic bone disease affecting the spine, in *The Spine,* R. Rothman and F. Simeone (eds.), Saunders, Philadelphia, 1975.

12 Dent, C. E., and T. C. B. Stamp: Vitamin D, rickets, and osteomalacia, in *Metabolic Bone Disease,* vol. I, L. V. Avioli and S. M. Krane (eds.), Academic, New York, 1977.

13 Krane, S. M., and H. F. Holick: Metabolic bone disease, in Harrison's *Principles of Internal Medicine,* 9th ed., K. J. Isselbacher et al. (eds.), McGraw-Hill, New York, 1980.

14 Harrison, H. E., and H. C. Harrison: Rickets and osteomalacia, in *Disorders of Calcium and Phosphate Metabolism in Childhood and Adolescence,* Saunders, Philadelphia, 1979.

15 Root, A. W., and H. E. Harrison: Recent advances in calcium metabolism. II. Disorders of calcium homeostasis, J. Pediatr., 88:177, 1976.

16 Jackson, R. L.: Maternal and infant nutrition and health in later life, Nutr. Rev., 37:33, 1979.

17 Barness, L. A.: Nutrition and nutritional disorders, in *Textbook of Pediatrics,* 10th ed., V. C. Vaughan III and R. J. McKay (eds.), Saunders, Philadelphia, 1975.

18 Lakdawala, D. R., and E. M. Widdowson: Vitamin D and human milk, Lancet, 1:167, 1977.

CHAPTER 15

NUTRITIONAL ASPECTS OF DISEASES OF THE GASTROINTESTINAL TRACT

CONTENTS

DISEASES OF THE SMALL INTESTINAL WALL
   Celiac-Sprue
   Tropical Sprue
   Crohn's Disease
   Radiation Enteritis
   Intestinal Bypass
   Small Bowel Resection
DISEASES OF THE COLON
   Nonspecific Ulcerative Colitis
   Colonic Diverticulosis
EXCLUSION DIETS IN FOOD INTOLERANCE AND
GASTROINTESTINAL ALLERGIES
   Enzyme Deficiency States
   Gastrointestinal Allergies
   Flatulence
GASTROINTESTINAL DISEASE IN THE AGED

INTRODUCTION

The gastrointestinal (GI) tract is essential for the digestion of ingested food and the absorption of the products of digestion. Almost all diseases of the GI tract result in some disturbance of nutrition, and consequent nutritional deficiency may in turn aggravate the malfunction.

Epidemiological studies have suggested that diet may be important in the pathogenesis of a number of GI diseases, including dental caries, cancer of the stomach and colon, and sigmoid diverticulosis. Causal relationships are frequently difficult to prove, however, and there is often more speculation than there are hard data. This chapter addresses mainly the nutritional problems which occur in association with those GI diseases most frequently encountered in North American and western European communities.

A major cause of nutritional deficiency is disease of the GI tract. The two most important consequences are the following:

1 *Loss of weight* due to inadequate intake of calories or to disturbed digestion or absorption
2 *Anemia,* most commonly due to iron deficiency

Anemia may be a consequence of chronic continuous, or intermittent, blood loss from the GI tract or of poor absorption of iron. Less common is anemia due to deficiencies of folacin or cobalamin that occur as a consequence of various malabsorptive diseases.

Loss of Weight

Loss of weight is most often due to reduction of caloric intake, which may occur for many different reasons. Much less common is loss of weight due to malabsorption or a metabolic disorder, such as hyperthyroidism or diabetes mellitus. The weight of an adult patient is the only anthropometric measurement commonly recorded. It is invaluable in following the patient's course and should be measured at every clinic visit; the same scales should be used each time to avoid technical error. Patients' stated weights should be confirmed whenever possible by objective records. Old photographs are sometimes useful as supporting evidence.

Proven loss of weight is not an indication for immediate diagnostic workup of absorptive function. A thorough clinical history is an essential first step. It should, but too often does not, include inquiry about diet and the amounts of food consumed and the reasons for any recent changes in intake. Reduction of intake of calories may be due to a large number of factors, some of which are listed in Table 15-1. Change is the important factor to establish. Change in dentition, onset of dysphagia, abdominal pain after food, nausea, diarrhea, and changes in medications should be included in the clinician's checklist. Some patients do lose weight voluntarily. Many people express anxiety about a change of environment or in their personal affairs by developing a change of appetite: some lose weight; some gain weight. Grief and bereavement are often causes of weight loss. The challenges and pressures of developing sexual maturity in the adolescent or young adult may induce, predominantly in females, reactions which can range from a minor to a full-blown case of anorexia nervosa (see Chapter 4).

TABLE 15-1
COMMON CAUSES OF REDUCED CALORIE INTAKE

Psychological	
Bereavement	Grief
Depression	Reactive states
	Anorexia nervosa

Physical	
Constipation	Pain due to:
Dysphagia due to:	Peptic ulcer
Painful lesions of	Gastric carcinoma
mouth or tongue	Ischemic bowel disease
Esophageal disease	Pancreatitis
Loss or perversion of	Poor dentition
taste	
Nausea due to:	
GI tract disease	
Liver disease	
Systemic disease	
Drugs	
Infections	

If there is doubt about whether loss of weight is occurring, the patient's weight should be recorded at weekly intervals for a month. Obviously this course is not appropriate for the very cachectic patient or a patient in whom a cause of weight loss can be established or is strongly suspected on the basis of symptoms and physical signs at the first encounter.

A calorie count of food consumed in the previous 24 hours is simple and inexpensive, compared with an elaborate diagnostic workup for malabsorption, and is too seldom done. Optimally, it should be done by an experienced dietitian in relaxed surroundings, but by using the approach outlined in Chapter 1, the physician or physician's assistant can perform a quick and adequate assessment, especially as he or she becomes more familiar with the rule-of-thumb conversions involved.

The possibility that a patient may falsify an account of the amount of food consumed cannot be ignored. It may occur as part of a general denial of sickness or in anorexia, for instance. Even careful observation on a metabolic ward may fail at first to detect concealment of food or induced postprandial vomiting.

Treatments of reduced caloric intake are discussed in Chapters 4 and 6.

Anemia

Deficiencies of iron, folacin, and cobalamin that result in anemia may occur as a consequence of GI disease. The main features of these different anemias are discussed fully in Chapter 10.

Iron deficiency is associated with a hypochromic, microcytic anemia. The tongue in iron deficiency is often depapillated and smooth and sometimes is sore; there may be angular stomatitis. The fingernails may be flattened or concave (koilonychia). Pharyngitis and a postcricoid web rarely occur.

The effects of prolonged iron deficiency will be discussed later in relation to its association with carcinoma of the upper GI tract.

When iron-deficiency anemia is diagnosed, possible sites of blood loss must be considered first. In women of childbearing age, menstruation and pregnancy, combined with insufficient ingestion of iron, are of prime importance and bleeding lesions in the GI tract are comparatively rare but must not be overlooked. Women often cannot quantify menstrual loss. The number of pads used is a very rough guide. In older women and in adult males of any age the GI trace is likely to be the site of blood loss. The common causes are listed in Table 15-2, and the uncommon causes in Table 15-3. Worldwide, the most common cause is probably hookworm disease due to infestation of the small bowel with *Ancylostoma*. Hookworm disease is no longer endemic in the continental United States, but small pockets of the disease may occur as the result of migration of infected persons into Europe and North America from endemic areas.

The treatment for iron deficiency due to blood loss is control of the site of bleeding, if possible. Often this is feasible. Peptic ulcers can be treated medically and surgically. Malignant lesions must be resected, if possible, and hemorrhoids must be resected if they are sufficiently severe. The need subsequently to restore

TABLE 15-2
COMMON CAUSES OF GASTROINTESTINAL
BLOOD LOSS

Site	Cause
Esophagus	Esophagitis Esophageal varices Gastroesophageal tears (Mallory-Weiss syndrome)
Stomach	Erosions Ulcer Carcinoma
Duodenum	Erosions Ulcers
Colon	Colorectal Polyps Carcinoma Diverticular disease Crohn's enterocolitis Ulcerative colitis Ischemic bowel disease Hemorrhoids
Systemic	Renal disease and uremia Blood dyscrasias

TABLE 15-3
UNCOMMON CAUSES OF GASTRO-
INTESTINAL BLOOD LOSS

Collagen diseases
Lymphoma
Meckel's diverticulum
Metastatic malignancies
Vascular malformations

depleted body stores of iron by prolonged oral administration or by intramuscular injection must be emphasized.

Gastroesophageal varices associated with high pressures in the portal venous system may be treated by diverting some or all of the portal blood flow from the liver or sclerosing the varices themselves. Some causes of bleeding are not amenable to treatment because a patient is too frail for surgery or the lesion is too diffuse, as in some vascular malformations of the GI tract. In these cases the continuing loss of iron is compensated for by the administration of oral iron, or if this is inadequate to meet the demands of hemoglobin synthesis, parenteral iron is given (see Chapter 10).

Deficiencies of both folacin and cobalamin cause a macrocytic megaloblastic anemia. Folacin deficiency occurs as a consequence of malabsorption in the small intestine and, to some extent, as a consequence of reduced intake associated with the anorexia of, for instance, inflammatory bowel disease. Diets which lack green vegetables or in which folacin-containing constituents are overcooked may be folacin-deficient. The major causes of folacin deficiency are listed in Table 10-9.

The conjunction of weight loss, abnormal fatty stools (which flush with difficulty), a sore, red, smooth tongue, and macrocytic anemia suggests folacin deficiency due to small intestinal malabsorption. Folacin deficiency may be documented by estimating folacin activity in peripheral red blood cells. Some degree of deficiency of cobalamin may also be present in such cases, and measurement of serum cobalamin provides a reliable index.

Cobalamin deficiency is seen typically in pernicious anemia, but there are other causes (Table 10-12). In addition to macrocytic, megaloblastic anemia, a sore, red, smooth tongue, and mild weight loss, there may also be peripheral neuritis, with glove-and-stocking anesthesia; long-tract damage of the spinal cord, causing motor weakness and loss of posterior column function (position and vibration sense and light touch); and, sometimes, mental disturbance and frank psychosis. The best estimate of cobalamin deficiency is the level in the serum, which is a reliable indirect measurement of body stores.

Associated with deficiency of both folacin and cobalamin is a dysplasia of cells other than those of the hematopoietic system. Cells of rapid turnover are especially affected. Thus bizarre "megaloid" cells are seen in the epithelium of the buccal, gastric, and small intestinal mucosal surfaces. In the small intestine these changes are associated with defective brush-border enzymes and absorption; enzyme activity and the structure and function of the enterocyte are restored to normal with repletion of the deficient vitamin.

Other Effects of Gastrointestinal Disease on Nutrition

Other important malnutritional consequences of GI disease are best considered under the categories of acute and chronic diseases. In acute diseases, loss of fluid and electrolytes, due to vomiting and diarrhea, is the predominant problem. The major cause of acute GI disease is infection with enteropathic microorganisms, such as pathogenic *Escherichia coli, Shigella, Vibrio cholera,* and some viruses, or ingestion of the toxic products of microorganisms such as staphylococci. Management consists of replacement of fluid and electrolytes, especially sodium and potassium and sometimes magnesium and chloride, and specific treatment of any continuing infection.

The consequences of chronic GI disease are usually more insidious. Prolonged malabsorption of fat (chronic steatorrhea) may occur principally because of failure of pancreatic enzyme secretion, lack of deconjugation of bile salts, and disease of the absorptive surface of the small bowel. The importance of this functional defect is threefold: (1) calories are lost in the stool; (2) fat-soluble vitamins are not absorbed normally; and (3) the excess fat in the lumen of the gut forms soaps, particularly with calcium, thereby grossly disturbing a delicate environmental balance. Normally, the major part of dietary calcium is not absorbed and is available for binding organic acids, which inhibits their absorption. If calcium is bound by fatty acids, other organic acids, of which oxalate is an important example, are not bound and excreted but are absorbed. Thus, persisting steatorrhea is associated with hyperoxaluria, and renal calculi consisting of calcium oxalate occur. These renal calculi are a recognized complication of short-bowel syndromes and of Crohn's disease of the small intestine.

DISEASES OF THE ORAL CAVITY

Lesions of the soft tissues of the mouth, such as glossitis, gingivitis, and pharyngitis, may interfere with eating and thus cause a deficiency of calories and nutrients, particularly in older people. The state of these tissues themselves may be determined by nutritional factors. The appearance of the lips, tongue, and gums provides a useful though not a consistently positive index of the deficiency of a number of nutrients, such as iron, cobalamin, folic acid, riboflavin, niacin, pyridoxine, and vitamin C. These changes are discussed, and some are illustrated, in Chapter 1. It should be emphasized that there is a limit to the variety of ways in which nutritional deficiencies and other pathogenic effects of whatever nature are expressed throughout the GI tract. This holds true for the tongue, buccal cavity, small intestine, and colon. Thus glossitis does not in itself permit diagnosis of a specific deficiency.

Diseases of the Teeth

The most common disease in the mouth is dental caries. *Caries* is derived from the Latin word for "decay." The changes involve demineralization of the tooth surface due to attack by organic (mainly lactic) acid produced by bacterial enzymes acting on the sugar-containing substrates. A study in Scandinavia suggests that high sucrose intake in the form of candy is the most important cause [1]. It seems reasonable that the frequency of exposure to sucrose rather than total consumption correlates with the prevalence of caries, but this correlation is as yet unproven.

A concentration of one to two parts of fluoride per million in drinking water confers significant protection in children up to the age of 13 years by a process of irreversible incorporation of fluoride into dental hydroxyapatite. Fluoride ions substitute for some hydroxyl ions. The relatively insoluble fluorohydroxyapatite is more stable and resists acid erosion better. Topical application of fluoride has a protective effect in both children and adults, for reasons which are not understood. It may be an expression of inhibition of acid-forming microorganisms [2].

To date no serious side effects either of fluoridation of water or of topical application of fluoride have been shown to occur, though fluorosis (Color Figure 20) is a potential hazard and might occur in those who ingest unusually high amounts of fluoride from other sources, such as tea.

In childhood, deficiency of vitamin A is associated with poor growth of enamel and dentin. Deficiency of vitamin D results not only in the faulty bone growth and mineralization of rickets, but also in defective calcification of dentin. Defective synthesis and depressed secondary calcification of dentin occur in scurvy, and in adults vitamin C deficiency also causes weakening or disruption of periodontal fibers with resultant loosening and loss of teeth. (See discussion of vitamin C in Appendix 6.)

Carcinoma of the Oral Cavity

Malignant lesions of the buccal cavity, including the tongue, are predominantly squamous cell carcinomas.

Epidemiology   The incidence of carcinoma of the tongue and buccal cavity varies widely in different populations. Together with malignancy of the pharynx, these lesions account for 2 percent of all deaths from cancer in the United States. The lesions occur in a male-female ratio of about 9:1.

When esophageal cancer occurs together with another primary cancer, the other primary cancer is oral in 50 percent of such cases [3], which suggests some causal association.

Etiology   The etiology of carcinoma of the oral cavity is still speculative. Chronic irritation from jagged teeth or from the mouthpieces of old pipes has been held responsible. There is a definite association with chewing tobacco or betel nut and probably with smoking tobacco and heavy consumption of alcohol. It is also possible that long-standing iron deficiency may be involved as a causal factor, as first suggested by Ahlbom [4], but since the lesions predominate overall in males, chronic iron deficiency is clearly not the only cause.

Clinical Manifestations   Nonhealing ulceration of the tongue or cheek is the common mode of presentation. Occasionally, the chance discovery of painless, enlarged cervical nodes is the first indication of tongue cancer.

Laboratory Tests   There is no laboratory test which offers a diagnosis early in the disease. Biopsy and histological examination of a suspected lesion must be done and as soon as possible.

Management   Surgical excision, often combined with x-irradiation, offers the best chance of cure. If the tumor has spread too widely for resection, irradiation alone is used. Curative surgery of cancer of the tongue often requires extensive block dissection of the mouth and neck. Eating may be significantly affected. Current approaches to maintaining good nutrition in such cases are discussed in Chapter 3.

Prevention   Since the cause is unknown, there is no valid preventive measure. Avoidance of tobacco chewing and excessive alcohol consumption and good dental care, together with the prevention or treatment of chronic iron deficiency in women, are the best recommendations that can be made.

DISEASES OF THE PHARYNX AND ESOPHAGUS

Chronic Pharyngitis

Epidemiology   Chronic pharyngitis is a condition which is difficult to define and about which little is known. The important change involved is mucosal atrophy. Difficulty in swallowing (dysphagia) is the usual symptom. In some communities in poorer parts of the United States it may occur in approximately 5 percent of the women between the ages of 40 and 75 years. It is sometimes dismissed as being of psychological origin. When it is associated with chronic iron deficiency, as many believe it usually is, it carries an increased risk of developing pharyngeal carcinoma, so that affected subjects should be examined carefully for this at regular intervals [5].

Etiology   In women chronic pharyngitis may be a consequence of chronic iron deficiency. It has been debated for 50 years whether there is a greater than chance association between iron deficiency and dysphagia. Over this period two eponymous syndromes, the Paterson-Kelly and Plummer-Vinson syndromes, have been instilled into the minds of generations of medical students. They are almost identical and consist of a postulated association of iron deficiency, glossitis, angular stomatitis, atrophic pharyngitis, and in some subjects, a pharyngeal web with dysphagia. However, an epidemiological survey [6] has suggested that there is no evidence for an association between dysphagia and anemia and that the Paterson-Kelly or Plummer-Vinson syndrome does not exist. Earlier reports were based, these authors believe, on patients seen in hospitals, and therefore, the population studied was highly selected. This may or may not be true, and there may, in addition, be regional and population differences. It is likely that the issue is not yet closed. Iron deficiency is far less prevalent in the United States and the United Kingdom now than it was 50 years ago, probably as a result of better diet and better control of menorrhagia, but the condition still occurs in both countries. Further studies of this condition, which is often ignored, should be feasible.

In men, alcohol and tobacco abuse are usually held responsible for chronic pharyngitis, but the relationship is far from clear.

There is some evidence to suggest that chronic pharyngitis carries the risk of developing pharyngeal carcinoma.

Clinical Manifestations   Difficulty in swallowing, particularly relatively large, poorly masticated pieces of meat and other solid foods, and a sensation of ingested food sticking behind the sternum are the common manifestations.

Diagnosis   Diagnosis requires epithelial biopsy and radiological examination, in which barium contrast medium is used and lateral views of the hypopharynx and upper esophagus are taken.

Treatment   Treatment consists of discontinuing the use of tobacco and hard liquor. If there is evidence of iron deficiency, it should be treated together with any other deficiencies that may be present, and the patient should be closely followed [7].

Esophageal Rupture

Rupture of the esophagus is fortunately a rare event. It may occur, however, especially in the frail and elderly, as a consequence of swallowing solid substances, such as poorly masticated, hard food; as a consequence of severe retching following ingestion of corrosives; or as a consequence of diagnostic and therapeutic procedures such as endoscopy and the passage of dilators of various types. Treatment of the condition is almost invariably surgical repair, with the timing and approach determined by the speed with which the diagnosis is made after the event and the extent of mediastinal and pleural involvement. No foods or liquids should be given orally from the time the diagnosis is suspected until it has been unequivocally excluded or surgery has been performed. Formerly, patients were given fluids and 5 percent dextrose intravenously and were fed by temporary gastrostomy or jejunostomy if their nutritional state was judged too poor to sustain them through the reparative surgery, which often involves extensive and prolonged drainage of the mediastinum and pleural cavity. Complete parenteral nutritional support or jejunostomy is now used. Figures expressing the impact that intravenous feeding has had on mortality compared with feeding by jejunostomy would be of value. At present, tube feeding via jejunostomy probably carries less risk of complications, especially in hospitals not especially equipped for total intravenous feeding techniques (see Chapter 3).

Esophagitis

Chronic Esophagitis   Chronic esophagitis is a subacute or chronic inflammation of the mucosal surface of the esophagus, especially of its lower end. The inflammatory infiltrate may be superficial, or it may involve the whole thickness of the lamina propria and underlying structures. There may be punctate erosions or widespread loss of epithelium, leaving surfaces which bleed on contact or spontaneously. Whether this common disease owes anything to diet in its causation is uncertain, though simple reasoning suggests the two might be associated in some way.

Epidemiology   There are no reliable figures of the prevalence of this condition, which must rank with peptic ulcer in its frequency. It is clearly one of the most common causes of nonulcer dyspepsia.

Pathogenesis   Although it is often termed *reflux esophagitis,* it is not clear on the basis of experimental studies whether gastric reflux is the primary cause of esophagitis or vice versa. Certainly gastric reflux can occur without esophagitis. Esophagitis is almost always associated with gastric reflux, which is best demonstrated with a pH electrode probe. According to Pope, who has written an excellent review of the subject [8], the observed data show no clear-cut relationship between a sliding type of hiatus hernia and acid reflux, let alone esophagitis, though of course all three may coexist in the same subject.

Some dietary components act as esophageal irritants. Citrus juices, chocolate, undiluted liquor (spirits), some nuts, and many spices are some of the items of which patients complain. There is marked individual variation. The way in which these substances cause symptoms requires further study. Undoubtedly, some irritants have a direct effect on the esophageal mucosa, perhaps as a consequence of an allergic response similar to that seen with certain specific foods that produce aphthous ulcers of the tongue or buccal mucosa. Others may exercise their effect by the indirect mechanism of lowering the lower esophageal sphincteric (LES) pressure, first described by Code and coworkers, which appears to play a major role in preventing gastric reflux [9]. Whether fluctuations in effective concentrations of some of the known GI hormones, in response to various ingested foods, is an important factor is unresolved, but the problem is a current, active research area. Pharmacologically active xanthines, such as caffeine and theobromine, which are found in coffee and chocolate for example, may affect LES pressure in experimental preparations and in humans, but other factors may exert opposite effects simultaneously.

Esophagitis with gastric reflux is common in the third trimester of pregnancy, possibly as a result of mechanical factors or hormonal effects or a combination of both. A decrease in LES pressure correlates with an increase in circulating progesterone activity.

The smoking of tobacco has been claimed to be an aggravating factor in chronic esophagitis [10, 11]. It is said to cause reduction of LES pressure.

Symptomatology and Diagnosis   The common complaints are a burning pain behind the sternum (heartburn), which may radiate anywhere in the chest, and regurgitation of acid or bilious material into the mouth after meals, on stooping forward or lying down. Stricture, carcinoma, and achalasia must be excluded by x-rays of the esophagus, using radiopaque material.

Management   As a general guide the patients should be questioned about specific foods, solid or liquid, which provoke symptoms. These should be rigorously excluded, and in addition, drinking hot liquids and swallowing poorly masticated solids should be proscribed. Large meals which fill the stomach are to be avoided, and no foods should be eaten for 3 hours before going to bed or lying down. Despite the failure to demonstrate an association between gastric reflux, extraabdominal pressure, and obesity, a short period of maintenance on a weight-reducing diet produces rapid relief of esophageal symptoms in many patients. Antacids help to relieve discomfort or pain and should be used continuously rather than intermittently, and in all but the mildest cases, the head of the patient's bed should be elevated on 6- to 8-inch blocks.

Some dietary manipulation and the use of antacids will partly or wholly relieve symptoms in pregnancy, but occasionally severe damage and stricture of the esophagus may occur.

Should a patient state that heartburn worsens after smoking, advice to reduce or stop smoking should reinforce the patient's own drive to do so, but he or she should also be advised to anticipate the likelihood of gaining weight as a consequence and to take precautions against doing so.

An undefined proportion of patients with reflux esophagitis develop esophageal stricture, and some may develop carcinoma of the esophagus, although this association has not been clearly established. Once stricture has occurred, only mechanical dilation or surgery can relieve the obstruction. The results of surgery are not good. Postoperatively, gastric reflux is likely to recur, in spite of procedures to reduce gastric secretion, such as vagotomy.

Many patients who require surgery have been managed inadequately for months or years and may be severely undernourished and emaciated. Restoration of a better nutritional state before surgery is then desirable and can be accomplished by continuous gastric tube feeding or by parenteral feeding if a patient cannot ingest adequate amounts of a fortified liquid diet.

Acute Esophagitis   Acute esophagitis is caused almost exclusively by ingestion of very hot fluids or corrosives. Where corrosive ingestion is known or suspected, nothing should be given by mouth until cautious endoscopy has been performed to assess the degree of injury. When only minor inflammation is seen, the patient is encouraged to eat a soft, bland diet for 2 or 3 days. When ulceration or hemorrhage is present, complete parenteral nutritional support alone should be given until the risk of perforation is deemed to have passed, usually a matter of 10 to 20 days [12]. Stricture of the esophagus or stomach may subsequently develop. Stricture of the esophagus may respond to mechanical dilation, and there is a good case to be made for early dilation, while the mucosal surface is still not fully healed. Severe strictures require colonic interposition. Gastric stricture, usually of the antrum, requires surgical correction. It is frequently stated that the risk of esophageal cancer developing after significant corrosive injury is about 1000 times greater than in age- and sex-matched controls. There is, therefore, a strong argument for early surgical resection of a severely damaged segment.

Achalasia

A much rarer condition than reflux esophagitis, achalasia is a disease of early middle age in which the circular muscles of the distal esophagus fail to relax because of an unexplained neurological disturbance. The proximal end of the esophagus becomes increasingly dilated and ultimately saccular. Regurgitation of food and aspiration pneumonitis may supervene. Ulceration of the esophagus occurs, and there is some evidence that esophageal carcinoma may be a late complication [13]. Treatment of the disease involves restoration of the patient's nutritional state, dilation by mechanical rupture of the circular muscle of the affected segment, or surgical myotomy of the muscles by a direct approach. Such patients frequently do not have sufficient attention paid to their weight loss and other nutritional deficiencies and show extreme degrees of cachexia.

Carcinoma of the Esophagus

Carcinoma of the esophagus is an important cancer of the GI tract and is responsible for 1 percent of all deaths from malignancy. It may arise in any part of the esophagus.

Epidemiology   Carcinoma of the esophagus occurs in about 12,000 Americans each year. The incidence is about four times higher in black males than white (6.0 per 100,000 versus 1.35 per 100,000). It occurs predominantly in males in a ratio of about 3:1, but there is a special type of hypopharyngeal or upper esophageal lesion associated with postcricoid webs and chronic iron deficiency in which the male-female ratio is about 1:19. Associations with smoking and alcohol consumption have been established epidemiologically, but any specific causal factor still eludes us. In a region in north China and in another region in Iran, the incidence is about 100 times higher than in white people in the United States. Although no local dietary or other factor has yet been implicated, it is difficult to ignore the possible role of food content, quality, or contamination.

Symptomatology   Difficulty in swallowing solids and, later, liquids and regurgitation are the presenting symptoms. There may be retrosternal pain and heartburn.

Diagnosis   Diagnosis is established by x-ray examination (barium swallow), esophagoscopy, and histological examination of tissue taken at esophagoscopy.

Treatment   The nutritional importance of esophageal cancer is its association, even at a symptomatically early stage, with loss of weight as a consequence of dysphagia, first for solid foods and later for liquid foods.

Treatment of cancer of the esophagus involves either surgical resection or radiotherapy. The results of both are, in the main, palliative. Part of the failure of either to achieve a high rate of cure is inherent in the site and nature of the neoplasm, part is a result of the delay in presentation of the patient to the physician, and part is possibly a consequence of the state of malnutrition of the patient at the time of diagnosis and treatment, as determined by the criteria of weight for height and of arm circumference and by clinical and laboratory evidence of a deficiency of protein, iron, and other specific nutrients and even of essential fatty acids [14].

This malnutrition is now amenable to a planned regimen of nasogastric tube feeding, tube feeding through a gastrostomy or jejunostomy, or parenteral feeding, before and after surgical resection or radiation therapy (see Chapter 3).

Esophagectomy and esophagogastrectomy are major insults to the body, and postoperative recovery is usually slow. Return of appetite is delayed or may never occur. Diarrhea persists, and sometimes intestinal malabsorption may occur [15]. The consequences of irradiation are similar. How much benefit will accrue to the patient in terms of quality of life and possibly higher rates of cure as a consequence of better nutrition that permits more extensive surgery or intensive irradiation may become apparent in the next decade.

DISEASES OF THE STOMACH

The major digestive role of the stomach is to serve as a container or "hopper" which mixes ingested food to a fluid consistency and then modulates its presentation to the small intestine for digestion and absorption. In chronic atrophic gastritis, in which gastric secretion of hydrochloric acid and proteolytic enzymes (pepsinogens) may be much reduced or absent, there may be no or minimal disturbance of digestive processes. By contrast, the management of patients after surgical procedures which significantly disturb the "hopper" function of the stomach is one of the major problems in clinical nutrition.

Gastritis

Gastritis is an inflammation of a part or the whole of the gastric mucosa. The inflammatory process may be localized or diffuse, and it may involve the body of the stomach, the pyloric antrum, or both. It is described as superficial when only the superficial layers of the lamina propria are infiltrated with mononuclear cells.

Acute Gastritis Acute gastritis is characterized by edema and hyperemia of the mucosa and sometimes of the submucosal structures and by infiltration with inflammatory cells, predominantly polymorphonuclear neutrophils. A variable number of eosinophils may be present. The body of the stomach and the pyloric antrum are both affected, the antrum usually more than the body.

Epidemiology There are no epidemiological data available.

Etiology The cause of acute gastritis is usually ingestion of some irritant or corrosive. Ethyl alcohol should probably take first place in terms of frequency, but various anti-inflammatory drugs, such as acetylsalicylic acid (aspirin) and phenylbutazone, are important. Staphylococcal toxin, a consequence of faulty handling of food, is another common cause. Ingestion of corrosives and irradiation tend to produce more damage and lesions which take longer to heal and which may sometimes be irreversible.

Symptomatology   The symptoms of acute gastritis are variable. Epigastric pain, anorexia, nausea, vomiting, hematemesis, and fever may occur. The lesions, however, may be symptomless.

Treatment   Treatment consists of maintenance of fluid and electrolyte balance, which sometimes requires parenteral fluids if vomiting is protracted, and a light diet as soon as the patient can tolerate food. Causal agents should be withheld, including aspirin-containing proprietary preparations for alcoholic hangover.

Acute gastritis usually resolves in a matter of days, and the mucosa may heal completely. Whether repeated insults to the mucosa result in chronic gastritis is not known.

In one study [16] it was shown that those who drink fluids very hot show a greater prevalence of chronic gastritis than those who drink fluids at a lower temperature. This suggests a link between repeated acute insults and the development of chronic disease. The claims that alcoholism is associated with chronic atrophic gastritis are not well substantiated.

Chronic Gastritis   Chronic inflammation of the gastric mucosa may be superficial or may involve the whole thickness of the lamina propria. In the latter condition a variable degree of atrophy, with loss of specialized glandular cells, is evident. The changes may be localized or diffuse. The mucosa of the whole of the acid-secreting part (body) of the stomach may be affected, while that of the antrum may be relatively spared. This result is seen frequently in pernicious anemia. Both antrum and body may be affected equally, or the antrum may be more severely affected than the body, as in active duodenal ulcer disease. The inflammatory cellular infiltrate is predominantly mononuclear, consisting of lymphocytes and plasma cells. Some polymorphs and eosinophils may be present.

Epidemiology   Although no satisfactory data are available, the diversity of distribution and the extent of the lesions strongly suggest that chronic gastritis consists of a number of conditions of different etiologies. This suggestion is reinforced by the variety of associations of chronic gastritis with other diseases. There is clear-cut evidence of chronic gastritis in peptic ulcer disease, which is associated with normal or excess gastric acid secretion. By contrast severe chronic gastritis is present in pernicious anemia, in which there is a complete absence of acid secretion. The occurrence of gastric autoimmune reactions in the chronic gastritis of pernicious anemia, and to a lesser extent in that associated with chronic iron deficiency, contrasts with the complete absence of such immune responses in the gastritis of peptic ulcer disease or in what is probably the most common form of chronic gastritis, that found increasingly with advancing age, which almost certainly does not progress to the functional lesion of pernicious anemia.

Chronic gastritis is commonly asymptomatic, and in consequence, its prevalence in any community is unknown. It is very likely that it is a cause of so-called nonulcer dyspepsia in some patients [17].

Etiology   There is currently no evidence that diet is a significant factor in the development of chronic gastritis, except possibly with regard to alcohol ingestion and hot fluids, previously referred to. Long-standing iron deficiency has been considered by some physicians to predispose a person to chronic gastritis. Others believe that the absorption of inorganic iron in the diet is impaired because of gastric anacidity associated with chronic gastritis. The evidence has been carefully reviewed [18]. In general, there is need for well-planned studies of the effects of diet on the gastric mucosa, a subject about which we have little information. Another important nutritional aspect of chronic gastritis is impaired absorption of cobalamin due to reduced or absent secretion by the gastric parietal cells of a glycoprotein termed *Castle's intrinsic factor*. The consequences of iron and cobalamin deficiencies and their treatment are discussed in Chapter 10.

Peptic Ulcer Disease

Peptic ulcers usually occur in the stomach (gastric ulcers) or in the first part of the duodenum (duodenal ulcers), but may be found in the lower part of the esophagus and the pyloric channel and the more distal segments of the duodenum. By definition, they occur wherever there is acid- and pepsin-containing gastric secretion. They may therefore occur in a Meckel's diverticulum of the terminal small intestine that contains heterotopic gastric acid–secreting mucosa.

When the lesion is so shallow that it involves only the mucosa, it is called an *erosion*. Erosions, unlike peptic ulcers, may occur in atrophic gastritis, even when acid and pepsin secretion is impaired or absent. Lesions involving submucosal structures as well are termed *ulcers*. Like erosions, ulcers usually tend to heal rapidly, but some may persist to become chronic ulcers in which fibrous scar tissue surrounded by inflammation is the important feature. Healing of ulcers may not occur or may be incomplete, and in long-standing cases the lesion is irreversible.

Peptic ulcers are usually associated with pain, but there is no general agreement as to its cause. It is agreed that neutralization of gastric acid with alkali, buffering of the acid by protein-containing foods, or a reduction in the amount of acid by drugs which inhibit acid secretion usually result in relief of pain.

Epidemiology   Peptic ulcer disease is found throughout the world. There are data which suggest regional and ethnic differences in the incidence of ulcer disease and the prevalence of chronic ulcers and in site of ulcers, viz., whether the stomach or duodenum is more affected.

Many believe that estimates of the incidence and prevalence in the United States of peptic ulcers of the stomach or duodenum are not yet reliable, mainly because of the lack of a confident diagnosis, which requires endoscopic visualization. A reasonable estimate is that at any time about 3 million subjects have a peptic ulcer, that about 2.4 million of ulcers are duodenal ulcers, and that the male-female ratio is about 3:1 for duodenal ulcer and much nearer 1:1 for gastric ulcer. The best estimates of the incidence of duodenal ulcer are 1.8 per 1000 men per year and 0.8 per 1000 women per year, and of gastric ulcer 0.5 per 1000 men and 0.4 per 1000 women.

Pathogenesis   The pathogenesis of duodenal and gastric ulcers does not appear to be the same. There are almost certainly significant genetic differences as well as differences in the ratio of duodenal to gastric ulcers in various populations throughout the world, familial differences, differences in incidence when acid hypersecretion occurs as a consequence of a gastrin-secreting tumor, and others. They have been reviewed by Sturdevant and Walsh [19]. It seems likely, but is currently unproven, that differences of diet alone must exert an influence, particularly on the stomach, as do many drugs. The influence of diet may in the future be a fruitful field for study, as suggested more than 60 years ago by McCarrison and recently reexamined [20].

Clinical Manifestations   The usual clinical features are epigastric pain occurring with some relationship to ingestion of food. The peak of the attack of pain coincides with the peak in the acid level of gastric contents, which is unbuffered by food in the stomach. Such pain may awaken ulcer patients soon after they have gone to sleep at night, especially if they have eaten late. It is usually relieved by antacids.

Diagnosis   Diagnosis is established by history and the variable finding of epigastric tenderness, but principally by radiological demonstration of an ulcer crater in the stomach or duodenum and by direct visualization through fiberoptic endoscopy.

Management
Diet   Does dietary management have a role in the prevention or treatment of peptic ulcers? Without any clear knowledge of causation it is impossible to say whether dietary management can *prevent* peptic ulcers. The cohort effect observed in men in the United Kingdom born between 1875 and 1900 strongly suggests involvement of environmental factors. Dietary ones seem likely, but to date no likely candidates have been uncovered. With regard to *treatment,* comparisons of bland and unrestricted diets in patients with duodenal ulcers have shown no differences in healing rates [21]. In consequence, the standard practice today is to encourage patients to eat anything they want that does not produce symptoms, to avoid foods that do, and to maintain a desirable weight. Despite such encouragement, some patients still select bland and even "white" diets as a consequence of their conditioning. If they do, they may need supplements of minerals, especially iron, and water-soluble vitamins, especially ascorbic acid.

Patients should avoid late-evening snacks, which stimulate nocturnal secretion of acid, and should reduce consumption of coffee and alcohol, or exclude both. Often it is more realistic to recommend reduction of intake than total abstinence. The latter sometimes strains compliance beyond the breaking point. Rather than impose arbitrary dietary restrictions, we believe patients should be encouraged to use personal judgment, experience, and responsibility.

Medication Use of large doses of antacids, which contain aluminum and magnesium salts in varying proportions, has been shown to be effective in relieving ulcer pain and also in accelerating the healing of ulcers.

In the past 5 years a family of drugs capable of inhibiting acid secretion in response to food or other stimuli such as gastrin or histamine has become available. They are called H_2 inhibitors, indicating the postulated parietal-cell surface receptors they block. Their use in the treatment of peptic ulcer disease has become routine, and despite minor side effects, is likely to displace surgery for the treatment of duodenal ulcer because of their efficacy. The evidence that they produce healing in gastric ulcer disease is less convincing.

Antacids are known to inhibit the absorption of phosphates, inorganic iron, and thiamine. It is highly possible but not proven that the absorption of some other essential nutrients, for instance trace elements, may be likewise inhibited. By analogy with the common practice when using D-penicillamine in Wilson's disease (Chapter 16), it is recommended that large-dose antacids be discontinued for the first part of 1 day each week and mineral and water-soluble vitamin supplements be given.

Complications Complications include bleeding, perforation, and pyloric obstruction. Bleeding may be acute, massive, and life-threatening, or it may be minor and intermittent. Much bleeding is probably undetected. It may be chronic, and iron loss may outstrip absorption of iron from the diet, so that an iron-deficiency anemia ensues.

The dietary regimen in acute, clinically significant upper GI bleeding was revolutionized by Meulengracht [22]. He fed patients after hematemesis as soon as they felt hungry, contrary to established practice, with the result that a mortality of up to 20 percent was converted to about 1 percent. Nearly 50 years later many patients are still fasted unnecessarily after upper GI bleeding.

Both the surgical and conservative management of perforated peptic ulcer require parenteral feeding and continuous gastric suction (see Chapter 3). It is impossible to maintain anabolism with intravenous infusions of 5% dextrose and normal saline, from which vitamin supplements are often omitted. Total parenteral nutrition is maintained until the patient's condition is stable, the return from nasogastric suction is minimal, and bowel sounds have returned.

Pyloric obstruction is also treated with total parenteral nutrition and continuous gastric suction both before and after surgery, until bowel sounds have returned and gastric emptying of liquids and soft food is restored.

Indications for Surgery The indications for acute surgical intervention are massive recurrent hemorrhage at the ulcer site or perforation of an ulcer. Elective surgery is performed in cases of nonhealing or recurrent gastric ulcers, in older subjects with gastric ulcers in whom there is a significant risk of gastric

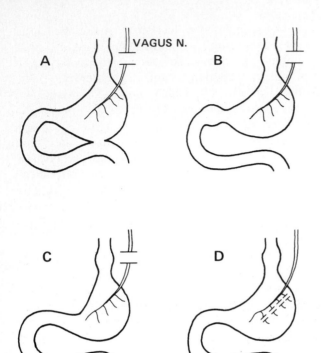

FIGURE 15-1
Selected gastric surgical procedures. (a) Truncal vagotomy and gastrojejunostomy; (b) truncal vagotomy and pyloroplasty; (c) truncal vagotomy and antrectomy; (d) highly selective vagotomy.

cancer, in cases of pyloric obstruction, and in subjects with intractable ulcer pain that is unresponsive to standard medical therapy with antacids and inhibitors of acid secretion. It is well to bear in mind that there is a very high chance that any form of gastric surgery will result in some permanent though often minor disturbance of GI function, and a decision to operate must be based on a thoughtful and individual appraisal of the patient. After surgery the patient may never be the same again.

Surgical Procedures Selected gastric surgical procedures are illustrated in Figure 15-1. In general those with the most favorable outcome in terms of postoperative status do not involve resection. Highly selective, or parietal cell, vagotomy is currently being evaluated as the best means of reducing acid-pepsin secretion without disturbing other gastric functions and is probably the best surgical treatment for a duodenal ulcer. For a chronic gastric ulcer, resection is mandatory.

Gastric Cancer

Gastric cancer lesions are almost always adenocarcinomas and arise from the gastric mucosa anywhere in the stomach.

Epidemiology   There are major differences in the incidence of gastric cancer in different countries and in different regions or population groups within national boundaries. In some countries, the higher risk in the lowest social classes is well established, and higher rates have been observed in urban populations than in rural populations. A significant fall in the incidence of gastric cancer has occurred in the past 50 years in the United States, England, Wales, and Norway. A similar trend has been noted in more recent years in Nisei Japanese in Hawaii and in California, and most recently in Japan itself. These observations have stimulated much speculation about the differences and effects of changes in the environment and particularly in the diet.

Diets high in salt and low in ascorbate, a high consumption of smoked foods, and a low consumption of dairy products have all been entertained as predisposing factors, but obviously no firm conclusions can be drawn [23].

Males are affected approximately twice as often as females in most of the populations that have been studied. If these figures are analyzed by age, the sex ratios in the youngest and oldest groups of those developing gastric cancer approach unity, a finding which suggests that the higher the total caloric consumption the greater the risk. This finding also suggests that dietary carcinogens are involved [24]. In the last 5 years there has been considerable interest in the possible action of N-nitrosamines as carcinogens in the GI tract. These substances may be formed as a consequence of bacterial action on inorganic nitrites present as preservatives in various processed animal products such as ham, bacon, and luncheon meats. The achlorhydric stomach is thought to be a site for these interactions, since it contains considerable bacterial flora capable of producing nitrosamines. This may explain the higher risk of gastric cancer observed in subjects with pernicious anemia.

Future studies of dietary factors in relation to the incidence of gastric cancer (and gastric ulcer) may yield rewarding information. It is heartening that in a world where many hazards to health seem to be increasing, we are, albeit unwittingly, getting something right!

Symptoms   Epigastric pain after meals that is unrelieved by antacids or inhibitors of acid secretion, anorexia, weight loss, and, in a more advanced stage, nausea and vomiting and gastric obstruction are the predominant symptoms. Occasionally, hematemesis or jaundice, due to metastatic spread to the porta hepatis and liver, may be the first manifestation.

Diagnosis   Diagnosis is made by radiological studies of the stomach using barium contrast techniques, and by direct inspection and biopsy using fiberoptic endoscopy.

Treatment   Surgical excision of the lesion offers the only chance of cure, and then only in some 20 percent of patients in whom the lesion is resectable because there is no local or metastatic spread. The usual operation is total or subtotal gastrectomy. The consequences are described below, under "Nutritional Problems Following Gastric Surgery." Malabsorption of cobalamin is invariable, and the vitamin must be given regularly by intramuscular injection.

When surgical cure is not feasible, various types of palliative surgery may be done to prevent GI obstruction.

Nutritional support is always important. Before surgery, total parenteral feeding may restore the cachectic patient, thus reducing the operative risks. When the nutritional impact has been less severe, the diet should be supplemented with protein, vitamins, and minerals. Iron deficiency occurs frequently, and occasionally body stores of cobalamin are found to be depleted. Both nutrients should be replaced by intramuscular injection.

Nutritional Problems Following Gastric Surgery

After gastric surgery total parenteral feeding is not used in the uncomplicated patient because feeding by mouth is usually restored in 3 to 7 days postoperatively, as soon as bowel sounds return and the patient feels hungry. Even when trauma to the lower esophagus during truncal vagotomy results in edema, causing dysphagia with substernal pain, which may persist for 10 to 15 days postoperatively, the patient is encouraged to eat a soft diet, usually successfully.

Enthusiasts recommend that when restoration of oral feeding is delayed beyond 3 or 4 days, parenteral feeding should be commenced. Others favor full parenteral feeding for the first 5 or 6 postoperative days. Lacking convincing data, we have restricted this route to patients who were clearly malnourished before surgery or in whom postoperative complications delayed oral feeding by more than 7 days. Assessment of individual patients is essential.

The majority of the nutritional deficiencies which occur after operations on the stomach develop insidiously over the course of years rather than months. In consequence we know much more about the nutritional sequelae of the earlier surgical procedures, such as gastroenterostomy, partial gastrectomy, and truncal vagotomy, and of drainage procedures such as pyloroplasty than about the long-term metabolic effects of highly selective vagotomy, which has been used widely for less than a decade.

Any operation which destroys or bypasses the pylorus renders the stomach incontinent. The consequences are dumping and diarrhea. Reflux of bile into the stomach may also occur and sometimes may be associated with nausea and vomiting.

Dumping, a term introduced by Mix in 1922, consists of nausea, abdominal bloating and cramping pains, and diarrhea, together with vasomotor imbalance, palpitations, sweating, weakness, drowsiness, and dyspnea, all occurring between 5 and 90 minutes after eating. Reactive hypoglycemia, sometimes referred to as *late dumping,* occurs between 60 and 180 minutes following a meal containing carbohydrate and expresses itself as sweating, palpitations, light-

TABLE 15-4
IMPORTANT NUTRITIONAL CONSEQUENCES OF
GASTRIC SURGERY

Change	Causes
Weight loss	Reduced caloric intake Malabsorption (minor)

Anemia	Iron deficiency due to
	  depressed intake,
	  depressed absorption,
	  or bleeding
	Cobalamin deficiency due to
	  lack of intrinsic factor
	Folacin deficiency (uncom-
	  mon except in alcoholics)

Osteomalacia and
  calcium deficiency
	Reduced absorption of cal-
	  cium and vitamin D due to
	  mild steatorrhea

headedness, confusion and, rarely, stupor. These phenomena are due to the too rapid passage of hyperosmolar gastric contents into the upper part of the small intestine and to the rapid absorption of glucose. Dumping is thought to be due to a combination of contracted blood volume, autonomic reflexes stimulated by duodenojejunal distention, and release of vasoactive hormones by the intestine. The consequence of dumping is that patients are discouraged from eating, and this is compounded by early satiety, which occurs in patients after partial gastrectomy. Loss of weight and nutritional deficiencies ensue (Table 15-4).

Weight Loss   Weight loss occurs invariably after total gastrectomy [25], in about a third of patients after a Billroth I partial gastrectomy, and more often after a Billroth II and similar procedures. It occurs in less than 5 percent of subjects after proximal gastric vagotomy, an operation now about 10 years old, which reduces gastric acid secretion without requiring a drainage procedure. Since the pylorus is left intact [26], the surgical treatment of duodenal ulcer disease is now much less prone to result in disturbed function. However, the surgical treatment of choice for gastric ulcer disease is still partial gastrectomy, so that nutritional problems following gastric surgery will persist and demand expert care.

Although there is a widely held belief that intestinal malabsorption is the major cause of weight loss after gastric surgery, it is clear that inadequate intake of food is the most important factor. Fecal fat values above 15 g per day after gastric surgery are rare, and excess nitrogen loss is minimal, except in those patients in whom small bowel disease is present coincidentally.

Treatment of weight loss requires persistent encouragement of the patient to eat and advice on ways to reduce dumping. It has been demonstrated that the average caloric intake of underweight postgastrectomy subjects averages 75 percent of the requirement for maintenance of normal weight. Successful persuasion to eat usually results in satisfactory weight gain [27]. It is important to reinforce dietary counseling given prior to discharge from the hospital by subsequent additional consultations as the patient resumes full activity and attempts to eat an adequate diet. Dumping can be mitigated or cured by eating frequent, small, dry meals and avoiding sugar and concentrated sweets. Fluids should be taken no less than 30 minutes before or 60 minutes after meals. If ingestion of whole milk causes bloating and diarrhea, the cause may be rapid gastric emptying and the inability of lactase in the upper intestine to achieve complete hydrolysis of the lactose-containing bolus. The consumption of milk should be reduced, or cheese should be substituted for milk.

It has been shown that recumbency slows gastric emptying after gastric surgery [28]. Patients are advised to lie down for half an hour after meals. A small dose of an anticholinergic, propantheline bromide, a few minutes before meals reduces symptoms.

Anemia   Following gastric surgery, anemia, defined as a hemoglobin level of less than 12.9 g/dl, occurs in up to 50 percent of patients. The most common type of anemia is that due to iron deficiency. GI bleeding prior to surgery may have depleted the iron stores of the body. Reduction of gastric acidity may result in depressed absorption of inorganic iron. Reduced consumption of food is a cause of inadequate intake of organic and inorganic iron. There may, in addition, be an intermittent or a continuous slow loss of blood following surgery, from gastritis, erosions, and sometimes recurrence of ulcer disease.

Not surprisingly, anemia is least likely to ensue after the least extensive surgery, namely, proximal gastric or highly selective vagotomy without pyloroplasty or gastroenterostomy.

Anemia is treated with oral inorganic iron, the absorption of which is much enhanced if given with 500 mg of ascorbic acid. If oral iron is poorly tolerated, it is given parenterally.

If megaloblastic anemia develops after gastric surgery, it does so usually many years later, except after total gastrectomy, in which a clinical deficiency of cobalamin occurs between 1 and 5 years later, since the removal of all intrinsic factor–secreting mucosa results in almost complete lack of absorption of dietary cobalamin and of reabsorption of endogenous cobalamin in the bile. The hepatic stores of cobalamin are steadily depleted. Following partial gastrectomy, the loss of intrinsic factor may be only partial, but chronic gastritis may in time cause loss of an increasing proportion of intrinsic factor–secreting cells, and deficiency of cobalamin will ultimately develop in about 4 to 6 percent of subjects within 10 years following gastric surgery. Folacin deficiency severe enough to produce anemia is much less common.

The important rule is to anticipate the clinical expression of cobalamin deficiency by an annual assessment of serum cobalamin activity. Red blood cell folic acid activity may be measured at the same time. If cobalamin deficiency is developing or is already present, 100 μg cobalamin is given intramuscularly each month. Oral folic acid may be given, if necessary, in a dose of 1 mg daily but only after cobalamin deficiency has been excluded or treated.

Steatorrhea   There is frequently a modest malabsorption of fat after gastric surgery, with the degree varying according to the surgical procedure; for example, steatorrhea appears to be minimal or absent after proximal gastric vagotomy. The degree of steatorrhea does not correlate with postoperative weight loss [29]. Possible causes of steatorrhea are incoordination of pancreatic and biliary secretions, proximal small intestinal bacterial overgrowth causing bile salt deconjugation, sometimes pancreatic disease, and, rarely, unmasking of a gliadin-sensitive enteropathy. The steatorrhea is very seldom of a degree that produces symptoms or requires restriction of dietary fat, but it persists indefinitely and sometimes increases with time and age. It is therefore a significant factor in inhibiting absorption of fat-soluble vitamins, including vitamin D, and, possibly more important, in forming insoluble soaps with dietary calcium. Calcium deficiency and osteomalacia occur in up to 25 percent of subjects after partial gastrectomy, and there is a positive correlation with the degree of steatorrhea [30]. There is need for more vigorous prophylaxis. If a postgastrectomy patient cannot tolerate a pint of low-fat milk daily or the equivalent in milk products, then 325 mg calcium lactate should be taken four times daily and 1250 μg vitamin D once daily. Urinary calcium should be measured at the end of 2 or 3 months to check that the patient is not becoming hypercalcemic.

A strong case can clearly be made for avoiding any sort of gastric or vagal surgery, but if some procedure is unequivocally indicated, as occurs especially in the case of gastric ulcer, there is no reason why postoperative life should not be compatible with sound nutritional status, provided the patient receives continuing nutritional surveillance. It should be emphasized that the effects of both cobalamin deficiency and calcium deficiency may be irreversible and prevention should be the goal.

Malabsorption   The causes of small intestinal malabsorption are numerous. We are mainly concerned with causes of chronic or persistent malabsorption, since it is in association with these that nutritional deficiencies are most likely to occur. Memorizing a long list of clinical rarities as possible causes of malabsorption has little to commend it. Table 15-5 is provided for reference. The most frequently encountered and, therefore, the most important diseases of malabsorption are diseases of the pancreas, those in which there is inflammation or infiltration of the small intestinal wall, and conditions in which the proximal small bowel becomes populated by a large number of microorganisms.

TABLE 15-5
CAUSES OF SMALL INTESTINAL MALABSORPTION

Chronic atrophic gastritis of pernicious anemia
Gastric resection
Pancreatic insufficiency
  Fibrocystic disease
  Chronic pancreatitis
  Pancreatectomy
Biliary deficiency
Gliadin-sensitive enteropathy (celiac-sprue)
Tropical sprue
Other enterocytic intolerance (soy flour,
  milk protein)
Small-bowel
  Resection
  Bypass
  Strictures
  Diverticulosis
  Fistulas (usually Crohn's disease)
Crohn's disease (regional enteritis)
Whipple's disease
Lymphoma
Amyloidosis
Hypogammaglobulinemias
Parasitic infestations
  Giardiasis
  Diphyllobothriasis
Circulatory disorders
  Blood vessels: Ischemic vasculitis and occlusions
  Lymphangiectasia
Endocrine disorders
  Addison's disease
  Zollinger-Ellison syndrome
  Werner-Morrison syndrome
  Diabetes mellitus
Drugs
  Colchicine
  Folacin antagonists
  Neomycin
  Phenindione

DISEASES OF THE PANCREAS

About 85 to 90 percent of pancreatic exocrine function must be lost before inadequate lipase and alkali secretion results in steatorrhea [31].

Cystic Fibrosis (Mucoviscidosis)

In cystic fibrosis, dysfunction of all exocrine glands occurs. Secretions of mucus are abnormally thick, and secretions of sweat have an abnormally high content of sodium, potassium, and chloride.

The pancreas ultimately becomes a small fibrosed organ as a consequence of obstruction of its ductular system by plugs of mucoid debris, leading to atrophy of exocrine structures. Endocrine secretions are also affected, usually as a late complication, so that diabetes mellitus occurs as a result of lack of insulin. Another problem is obstructive pulmonary disease, which results from mucoid pulmonary secretions. Later complications are focal biliary and parenchymal hepatic cirrhosis leading to postsinusoidal portal hypertension. Duodenal ulceration occurs more frequently in cystic fibrosis.

Epidemiology   The disease is an inherited one. The mode of inheritance is as an autosomal recessive allele, which has a frequency of 5 percent. The prevalence rate is consequently about 1:2000. The pancreas is involved in 80 to 90 percent of homozygotes.

Symptomatology   The disease usually declares itself in childhood. Affected subjects fail to thrive, are underweight in spite of enormous appetite, pass fatty, foul-smelling stools, and have recurrent pulmonary infections and lung collapse. Increasing numbers of affected children survive to adult life as a consequence of better management of nutritional problems and of the obstructive pulmonary disease.

Diagnosis   The volume and pH and the lipase, amylase, trypsinogen, chymo-trypsinogen, and carboxypeptidase contents of the pancreatic secretions are much reduced. Consequently, malabsorption of fat, protein, complex carbohy-drates, water- and fat-soluble vitamins, and many minerals results.

Treatment   Treatment consists of adequate oral supplements of pancreatic enzyme extracts, such as Viokase or Cotazym, a high-carbohydrate diet with moderate fat restriction, and supplements of all vitamins, if necessary by injection. Hydrolyzed protein supplements that contain short-chain peptides (see Chapter 3) and medium-chain triglycerides in a palatable form may be especially valuable in children with the disease who fail to grow. The peptides are absorbed without need of pancreatic proteolytic enzymes, and absorption of medium-chain triglycerides does not require bile salts; approximately 30 percent of a single dose is absorbed without predigestion by pancreatic lipase.

In hot weather, sodium chloride supplements may be necessary because control of the amount of these ions lost through the sweat glands is lacking. Oral supplements of magnesium and calcium may also be required. Estimations of serum concentrations provide an indication for such supplements.

Pancreatitis

In early attacks of acute pancreatitis, inflammation, edematous swelling, and sometimes hemorrhagic changes in the gland occur. With repeated attacks chronic pancreatitis ensues, with variable scarring and fibrosis of the exocrine pancreas.

Epidemiology There are no reliable data on chronic pancreatitis for any population.

Etiology Alcohol is the most common cause of chronic pancreatitis in the United States, followed by biliary tract disease. Spontaneous forms also occur, viral infections or drugs may sometimes be implicated, and there is a familial type.

Symptomatology Attacks of epigastric pain, nausea, and vomiting after ingestion of excess alcohol are typical of acute pancreatitis, and the pancreas at the time of the first attack already shows evidence of chronic disease. As the disease progresses, pain may become persistent.

The loss of pancreatic function may finally be as severe as in cystic fibrosis. However, nutritional problems arise less commonly because chronic pancreatitis, from whatever cause, is rare below the age of 30, the progression of the disease may be slow, and years may ensue before more than 85 to 90 percent of the exocrine pancreas is destroyed. When malabsorption develops, weight loss occurs.

Treatment Oral supplementation with a pancreatic extract (3 to 5 tablets of Cotazym with each meal) and vitamins provides adequate treatment. If severe steatorrhea persists, the dose of Cotazym is increased. Pain may require heavy doses of analgesics, and habituation to narcotics may occur.

It has been shown that antacids and H_2 inhibitors of secretion of gastric acid enhance residual pancreatic enzyme activity by elevating duodenal pH. In a small number of patients pancreatic extracts are poorly tolerated or ineffective. Medium-chain triglycerides and mixtures of short polypeptides are very useful in maintaining weight and lean body mass in these cases.

Malabsorption or cobalamin is an uncommon but well-documented complication of exocrine pancreatic failure. The ingenious suggestion that it is due to a failure in the release of cobalamin from a non-intrinsic factor cobalamin binder (the R protein present in saliva and other upper GI secretions) prior to binding of the vitamin to intrinsic factor [32] awaits confirmation. When deficiency of cobalamin occurs, 100 µg of the vitamin is given monthly by intramuscular route.

Carcinoma of the Pancreas

The usual type of pancreatic carcinoma is an adenocarcinoma of ductal origin. These carcinomas arise in the head of the pancreas in about 70 percent of the cases, in the body in 20 percent, and in the tail in about 10 percent.

Epidemiology These lesions constitute 2 to 4 percent of all carcinomas. Mean age of onset is 55 years. The male-female ratio is about 2:1.

Associations with alcoholism, smoking, coffee drinking, and diabetes mellitus are claimed, but none is unequivocally established.

Symptoms Pain, weight loss, and jaundice are relatively late manifestations of pancreatic carcinoma. Ill-defined abdominal discomfort after meals, slight anorexia, and some depression are early symptoms, but these symptoms are so nonspecific that they have little value in establishing an early diagnosis.

Diagnosis Earlier diagnostic techniques have been displaced by endoscopic retrograde cholangiopancreatography (ERCP), ultrasonography, and computerized tomography. It is too early to determine whether these methods will provide the means of making earlier diagnosis and thus improve the prognosis, which currently is very poor, the usual figure being less than 1 percent surviving more than 5 years.

Treatment Surgical excision of the pancreas provides the only chance of cure. The standard operations are pancreaticoduodenectomy or bypassing cholecystojejunostomy. The latter is favored, since the metabolic effects of pancreatectomy are profound in that both exocrine and endocrine functions are lost. Total parenteral feeding has had a major impact on the immediate postoperative course, in which there was as high as 50 percent mortality after pancreatectomy. Increasingly, radical surgical procedures are now possible, and if coupled with earlier diagnosis, some improvement in survival can be anticipated.

Nutritional support comprises insulin injections, frequent high-protein and high-carbohydrate meals with Cotazym or Viokase added, medium-chain triglycerides to substitute for long-chain fatty acids, and vitamin and mineral supplements. Gastric acid secretion must be reduced with an H_2 inhibitor drug. If there is biliary obstruction with unrelenting pruritus, cholestyramine is given to chelate bile salts in the small intestine.

DISEASES OF THE SMALL INTESTINAL WALL

The absorptive surface of the healthy small intestine is very large and greatly exceeds what is needed for the absorption of adequate amounts of all known nutrients. Inflammatory diseases of the small bowel disrupt and reduce the absorptive surface. Specific receptor sites, such as those for the cobalamin–intrinsic factor complex, and the activity of brush border enzymes, which play an essential role in the absorption of disaccharides, polypeptides, and folacin, may be significantly disturbed. Sites of absorption for various nutrients are shown in Figure 15-2.

The important inflammatory diseases are celiac-sprue (gliadin-induced enteropathy), tropical sprue, and Crohn's disease, and the important iatrogenic cause of malabsorption is radiation enteritis.

Celiac-Sprue

In celiac-sprue the mucosa of the duodenum and proximal jejunum is affected, with the changes extending to a varying distance caudally. The villi become atrophic, and a major reduction in the absorptive surface occurs as a

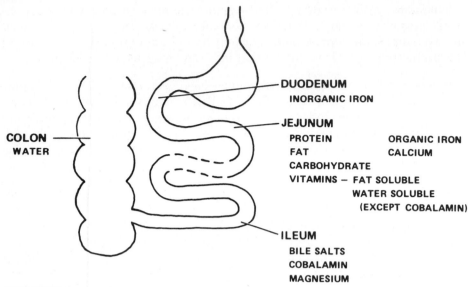

FIGURE 15-2
Sites of intestinal absorption.

consequence. The brush border of microvilli is disrupted, since the microvilli are stunted and misshapen, and the activity of brush-border enzymes is markedly reduced. The lamina propria is infiltrated with inflammatory cells, mainly mononuclear B lymphocytes and plasma cells.

Epidemiology   Celiac-sprue has been recognized for more than 100 years. More than 40 years ago in the Netherlands Dicke concluded that the major cause was intolerance of wheat products [33], and more recently it has been demonstrated that it is the α-gliadin fraction of the proteins of wheat, rye, and barley which exert this damaging effect on the gut wall, but only in a relatively few subjects. Data on the prevalence of susceptible individuals are currently inadequate because reliable diagnosis of the disease requires procedures such as small bowel biopsy and rigorous exclusion and reintroduction of dietary α-gliadin. Thus some populations have been intensively studied and others hardly at all. In parts of Eire the prevalence may be between 1 in 200 and 1 in 500, the highest prevalence recorded. In the United States it is generally thought to be on the order of 1 in 3000. The disease may express itself in infancy after the age of 6 months or in childhood, as failure to thrive and grow, or in adult life, especially at times of special nutritional demand, such as pregnancy.

Etiopathogenesis   The cause of celiac-sprue remains uncertain, but two theories currently are under consideration. One theory is that the basic lesion is a lack of a brush-border enzyme which normally takes part in the digestion of α-gliadin or a product of its breakdown. Such a product exerts a damaging effect on the epithelial cell, possibly by forming a complex with some membrane component of the cell, thereby disrupting its integrity. The other theory is that immunological hypersensitivity to α-gliadin or one of its products is the primary lesion. Immune reactivity to α-gliadin is demonstrable in subjects with the disease, but some believe this is a secondary phenomenon.

Clinical Aspects   The consequences of the disease are impairment of absorption of all nutrients, even of cobalamin, although this vitamin is absorbed in the distal ileum, unlike most other nutrients, which are absorbed in the jejunum. The daily fat excretion in the untreated adult may be 60 g or more, and this malabsorption of fat is associated with failure of absorption of essential fatty acids, fat-soluble vitamins, and such divalent cations as calcium and magnesium, which form insoluble soaps with the fats.

Milk intolerance may occur as a consequence of inadequate lactose digestion by brush-border lactase, and bloating, flatulence, and diarrhea result.

In severe disease, hypoalbuminemia occurs because of excessive loss of protein from the bowel wall (protein-losing enteropathy) and because of malabsorption of dietary proteins. It is rare for the disease to progress to this stage, since diagnosis is usually made earlier and appropriate treatment instituted.

Electrolytes, even water, water-soluble vitamins, and trace elements, such as zinc, are all poorly absorbed. Some of the important deficiencies which are found in untreated celiac-sprue are of vitamin K, vitamin D, calcium, folacin, and possibly other water-soluble vitamins. Deficiency of cobalamin may occur, but it is rarely the cause of hematological or neurological change.

Treatment   The treatment of the underlying mucosal disease is complete exclusion of wheat, rye, and barley gluten from the diet. Functional and structural improvement occurs quite rapidly if the diagnosis is correct and if the exclusion is complete. However, even traces of gluten may inhibit mucosal recovery or precipitate a relapse. Wheat flour is used extensively as an extender in processed foods such as soups and salad dressings (see Table 15-6) and may be difficult to avoid. The American Celiac Society provides very detailed information about the gluten content of foods, which should be available to every celiac patient. When one member of a family is found to be affected, it is usually more convenient and less demanding of the patient if the whole family, when eating at home, adopts a gluten-exclusive regimen. This ensures too that there is less chance of the inadvertent ingestion of gluten by the affected member.

In the more severely ill celiac patient, vigorous nutritional support may be needed during the time that the effects of gluten exclusion are being achieved. Untreated patients may be deficient in electrolytes, especially potassium, calcium, and magnesium, in fat- and water-soluble vitamins, in iron, and possibly in trace elements such as zinc. The majority of such patients respond to oral supplements of these nutrients (Table 15-7). Medium-chain triglycerides

TABLE 15-6
A GLUTEN-FREE DIET

Foods allowed	Foods not allowed
Beef, lamb, pork, veal, fish or poultry	Breaded meat or fish
	Creamed meat thickened with wheat flour
	Luncheon meats, sausage, frankfurters, bologna
	Commercial ground beef with cereal fillers
	Croquettes
Cheese	Processed cheese products unless known to be wheat-free
	Cheese sauces
Eggs	Egg dishes thickened with wheat flour
Fruits	
Vegetables prepared plain or creamed	Creamed or escalloped vegetables if thickened with wheat flour or topped with bread crumbs
Bread and cereal products made from allowed flours	Whole wheat, white, or gluten flours
	Bread, biscuits, rolls, muffins
	Crackers, pretzels, corn chips, and other snack foods
	Rusks, zwieback
	Rye krisp
	Doughnuts, pancakes, waffles, or any product made from wheat, rye, barley, or oat grains
	Bran or bran cereals, farina, grapenuts, oatmeal, shredded or puffed wheat, buckwheat, pablum, or other cereals made from wheat, rye, barley, or oat grains
	Prepared flour mixes
	Macaroni, noodles, spaghetti, and other pastas
Soups made with allowed foods, thickened	Soups containing commercially prepared noodles, macaroni, spaghetti
	Soup mixes and bases
	Bouillon cubes
Fats (butter, margarine, cream) corn oil	Commercial salad dressing
Desserts containing cornstarch, tapioca, or rice	Commercial ice cream with cereal additives; cakes, pastries, cookies, and puddings unless prepared with allowed flours; ice cream cones
Sweets containing white, brown, or maple sugars	Candies of unknown composition
Milk, as tolerated; carbonated beverages	Malted milk or drinks; Ovaltine; commercial chocolate milk; Postum; instant coffee; ale and beer; fruit punch powders
Gravies and sauces thickened with rice	Sauces and seasonings made with disallowed cereal products; commercial meat sauces; prepared mustard; soy sauce; horseradish

TABLE 15-7
SUGGESTED DAILY ORAL SUPPLEMENTS IN GLUTEN-SENSITIVE ENTEROPATHY BEFORE A RESPONSE TO GLUTEN EXCLUSION IS OBTAINED

Potassium chloride	Vitamin K_1
Calcium gluconate	Cobalamin
Vitamin A	Folic acid
Vitamin D	Vitamin C
Vitamin B complex tablets containing daily requirements of thiamine, riboflavin, and niacin	

and amino acid mixtures (see Chapter 3) have been used, but there is no clear evidence that they confer benefit, and the latter particularly are unpalatable and may cause nausea and diarrhea because of their hyperosmolarity. Intolerance of whole-milk and lactose-containing products may persist until the mucosa reverts to normal function and brush-border enzyme activities are restored.

Some children and older adults with untreated celiac disease become severely ill with anorexia, persistent diarrhea, and an inability to tolerate oral feeding. This malignant form of malnutrition can be treated successfully by complete parenteral feeding, and oral gliadin-free feeding can be reestablished gradually. Diarrhea can be partly or wholly controlled with drugs, such as loperamide or opium preparations.

Tropical Sprue

Tropical sprue is a disease of tropical or subtropical areas. The small intestinal pathology is very similar to that in gliadin enteropathy but involves the whole length of the small bowel.

Epidemiology The disease has a definite but unexplained geographical distribution. It is endemic but may assume epidemic frequency, and the onset of clinical disease is sometimes explosive. The current view is that tropical sprue, subclinical tropical enteropathy, and postinfective malabsorption in the tropics are probably all expressions of population of the upper small bowel with enteropathogenic coliform organisms. The chronicity of sprue, as compared with postinfection malabsorption, may be due to a prolonged small-bowel transit time in sprue, a condition which favors persistence of bacterial flora but which responds to antibiotics. Another theory is that dietary fat plays an important role, with long-chain fatty acids having an inhibitory effect on coliforms in the jejunum. According to this theory, the geographical distribution of the disease can be viewed as an expression of differences in fats consumed.

Clinical Picture   Depression or irritability, abdominal bloating and cramping pains, and diarrhea are common manifestations. Signs of some nutrient deficiencies appear early. Treatment consists of oral tetracycline and folic acid and intramuscular cobalamin. Improvement occurs within 2 to 3 weeks. Folic acid, 5 mg daily, is given for at least 2 years to achieve full restoration of small intestinal structure and function. It is more effective when it is commenced in the early stages of the disease [34].

Crohn's Disease

Crohn's disease is an inflammatory disease of unknown etiology that may affect any part of the GI tract but has a special predilection for the terminal ileum and, to a lesser extent, the proximal colon. The lesions involve segments of bowel and consist of inflammation of the full thickness of the bowel wall, infiltration with mononuclear inflammatory cells, formation of noncaseating granulomas, deep linear ulceration of the mucosa, and lymphatic obstruction.

Epidemiology   The disease is of world wide distribution. The incidence in the United States and northern Europe is variously found to be between 1 and 4 per 100,000 per year with males somewhat more prone to the disease. The peak age of onset is in the third decade.

The disease sometimes shows evidence of clustering in families, and both Crohn's disease and ulcerative colitis may occur in siblings, but no clear genetic pattern has emerged.

Clinical Picture   Diarrhea, malabsorption, and intestinal bleeding are the predominant features. Obstruction may result from stricture formation, and fistulous tracts from affected bowel to other structures, including the bowel, bladder, vagina, and skin, occur in probably less than 50 percent of patients.

Important nutritional implications are anorexia, which occurs in the active phases of the disease, partly due to the occurrence of abdominal cramping pain on eating; a variable degree of general malabsorption; protein-losing enteropathy; and iron deficiency due to poor diet, poor absorption, and continuous or intermittent blood loss. The terminal 90 cm of the ileum is essential for the absorption of both exogenous and biliary cobalamin and the reabsorption of bile salts. Deficiency of cobalamin occurs in about 50 percent of the patients with Crohn's disease involving the small intestine, unless they are treated with intramuscular injections of the vitamin.

Management   Careful studies, particularly of children with Crohn's disease, have shown that their failure to grow is due in part to inadequate consumption of food as well as malabsorption of food [35]. During the active phase of the disease, affected children are in negative nitrogen balance. Anorexia, abdominal cramping pain, and postprandial diarrhea inhibit intake, and it has been well demonstrated that a period of parenteral feeding reverses the nitrogen imbalance, corrects other nutritional deficiencies, and allows growing children to achieve a reasonable weight and height for their age. After 4 weeks of parenteral feeding, patients have sometimes been successfully fed once again by mouth because the underlying disease is less active, but relapse does occur. A combination of oral and parenteral feeding, particularly in the prepubertal phase of maximal potential growth, may become an important part of treatment. Recently, a deficiency of zinc has been demonstrated in some patients with Crohn's disease [36]. In patients who develop skin lesions and growth retardation, the serum zinc level should be estimated or 220 mg zinc sulfate may be given orally on an empirical basis twice daily.

In Crohn's disease, low-residue and elemental diets and parenteral feeding have been used in attempts to reduce abdominal pain, the risks of obstruction, and the volume of diarrhea and to allow healing of enteroenteric and enterocutaneous fistulas. There are no controlled trials to support general applications of these diets, and there is much uncritical enthusiasm, now somewhat on the wane.

Reduction of bulk in the lumen may reduce smooth muscle activity in the bowel, but the concept of "resting the bowel" demands critical appraisal. Relief of pain and reduction in diarrhea certainly occur. Permanent, spontaneous healing of fistulas has not occurred in our experience. It is probably rare. Complete exclusion of nutrients by mouth does induce changes in the intestinal mucosa. Experiments in dogs have shown some atrophy of small intestinal villous structure when the animal is fed exclusively by the enteric route. The same changes probably occur in humans and may underlie the temporary failure of function and the occurrence of diarrhea on resuming oral feeding. Intermittent oral administration of an elemental diet has been advocated to mitigate this effect [37].

Surgical bypass of the segments of the bowel affected by Crohn's disease does seem in some cases to be associated with a reduction in the inflammatory response in the bowel wall. This has certainly been so in subjects with Crohn's disease of the colon.

Our policy in adults is to use total parenteral feeding only when anorexia, nausea, or vomiting after meals is protracted and a state of nutritional deficiency is likely to ensue or when diarrhea is uncontrollable. Other aspects of nutritional support in Crohn's disease are similar to those described following intestinal resection.

Radiation Enteritis

The acute response of the small bowel to doses of radiation above 5000 rads is expressed as nausea, diarrhea, and malabsorption within 10 to 20 days of radiation treatment. It has become one of the more common diseases of the wall of the small gut in temperate areas where advanced medical treatment is available. Supportive treatment includes maintenance of a satisfactory nutritional state. Oral feeding, intragastric hyperalimentation, and parenteral feeding all have a place, and the choice depends on the patient's nutritional status, the outcome of radiotherapy (always for malignant disease), and the duration of symptoms. Systemic steroids may help to reduce diarrhea and malabsorption.

The delayed effects of radiation enteritis may appear months or years later. The acute changes of inhibition of epithelial cell turnover, ulceration of the epithelium, infection, inflammation, and edema are succeeded by ischemic changes throughout the whole thickness of the bowel wall, due to obliterative endarteritis. Fibrosis and stricturing may supervene.

Intestinal Bypass

The intestinal bypass operation was introduced about 15 years ago for the treatment of gross and life-threatening obesity that was unresponsive to medical and behavioral management. The usual practice has been to exclude surgically all but 30 cm of proximal small bowel and 10 cm of distal ileum. After surgery, patients behave similarly to those in whom extensive small bowel resection has been performed, and they must be treated (see below) according to the regimen outlined by Wright and Tilson [38]. Subsequently, persistent diarrhea is usual and, in a small proportion of patients, impossible to control and sometimes intolerable. The metabolic consequences of this operation are extremely severe and serious, and sometimes lethal nutritional complications have occurred. There are patients in our experience over the past 12 years who have received virtually no proper nutritional assessment after surgery, the only concern evident in their management being loss of weight. We have seen irreversible hepatic parenchymal, central nervous system, and bone disease and clinical evidence of deficiency of protein, ascorbate, thiamine, folic acid, cobalamin, essential fatty acids, and possibly zinc and hyperoxaluria with urinary calculi. Whether this surgical approach should be used at all is questionable, although it may have been life saving in some very obese patients. The procedure is now being displaced by gastric stapling. If intestinal bypass is done, careful monitoring of the patient at frequent intervals subsequently is essential. Patients who have had an intestinal bypass for many years should be screened for hepatic and bone disease. Some of the complications are listed in Table 15-8.

Metabolic studies and the pattern of weight loss after bypass [39,40] make it clear that the major cause of the initial calorie deficit is not malabsorption but anorexia, which in many subjects subsides in 10 to 18 months. Thus inadequate intake of essential nutrients and some malabsorption occur together.

Small Bowel Resection

Immediate Postoperative Management   Crohn's disease, ischemia due to thrombosis or embolism, trauma, and malignant infiltration are some of the conditions treated by resection.

Wright and Tilson [38] recommend that after resection of the small bowel, fluid and nutrient requirements be supplied entirely by parenteral route until the postoperative diarrhea has fallen below eight bowel movements or 2 liters of

TABLE 15-8
COMPLICATIONS OF SMALL INTESTINAL BYPASS

Immediate	
Infection	Renal failure
Pulmonary emboli	Wound dehiscence

Late	
Acute cholecystitis	Incisional hernia
Anemia	Intestinal obstruction
Electrolyte Imbalance	Liver injury
Hair loss	Trace element deficiencies
Immune disturbance	Urinary tract calculi
Arthralgias	Vomiting
Fever	
Rashes	

daily fecal output. Feeding small quantities by the oral route or by nasogastric tube is then commenced. If feeding is by the nasogastric route, a slow continuous drip of solution is used; it is initially isotonic, and its osmolarity is gradually increased. Carbohydrate is used first, and when 50 to 100 g is absorbed in 24 hours, protein hydrolysates are added and finally small but increasing amounts of fat. If these fats cause significant steatorrhea, medium-chain triglycerides, which are more easily absorbed, are substituted.

Long-Term Management Provided the duodenum, distal ileum, and ileocecal valve are spared, up to 40 percent of the small intestine may be removed without long-term sequelae. More extensive resection (50 percent or more, or resection of the distal ileum and ileocecal valve) results in variable malabsorption, the severity of which depends on three factors: (1) the extent of resection, (2) the site of resection, and (3) the presence of retained, diseased segments of bowel.

Small meals that are low in fat content should be given every 2 or 3 hours. We do not use so-called elemental diets routinely; they are hyperosmolar and increase diarrhea, as well as being unpalatable, but occasionally they are well tolerated. Long-chain triglycerides are added by degree but should be restricted to an intake which does not increase steatorrhea, usually in the range of 25 to 75 g daily. Medium-chain triglycerides can be added as a source of energy. Usually 25 to 40 g daily are tolerable; larger amounts cause diarrhea. The cutaneous application of sunflower-seed oil has been advocated as a source of essential fatty acid. If long-chain triglycerides are poorly absorbed, this procedure, which is too little employed, is worth a trial.

When the patient's bowel has achieved stable function, some or all of the supplements listed in Table 15-9 should be given according to need, as judged by

TABLE 15-9
NUTRITIONAL SUPPLEMENTS FOLLOW-
ING RESECTION OF SMALL BOWEL

Minerals
  Calcium gluconate, 15 g (1365 mg Ca)
    daily (oral)
  Magnesium sulfate, 1-6 g daily (oral)
  Iron as ferrous gluconate, 600 mg
    daily (oral)
  Zinc sulfate, 250 mg daily (oral)

Vitamins
  Vitamin B complex plus vitamin C
    preparations, 5 times RDA (oral)
  Folacin, 5-10 mg daily (oral)
  Cobalamin, 100 μg IM, monthly
    after resection of significant
    length of ileum
  Vitamin A, 25,000-50,000 units
    daily and Vitamin D, 30,000 units
    daily (give orally as combined
    preparation)
  Vitamin K_1, 10 mg daily (oral)

Caloric supplements
  Medium-chain triglycerides as
    Portagen or other preparation

Protein
  Flexical

the patient's laboratory data, since malabsorption of fat, fat-soluble vitamins, calcium, magnesium, iron, and water-soluble vitamins may persist. Intramuscular cobalamin must be given, 100 μg every 3 or 4 weeks, if the terminal ileum has been resected.

Hyperoxaluria occurs in nearly 75 percent of subjects with ileal resection. It is believed to be due to calcium being unavailable to form insoluble calcium oxalate in the lumen, since an increased amount forms calcium "soaps" with unabsorbed fat. Free oxalic acid is consequently absorbed in the colon. Treatment consists of avoidance of oxalate-containing foods, especially many green vegetables, beets, rhubarb, nuts, and chocolate (Table 15-10). Calcium lactate or carbonate given orally should bind oxalate in the lumen. However, oral calcium compounds have not clearly been shown to be effective and theoretically may exert a stimulating effect on gastric acid secretion, which is often high after small-bowel resection, possibly because of a reduced amount of a hormonal inhibitor. Avoidance of dietary oxalate may be preferable.

Hofmann suggested that bile salts, which are not absorbed when the distal ileum has been resected, pass into the colon and inhibit water absorption, thus adding to the diarrhea. There is evidence now that bile salts stimulate the colonic

TABLE 15-10
OXALATE CONTENT OF COMMON FOODS

Foods containing more than 100 mg oxalate per 100 g	
Beets (leaves and roots)	Rhubarb
Cocoa butter	Spinach
Parsley	Swiss chard
Peanuts and peanut butter	Wheat germ

Foods containing 70–100 mg oxalate per 100 g	
Collards	Okra
Leeks	

Foods containing 40–70 mg oxalate per 100 g	
Celery	Potatoes, sweet
Ovaltine	Raspberries, black

Source: Geigy Scientific Tables of Composition of Foods, 7th ed., 1973.

mucosa to secrete water. Administration of cholestyramine, a bile salt chelating agent, improved the diarrhea in many patients if less than 100 cm of small intestine had been resected [41]. After more extensive resection, cholestyramine may be ineffective, and diarrhea is probably due to increased fat content of the stool. Diphenoxylate or loperamide serve to control diarrhea; occasionally opiates, which are more effective, must be used.

DISEASES OF THE COLON

Nonspecific Ulcerative Colitis

Nonspecific ulcerative colitis appears to be a disease entity involving only the colon and rectum. The basic lesion is inflammation of the mucosa, and the submucosal structures are involved only when the disease is very severe or of long duration. Diarrhea and rectal bleeding are the main symptoms. Abdominal pain may be completely absent; if it is present, it is usually mild and may be no more than ill-defined suprapubic discomfort. The pattern of onset of the disease ranges from insidious to fulminating. The latter constitutes one of the major medical emergencies and has a mortality of 5 to 10 percent. Fortunately, it is rare.

The etiology of this disease is unknown, and speculation and research currently invoke an infectious or immunological cause.

Epidemiology   Ulcerative colitis appears to be a disease of areas with a temperate climate. This pattern of distribution is possibly due to masking of ulcerative colitis by other more common diarrheal diseases in the tropics and subtropics. It affects both sexes almost equally. It is much more common in people of Jewish ancestry than in others. It occurs at any age, but the peak decades are the second and third, and in some surveys, a second peak has been noted in the sixth decade, though the reasons are unexplained.

The incidence in the United States is on the order of 5 per 100,000 per year, and the prevalence rate is 40 to 100 per 100,000.

Clinical Picture   Diarrhea and bleeding per rectum are the outstanding features. Weight loss sufficient to cause concern occurs only when the disease is severe enough to produce anorexia, since a major degree of malabsorption is not a feature of the disease. However, when the disease is active, a deficiency of jejunal brush-border enzymes has been convincingly demonstrated, so that intolerance of whole milk due to its lactose content, may occur with abdominal bloating and flatulence. There is also good reason to suspect that immune hypersensitivity to cow's milk proteins may occur in some subjects with the disease, and significantly reduced relapse rates have been observed in 15 percent of subjects with ulcerative colitis who consume a milk-exclusion diet [42].

Treatment   Apart from poorly substantiated claims of the value of treatment by dietary means alone, therapy in ulcerative colitis comprises oral or intravenous corticosteroids in the acute attack, corticosteroids by enema, and for the prevention of relapses, salazosulfapyridine (Azulfidine).

In a severe attack in which toxic megacolon may occur, oral feeding is suspended and effective intravenous nutrition is instituted. However, if the patient is less sick and can tolerate food by mouth, the diet should be designed to stimulate the patient's appetite and to provide high nutritional value. Protein loss from the diseased colon can be great. Only well-tolerated foods should be given. A history of intolerance of cow's milk justifies its exclusion from the diet. The intolerance may be a consequence of hypersensitivity to the protein content or of primary or secondary hypolactasia and lactose intolerance. Our own practice is to advise milk exclusion for those patients, in addition, who fail to respond favorably to a proven medical regimen. When necessary, a soy protein substitute for cow's milk may be used. As regards supplementation with amino acid diets, our own experience has been to avoid them. They are unappetizing as well as hyperosmolar, and since there is no evidence of significantly impaired small intestinal proteolysis in ulcerative colitis, there is no rationale for their administration. High protein intake can be designed around egg or meat protein, with some vegetable proteins included. If, as rarely happens, normal dietary fats can be tolerated in only very limited amounts, minor supplementation with medium-chain triglycerides in a palatable form, e.g., mayonnaise, and in cooking, is worth testing.

Citrus fruits and other foods and beverages with a laxative effect should be

TABLE 15-11
DIETARY MANAGEMENT IN ULCERATIVE COLITIS

Degree of disorder	Aliments and nutrients
Mild or moderate	Give high-protein and vitamin supplements
	Exclude cow's milk if history of intolerance
	or failure to respond to medical treatment
	Avoid citrus fruits and other laxative foods
	and beverages
	Treat iron deficiency by intramuscular route
Severe	Use parenteral fluid replacement and steroids
	Use total parenteral nutrition until controlled

excluded during an attack but can be taken during remissions with caution and moderation if the patient feels seriously deprived. The major points of the diet in inflammatory disease of the large bowel are tabulated in Table 15-11.

Colonic Diverticulosis

Colonic diverticulosis is a condition which consists of small berrylike outpouchings of the colonic mucosa at the sites of passage of mesenteric vessels through the circular muscle of the colon and between the longitudinal muscles. The common site in western populations is the sigmoid colon, but the outpouchings may extend proximally in the descending colon and even involve the whole colon.

The outpouchings may be present without symptoms, or may be associated with mild symptoms like those of an irritable bowel. The important complication is diverticulitis, acute inflammation of a diverticulum. The cause of this inflammation is unknown, but the consequences, which can be serious, are severe bleeding, abscess formation, and local or generalized perforation.

Epidemiology Diverticulosis is a disease of advancing age. Studies in the United States and in the United Kingdom have shown that 33 percent of people over the age of 60 years have demonstrable diverticula. There are data which suggest that in groups of subjects living as far apart as South Africa and South Korea, where diets have a much higher fiber content than standard western diets, diverticulosis is unknown.

Treatment There is a growing body of evidence that diverticular disease is better managed by use of diets of high-fiber content plus stool bulk producers (bran, psyllium, methylcellulose, and polycarbophil) than by traditional low-residue diets. Trials have shown significant reduction in attacks of supervening diverticulitis in subjects ingesting bran regularly [43].

Patients are usually advised to avoid ingesting the seeds of various fruits such as raspberries, figs, and tomatoes, as it is believed that these may somehow become incarcerated in a diverticulum and trigger diverticulitis. This theory has not been proved.

Whether diverticular disease can also be prevented by high-fiber diets is also unproven and rests on inadequate epidemiological evidence gleaned from African and Asian populations. A long-term prospective trial is required to test this speculation.

EXCLUSION DIETS IN FOOD INTOLERANCE AND GASTROINTESTINAL ALLERGIES

A full treatment of exclusion diets is beyond the scope of this chapter. Many patients with irritable bowel syndromes have been committed to long periods of rigid and unappetizing diets from which some essential nutrients have in many cases been partly or wholly excluded on the basis of medical superstition and inadequate empirical testing. However, this should not be interpreted as implying that all exclusion diets are unnecessary.

Enzyme-Deficiency States

Congenital absence of certain intestinal enzyme systems, such as the lactose-splitting enzyme of the intestinal brush border, lactase, may be an indication for the exclusion of a specific sugar. Subjects with alactasia or hypolactasia, may complain of bloating, flatulence, and diarrhea after ingesting 500 ml or more of cow's milk (containing 20 g of lactose). This is due to failure to break down lactose to its constituent monosaccharides, glucose and galactose, at the brush border. Very little of the unhydrolyzed lactose is absorbed; instead it is transported to the distal ileum and colon, where it is fermented by bacteria and is converted to organic acids and carbon dioxide. Another example is sucrase-isomaltase deficiency present in infancy.

In rare cases intolerance of carbohydrate is due to a congenital and isolated defect in intestinal transport, as in glucose-galactose malabsorption, so that osmotic diarrhea occurs when these sugars are ingested. Replacement of dietary glucose and sucrose with fructose results in relief of symptoms.

Gastrointestinal Allergies

Hypersensitivity to other foodstuffs has been well documented ever since the observations of Prausnitz and Küstner [44]. It has been estimated that about 0.5 percent of infants are hypersensitive to cow's milk protein. This hypersensitivity may express itself as a failure of the child to thrive, as fretfulness and flatulence in the child, or in extreme cases, as hemorrhagic colitis with secondary iron-deficiency anemia.

The suspected but less severe and less acute GI allergies create greater therapeutic problems. Patients in this group may present in the clinic seriously underweight and overanxious, sometimes displaying symptoms and signs of specific nutritional deficiency. They may, by a reductive process, have adopted a diet of overcooked lamb and rice or something similar. They are often desperate but initially impervious to rational management. Inquiry elicits the fact that their original symptoms may have been only a transient bout of nausea or of diarrhea, sometimes associated, although this was not initially recognized, with some medication, often an oral antibiotic for intercurrent infection. Many subjects believe themselves, for the above or other reasons, to be allergic to a specific food or a number of foods. To prove an allergy is almost always difficult and often impossible. It is likely that informative tests that are more permissible in this hepatitis-ridden age than the original Prausnitz-Küstner test, which requires transfer of human serum, may shortly become available. The addition of suspected allergens to amino acid diets, which are to a large extent allergen-free, for testing on a double-blind basis has in our hands proved disappointing, since these diets are unappetizing and are so poorly tolerated that most test subjects fail to stay on them the required 10 to 14 days.

Earlier claims by Rowe and others that inflammatory bowel diseases, such as nonspecific ulcerative colitis, are an expression of a chronic dietary allergy have never been fully substantiated. Some observations by Wright and Truelove [42] strongly reinforced this possibility, and since cow's milk cheese was the triggering food, lactose intolerance cannot have been implicated. β-Lactoglobulin sensitivity has been well documented in infants, and rectal mucosal inflammation indistinguishable from ulcerative colitis has been reported in children allergic to cow's milk [45].

In managing GI allergies a thorough, probing history must be taken. Skepticism should never be expressed. The patient's confidence should be gained if possible, and a dietary regimen of exclusion and addition of foodstuffs, one by one, should be devised. The help of a dietitian is valuable here. Experience of success is still uncommon, however.

Since 1973 there have been some reports of benefit being derived from oral disodium cromoglycate, which is thought to stabilize cells in the mucosa which release pharmacologically active substances when involved in some immune reactions. Development of this drug or similar ones may be so successful as to obviate wholly the need for identification of suspected allergens and their exclusion. Another approach may develop from studies currently being conducted of the relationship between the time of first presentation of various foods to the weanling infant and subsequent development of hypersensitivity.

Two principles should be kept in mind. First, as far as it is consonant with achieving and maintaining satisfactory nutrition, the aim should be to devise an attractive diet. Second, as with other therapeutic components, diet should be regularly reviewed. The value of the assistance of trained dietitians cannot be exaggerated in achieving these aims, and it is regrettable that their aid is not solicited more by medical practitioners, since they possess the expertise and the opportunity to apply themselves single-mindedly to these matters.

TABLE 15-12
FOODS OF VARIABLE FLATULENCE

Normal levels
   Meat, fowl, fish
   Lettuce, cucumber, broccoli
   Peppers, avocado, cauliflower
   Tomato, asparagus, zucchini
   Okra, olives
   Cantaloupe, grapes, berries
   Rice, corn, corn chips
   Potato chips, popcorn
   Graham crackers
   All nuts, eggs, Non-milk chocolate
   Jello, fruit ice
   Water (probably the safest of all)
Moderately flatulent
   Pastries, potatoes, eggplant
   Citrus fruit, apples, bread
Extremely flatulent
   Milk, milk products, onions
   Beans, celery, carrots
   Raisins, bananas, apricots, prune juice
   Pretzels, bagels, wheat germ, brussel sprouts

Source: L. O. Sutalf and M. D. Levitt, Follow-up of a flatulent patient, Dig. Dis. Sci., 24:652, 1979.

Flatulence

It is well known that ingestion of certain foods is associated with the passage of abnormal amounts of gas from the bowel. Various beans have such a reputation, and for some, this is a serious handicap to adopting a nutritionally adequate vegetarian diet. A list of variably flatulent foods is shown in Table 15-12, based on studies of a singularly cooperative excessively flatulent patient [46]. These studies provide a valuable model for future studies of large numbers of subjects, from which it should be possible to draw some general conclusions.

GASTROINTESTINAL DISEASE IN THE AGED

The prevalence of GI symptoms and diseases increases with age. In patients over the age of 70 years carcinoma of the stomach or large bowel, peptic ulcer, and intestinal obstruction due to hernias and colonic diverticular disease constitute the major part of the 20 percent of all deaths attributable to GI disease. Such disorders in the older patient require the same modalities of management, including attempts to maintain caloric and nitrogen balance, as in younger patients. More important as special problems of the elderly are (1) anorexia, (2) nausea and vomiting associated with extraintestinal diseases and their treatment,

(3) diarrhea, with or without fecal incontinence, and (4) constipation. These are discussed in Chapter 4. The impact of therapeutic agents on nutritional status, an especially important topic in relation to the aged, is reviewed in Chapter 6.

REFERENCES

1 Gustaffson, B. E.: Vipeholm dental caries study: survey of literature on carbohydrate and dental caries, Acta Odont. Scand., 11:207, 1954.

2 Holloway, P. J., P. M. James, and G. O. Slack: Dental caries among the inhabitants of Tristan da Cunha, Roy. Soc. Health, J82:139, 1962.

3 Goodner, J. T., and W. L. Watson: Cancer of the esophagus, its association with other primary cancers, Cancer, 9:1248, 1956.

4 Ahlbom, H. E.: Simple achlorhydric anaemia, Plummer-Vinson syndrome, and carcinoma of the mouth, pharynx and oesophagus in women, Br. Med. J., 2:331, 1936.

5 Richards, S. H., D. Kilby, and J. D. Shaw: Postcricoid carcinoma and the Paterson-Kelly syndrome, J. Laryngol. Otol., 85:141, 1970.

6 Elwood, P. C., A. Jacobs, R. G. Pitman, and C. C. Entwistle: Epidemiology of the Paterson-Kelly syndrome, Lancet, 2:716, 1964.

7 Chisholm, M., G. M. Ardran, S. T. Callender, and R. Wright: A follow-up study of patients with postcricoid webs, Q. J. Med., 40:409, 1971.

8 Pope, C. E., II: Pathophysiology and diagnosis of reflux esophagitis, Gastroenterology, 70:445, 1976.

9 Castell, D. O.: Diet and the lower esophageal sphincter, Am. J. Clin. Nutr., 28:1296, 1975.

10 Dennish, G. W., and D. O. Castell: Inhibitory effect of smoking on the lower esophageal sphincter, N. Engl. J. Med., 2:1136, 1971.

11 Stanciu, C., and J. R. Bennett: The effect of smoking on gastro-oesophageal reflux, (abstract), Gut, 13:318, 1972.

12 DiCostanzo, J., M. Noirclerc, J. Jouglard, J. M. Escoffier, N. Cano, J. Martin, and A. Gauthier: New therapeutic approach to corrosive burns of the upper gastrointestinal tract, Gut, 21:370, 1980.

13 Just-Viera, J. O., and C. Haight: Achalasia and carcinoma of the esophagus, Surg. Gynecol. Obstet., 128:1081, 1969.

14 Wapnick, S., D. A. Norden, and D. J. Venturas: Essential fatty acid deficiency in patients with lesions of the gastrointestinal tract, Gut, 15:367, 1974.

15 Shils, M. E., and T. Gilat: The effect of esophagectomy on absorption in man: clinical and metabolic observations, Gastroenterology, 50:347, 1966.

16 Edwards, F. C., and J. H. Edwards: Tea drinking and gastritis, Lancet, 2:543, 1956.

17 Edwards, F. C., and N. F. Coghill: Clinical manifestations in patients with chronic atrophic gastritis, gastric ulcer, and duodenal ulcer, Q. J. Med., 37:377, 1968.

18 Witts, L. J.: *The Stomach and Anaemia*, Athlone Press, London, 1966.

19 Sturdevant, R. A. L., and J. H. Walsh: Duodenal ulcer, in *Gastrointestinal Disease*, vol. 1, M. H. Sleisinger and J. S. Fordtran, (eds.), Saunders, Philadelphia, 1978.

20 Jayaraj, A. P., F. I. Tovey, and C. G. Clark: Possible dietary protective factors in relation to the distribution of duodenal ulcer in India and Bangladesh, Gut, 21:1068, 1980.

21 Buchman, E., D. T. Kaung, K. Dolan, and R. N. Knapp: Unrestricted diet in the treatment of duodenal ulcer, Gastroenterology, 56:1016, 1969.
22 Meulengracht, E.: Treatment of haematemesis and melaena with food, Acta Med. Scand. Suppl., 50:375, 1934.
23 Wynder, E. L., J. Kmet, M. Dungal, and M. Segi: An epidemiological investigation of gastric cancer, Cancer, 16:1461, 1963.
24 Griffith, G. W.: The sex ratio in gastric cancer and hypothetical considerations relative to aetiology, Br. J. Cancer, 22:163, 1958.
25 Everson, T. C.: Nutrition following total gastrectomy, with particular reference to fat and protein assimilation (abstract), Int. Surg., 95:209, 1952.
26 Kennedy, T.: A critical appraisal of surgical treatment, in *Topics in Gastroenterology,* S. C. Truelove and C. P. Willoughby (eds.), Blackwell, Oxford, 1979.
27 Johnson, I. D. A., R. D. Welbourn, and K. Acheson: Gastrectomy and loss of weight, Lancet, 1:1242, 1958.
28 Hancock, B. D., E. Bowen-Jones, R. Dixon, T. Testa, I. W. Dymock, and J. S. Cowley: The effect of posture on the gastric emptying of solid meals in normal subjects and patients after vagotomy (abstract), Br. J. Surg., 61:326, 1974.
29 Lawrence, W., P. Vanamee, and A. S. Peterson: Alterations in fat and nitrogen metabolism after total and subtotal gastrectomy, Surg. Gynecol. Obstet., 110:610, 1960.
30 Eddy, R. L.: Metabolic bone disease after gastrectomy, Am. J. Med., 50:442, 1971.
31 DiMagno, E. P., V. L. W. Go, and W. H. Summerskill: Relations between pancreatic enzyme outputs and malabsorption in severe pancreatic insufficiency, N. Engl. J. Med., 28:813, 1973.
32 Allen, R. H., B. Seetharam, E. Podell, and D. H. Alpers: Effect of proteolytic enzymes on binding of cobalamin to R protein and intrinsic factor, J. Clin. Invest., 61:47, 1978.
33 Dicke, W. K.: Therapy of coeliac disease, Ned. Tijdschr. Geneesk., 95:124, 1951.
34 Klipstein, F. A.: Tropical sprue, in *Gastroenterology,* vol. 2, H. L. Bockus (ed.), Saunders, Philadelphia, 1976.
35 Kirschner, B. S., O. Voinchet, and I. H. Rosenberg: Growth retardation in inflammatory bowel disease, Gastroenterology, 75:504, 1978.
36 Solomons, N. W., I. H. Rosenberg, H. H. Sandstead, and K. P. Vo-Khactu: Zinc deficiency in Crohn's disease, Digestion, 16:87, 1977.
37 Driscoll, R. H., Jr., and I. H. Rosenberg: Total parenteral nutrition in inflammatory bowel disease, Med. Clin. North Am., 62:185, 1978.
38 Wright, H. K., and M. D. Tilson: *Postoperative Disorders of the Gastrointestinal Tract,* Grune & Stratton, New York, 1973.
39 Pilkington, T. R. E., J. C. Gazet, and L. Ang: Explanations for weight loss after ileojejunal bypass in gross obesity, Br. Med. J., 1:1504, 1976.
40 Bray, G. A.: UCLA Conference on intestinal bypass operation as a treatment for obesity, Ann. Intern. Med., 85:97, 1976.
41 Hofmann, A. F., and J. R. Poley: Role of bile salt malabsorption in pathogenesis of diarrhea and steatorrhea in patients with ileal resection, Gastroenterology, 62:918, 1972.
42 Wright, R., and S. C. Truelove: A controlled therapeutic trial of various diets in ulcerative colitis, Br. Med. J., 2:138, 1965.
43 Broadribb, A. J.: Treatment of symptomatic diverticular disease with a high fiber diet, Lancet, 1:664, 1977.

44 Prausnitz, C., and H. Küstner: Studiern über die Ueberemphindlichkeit, Zentralbl. Bakteriol. (Orig.), 86:160, 1921.

45 Gryborski, J. D., F. Burkle, and R. Hillman: Milk-induced colitis in an infant, Pediatrics, 38:299, 1966.

46 Sutalf, L. O., and M. D. Levitt: Follow-up of a flatulent patient, Dig. Dis. Sci., 24:652, 1979.

CHAPTER 16

NUTRITIONAL ASPECTS OF LIVER AND BILIARY DISEASE

CONTENTS

INTRODUCTION

The liver plays an essential and, in many ways, central metabolic role. It controls the utilization of exogenous and endogenous amino acids and is the sole site of synthesis of many plasma proteins. It is the major regulator of blood glucose, serving as a store of readily mobilizable carbohydrate in the form of glycogen. It synthesizes cholesterol, plasma lipids, and lipoproteins, oxidizes fatty acids, and provides a store of mobilizable fat. It elaborates prothrombin and other factors essential for blood coagulation, converts precursors of vitamins and hormones to their active forms, and is also responsible for the degradation of other vitamins and hormones.

The liver is a remarkable organ. It has two blood supplies, the hepatic artery and the portal vein. It possesses remarkable resistance to traumatic insults, impressive regenerative powers following partial destruction or surgical extirpation, and an enormous reserve of function. An 80 percent reduction in parenchymal liver mass is consonant with survival and unimpaired intermediary metabolism. The liver receives portal blood directly from the intestine, so that nutrients and absorbed toxic substances reach the liver on first pass through the body at higher concentrations than occur in any other organ. It plays a vital role in the detoxication and excretion of many drugs and natural products of metabolism. One vehicle for the excretion of these substances is bile, which the liver secretes. Bile is also an essential factor in the absorption of fat from the intestine.

It is appropriate to consider hepatic and biliary diseases in concert rather than in separate chapters because of the close interdependence of function of the two systems. Since the primary aim of this text is to emphasize the practical and clinical aspects of nutrition, in this chapter only a short general review of the metabolic implications of hepatobiliary disease is presented. It is followed by an examination of the impact of diseases of the liver and biliary system on nutritional status and of the role of dietary management, if any, in each one. The chapter also includes a short summary of what is currently known about dietary factors in the causation of diseases of the liver, emphasizing the order of importance of these different topics for the practicing physician.

EFFECTS OF HEPATIC AND BILIARY DISEASES ON NUTRITIONAL STATE

It must be a measure of the liver's functional reserve that in neither acute nor chronic liver disease is any consistent disturbance of the patient's nutritional state observed using current probes, unless the degree of hepatic injury is so severe that it threatens survival of the patient.

However, acute and chronic disease of the liver and biliary tract may induce intolerance of some foods, anorexia, nausea, and vomiting, and some of these diseases may be associated with a degree of malabsorption. In acute hepatitis these changes are usually transient, and few nutritional effects ensue of importance sufficient to require special attention. Hypoglycemia may occur as a consequence of failure to store adequate liver glycogen, and there may be some disturbance of plasma amino acid and lipid levels. In acute hepatic failure, for instance, there is an elevation in the concentration of all plasma amino acids except the branched-chain ones, leucine, isoleucine, and valine [1]. But in general, these metabolic upsets are so short-lived that no special supplementary nutritional measures are deemed necessary. This course of treatment is reinforced by the results of studies done in the United States more than 30 years ago which showed that force-feeding patients who had acute viral hepatitis 3000 kcal daily had a marginal beneficial effect on the course of the disease, shortening it by a few days [2].

In chronic liver diseases a deficiency of fat-soluble and, to a lesser extent, water-soluble vitamins has been documented in a significant number of subjects [3]. The causes are unclear. The patients studied were not alcoholics in whom deficient dietary intake frequently occurs. It is likely, however, that an important factor was reduced consumption of food.

When intrahepatic or extrahepatic obstructive biliary disease is present, a situation which occurs in a significant number of cases of hepatic cirrhosis, there may be superadded intestinal malabsorption of fats and consequent deficiency of exogenous and endogenous fat-soluble vitamins or provitamins.

The effects of inhibition of nutrient intake may be aggravated by damage to hepatic cells (hepatocytes) which, when the damage is sufficiently severe, results in a reduction of the storage and synthetic functions of the liver.

Lipid Metabolism

Acute or chronic damage to the liver or biliary tracts may disturb the plasma levels of lipids and lipoproteins. Extrahepatic obstruction as a consequence of gallstones or carcinoma of the head of the pancreas results in marked hypercholesterolemia, the major increase being in the *free* cholesterol component. Cutaneous xanthomas (Color Figure 17), and sometimes peripheral neuropathies due to xanthomatous infiltration, may appear. *Esterified* cholesterol levels are less elevated in biliary obstruction and, if liver parenchymal disease is present, may actually be subnormal as a result of a lack in the plasma of a specific liver-derived enzyme, lecithin cholesterol acyltransferase. This enzyme deficiency is associated with the appearance of qualitatively abnormal low-density lipoprotein (LDL) and high-density lipoprotein (HDL) in the plasma. Serum triglyceride levels are usually elevated in obstructive jaundice, whereas in acute and chronic hepatitis they may be normal or only slightly elevated. Serum phospholipids are disturbed in both biliary obstructive disease and in parenchymal liver disease. Although the total level of phospholipid remains within the normal range, the plasma lecithin-lysolecithin ratio is increased, sometimes dramatically.

The largest elevations of plasma concentrations of both cholesterol and phospholipid are found in patients with primary biliary cirrhosis, a chronic unremitting disease in which intrahepatic biliary obstruction is the major factor.

Even when they persist for years, these changes in lipid metabolism do not appear to be associated with highly significant extrahepatic pathology. There is no good evidence of increased cardiovascular disease; the risk of ischemic heart disease is certainly not greatly increased and is probably not increased at all. It should be emphasized that the lipoprotein abnormalities associated with hepatic disease and biliary obstruction are not the same as those occurring in the hyperlipoproteinemias discussed in Chapter 8.

The changes which occur in red blood cells in chronic hepatobiliary disease do have significance. In chronic hepatitis the red cell membrane contains greater amounts of cholesterol and phospholipid than normal and its physical properties undergo change. In consequence the surface area of the cell is increased, and this increase leads to the appearance of so-called target cells and a reduced red cell survival, which may sometimes result in a significant hemolytic anemia if spontaneous or ethanol-induced acute exacerbation of the underlying parenchymal disease occurs.

Albumin Synthesis

The protein synthetic activity of the liver is usually assessed clinically by measuring the concentration of plasma albumin and the activity of plasma prothrombin. Albumin is quantitatively the most important protein synthesized by the liver. In the healthy 70-kg adult the daily contribution is approximately 12 g to a total albumin pool of 500 g. The stimulus for albumin synthesis is reduction in the extravascular colloid osmotic pressure. Since the half-life of plasma albumin is of the order of 20 days, the plasma concentration is a poor indicator of acute hepatic dysfunction when it is followed by early recovery. In chronic liver disease, either chronic active hepatitis or terminal alcoholic cirrhosis, a significant fall in albumin level is a marker of liver failure. Malnutrition may of course contribute to inadequate synthesis, and significantly increased loss of albumin into the gastrointestinal tract may occur rarely as a consequence of erosive gastritis or of portal hypertension, each of which can cause a protein-losing gastroenteropathy.

The half-life of injected radioiodine-labeled albumin is prolonged in subjects with parenchymal liver disease. This increase in half-life is presumably a compensatory phenomenon to minimize the effects of reduced synthesis of albumin. It must be emphasized that in early alcoholic cirrhosis, even when hypoalbuminemia and ascites are present, isotopic techniques that utilize [^{14}C]carbonate reveal normal or increased albumin synthesis. In these patients the hypoalbuminemia is dilutional and acts as an osmotic stimulus for albumin synthesis.

A marked reduction in the resting and postdigestive rates of urea synthesis occurs in significant hepatic parenchymal disease, and in consequence, elevated levels of aromatic amino acids and ammonia occur in the plasma. The plasma concentrations of branched-chain amino acids (valine, leucine, and isoleucine) are normal or even reduced. This is probably an expression of the fact that muscle metabolism is less disturbed than hepatic function. It may in part be due also to the hyperinsulinemia which occurs in cirrhosis.

These elevated plasma levels are seen in acute hepatic failure even when no protein has been ingested and reflect release of amino acids from tissues, including the damaged liver, and failure of the liver to utilize them.

In chronic hepatic failure, circulating levels of methionine and the aromatic amino acids tyrosine and phenylalanine are elevated and those of the branched-chain amino acids are depressed.

It is often inferred from animal experiments that ethanol has an inhibitory effect on synthesis of hepatic protein in the liver in humans. This inhibitory effect is currently thought to be caused by one of the products of ethanol oxidation, but not by the first product in the oxidative process, namely, acetaldehyde.

Carbohydrate Metabolism

The liver serves as the main homeostatic control of the blood glucose level. A physiologically efficient range of about 10 percent of the mean blood level is maintained in the face of surges of glucose concentrations in the portal blood after carbohydrate meals and steady utilization of glucose by the central nervous system and other tissues. The hepatic parenchymal cells share with the kidney the enzyme glucose-6-phosphatase, which is essential for the intracellular formation of glucose and its release into the bloodstream for use by other tissues of the body. The glucose is derived in part from glycogenolysis and in part from gluconeogenesis; the contribution from glycogen decreases as an overnight fast extends to 24 hours from the last meal, and the proportion from gluconeogenesis increases. Pyruvate, lactate, glycerol, and some so-called glucogenic amino acids such as alanine are the principal precursors of glucose. The regulation of blood glucose involves coordination of glycogenolysis and gluconeogenesis. Glucose precursors and hormones play essential roles in these interconversions. Hepatic parenchymal cells are very sensitive to circulating insulin; a twofold increase in portal venous insulin concentration in a fasted subject results in complete inhibition of gluconeogenesis. These cells are also responsive to glucagon, which stimulates glycogenolysis and gluconeogenesis.

In acute disease of the liver serious disturbance of carbohydrate metabolism occurs only if the damage to the organ is very severe, as in fulminant hepatitis, fortunately rare, and acute yellow atrophy associated with poisoning by paracetamol, carbon tetrachloride, and other hepatotoxic drugs. In these conditions the hypoglycemia is a consequence of failure of glycogen storage and of gluconeogenesis. It may be profound, resulting in confusion or coma. Hypoglycemia is comparatively infrequent in the chronic parenchymal failure of cirrhosis. Its absence is currently ascribed to the very large reserve capacity of the liver and also to renal gluconeogenesis, which may compensate for the inadequate metabolic activity of the liver.

The hypoglycemia which may complicate acute ethanol intoxication in fasting subjects occurs in the presence or absence of liver dysfunction. It is discussed in Chapter 17.

Abnormal oral glucose tolerance of a diabetic type has been observed in cirrhosis, chronic active hepatitis, and acute viral hepatitis. In many subjects in whom there is an abnormal response in the oral test the pattern of the intravenous test may be normal. Portosystemic shunting of glucose, hypokalemia, and failure of release of a putative gut hormone offer partial but not completely satisfactory explanations of this phenomenon. There may be impaired synthesis and storage of glycogen, possibly as the result of decreased sensitivity to insulin by hepatocytes or by cells of peripheral tissues.

The Metabolism of Fructose   Fifty percent of ingested sucrose is fructose and is absorbed unchanged as fructose. Of this, 70 percent is converted in the healthy liver to lactate, which is rapidly metabolized after conversion to pyruvate. In cirrhosis there may be some decrease in the rate of metabolism of fructose-derived lactate, and it may accumulate in the blood. Lactate is potentially toxic and is associated with hyperuricemia.

Vitamins

Water-Soluble Vitamins   There is not much evidence of significant deficiencies of water-soluble vitamins in patients with any type of liver disease, except in association with chronic alcoholism. Even in chronic alcoholism only thiamine, folacin, and possibly pyridoxine are found in some subjects to be deficient to a degree which may have significant metabolic and functional implications.

Thiamine (vitamin B_1), as thiamine pyrophosphate, is the prosthetic group in several enzymatic reactions involved in pathways through which tissues derive their energy needs. The metabolism of glucose to pyruvate and the metabolism of ethanol to acetaldehyde join beyond the pyruvate dehydrogenase step, where acetaldehyde from pyruvate is then transferred to lipoic acid by the action of lipoate transacetylase. The integrity of the pyruvate dehydrogenase complex, of which thiamine pyrophosphate is an integral part, is essential for these reactions.

A nutritionally important degree of thiamine deficiency is seen in severe alcoholics with or without alcoholic liver disease and is a consequence of deficient dietary intake and, presumably, increased utilization. The most severe clinical manifestations are neurological, and are termed Wernicke's encephalopathy and Korsakoff's psychosis (discussed in Chapter 17). Peripheral neuropathy is seen in alcoholic cirrhosis. It may respond to treatment with thiamine. Transketolase activity in red blood cell hemolysates is the most reliable laboratory test of thiamine deficiency. This enzyme is thiamine pyrophosphate–dependent, and in thiamine deficiency the activity of the enzyme in vitro should increase when exogenous thiamine pyrophosphate is added. This result is observed in the red blood cell hemolysates from many alcoholic cirrhotic patients but rarely in hemolysates from patients with nonalcoholic liver diseases.

Pyridoxine   The active coenzyme form of pyridoxine (vitamin B$_6$) is pyridoxal 5-phosphate. The enzyme reactions in which it plays an essential role are transaminations and decarboxylations. One of the first steps in the synthesis of porphyrins from glycine is the decarboxylation of α-amino-β-ketoadipic acid to form δ-aminolevulinic acid; this reaction requires pyridoxal 5-phosphate. Serum and red cell transaminase activities are reduced in pyridoxine-deficient states and restored in vitro by adding pyridoxal 5-phosphate. In liver disease, in which these serum enzyme activities are very frequently elevated as a consequence of parenchymal damage, variable increases in laboratory values may result from adding pyridoxal 5-phosphate to the in vitro reactant mixture. Plasma levels of pyridoxal 5-phosphate have frequently been found to be low in patients with cirrhosis or obstructive biliary disease. Intravenous administration of pyridoxine does not produce as great an increase as in healthy controls. Both increased rates of clearance and decreased rates of phosphorylation have been held responsible for these findings. Deficiency of pyridoxal 5-phosphate may underlie the uncommon pyridoxine-responsive sideroblastic anemia, which rarely occurs in alcoholic liver disease.

Folacin   Folacin is discussed in Chapter 10.

Fat-Soluble Vitamins

Vitamin A   Absorption of retinyl palmitate from the gastrointestinal tract is dependent on the normal absorption of lipids. The ester is hydrolyzed before entering the enterocyte and then reesterified before leaving the intestine. When bile salts are inadequate for normal micellar synthesis, the absorption of vitamin A and of carotenoids is impaired.

The liver is the main site of storage of vitamin A. Hepatic retinyl esters are hydrolyzed before release into the circulation, and the free retinol is bound to a specific α$_1$-globulin, which is associated with circulating prealbumin.

Retinol in the liver is also conjugated to form a glucuronide, which is excreted in the bile. If no supplements are given, chronic biliary obstruction results in vitamin A deficiency as a consequence of continuing malabsorption. This develops only after a period of a year or more, since body stores in the liver are large in relation to the catabolic rate. Thus it is likely to occur mainly in primary biliary cirrhosis. Severe hepatic parenchymal disease may result in reduced storage and failure of release of retinol into the circulation. Signs of deficiency in peripheral tissue appear very late in chronic progressive liver failure; the most common manifestation is follicular hyperkeratosis (Color Figure 4).

Vitamin D   Calciferol (vitamin D$_2$) and cholecalciferol (vitamin D$_3$) are absorbed in conjunction with lipids from the small intestine, and their absorption requires adequate formation of micelles. Absorption is impaired in biliary obstructive disease and sometimes in severe parenchymal liver disease.

In hepatic parenchymal disease there may also be impaired hydroxylation of cholecalciferol to 25-hyroxycholecalciferol, and plasma levels of the latter tend to be low. However, the plasma levels correlate poorly with evidence of depressed calcium absorption and osteomalacia. The blood concentration of

1,25-dihydroxycholecalciferol formed from 25-hydroxycholecalciferol in the kidney determines calcium absorption by the small intestine.

The liver excretes vitamin D in the bile and also metabolizes it through the microsomal enzyme pathway. Barbiturates and some other anticonvulsants induce increased activity in the microsomal enzyme pool. In consequence vitamin D is more rapidly metabolized, and failure of calcium absorption may result in osteomalacia in adults and rickets in children. Both of these conditions respond to relatively large doses of vitamin D.

Vitamin K Both vitamin K_1 (phylloquinone), found in vegetable foods such as spinach and cereals, and vitamin K_2 (menaquinone), produced by gastrointestinal bacteria, are absorbed in the small intestine together with triglycerides. Their absorption therefore requires bile salts and formation of micelles. In obstructive biliary disease absorption is impaired because of lack of bile salts, and deficiency of the K vitamins may occur. This results in a drop in plasma prothrombin and three other circulating blood coagulation factors, namely, factors VII, IX, and X, of which vitamin K is a precursor.

In severe hepatic parenchymal disease similar deficiencies may occur as a consequence of inadequate dietary intake, defective hepatic storage of vitamin K, and defective hepatic synthesis of the clotting factors. Whereas injections of vitamin K or oral administration of the water-soluble menadione congeners (vitamin K_3) will restore prothrombin activity in obstructive biliary disease, in severe parenchymal disease of the liver there is failure to respond. This is interpreted as an indication of irreversible liver failure and carries a poor prognosis. It is important to establish that such patients are receiving vitamin K. The parenteral route is preferred in order to ensure that the drug is being made available to the liver.

Vitamin E (Tocopherols) The absorption of tocopherols is determined by the same mechanisms as the absorption of other fat-soluble vitamins. The tocopherols are antioxidants and may conserve essential fatty acids. That deficiencies occur to a degree causing any symptomatology or clinical signs in adults is uncertain; a hemolytic anemia responsive to α-tocopherol has been well documented in low-birth-weight infants [4]. There is some evidence that in adults in whom intestinal absorption is depressed, as in biliary obstructive disease, red blood cells have a shortened half-life which can be prolonged by α-tocopherol supplements.

Minerals

Iron The liver is a major iron-storage organ, containing in a healthy 70-kg male approximately 300 mg, or one-twelfth, of the total body iron. The iron in the liver is in the form of hemosiderin in the Kupffer cells and ferritin in the hepatocytes. Acute hepatic damage, as in viral hepatitis, is associated with an increased concentration of serum iron and with saturation of serum transferrin, but these effects are transient and appear to have no functional significance.

Abnormalities of iron metabolism in diseases of the liver and biliary tract are mainly secondary to blood loss or to reduced red cell life span. The former commonly occurs in the upper gastrointestinal tract from recurrent erosive gastritis, peptic ulcer, or recurrent bleeding from esophageal varices. An iron-deficiency anemia results (see Chapter 10). In the absence of bleeding the available data suggest that some minor enhancement of absorption of iron occurs, resulting in iron overload in subjects with chronic hepatic parenchymal disease. There is an increased content of iron in the cirrhotic liver.

The picture is very frequently complicated by alcoholism. Inadequate dietary intake of iron may occur and result in a hypochromic microcytic anemia. There may be a block in heme synthesis as a consequence of pyridoxal 5-phosphate deficiency, so that excess iron appears in red cells or their precursors in bone marrow, which are termed *sideroblasts*. There is also a direct toxic effect of ethanol on the bone marrow, suppressing the production of red and white blood cells and platelets.

Calcium   The absorption of calcium may be depressed in hepatic or biliary disease if there is inadequate 1,25-dihydroxycholecalciferol available. In addition the effects of impaired lipid absorption on calcium absorption are more direct, long-chain fatty acids forming insoluble soaps with available dietary calcium. The consequences are most manifest in primary biliary cirrhosis but may also be seen in other long-standing hepatobiliary disease. The response to vitamin D supplementation in the early stages of calcium depletion is excellent.

NUTRITIONAL MANAGEMENT OF SPECIFIC HEPATIC AND BILIARY DISEASES

Acute Hepatitis

The important nutritional aspects of acute hepatitis from whatever cause are some degree of loss of appetite, nausea and vomiting, and hepatic failure due to damage to the hepatocyte population.

The causes are, in order of frequency, infection with types A, B, and non-A, non-B viruses, ethanol poisoning, and sensitivity to or intoxication by drugs. Other rarer causes are poisoning by *Amanita phalloides* and other poisonous fungi of the same family, chlorinated hydrocarbons such as carbon tetrachloride, surgical shock and septicemia, and acute hepatic failure associated with fatty liver in the late stages of pregnancy.

Viral Hepatitis   Viral hepatitis is an acute or subacute inflammatory disease of the liver caused by infection with different viruses, of which two, termed *types A* and *B*, have been well characterized. Other viruses are suspected on epidemiological and clinical grounds and are currently referred to as *non-A, non-B*.

Epidemiology   The agents are transmitted by blood, urine, feces, semen, and possibly saliva. Outbreaks of type A disease may occur from fecal contamination of water supplies and shellfish, and cases of type B occur as a consequence of transfusion of blood or blood products, use of unsterilized needles and syringes by narcotics addicts, contamination of equipment (which may occur in renal dialysis units), sexual exposure, and accidental penetration of the skin in surgery or during an autopsy. Human plasma derived from a large pool of subjects has in the past been an important hazard.

Pathology   The whole liver is involved in an acute inflammatory response, with variable degrees of necrosis of hepatocytes, especially in the centrilobular zone. Sometimes cholestasis may be a dominant feature, occurring as a result of edema and inflammatory swelling.

The most extreme form of the disease is massive necrosis, which involves a whole lobe of the liver and results in fulminant hepatic failure.

Symptoms   The disease may be very mild and detectable only by serum findings of elevated transaminase enzymes. There may be mild gastroenteritis or an influenzal type of illness. Moderately severe disease is marked by jaundice, loss of appetite, nausea, sometimes vomiting, light-colored stools and dark urine, and a heavy feeling in the region of the liver, which is usually tender to palpation and percussion. The severest attacks are those in which acute hepatic failure occurs, often associated with development of dependent edema or ascites and disturbance of consciousness that progresses to coma and frequently to death.

Diagnosis   Leukopenia (both lymphopenia and neutropenia) occurs in the preicteric phase. The serum bilirubin concentration is elevated, and when it is raised to about 3 to 4 mg/dl, the patient becomes icteric. Bilirubin appears early in the urine. Damage to liver parenchyma results in increased serum levels of hepatocyte-derived enzymes, such as transaminases. Hyperglobulinemia and hypoalbuminemia occur. In some patients a definite intrahepatic cholestatic picture occurs. The serum alkaline phosphatase level may be markedly elevated, and the stools become acholic.

In type A viral hepatitis detection of the virus is still not a routine procedure, but detection of type B virus in serum is now widely practiced. When patients with type B viral hepatitis are checked within a week of the outset of the disease, the sera from a large majority of these patients are positive for the so-called surface antigen (HBsAg) and the e antigen (HBeAg).

Treatment   In all but the most severely affected patients, recovery is the rule and is rapid, especially in children.

Mortality in the acute illness is about 1 per 1000 in type A hepatitis and as high as 1 in 10 in clinically significant type B hepatitis. Some patients, particularly those with type B (and with possible non-A, non-B) disease, make only a partial recovery and develop a chronic inflammatory disease of the liver. In some this chronic inflammation progresses to cirrhosis and liver failure (chronic active hepatitis), and in others it appears to be chronic but nonprogressive and is associated only with variable abnormalities in hepatic enzyme activities in the serum (chronic persistent hepatitis).

Nutritional Aspects   Because of the anorexia and malaise which are striking features of acute viral hepatitis, some loss of weight is the rule by the end of the acute illness and in adults may be as much as 5 to 6 kg.

In an attempt to combat this and possibly accelerate recovery, comparisons of patients with viral hepatitis eating low- and high-fat diets have been made [5] and have shown that higher fat intake is associated with more rapid regaining of weight and improvement in liver function. In 1955 Chalmers and coworkers [2] reported the results of feeding servicemen with viral hepatitis 3000 kcal daily. Their intake included 150 g of fat or more and similar amounts of protein. When their recoveries were compared with those of controls who ate ad libitum and much less than 3000 kcal daily, the force-fed subjects recovered sooner by an average of 6 days.

Such measures have not subsequently been recommended or practiced. However, it is clearly sensible to encourage patients to eat a diet as high in calories as they can tolerate, which provides the Recommended Daily Allowances (RDAs) of essential nutrients and thus ensures that no significant deficiency will occur. A few patients develop intractable vomiting and require parenteral fluid and electrolytes during the acute phase of the disease.

Bucher and coworkers [6] have experimental evidence from mice with murine hepatitis that injections of insulin and glucagon together enhance hepatic healing. Now that total parenteral nutritional support of humans is possible, comparable observations in patients with acute viral hepatitis who are intravenously fed different mixtures of nutrients, including amino acids, and hormones are likely to become available in the future.

In convalescence two recommendations have become traditional but are not reinforced by data. These are to eat a low-fat diet, which runs counter to Hoagland and coworkers' studies [5], and to abstain from ethanol. The best advice, since there is wide individual variation in tolerance of both fat and ethanol following acute hepatitis, is to eat as much of a habitual diet as possible and to ingest ethanol in moderation, if it is desired.

The nutritional management of fulminant hepatic failure is discussed later in this section.

Alcoholic Hepatitis   Alcoholic hepatitis may or may not be a precursor to alcoholic cirrhosis. We consider here an illness characterized by weakness, marked fatigue, fever, variable icterus, and heavy ingestion of ethanol for months or years prior to its onset. The peripheral neutrophil count is usually elevated, but on occasion, the bone marrow is temporarily depressed by the direct effect of ethanol and there may be pancytopenia. When absence of a coagulopathy or prolonged bleeding time permits liver biopsy, the liver is found to display patchy infiltration with neutrophils, variable amounts of fatty infiltration, and the presence of alcoholic hyaline. Blood studies reveal moderate increases in liver transaminase activities, the SGOT (serum aspartate aminotransferase) level is almost always higher than the SGPT (serum alanine aminotransferase) level, and there is a moderate to major elevation of plasma bilirubin.

If there is advanced hepatocellular disease, the concentration of albumin in the serum may be reduced, as may the prothrombin activity. Recovery follows withdrawal of ethanol in over 90 percent of subjects [7]. Many patients with this condition have become chronically malnourished over the course of years, and since laboratory assessments of individual nutrient deficiencies are rarely made, full vitamin and mineral supplementation must be provided, with particular attention directed to deficiencies of phosphate or magnesium, of vitamin K as a precursor of prothrombin and factors VII, IX, and X, and of thiamine and other B vitamins. A failed response in prothrombin activity to parenteral vitamin K is an ominous indication of liver failure, which is usually irreversible.

Clinical recovery may be delayed for days and sometimes weeks despite exclusion of ethanol. It is essential to counsel the patient to abstain completely from alcohol, and if there is to be any chance of compliance, he or she should join some supportive program. It is a matter of common knowledge that success is uncommon. The complication of a clinically important amount of ascites in alcoholic hepatitis is discussed in the section on cirrhosis.

Hepatic Damage Due to Toxins

Drugs   The more commonly encountered hepatotoxic drugs are listed in Table 16-1 according to the type of lesion produced and whether it is dose-related or a consequence of idiosyncrasy or hypersensitivity. Clinically those drugs which produce hepatocellular damage may present symptoms, signs, and laboratory changes similar to or indistinguishable from those seen in viral hepatitis. Withholding the drug results in apparently complete recovery. Occasionally, massive necrosis and fulminant hepatic failure and death may ensue. In the case of some of the drugs which have been implicated, early recognition of hepatic damage and drug withdrawal are important and sometimes lifesaving. This is true in the case of isoniazid. Some drugs, such as methyldopa, produce not only a reversible hepatitis but also a chronic active hepatitis.

Mushroom Poisoning   Serious liver damage or failure may follow ingestion of certain mushrooms, of which *Amanita phalloides* is one of the most important and deadly examples.

Epidemiology. Sporadic cases or groups of poisoned subjects who have shared a meal of mushrooms are seen in season in all areas where *Amanita* grow.

Pathology. The toxic effects are due to the amanitidine cyclopeptides, which bind irreversibly to proteins of the central nervous system and liver and cause cell death by currently unknown mechanisms. At autopsy the liver shows acute yellow atrophy and the kidneys show necrotic changes. There are areas of acute degeneration and hemorrhages in the central nervous system.

Symptoms. The first symptoms of mushroom poisoning are abdominal cramps, nausea, vomiting, and diarrhea, which occur 10 to 20 hours after ingestion. There may be an apparent partial improvement in the patient's condition, but this is transient. Thirst and depression of urine formation follow.

TABLE 16-1
HEPATOTOXIC DRUGS MOST COMMONLY ENCOUNTERED

	Cause
Drugs causing hepatocellular damage	
Halothane	Hypersensitivity
Acetaminophen (paracetamol)	Dose-related
Thiopentone	Dose-related
Ampicillin	Hypersensitivity
Sulfamethoxazole	Dose-related
p-Aminosalicylate*	Dose-related
Isoniazid†	Dose-related
Rifampin	Dose-related
Methyldopa	Hypersensitivity
Tetracycline	Dose-related
Drugs causing cholestasis	
Phenothiazines‡	Hypersensitivity
Methyltestosterone	Dose-related
Estrogens	Dose-related
Amitriptyline‡	Uncertain
Imipramine‡	Uncertain

*Some cholestatic properties.
†More common or severe in rapid acetylators.
‡Sometimes causes hepatocellular damage.

Onset of coma and of hepatic failure occurs hours or days later. In fatal cases death occurs in 72 to 120 hours.

Diagnosis. Diagnosis is based on the history, the clinical course, and the conjunction of hepatic and central nervous system damage.

Treatment. The outcome of *Amanita* poisoning depends largely on the dose. In typical outbreaks, several people have shared the poisonous mushrooms but have eaten varying amounts, so that one or two may succumb but the rest survive after illnesses of variable severity. There is currently no effective treatment except to induce emesis or to evacuate the stomach shortly after ingestion and restore fluid and electrolytes and correct hypoglycemia.

Fulminant Hepatic Failure Massive hepatic necrosis results in fulminant failure. The causes may be viral agents, toxic drugs, ethanol, and septicemic shock. In toxemia of pregnancy an unknown factor produces acute yellow atrophy, or what has been termed *pernicious steatosis*. This is a rare event and affects mainly obese, young primiparous subjects, who present with severe headache, muscle pain, abdominal pain, vomiting and hematemesis, somnolence, and renal failure. Mild jaundice may also be present.

The problems presented by fulminant hepatic failure include alterations of behavior and consciousness, a bleeding coagulopathy, electrolyte disturbances (especially hypokalemia), renal failure, hypoglycemia, and respiratory instability.

The patient's breath has a characteristic odor described as fetor hepaticus, a sweet feculent smell reminiscent of mice or acetamide.

Laboratory values are of little diagnostic help. Serum transaminase levels are invariably elevated, sometimes very high. Conjugated serum bilirubin may become very high if the patient survives long enough or finally recovers, but initially it is only slightly elevated.

Management Intravenous support is directed particularly to preventing hypokalemia. Calcium and magnesium levels are monitored, and both are infused if necessary. If hypoglycemia develops, glucose is given intravenously to maintain blood glucose levels within the normal range. Patients are given no proteins by mouth, since these may increase the likelihood of developing hepatic encephalopathy. α-Keto analogues of essential amino acids given intravenously or orally have been only partly evaluated. The results are promising in the treatment of encephalopathy, but there is no evidence that they decrease the metabolic load on the seriously damaged liver.

Vitamin K is always given intravenously (not intramuscularly because of the risk of hematoma production), but it rarely restores prothrombin activity. Therefore, 3 units of fresh-frozen plasma is given daily. This may to some extent mitigate the disseminated intravascular coagulation which often develops.

An H_2 histamine-receptor inhibitor, cimetidine, has been shown to be effective in reducing the incidence of upper gastrointestinal bleeding and should always be given as soon as the onset of liver failure is recognized, since severe bleeding may be the final, fatal event.

To date no manipulations of nutritional factors, such as specific amino acids, lipids, or specific essential nutrients, have been shown to confer benefit. It is remarkable that when recovery occurs, the liver may show no evidence of damage. This observation has been reported in many of the cases studied. The overwhelming impression is that if the patient could only be supported for a long enough period, then the liver, which is known to have remarkable powers of regeneration, would recover.

Because of the possibility of eventual hepatic recovery, techniques for providing temporary substitutes for the patient's own hepatic function have been devised. These have included exchange transfusion, plasmapheresis, cross-circulation with suitable humans or baboons in which previous total exchange of simian with human blood has been effected, and extracorporeal hepatic perfusion using hog liver. None has proved of value.

Experimental studies in rodents have suggested that insulin and glucagon injections together may provide a regenerative stimulus to the liver [8]. Other hormonal factors and various amino acids may also support hepatocyte proliferation, but no convincing studies in humans have been reported. Until preventive immunization becomes an effective protection against viral hepatitis, efforts to protect the liver against harmful agents and to encourage regeneration are clearly worthwhile.

Corticosteroids have no place in the management of acute hepatic failure. In conclusion, it is clear that we lack the means to do more than provide the simplest forms of supportive treatment to patients with acute hepatic failure. The mortality remains depressingly high, ranging from about 30 to 80 percent in recent publications.

Chronic Hepatitis

Cirrhosis Posthepatitic cirrhosis, chronic active hepatitis, and alcoholic (Laennec's) cirrhosis are all characterized by chronic inflammation of the liver, bridging fibrosis, collapse of normal architecture, nodular regeneration, and a variable degree of functional impairment which, as measured by the tests applied today, may be minimal until the terminal phase of the disease.

The causes are chronic infection with hepatitis B virus, an induced autoallergic state, chronic ethanol consumption, and deposition of toxic amounts of iron or copper. These last two conditions are discussed separately because of the special problems of dietary management they pose in their early and reversible stages, but in their advanced stages, when the liver has developed cirrhosis, which is irreversible, management is no different from that recommended for other cirrhotic patients.

Nutritional management is entirely nonspecific. Usually 60 to 80 g of protein of high biological value is recommended daily if the cirrhosis is well compensated. If the subject is clearly malnourished, larger amounts are given. The patient should be kept under observation since there is a possibility of precipitating encephalopathy. Should behavior or mental status change significantly, protein intake is reduced. This and other problems relating to hepatic encephalopathy are discussed below.

Few restrictions of diet should be applied. Most physicians insist on complete abstinence from ethanol. This is sensible advice for the covert as well as overt alcoholic, though compliance is probably poor, but it may impose hardship on the patient of moderate habits who does comply with medical advice but to whom a glass of wine with a meal is one of life's pleasures. There is a need here for designing an individual regimen.

Carbohydrate should be consumed in relatively large amounts, aproaching 60 percent of calorie intake, provided it is tolerated. However, in some cirrhotic patients there is impairment of glucose tolerance due to peripheral insulin resistance, since some degree of hyperinsulinemia is the rule. If glucosuria occurs, carbohydrate intake should be modified to less rapidly digested forms (starch), and if it still persists, the total intake should be reduced. There is no need to restrict fat unless the patient is intolerant of fat or has a defect of fat absorption. In the latter case, there is a risk of malabsorption of all lipids and fat-soluble vitamins. Some patients become aware that certain foods, usually those high in fat content, upset them. They should avoid these.

There is good reason to give supplements of all water-soluble vitamins, since it has been shown that deficiencies may occur in cirrhosis that are not alcohol-related. In the alcoholic, thiamine and folacin deficiencies occur frequently. Vitamins A, D, and K should also be given, since some malabsorption is likely to be present. In the past it has been common practice to restrict the intake of salt only when sodium overload occurs with ascites. A strong argument can be made for guiding the patient toward a reduction in sodium chloride intake to 3 g, 60 percent of the amount recommended in the current prudent United States diet. There are no published studies which show whether this practice will delay the onset of ascites, but since there is clear evidence that adaptation to a lower salt intake can be achieved in a relatively short time, the hardships of a very low salt diet, which is recommended when ascites does develop, will be in part mitigated.

Cirrhosis with Ascites   The onset of ascites is heralded by an increase in girth. Males note it especially because of tightness of the waistband of their trousers.

The development of ascites represents a milestone on the road to liver failure. Twenty-five to fifty percent of cirrhotic patients die within a year of onset of ascites, but it is not necessarily a terminal event. Proper management may be rewarded by years of active life.

The cause of ascites is not well understood, but the factors operating in concert are portal hypertension, a reduction of plasma oncotic pressure (usually as a consequence of hypoalbuminemia), and sodium retention by renal tubules (due to activation of the renin-angiotensin-aldosterone system) and possibly other mechanisms as well.

The kidneys of some patients with ascites are capable of excreting relatively large amounts of sodium. In current jargon, they can generate "free water." These patients are *water-tolerant* and respond well to a salt-restricted diet. The kidneys of another group of cirrhotic patients with ascites excrete only very small amounts of sodium and do not generate free water easily. They are termed *water-intolerant* and will not respond to even a severely sodium-restricted diet. Treatment of the latter group of patients includes diuretics, low salt intake, and restriction of water intake to 1 liter. Despite these measures patients become hyponatremic, ascites often persists, and survival is often short.

Low-salt diets using conventional foods are limited by the restriction of protein and the patient's tolerance. The majority of patients will adapt to a low-salt diet with ease, but some do not. Of the latter, some find a potassium chloride substitute palatable, but a few hard-core salt lovers must be treated with a lesser degree of salt reduction and increased diuretics to achieve negative sodium balance. It has already been pointed out that a gradual adjustment to a low salt intake may avert the problem.

The practice of not adding salt at the table and avoiding salty foods achieves a daily intake of less than 50 meq of sodium chloride. In order to reduce the intake to 20 meq or less, salt-free bread and butter and cooking without salt are essential. Some medications, particularly antacids, contain substantial amounts of sodium and must be eliminated (Table 9-2).

Hypokalemia may occur during treatment with thiazides or loop diuretics such as furosemide and ethacrynic acid. The patient should be monitored, and potassium replaced if necessary. Occasionally the hypokalemia is a consequence of magnesium depletion and can only be effectively treated if the magnesium depletion is corrected.

Since hypoalbuminemia is one factor in the formation of ascites, it would be desirable to correct it. Unfortunately, increasing dietary protein does not result in increased albumin synthesis because the synthetic capability of the liver is usually already fully extended, the exception being a number of malnourished alcoholics. Infusions of salt-free albumin are occasionally effective in precipitating natriuresis.

Hepatorenal Syndrome   Renal failure may occur in patients with liver disease. Numerous conditions may be responsible. Those which are seen most commonly are fulminant hepatic failure and cirrhosis with uncompensated failure, especially in alcoholics; those seen less frequently occur after exposure to toxic drugs and after surgery for obstructive jaundice, especially if it is associated with septic shock. Ascites is often present.

The cause of hepatorenal syndrome is unknown. Treatment is the standard one for acute renal failure, including careful control of fluid intake, monitoring of serum electrolytes and avoidance of hyperkalemia, and a low-protein or no-protein diet. The prognosis is very poor, the mortality rate being in excess of 95 percent.

Hepatic Encephalopathy   Important complications of chronic progressive failure of the liver or of portal systemic bypass of the liver are altered consciousness or patterns of behavior. Minimal changes may be an alteration of sleep rhythm or loss of mental energy, and these frequently go unnoticed. In more severe cases stupor or coma occur, and in extreme cases, death.

These expressions of disturbed cerebral function may be chronic, intermittent, or fluctuant. The changes in function of the central nervous system (i.e., stupor, convulsions, and coma) which occur in fulminant hepatitis are thought to be of similar or identical nature, but the evidence is not convincing.

The causes of hepatic encephalopathy have not been completely identified. In chronic liver disease the association of onset of cerebral disturbance with ingestion of protein or upper gastrointestinal bleeding, which also presents a load of protein for digestion and absorption, strongly suggests that the products of protein digestion are responsible. The current view is that ammonium ions overwhelm or bypass, via portosystemic collaterals, the metabolic resources of the diseased liver and have a direct toxic effect on the brain. However, correlation of circulatory ammonium concentrations and the degree of encephalopathy is only approximate. In about 10 percent of patients with clinical encephalopathy the ammonium concentration in arterial blood, which is thought to be a more reliable source than the concentration in venous blood, is within the normal range. Evidence for abnormalities of other constituents of the blood has been sought, and measurements of concentrations of various substances in cerebrospinal fluid (CSF) and brain tissue in encephalopathic and control subjects have been made.

The concentrations of aromatic amine precursors, namely phenylalanine, tyrosine, and tryptophan, are elevated in the plasma in hepatic encephalopathy, and there may sometimes be depressed plasma concentrations of branched-chain amino acids. Published data are not consistent on this point. It has been claimed that the plasma-CSF ratios of most amino acids are unaltered in hepatic encephalopathy but the CSF and brain concentrations of branched-chain amino acids are elevated, though the plasma concentrations are within normal limits.

Fischer and coworkers have advocated infusion of amino acid mixtures high in branched-chain amino acid content [9], and Walser and colleagues have used α-keto analogues of essential amino acids orally or intravenously to reduce the concentration of glutamine, which serves as the amino donor [10]. Currently no regimen with a predictable outcome that uses these preparations has been devised, and we continue to apply the following standard procedures.

At the onset of encephalopathy protein should be totally excluded. If the patient is conscious, glucose drinks are given. Otherwise fluid and electrolytes are administered intravenously together with 10% glucose. Since the origins of "ammonia" are at least in part the bowel flora, enemas are used to wash out colonic contents.

If bleeding is the precipitating cause, treatment is directed to its control. Many centers still use neomycin or some other nonabsorbed antibiotic to suppress urea-splitting organisms. We have found lactulose, given in divided oral doses totaling 60 to 100 g daily, an effective treatment. Lactulose is a synthetic disaccharide which is not hydrolyzed by the mammalian brush-border enzymes. It therefore passes down the small intestine unmetabolized until it reaches the bacterial flora of the terminal ileum and colon. It constitutes a hyperosmolar load and produces diarrhea. Bacterial enzymatic action splits some of the molecule into lactic and other organic acids, the luminal pH is lowered, and ammonium ions are trapped. Following recovery of consciousness, protein is introduced into the diet in increments of 20 g per day every 3 days, the protein being distributed evenly through the day. Lactulose administration is continued, the dose being adjusted to produce about three bowel movements per day. This regimen permits higher protein intake than would be possible if it were given alone, and many patients are able to consume 60 to 100 g or more of protein daily, an amount consonant with positive nitrogen balance. However, as deterioration of liver function proceeds, tolerance of ingested protein gradually diminishes, or upper gastrointestinal bleeding from esophageal varices, gastric erosions, or ulcers precipitates increasingly frequent attacks of coma and death eventually occurs.

Primary Biliary Cirrhosis

Epidemiology   Primary biliary cirrhosis is an uncommon disease of unknown etiology predominantly affecting middle-aged women. The female-male ratio is 9:1. It constitutes between 0.6 and 2 percent of all deaths from cirrhosis.

Pathology   Progressive intrahepatic cholestasis occurs as a consequence of patchy inflammatory infiltration of the portal triads. Plasma cells and lymphocytes predominate in the lesions, and granulomas may be seen, with giant-cell formation, in the region of the biliary ductules which undergo lysis. Later in the course of the disease the changes in the liver increasingly approximate postnecrotic cirrhosis. There are autoallergic components to the disease.

Symptoms   The onset is insidious. Fatigue or pruritus may be the first evidence of the disease. Jaundice is at first absent or minimal. The urine becomes darker, and the stools lighten. Cutaneous xanthomas develop in the skin flexures of the hands later in the course of the disease (Color Figure 18), and yellow-brown pigmentation of the skin becomes increasingly deep. The liver is enlarged and firm, and the spleen is often palpable. Weight loss and steatorrhea occur as a result of cholestasis, and lipid-soluble nutrients are depleted. Hypoprothrombinemia occurs as a result of deficiency of vitamin K, and pathological fractures and vertebral compression occur as a consequence of calcium and vitamin D deficiency. Osteoporosis is found, as well as osteomalacia, reflecting both protein wasting, as a consequence of the liver disease, and the effects of treatment with corticosteroids.

Treatment   Nutritional support of this chronic, inexorably progressive disease is assuming increasing importance. It is essentially the same as that for patients with chronic biliary stricture or atresia, since the basic disturbance is a deficiency of intestinal bile salts, and consists of the following:

1 Restriction of long-chain fatty acid intake. These are poorly absorbed, and in consequence malabsorption of calcium, magnesium, and fat-soluble vitamins occurs. Restriction to less than 40 g daily is achieved by drinking low-fat milk, avoiding butter and cheese and all visible fat on meat or poultry, and adding medium-chain triglycerides in the form of Portagen (Mead Johnson) to the diet.

2 Supplementation with 1 g of calcium daily, most commonly as calcium gluconate. Magnesium is not given routinely, but magnesium deficiency may occur. In this event 1 g magnesium carbonate is given daily.

3 Supplementation with the following vitamins monthly by intramuscular injection: vitamin A, 100,000 units; vitamin D, 100,000 units; and vitamin K (as Phytomenadione), 10 mg.

Cholestyramine is often given before each meal to prevent bile salt reabsorption and to reduce pruritus. It is important not to give calcium with cholestyramine in order to avoid chelating the calcium, which makes it unabsorbable.

In advanced disease, bone pain and fractures may not be prevented by the above regimen, and intravenous calcium gluconate (15 mg of calcium per kilogram of body weight in 5% dextrose each day for 7 days) is recommended [11]. It is claimed that 15 to 30 μg of 1,25-dihydroxycholecalciferol given intramuscularly each month may improve the symptoms of the bone disease and the myopathy which is sometimes seen in primary biliary cirrhosis.

Hepatic retention of copper as a consequence of diminished biliary excretion of the metal is high in primary biliary cirrhosis. Trials of D-penicillamine, which mobilizes hepatic copper by chelation and takes it out of the body through the kidney, have been reported but there is no evidence to date of a beneficial effect on the course of the disease. D-Penicillamine is a drug with significant toxicity. Copper is widely distributed in foodstuffs; nuts, liver, kidney, chocolate, corn oil margarine, mushrooms, shellfish, and dried legumes have a particularly high content of copper. Avoidance of such foods, which does not constitute a major hardship or health hazard, should be recommended as soon as a diagnosis of primary biliary cirrhosis is made.

Chronic Biliary Obstruction

In patients in whom surgical correction is planned, no special nutritional support is necessary other than preoperative measures to restore prothrombin and other blood coagulation factors with intramuscular injections of vitamin K (10 mg Phytomenadione).

In cases in which obstructive disease is not remediable, the nutritional problems are the same as those in primary biliary cirrhosis.

Congenital Biliary Atresia The surgically untreatable or unsuccessfully surgically treated infant or child with congenital biliary atresia is treated with a low intake of long-chain fatty acids as triglycerides, medium-chain triglyceride supplementation in low-fat milk shakes and other palatable forms (see Chapter 3), high protein and high-carbohydrate intake, and monthly intramuscular injections of fat-soluble vitamins. Oral supplementation of calcium and magnesium is also given, and it is recommended that levels of both be monitored regularly every 2 weeks until a stable regimen has been established. At best the child will lead a relatively normal life for some years, but ultimately portal hypertension, ascites, and liver failure supervene. Whether retention of copper or other metal has a toxic effect on the liver has not been studied. It would seem to be a relatively simple and prudent matter to adopt a diet low in copper content.

Acquired Biliary Obstruction The dietary management of a patient with acquired biliary obstruction is the same as that for primary biliary cirrhosis.

Hepatolenticular Degeneration (Wilson's Disease)

Epidemiology Wilson's disease is a rare disease in which copper accumulates steadily to toxic concentrations in the liver, brain, eye, and kidney. Prevalence is believed to be about 1 in 200,000, and there have been a total of about 1100 known cases in the United States. It is the product of autosomal recessive inheritance.

Symptoms   The presenting symptoms are hepatic or neurological. The liver disease (cirrhosis and progressive hepatic failure) tends to declare itself earlier than that of the central nervous system. Portal hypertension may develop, splenomegaly may appear, and death may occur as a consequence of variceal bleeding.

Biochemical studies reveal a significant reduction in the plasma concentration of a blue copper-binding glycoprotein called *ceruloplasmin* in all but 5 percent of subjects homozygous for Wilson's disease. A similar reduction is found in 10 percent of heterozygotes. As with primary biliary cirrhosis or chronic biliary obstruction, the liver contains increased amounts of copper, distributed unevenly through the parenchyma.

Dietary Management   Treatment of Wilson's disease is aimed at the following:

1 Reducing copper absorption and mobilizing copper in the liver, brain, and other organs.

2 Providing nutritional support for liver failure, of which ascites may be a late expression.

Low-copper diets may be of value, although the mainstay of treatment is D-penicillamine. Foods of high copper content, such as nuts, chocolate, mushrooms, liver, kidney, corn oil margarine, dried legumes, and shellfish, should be avoided. The diet should be low in salt (40 to 80 meq) and provide adequate protein and calories. Although D-penicillamine is an effective drug for inhibiting copper absorption, it may cause ageusia (loss of taste), anorexia, and nausea. Since it is now recommended that D-penicillamine be taken indefinitely, there may be some difficulty in maintaining good nutritional status in patients. A practical way to combat this is to withhold the drug for 1 day every 2 weeks and have the patient ingest essential nutrients in large amounts that day. The patient's weight should be checked every 2 weeks, and evidence of nutritional deficiency should be looked for. Iron deficiency is likely to occur in young women and children being treated, and regular oral supplementation with iron should be given. If liver failure or portosystemic bypass occurs, the patient may develop encephalopathy as a consequence of too high a dietary protein intake or upper gastrointestinal bleeding.

Recent data suggest that treatment to reduce the copper load of the liver and brain is effective.

It is recommended that the pyridoxine antagonistic effect of D-penicillamine should be countered by giving 25 mg of pyridoxine orally each day. Wilson's disease is also discussed in Chapter 18.

Hemochromatosis and Iron-Storage Diseases

As a consequence of a persistent, slightly abnormal elevation of intestinal iron aborption, prolonged exposure to high dietary iron content, or repeated transfusions with red blood cells, many organs of the body develop iron overload. Only the first of these three categories, termed *primary hemo-chromatosis,* is discussed here.

Primary Hemochromatosis

Epidemiology   Primary hemochromatosis is an inherited defect. The overt disease displays a male-female ratio of about 5:1. Family studies, the increased frequency of HLA-A3 and HLA-B14 histocompatibility antigens, and the frequent negative history of alcohol consumption in primary hemochromatosis help to separate the disease as an entity from alcoholic cirrhosis, in which an accumulation of hepatic iron as a secondary event seems to occur.

Pathology   The presence of high concentrations of intracellular iron for prolonged periods causes cell damage in many organs such as the liver, heart, and pancreas, possibly through a mechanism of induction of increased lysosomal fragility and increased concentrations of acid hydrolases. The total body load of iron may be as much as 20 to 40 g, as compared with the normal iron load of 4 to 5 g.

Symptoms   The clinical picture is progressive liver and cardiac damage, which, if untreated, terminate in irreversible cirrhosis and progressive heart failure. Primary liver cancer may be a terminal event. The earliest symptoms are bronze pigmentation of the skin, some loss of energy and libido, and an enlarged liver. Diabetes mellitus occurs as a consequence of pancreatic involvement.

Diagnosis   A liver biopsy showing increased iron content without cirrhotic changes in the early stages but with a variable degree of cirrhosis later in the course of the disease is the best diagnostic test. Serum iron levels are elevated, the concentration of the β_1-globulin iron-binding protein, transferrin, is reduced, the transferrin is completely saturated, and the amount of circulating ferritin is increased.

Treatment   Treatment is based on regular phlebotomy, by which means about 15 g of iron can be removed annually.

There is no proven advantage to adopting a special diet.

When irreversible damage to the liver has become established, the treatment, including dietary management, is the same as in other chronic liver diseases.

Two current areas of concern are worth addressing in the context of iron overload and its consequences. The first is whether the currently widespread practice of consuming 500 to 2000 mg of ascorbic acid daily carries a risk of inducing iron overload because of the ability of ascorbic acid to enhance significantly the absorption of inorganic iron or, as appears possible from recent observations of a thalassemic patient who already had an iron overload, to induce tissue damage by causing some hitherto unsuspected translocation of tissue iron [12].

Currently there are insufficient data on which to base any recommendation other than a clear contraindication to the ingestion of massive doses of ascorbic acid or ascorbate-containing foods by subjects with iron-overload disease or by their relatives.

The second, related problem is whether wheat flour should be fortified with iron at all or at a relatively high level. Crosby [13] has criticized fortification of bread on the grounds that it constitutes a hazard to subjects with latent hemochromatosis. His argument is supported by the observed rarity of overt hemochromatosis in women during their menstrual lives. The male-female ratio is approximately 5:1. Currently in Sweden there has been a progressive decrease in iron-deficiency anemia in females concurrent with a stepwise increase in degree of iron fortification of flour; there has been no reported increase in hemochromatosis in either males or females [14].

Since hemochromatosis is a disease with a prolonged incubation period, this problem is not likely to be settled for some years.

Nonhemolytic Hyperbilirubinemic Syndromes

There are a number of nonhemolytic hyperbilirubinemic syndromes. Those in which unconjugated bilirubin levels are elevated are expressions of a deficiency of an hepatic enzyme called *glucuronyl transferase* (Gilbert's syndrome; Crigler-Najjar syndrome), which catalyzes the conjugation of bilirubin. Those in which conjugated bilirubin is elevated (Dubin-Johnson syndrome; Rotor syndrome) are expressions of decreased secretion of conjugated bilirubin into the bile for reasons currently not well understood. In some of these, treatment with phenobarbital has been shown to lower circulating bilirubin concentrations. In Gilbert's syndrome this effect is due to induction by phenobarbital of more glucuronyl transferase activity, but the reason for the effect in Dubin-Johnson syndrome is unclear. In Gilbert's syndrome fasting produces a major elevation of unconjugated bilirubin; it reaches a peak at 48 hours. A minor elevation occurs in normal subjects. A lipid-free diet has a similar effect in Gilbert's syndrome. It is postulated that bilirubin sequestered in adipose tissue is mobilized under these conditions [15], and on the basis of this study the authors suggest that infants with neonatal hyperbilirubinemia should be given increased amounts of fat.

DIETARY FACTORS AND HEPATOBILIARY DISEASES

The liver receives everything that is absorbed from the small bowel and is also the major detoxicating organ of the body. These properties render it especially vulnerable to toxic substances which have been ingested or have been produced as a consequence of metabolic processes. (The hepatotoxic effects of some drugs have been discussed earlier in this chapter under "Hepatic Damage Due to Toxins.")

A question that is still unresolved is whether dietary deficiencies can produce permanent liver damage. In kwashiorkor the development of a fatty liver, similar to that associated with exposure to ethanol, has been observed, but there is no clear evidence that hepatic fibrosis occurs. The accumulation of fat is believed to be due to diminished production of apolipoproteins needed to transport triglycerides as very low density lipoproteins (VLDL) in the plasma. Ramalingaswami and Nyak have shown in rhesus monkeys that deficiency of dietary protein may inhibit rather than induce hepatic fibrosis and nodular regeneration [16].

Earlier experiments in rats, in which prolonged fatty livers induced by feeding low-protein diets and especially by feeding diets low in methionine or cystine appeared to predispose the rats to fibrosis, have not shed light on the situation in humans. The high prevalence rates of cirrhosis observed in tropical and subtropical countries where protein deficiency, especially in childhood, is also common seem to be associated more significantly with a high frequency of hepatitis B antigenicity. The key to the cause of irreversible hepatic fibrosis in humans is still to be found, and it must be concluded that, in the light of current knowledge, there is no good evidence that nutritional deficiency alone results in progressive liver damage, except possibly in bypass of the small intestine, which is discussed below.

Obesity

Fatty infiltration of the liver is found in association with obesity, but there is no evidence of significantly disturbed function. However, attention has recently been focused on hepatic steatosis, a condition occurring in obese adults in which there seems to be focal fatty change in the liver, which is sometimes diagnosed mistakenly as metastatic tumor. The condition is not confined to the obese and has been observed in patients who are undernourished, who have congestive heart failure, or who are receiving corticosteroid therapy [17].

Jejunoileal Bypass

Jejunoileal bypass surgery for severe obesity that is resistant to other means of treatment has had a checkered career. After 15 years it is now falling into disrepute and is being displaced by gastric stapling as a means of producing loss of adipose stores. The initial weight loss after bypass has been shown to be due more to marked reduction in intake of calories as a consequence of reduction of appetite than to malabsorption [18]. Why this happens is not known.

A significant number of subjects develop hypertriglyceridemia and severe fatty infiltration of the liver, and a number of deaths from hepatic failure have been reported. Cirrhosis may also occur. Autopsies have revealed both acute inflammatory changes and intrahepatic cholestasis. It seems likely that at least one factor is severe deficiency of protein, which may be due both to inadequate intake and to malabsorption. Reduced concentrations of plasma amino acids are found in the first 1 or 2 years after the operation [19]. Other possible causes are a toxic effect on the liver of bile salts, such as lithocholate, which may be formed in the colon as a consequence of bacterial action on chenodeoxycholate, which would normally be absorbed in the small intestine, and hepatotoxicity due to failure to ingest or absorb some presently unidentified nutrient or nutrients essential for normal liver function or due to excess absorption of some toxic agent. If intestinal continuity is restored, the liver usually recovers.

It must be emphasized that patients in whom jejunoileostomy has been done should be kept under careful, continuing clinical and laboratory surveillance.

Continuous Nasogastric and Parenteral Feeding

A recognized complication of continuous parenteral feeding, even when the preparations used appear to be nutritionally adequate, is intrahepatic cholestasis together with fatty infiltration. This occurs particularly in the infant but is also seen in adults. The reasons for the cholestasis are unclear. Intravenous lipids or disturbances of amino acid intake have been held responsible, but intravenous infusions of glucose and amino acids result in hyperbilirubinemia and elevations of serum alkaline phosphatase and transaminases in infants, so that lipid infusions are probably not responsible [20]. Similar disturbances have been reported in patients receiving continuous enteral nutrition.

In summary, it is still quite uncertain how important dietary components or lack of essential nutrients are in the development of diseases of the liver, with the exception of the effects of ethanol, iron, and copper. Fatty infiltration of the liver occurs in young children with kwashiorkor, but there is no good evidence that cirrhosis may ensue. Currently it is widely held that development of ethanol-induced liver disease does not depend also on nutritional deficiencies, although such deficiencies are frequently present with alcoholic cirrhosis.

GALLBLADDER AND GALLSTONE FORMATION

Much has been written about the relationship of diet to the formation of gallstones. Gallstones, which are found in the gallbladder or some part of the biliary ductular system, are of two types, pigment and cholesterol stones, classified according to their major constituent. Pigment stones are composed of bile pigments derived from the catabolism of heme and occur in conditions characterized by chronic hemolysis, such as some genetically determined hemolytic anemias. Cholesterol stones are the common gallstones of North and South America. In the United States 12 million women and 4 million men have gallstones, 800,000 new cases appear annually, and a half million subjects are hospitalized each year. It is noteworthy that, unlike most diseases of unknown etiology, cholelithiasis cannot be considered a disease of civilization due to faulty diet or lifestyle associated with industrial societies, since it is particularly common in American Indians living in their native habitat; but there are significant racial differences in incidence.

There is currently little illumination of this area, which is surprisingly gloomy, in spite of the very high prevalence of gallstones and the distinguished studies by Small and others of physicochemical factors involved in differentiating lithogenic bile (conducive to stone formation) from nonlithogenic or micellar bile. Briefly, in lithogenic bile the proportions of the three main constituents, bile salts, cholesterol, and lecithin, differ from those in nonlithogenic bile in that there is supersaturation with cholesterol, which predisposes to the formation of cholesterol stones. What factors are known to affect these proportions?

An accepted and potentially useful fact is that overnight or fasting bile is lithogenic [21]. This has led, surprisingly late, to a recommendation that frequent meals, and particularly eating breakfast, may be a practical measure for preventing the formation of gallstones [22]. This may be the only useful diet-related feature of gallstones. Certainly there is no evidence that dietary lipid is of importance. There is also no correlation, contrary to a widely held belief, between obesity and the presence of gallstones, and since dietary fats are powerful releasers from the wall of the duodenum of the hormone cholecystokinin, which stimulates gallbladder contraction, a fatty meal may exercise a beneficial effect by preventing stasis of bile in the gallbladder. Also, attempts to reduce levels of serum cholesterol in subjects with atherosclerosis have resulted in an increased formation of gallstones for reasons which are unclear [23]. In addition, consumption of a diet of high fiber content has not been shown to reduce cholesterol supersaturation of bile, in spite of some evidence that some depression of cholesterol synthesis occurred [24].

Thus, in the light of current knowledge, it might appear that quality of diet has no known influence on the formation of cholesterol gallstones and that frequency of meals may be a significant factor.

REFERENCES

1 Record, C. O., B. Buxton, R. A. Chase, G. Curzon, I. M. Murray-Lyon, and R. Williams: Plasma and brain amino acids in fulminant hepatic failure and their relationship to hepatic encephalopathy, Eur. J. Clin. Invest., 6.387, 1976.

2 Chalmers, T. C., R. D. Eckhardt, W. E. Reynolds, J. G. Cigarroa, N. Deane, R. W. Reifenstein, and C. W. Smith: The treatment of acute infectious hepatitis: studies of the effects of diets, rest and physical reconditioning on the acute course of the disease and on the incidence of relapse and residual abnormalities, J. Clin. Invest., 34:1163, 1955.

3 Morgan, A. G., J. Kelleher, B. E. Walker, and M. S. Losowsky: Nutrition in cryptogenic cirrhosis and chronic aggressive hepatitis, Gut, 17:113, 1976.

4 Ritchie, J. H., M. B. Fish, V. M. McMasters, and M. Grossman, Edema and hemolytic anemia in premature infants: vitamin E deficiency syndrome, N. Engl. J. Med., 279:1189, 1968.

5 Hoagland, C. L., D. H. Labby, H. G. Kunkel, and R. E. Shank: An analysis of the effect of fat in the diet on recovery in infectious hepatitis, Am. J. Public Health, 36:1287, 1946.

6 Bucher, N. L. R., U. Patel, and S. Cohen: Hormone factors concerned with liver regeneration, in *Hepatotrophic Factors*, Ciba Foundation Symposium no. 55, Elsevier Excerpta Medica, Amsterdam, 1978.

7 Lischner, M. W., J. F. Alexander, and J. T. Galambos: Natural history of alcoholic hepatitis. I. The acute disease, Am. J. Dig. Dis., 16:481, 1971.

8 Bucher, N. L. R., and M. N. Swaffield: Regulation of hepatic regeneration in rats by synergistic action of insulin and glucagon, Proc. Natl. Acad. Sci. U.S.A., 72:1157, 1975.

9 Fischer, J. E., H. M. Rosen, A. M. Ebeid, J. H. James, J. M. Keane, and P. B. Soeters: The effect of normalization of plasma amino acids on hepatic encephalopathy in man, Surgery, 80:77, 1976.

10 Maddrey, W. C., R. L. Weber, A. W. Coulter, and M. Walser: Effects of ketoanalogues of essential amino acids in portal systemic encephalopathy, Gastroenterology, 71:190, 1976.

11 Sherlock, S.: Primary biliary cirrhosis, in *Liver and Biliary Disease,* R. Wright et al. (eds.), Saunders, Philadelphia, 1979.

12 Cohen, A., I. J. Cohen, and E. Schwartz: Scurvy and altered iron stores in thalassemia major, N. Engl. J. Med., 304:158, 1981.

13 Crosby, W. J.: Improving iron nutrition (Editorial), West. J. Med., 122:499, 1975.

14 Hallberg, L., C. Bengtsson, L. Garby, J. Lennartsson, L. Rossander, and E. Tibblin: An analysis of factors leading to a reduction in iron deficiency in Swedish women, Bull. WHO, 57:947, 1979.

15 Gollan, J. L., C. Bateman, and B. H. Billing: Effect of dietary composition on the unconjugated hyperbilirubinaemia of Gilbert's syndrome, Gut, 17:335, 1976.

16 Ramalingaswami, F., and N. C. Nyak: Liver disease in India, Prog. Liver Dis., 3:222, 1970.

17 Brawer, M. K., G. E. Austin, and K. V. Lewin: Focal fatty change of the liver, a hitherto poorly recognized entity, Gastroenterology, 78:247, 1980.

18 Pilkington, T. R. E., J. C. Gazet, and L. Ang: Explanations for weight loss after ileojejunal bypass in gross obesity, Br. Med. J., 1:1504, 1976.

19 Moseley, R., T. Pozefsky, and D. Y. Lockwood: Protein nutrition and liver disease after jejunoileal bypass for morbid obesity, N. Engl. J. Med., 290:921, 1974.

20 Rodgers, B. M., J. I. Hollenbeck, W. H. Donnelly, and J. L. Talbert: Intrahepatic cholestasis and parenteral hyperalimentation, Am J. Surg., 131:149, 1976.

21 Holzbach, R. T., M. Marsh, and M. Olszeroski: Cholesterol solubility in bile. Evidence that supersaturated bile is frequent in healthy man, J. Clin. Invest., 25:1467, 1973.

22 Capron, J. P., J. Delamore, M. A. Herve, J. L. Dupas, P. Poulain, and P. Descombes: Meal frequency and duration of overnight fast: a role in gallstone formation? Br. Med. J., 283:1435, 1981.

23 Sturdevant, R. A. L., M. L. Pearce, and S. Dayton: Increased prevalence of cholelithiasis in men ingesting a serum-cholesterol-lowering diet, N. Engl. J. Med., 288:24, 1973.

24 Tarpila, S., T. A. Miettinen, L. Metsaranta: Effects of bran on serum cholesterol, faecal mass, fat, bile acids and neutral sterols, and biliary lipids in patients with diverticular disease of the colon, Gut, 19:137, 1978.

CHAPTER 17

NUTRITIONAL ASPECTS OF ALCOHOL CONSUMPTION

CONTENTS

INTRODUCTION

Alcoholism has a major impact on medical practice. Overtly or covertly it is a primary cause of disease or a major secondary complication which threatens a successful outcome from the disease. It is a good practice to anticipate special problems when confronted by an apparently alcoholic patient. The mental checklist should include the following:

1 Is the patient intoxicated at the time of the interview?

2 Is the patient fabricating? This may include denial of alcohol (ethanol) consumption.

3 Does the patient show evidence of malnutrition? Particularly important are deficiencies of some electrolytes, e.g., potassium and magnesium, and of some nutrients, e.g., folacin and ascorbic acid.

4 Does the patient show evidence of liver failure, particularly liver failure that might cause failure of blood coagulation and hemostasis? If so, parenteral and oral treatment with vitamin K should be commenced as soon as possible and the prothrombin response should be checked daily. Failure of prothrombin response is evidence of severe hepatic damage and carries a bad prognosis.

5 Is the patient metabolizing drugs abnormally?

6 Will the patient respond in a predictable way to therapy and comply with any potentially hazardous long-term therapy, e.g., anticoagulants?

7 Does the patient show evidence of an opportunistic infection including tuberculosis?

8 Is the patient likely to respond to withdrawal of alcohol, with or without the added complication of surgery, with delirium tremens?

Clues to occult alcoholism may be obtained by taking a medical history. Direct questions about alcohol consumption are posed most naturally among those relating to other habits, such as smoking and use of over-the-counter medications. Patients may become evasive or defensive when questioned about alcohol consumption; some deliberately underestimate the amount, a few exaggerate. Any hostility or defensiveness should arouse suspicion, which may sometimes be confirmed by unequivocal physical findings or by questioning a spouse or others who live with the patient. Formal screening interview tests have been devised such as the Michigan Alcoholism Screening Test (MAST) [1] and may give as high as 98 percent positive identification if subjects are compliant. Many experienced physicians hold that there is no substitute for the alert doctor who is suspicious of alcoholism and is able to take a probing history of alcohol consumption without alienating the patient. The smell of alcohol on the breath or detection of significant amounts in blood or urine may be confirmatory. Useful laboratory tests are listed in Table 17-1.

Alcoholism is a disease. The adoption of a moralistic or punitive attitude by the clinician has not been shown to have value in management and usually alienates the patient. But it is hard to keep this in mind when faced with the need to make clinical decisions in an emergency room at 2 A.M., particularly when dealing with a repeat performer.

Ethanol might logically be regarded as just one of many drugs which affect nutritional status. It deserves special treatment, however, because of the enormous amounts consumed and its addictive properties.

It is a source, sometimes a major one, of calories but not of essential

TABLE 17-1
LABORATORY TESTS TO IDENTIFY ALCOHOLISM

Test	Comment
Blood alcohol level	Decays rapidly. Still very valuable
Serum aspartate aminotransferase (transaminase) (SGOT)	Elevated in acute or chronic alcoholic liver disease; usually SGOT > SGPT. But SGPT > SGOT in viral hepatitis
Serum alanine aminotransferase (transaminase) (SGPT)	Elevated in acute or chronic alcoholic disease; SGOT > SGPT
Serum γ-glutamyl transpeptidase* (GGTP)	Elevated in 60–80% of alcoholics, but may be elevated in subjects with other liver disease and in barbiturate users
Red cell macrocytosis without anemia[†]	Not associated necessarily with folacin deficiency or responsive to folacin therapy
Serum transferrin heterogeneity[‡]	Is still under development

*D. J. Boone, N. W. Tiety, and A. Weinstock, Significance of gamma-glutamyl transferase (GGT) activity measurement in alcohol-induced hepatic injury, Ann. Clin. Lab. Sci., 7:25, 1977.

†A. Wu, I. Chanarin, and A. J. Levi, Macrocytosis of chronic alcoholism, Lancet, 1:829, 1974.

‡H. Stibler, S. Borg, and C. Allgulander, Clinical significance of abnormal heterogeneity of transferrin in relation to alcohol consumption, Acta Med. Scand., 206:275, 1979.

nutrients. Its use in large quantities will displace a more nutritious diet and impair the absorption of some nutrients, and its metabolism requires essential nutrients, so that deficiencies may occur.

In clinical practice it is important to recognize that alcohol damages many organs directly. These include liver, pancreas, heart, gastrointestinal tract, and brain and also bone marrow. A background of chronic alcohol abuse may also have an important influence on the outcome of diseases not primarily caused by alcoholism as a consequence of its effects on these organs.

Alcohol is the most common cause of intoxication. Its excessive use is associated with trauma. Bruising, fractures, damage to the face and the eyes, subdural hematomas, burns, and death from burning are some of the well-recognized hazards of its use. A significant proportion of automobile accidents is associated with alcohol ingestion, and these accidents have become the most common cause of death in young people between the ages of 17 and 24 years. Innocent bystanders may suffer physical trauma. The extent of psychological trauma due to alcoholism cannot be estimated. Clearly no other drug has caused so many deaths and so much physical and mental morbidity for so many; nor, in moderation, provided so much pleasure. The dividing line between benefit and abuse is poorly defined and subject to the whole gamut of human attitudes and prejudices.

The subject of alcohol abuse is a vast one and presents problems to which no solutions appear yet to have been found. Fiscal policy and restriction of advertising have been shown to have significant effects on consumption [2], but governments tend to run scared, and there is little sign of resurgent support for another Volstead Act banning alcohol manufacture and sale in either the United States or abroad. Since solutions or even a consensus about means of prevention are lacking and since in the real world, supplies of alcohol will continue to flow and people will continue to drink them, it is essential that doctors, nutritionists, and paramedical personnel be able to anticipate, to recognize, and to treat the various aspects of malnutrition associated with ethanol.

Alcoholism is not always obvious to even the trained observer. Consequently, life-threatening situations such as delirium tremens with convulsions may occur without warning as a result of acute withdrawal, or Wernicke's encephalopathy, a disease which is almost invariably due to alcoholism and is responsive to thiamine, may go untreated too long and death ensue.

Alcoholism and nutritional deficiencies are not invariably associated. Comparisons of indigent and affluent alcoholics have made this clear. However, since many tests for nutritional deficiencies are still experimental or not widely obtainable, it is wise to consider the possibility of deficiencies and treat the alcoholic patient (whether he or she is being treated for a medical, surgical, or psychiatric problem) as if they were present until proven otherwise.

EPIDEMIOLOGY OF ALCOHOLISM

Many countries provide figures for rates of alcoholism and data on national consumption of alcohol. The sources of error are formidable. Illicit production or importation, wide variations in individual consumption and patterns of consumption, and the differing nature of alcoholic beverages make it difficult to establish reliable figures. Neither is there good agreement about the definition of alcoholism. Subdivision into alcohol dependency and alcohol-related disabilities has been recommended, but the distinction is blurred. We prefer to use the term alcoholism and define it as the intermittent or continued ingestion of alcohol leading to dependence or harm or both [3].

The Department of Health, Education, and Welfare 1971 report [4] states that 7 percent of the adult U.S. population manifests evidence of alcohol abuse or alcoholism; that is, 9 million out of an estimated 95 million consumers of alcohol, or 10 percent, show evidence of alcohol abuse or alcoholism.

More than 250,000 deaths in the United States annually are attributed to alcohol use, including at least 50 percent of fatal automobile accidents. Estimates of alcoholism in patients admitted to county and Veterans Administration hospitals are of the order of more than 50 percent having health problems directly or indirectly attributable to alcohol. In the United Kingdom, it has been reported that 19.5 percent of patients admitted to a London teaching hospital have a drinking problem [5].

In the United States, at least two-thirds of cirrhosis is due to alcohol. The prevalence of cirrhosis in different countries shows good direct correlation with per capita alcohol consumption. Another epidemiological finding which reinforces the importance of alcohol in causing cirrhosis is the observed dramatic reduction in autopsy-proven cirrhosis which occurred toward the end of the Prohibition era in the United States. The incidence of deaths from cirrhosis is now increasing in North America and in western European countries. In the United States today, cirrhosis is twice as common in men as in women, and twice as common in black men and women as in white men and women. [6]. There is recent evidence suggesting that exposure to alcohol is more likely to result in liver disease in women than in men [7]. In the United Kingdom alcohol has become the major cause of liver damage, in spite of the increase of type B viral hepatitis. The rate of increase is greater in women than in men [8].

The major dangers of alcoholism are listed in Table 17-2.

It has yet to be established whether genetic or cultural factors play the bigger role in alcoholism. The differences in prevalence rates among different ethnic groups in the United States do not help resolve the matter. The claims that Orientals are especially prone to developing histamine-release-like reactions of flushing and throbbing headaches after ingesting moderate amounts of alcohol

TABLE 17-2
THE DANGERS OF EXCESSIVE ETHANOL INGESTION

Acute	Intoxication and its consequences
	Hypoglycemia
	Gastrointestinal bleeding
	Interaction with drugs
	Alcoholic hepatitis
	Acute or chronic pancreatitis
	Wernicke's encephalopathy
	Korsakoff's psychosis
	Peripheral neuropathies
	Chronic gastritis
	Nutritional deficiencies
	Anemia:
	Marrow suppression
	Hemolysis
	Hemorrhage
	Thrombocytopenia
	Cirrhosis and its consequences:
	Portal hypertension
	Varices
	Encephalopathy
	Coagulopathies:
	Vitamin K deficiency
	Disseminated intravascular
Chronic	coagulopathy
Pregnancy	Fetal abnormalities (if ingested during pregnancy)

are not well substantiated, but the possibility that there may be genetically determined differences in the metabolism of ethanol should not be dismissed. Even a preference for alcohol may be an expression of a phenotype.

Studies suggest that both environment and genetic factors are identifiable in the greater risk of becoming an alcoholic that family members of alcoholics display.

EFFECTS OF ALCOHOL ABUSE

General Principles

Since it is currently impossible to define the etiology of alcoholism, we should address the matter of what damage alcohol does and how it does it. This approach permits a definition of alcoholism as the continuing or intermittent consumption of alcohol in amounts which produce intoxication, either acute, which may result in damage to the alcoholic or those in contact with him or her, or chronic, to a degree resulting in either reversible or irreversible damage to a range of tissues. Tolerance to the intoxicating effects of alcohol is very variable; habituation plays a major role in the metabolic handling of ethanol, mainly by the liver, and the rate of change of concentration of ethanol in the blood is a major determinant of mental status, i.e., sobriety or intoxication. Individual variation in the amount of alcohol necessary to produce tissue damage is probably large, and most quantitative estimates that have been published are of little value in providing useful guidelines. A study in France suggests that cirrhosis of the liver will occur in 20 percent of subjects consuming 180 g of ethanol per day for 25 years (equivalent to about one-tenth of a gallon of hard liquor), whereas a daily consumption of 30 g or less is innocuous [9].

The liver of the chronic alcoholic metabolizes ethanol to acetaldehyde more rapidly than that of the nonconsumer. Acetaldehyde concentrations in the blood and tissues rise higher than normal and cause damage to the liver, brain, heart, and other organs. It is generally agreed that when ethanol consumption constitutes more than 20 percent of total calories, damage to some part of the body will ensue in a matter of years. The difficulty lies in recognizing that such a situation exists.

Many subjects, particularly in upper-income groups, consume alcohol well in excess of 20 percent of total calories (for a comparison of the effective caloric content of ethanol, see Appendix 1, Table 1, and of alcoholic beverages, Table 11-6) and remain apparently functional and well-compensated for many years. They are not recognized to be in need of therapy, and most do not perceive the need. Chronic consumption of alcohol produces a state of mental and physical dependence. The relation between degree of dependence and duration of exposure to ethanol is unclear. However, at least some of the early pathological changes induced by alcohol are reversible [10], and for this reason alone, early correction of alcoholism is desirable. This view is reinforced by consideration of the impact of alcohol on affective life. Familial and societal damage may occur early and may be cumulative. The breakdown of interpersonal relationships is a major factor in subsequent mental and physical decompensation.

The consequences of physical dependence appear on withdrawal of alcohol. The pattern of symptoms and signs is reproducible, the intensity possibly dependent in part on duration of prior consumption and dosage.

Symptoms range from shakiness to delirium tremens. Tremulousness occurs 10 to 12 hours after withdrawal. The subject may sweat, and the pulse rate, respiratory rate, and blood pressure rise. The subject may feel anxious; nausea and vomiting may supervene. These symptoms and signs usually resolve in 24 to 48 hours but may last several days. The state of delirium tremens is far more severe and is life-threatening. About 10 percent of alcoholics may develop part or all of the syndrome during alcohol withdrawal. Usually it is heralded by exacerbation of the earlier symptoms. Trauma or major surgery may precede the onset. The patient may become extremely agitated and hyperthermic and may hallucinate. The hallucinations are usually terrifying. Seizures occur, and these are life-threatening. A mortality of nearly 50 percent was common for delirium tremens 50 years ago. The use of oral, intravenous, or intramuscular benzodiazepines and better supportive measures have revolutionized treatment of alcohol withdrawal, but a small number of subjects still die in delirium tremens. It has been shown that the oral route is preferable to the intramuscular route for achieving higher blood concentrations of benzodiazepines and should be used if swallowing or retention is not a problem.

Gastrointestinal Tract

Acute Effects   The acute effects of alcoholic beverages on the esophagus and stomach vary with the beverage's concentration of ethanol. Wines and beers are without demonstrable effect, whereas Palmer's studies [11] have shown gastric mucosal hyperemia and erosions in the stomachs of young men acutely intoxicated with distilled liquors. Decreased gastric emptying, nausea, and vomiting may occur. Vomiting may be violent and protracted. Tears of the mucosa around the gastroesophageal junction may result, and bleeding may be heavy and occasionally life-threatening (Mallory-Weiss syndrome). Consumption of ethanol and aspirin together is associated with greater risk of gastrointestinal bleeding than after either alone. Anorexia often follows excessive alcohol ingestion.

Chronic Effects   Epidemiological studies have associated chronic alcoholism with cancer of the tongue and esophagus but have not established that these lesions are due to a direct effect of alcohol. This association does not hold for cancer of the stomach. There is some lack of agreement whether continuing excessive alcohol consumption is associated with chronic atrophic gastritis. This may reflect in part differences between the populations studied. In theory it might occur as a consequence of repeated insults to the gastric mucosa, which has also been postulated in the case of drinking hot fluids, or it might be due to secondary nutritional factors. If there is an association, the gastric lesion does not progress to pernicious anemia. There are some studies suggesting that it may be reversible following alcohol withdrawal [12].

Experimental isocaloric replacement of carbohydrate by ethanol for 2 months in human subjects is associated with changes in the cytoplasm, mitochondria, and endoplasmic reticulum of small intestinal epithelial cells (enterocytes), and these changes are similar to those occurring in the liver cells of such subjects.

Halstead has produced evidence of abnormalities of nuclear maturation in the enterocytes of the small intestine in alcoholic subjects who are severely deficient in folacin. These changes do not occur in folacin-replete alcoholics or in nonalcoholic folacin-deficient subjects [13].

Functional changes in the gut are induced by ingestion of intoxicating amounts of ethanol. They have also been noted in as many as one-third of a group of chronic alcoholics. Malabsorption of d-xylose, glucose, fat, amino acids, vitamin B_{12}, and folacin has been documented. After acute alcohol ingestion, synthesis of triglycerides by the intestinal mucosa is increased. Nutritional deficiency accompanying chronic alcoholism appears to aggravate malabsorption, especially of folacin.

Pancreas

Chronic excessive ethanol ingestion is the most common cause of pancreatitis in the United States. The nature of the causal relationship is unknown, and there is no experimental animal model. The progress of the disease is marked by attacks of acute pancreatitis following alcoholic binges. The pancreas shows chronic structural damage at the time of the first attack of acute pancreatitis. Patients present 12 to 48 hours after a bout of drinking with severe abdominal pain (often it is epigastric or periumbilical and radiates to the back), nausea, and vomiting. There may be a leukocytosis, some fever, and elevated serum and urinary amylase activities. The attacks usually become less eloquent clinically as the inflamed pancreas becomes increasingly replaced by fibrous tissue in which calcification occurs to a variable degree. When about 90 percent of functioning exocrine pancreatic glandular tissue has been lost, failure of secretion of adequate pancreatic digestive enzymes occurs. The loss of lipase results in steatorrhea which leads in turn to inadequate absorption of calcium, magnesium, and fat-soluble vitamins. At this point, nutritional deficiencies may become evident as well as significant loss of weight.

Liver

The liver receives high concentrations of ethanol via the portal venous system and is the major site of ethanol metabolism. Ethanol appears to have direct effects on the hepatic parenchymal cells; it causes changes in the cytoplasm, endoplasmic reticulum, and mitochondria and increases in intracellular triglyceride leading to the appearance of a fatty liver. Fatty livers occur in well-nourished nonalcoholic individuals within 48 hours of ingesting alcohol at a level of 36 percent of total caloric requirements in place of carbohydrate in an otherwise balanced diet [10].

The phenomenon of fatty liver is not peculiar to ethanol intoxication. It occurs also in protein-calorie malnutrition, following small intestinal bypass for obesity, and in diabetes mellitus. The metabolic abnormality in each of these may be different.

The liver is the only site of detoxification of ethanol. The first step is oxidation to acetaldehyde (Figure 17-1). The major pathway uses the enzyme alcohol dehydrogenase, present only in the liver. In nonalcoholics the alcohol dehydrogenase–mediated step is the rate-limiting one in removal of ethanol from the circulation. Two other pathways are available (Figure 17-1). The catalase-mediated conversion is not important, but the microsomal ethanol-oxidizing system (MEOS) may be quantitatively important in the chronic alcoholic, since alcohol induces this system. The two alcohol dehydrogenase coenzymes are nicotinamide adenine dinucleotide (NAD) and thiamine pyrophosphate (TPP). Acetaldehyde is converted into acetyl coenzyme A (acetyl-CoA) via hydroxyethyl TPP, which then enters the Krebs tricarboxylic acid cycle. Pyruvate oxidation shares the same pathway at the hydroxyethyl TPP step. During high rates of ethanol oxidation, NAD^+ is depleted and NADH accumulates. The Krebs cycle is blocked in consequence. Some pyruvate may be

FIGURE 17-1
Pathways of formation of acetaldehyde from ethanol.

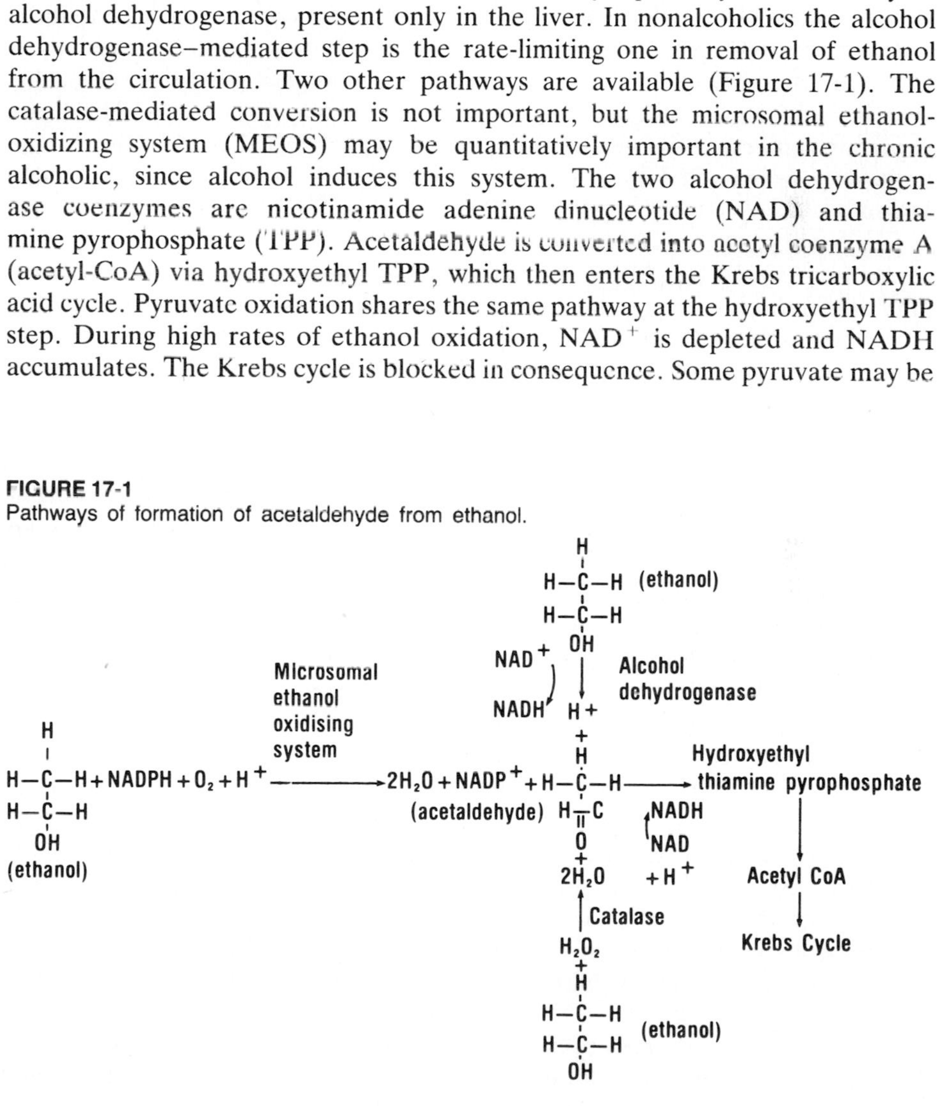

reduced to lactate, which regenerates NAD^+. Thus during alcoholic intoxication lactate may accumulate in the liver and its concentration may increase in the blood, producing an anion gap, and ketoacidosis may occur. Metabolic acidosis inhibits renal excretion of uric acid, which accumulates and which may precipitate an attack of gout.

The 2-carbon molecules cannot be oxidized further and are built up into fatty acids. These fatty acids are not oxidized, the synthesis by the liver of the protein moieties of lipoproteins is depressed, and fatty acids accumulate in the liver. In humans and other primates this is probably the first step in the development of cirrhosis, but it is a reversible one. If ingestion of ethanol ceases, the excess fat in the liver disappears in days, weeks, or less commonly, months. The accumulation of fat usually interferes with the functioning of the liver, causing a variable degree of intrahepatic cholestasis. Serum alkaline phosphatase activity is elevated, the bilirubin level may be increased, and hepatic parenchymal damage is indicated by elevated activities of serum transaminase enzymes. The serum aspartate aminotransferase (SGOT) level is typically higher than the alanine aminotransferase (SGPT) level in alcohol-related liver disease, for unknown reasons.

Acute Alcoholic Hepatitis   A much more serious liver disease may occur in a small proportion of heavy ethanol abusers after many years of drinking. It is termed *acute alcoholic hepatitis* and probably represents a more severe reaction of the liver to ethanol. The amount consumed, the duration of alcohol abuse, and individual susceptibility are important factors.

A biopsy of the liver will show patchy infiltration of the parenchyma and the portal tracts with polymorphonuclear leukocytes, ballooning, and some necrosis of parenchymal cells, particularly in the centrilobular areas. Eosinophilic inclusion (Mallory) bodies appear sporadically in the cytoplasm of dying cells. There will be a varying degree of cholestasis and fibrosis.

Clinical Picture   When patients with this disease are first seen, their conditions show remarkable variation. The patients may be asymptomatic or complain only of fatigue and chills, symptoms suggestive of the prodrome of influenza. At the other end of the spectrum they may be very sick, complaining of nausea and vomiting, fever, a distended abdomen, and marked icterus (jaundice). There is usually discomfort and sometimes pain in the right upper quadrant of the abdomen over the liver, and the liver is enlarged and tender to touch.

Laboratory Findings   There is usually a significant circulating leukocytosis and elevation of serum transaminases, the activity of SGOT being almost always higher than that of SGPT. Serum γ-glutamyl transpeptidase activity is almost invariably elevated. Serum albumin may be reduced, and the prothrombin time may be prolonged. Serum bilirubin concentrations range from normal to high levels.

Treatment   The treatment consists of withdrawal of alcohol, a diet containing sufficient protein and calories, and supplements of all vitamins and essential minerals. The possibility of the patient's developing delirium tremens must be entertained during the first week of alcohol withdrawal, and the sicker patients may develop the hepatorenal syndrome, with kidney failure and retention of waste products and potassium. This condition, of unknown etiology, has a grave prognosis. Ascites is treated with a low salt intake and diuretics.

Controlled trials have shown that there is no value in treatment with corticosteroids.

Prognosis The immediate mortality from acute alcoholic hepatitis is far less than that reported 25 years ago. It should not be more than 10 percent if the patient receives good supportive care. Ascites and failure of a prolonged prothrombin time to respond to vitamin K supplementation carry a poor prognosis. The clinical manifestations of the disease disappear over the course of 2 to 6 weeks in those who recover. The long-term prognosis depends on whether the patient continues to abuse alcohol [14].

Alcoholic Cirrhosis Alcoholism is the most common cause of cirrhosis in western countries. Its development is insidious, and it may proceed for many years before becoming symptomatic.

Epidemiology Some aspects of the epidemiology of acute alcoholic hepatitis have been discussed earlier. The prevalence of cirrhosis in some parts of the United States is of the order of 30 to 40 per 100,000 white males and 15 to 20 per 100,000 white females. For nonwhite males the figure is approximately double that for white males and for nonwhite females about 30 percent more than for white females [15].

Pathology The liver in alcoholic cirrhosis varies widely in size. In the early stages the liver tends to be large, may weigh 3 to 4 kg, and displays considerable fatty infiltration (steatosis). When the process has been continuing for many years, the liver may become smaller than normal and hard. The early appearance is of micronodular (Laennec's) cirrhosis, but in the late stages fibrosis and attempts at nodular regeneration may produce a macronodular appearance indistinguishable from postnecrotic cirrhosis of severe postviral hepatitis or chronic active hepatitis. Fibrous "bridging" occurs as a consequence of hepatocytic death and attempts at repair with collagen laid down by fibroblasts. Ultimately, this results in an impaired blood supply to the hepatocytes. Variable amounts of inflammation and fatty infiltration are found. There is usually an excess of stainable iron present, unless the patient suffers from recurrent gastrointestinal bleeding.

Clinical Presentation The usual presentation is an expression of one of the complications of cirrhosis, such as jaundice, bleeding esophageal varices, ascites, or less commonly, encephalopathy or severe bruising as a consequence of a coagulopathy. Anorexia and weight loss are common.

Physical findings are of hepatomegaly, splenomegaly, any of the changes noted above, and gynecomastia and testicular atrophy in males. There may be peripheral edema. About two-thirds of patients are jaundiced, usually not very severely. There may be ascites. Loss of lean body mass is often very striking.

Spider angiomas are common, and there may be redness of the palms of the hands due to increased circulation (palmar erythema).

Diagnosis   The patient's general condition and especially abnormalities of the blood clotting mechanisms very often preclude early diagnostic liver biopsy. The presumptive diagnosis is then made from the history and from physical and laboratory findings.

Laboratory Findings   Low serum concentrations of potassium and magnesium due to renal loss are frequently found in patients who have been drinking alcohol recently. Prolonged increased renal tubular loss of phosphate, which is linked with magnesium loss, may sometimes result in severe hypophosphatemia, sometimes manifest during nutritional repletion.

A variable degree of hyperbilirubinemia occurs. Values range from less than 1 to 30 mg/ml or more. With advancing liver damage the serum albumin and prothrombin levels tend to fall and the β- and γ-globulin levels tend to rise. Serum transaminase levels are only moderately elevated, and serum alkaline phosphatase may be slightly elevated or within normal limits.

Management   Treatment involves abstention from alcohol, a nutritious diet, a low-salt regimen and diuretics if ascites is present (see Table 9-6), and supplementation with essential nutrients and minerals. Of these, folacin and vitamin K are most likely to be deficient, sometimes to a degree that produces hematologic abnormalities. Thiamine levels may be low, with consequent disturbances of peripheral or central nervous function. In a few rare cases signs of mild scurvy or pellagra are observed, often being initially overlooked. Pyridoxine deficiency also occurs in a few rare cases, producing a sideroblastic anemia that is responsive to pyridoxine therapy (see Chapter 10). Recent evidence suggests the deficiency may be due in part to dephosphorylation of pyridoxal 5-phosphate in the presence of elevated levels of plasma and tissue alkaline phosphatase [16].

In order to ensure that deficiency of B vitamins and ascorbate are not adding to the patient's symptoms, our practice is to give one daily multivitamin capsule containing at least the recommended daily allowance (RDA) of all the B-complex vitamins and vitamin C.

Iron supplements should only be given if there is clear evidence of iron deficiency due to poor diet or recurrent gastrointestinal bleeding, since in the cirrhotic subject there is a tendency for iron overload of the liver to occur, which may add to parenchymal damage. Low levels of zinc due to increased renal excretion have been described, but the clinical importance of this has not been established.

The prognosis is good if the cirrhotic patient survives the first year after diagnosis and inception of treatment that includes abstinence from alcohol. Approximately 85 percent survive the following 4 years. Jaundice, vomiting of blood (hematemesis), ascites, and the failure of low prothrombin levels to respond to vitamin K are bad prognostic signs.

If disseminated infection or bacterial peritonitis supervene, the patient is likely to become febrile and develop a leukocytosis. Peritonitis is accompanied usually by generalized abdominal discomfort or pain, but it may be silent. Blood and ascitic fluid cultures should be done. Any such infection must be treated vigorously with antibiotics. In spite of intensive treatment, the chances of complete recovery, especially in the case of bacterial peritonitis, are slender.

Heart

Alcohol damages the heart. This has been demonstrated by light and electron microscopic studies of heart muscle obtained in vivo by biopsy from alcoholics [17] and of heart muscle obtained from mice fed alcohol [18].

The term *cardiomyopathy* is now replaced by *alcoholic heart muscle disease,* since the cause is now clear. In chronic alcoholism a direct toxic action of alcohol and the effects of thiamine deficiency may both damage the heart. Thiamine deficiency may occur when the amount ingested falls below 0.3 mg per 1000 kcal (other than from fat). A third complication is the hypertension associated with chronic alcoholism, the cause of which is still speculative.

When heart failure is present in any patient likely to be an alcoholic, alcohol should be withdrawn and a 1 week course of thiamine, 100 mg orally twice daily, should be given plus 50 mg IM daily in addition to any appropriate cardiac drugs to achieve as favorable a base line of cardiac performance as possible. The degree of reversibility possible is unclear, since some permanent muscle damage and scarring seem to occur.

Nervous System

The central and peripheral nervous systems are both affected by alcohol.

Acute Intoxication Drunkenness is due to the direct effect of ethanol on the central nervous system. The patterns of deranged function show considerable individual variation so that no two intoxicated subjects behave in exactly the same way. The blood alcohol concentration at which signs of intoxication appear also varies widely. The rate of increase of concentration in the blood is an important factor in determining the effect on the central nervous system, so that not only the amount of alcohol ingested but also the rate at which it is absorbed are important. Studies of changes in blood alcohol levels in relation to ingestion of alcohol with and without food have confirmed what is well known; drinking while eating food is less likely to cause intoxication [19].

Polyneuritis It has been stated that in nearly 10 percent of hospitalized alcoholics there is evidence of a peripheral neuropathy [20]. Involvement of the nerves is symmetrical. Symptoms are tingling and numbness in the feet and hands and weakness which tends to cause foot-drop. The ankle jerk reflex is diminished or absent, fine movements of the hands are lost, vibratory and position sense are impaired, and glove-and-stocking anesthesia may develop. The usual cause is deficiency of thiamine, as in classical "dry" beriberi, and many patients respond favorably, though not always completely, to thiamine therapy. Deficiencies of pyridoxine, cobalamin, and niacin may occasionally occur in chronic alcoholics and present as a peripheral neuropathy.

Wernicke's Encephalopathy Wernicke's encephalopathy is a disease of the central nervous system. Typically it occurs in male alcoholics but is seen occasionally in nonalcoholic subjects suffering from severe wasting diseases and nutritional deficiences. The major features are weakness or paralysis of extraocular movements, especially of lateral paired (conjugate) gaze; horizontal and vertical nystagmus; ataxia (unsteadiness) of gait; and confusion.

The pathological lesions are nerve cell necrosis and punctate hemorrhages in the mamillary bodies of the midbrain around the aqueduct of Sylvius.

The response to large intravenous doses of thiamine is dramatic with regard to the ophthalmoplegia (paralysis of eye muscles), but the ataxia and confusion may persist and show slow and only partial recovery. If the disease is left untreated, it is often fatal.

Recently a defect in transketolase, a thiamine-requiring enzyme, has been demonstrated in cultured epithelial cells from four patients with Wernicke's encephalopathy [21]. The enzyme in the patients' cells had a much lower avidity for thiamine pyrophosphate than the cells of controls. Should these studies be confirmed, they may herald a new understanding of the variable impact of nutrient deficiencies and possibly of alcohol on different individuals.

Korsakoff's Psychosis Korsakoff's psychosis is often linked with Wernicke's encephalopathy, since it occurs frequently in chronic alcoholics who manifest clinical signs of Wernicke's encephalopathy. Amnesia, loss of sense of time, confabulation, and confusion are seen in Korsakoff's psychosis, and they do not respond well to treatment with thiamine or multiple B vitamins. Further, Korsakoff's psychosis occurs only in alcoholism and not in other nutritionally impaired states.

There are other diseases of the central nervous system associated with chronic alcoholism such as cerebellar degeneration and the pontine lesions of Marchiafava-Bignami disease, but they are rare in the United States, their etiopathogenesis is unknown, and they are untreatable.

Bone Marrow

The most common cause of anemia in chronic alcoholics is iron deficiency [22]. Megaloblastic anemia associated with folacin deficiency is less common but is seen quite frequently in an alcoholic population. The deficiency may be due to dietary deficiency, malabsorption of folacin, or possibly poor hepatic storage of folacin and must often be a consequence of all three.

There is, in addition, in acute alcoholism a depression of hematopoiesis which is associated with vacuolization of red cell precursors and subsequent megaloblastic changes in the marrow, with a peripheral red cell macrocytosis, neutropenia, and thrombocytopenia. Reticulocytosis heralds recovery after abstention from alcohol for several days [23]. The hematological changes can be produced repeatedly in some individuals, on exposure to alcohol.

FETAL ALCOHOL SYNDROME

There is increasing concern in western countries about the harmful effects on the developing fetus of alcohol in the maternal blood stream. It has been emphasized elsewhere (Chapter 4) that pregnant women should avoid exposure to potentially harmful agents. These include tobacco, marijuana, alcohol, and any therapeutic drug that is not absolutely necessary. The most vulnerable period in terms of teratogenesis for the fetus is the first 2 months after conception.

The first substantiated report of the fetal alcohol syndrome came from France in a paper which presented observations of 127 affected children. In the United States early reports from Seattle [24] confirmed and extended the French observations. Between 30 to 50 percent of children of chronic alcoholic mothers show some evidence of the fetal alcohol syndrome. The neonatal death rate is increased nearly tenfold in some studies. The stigmata which have been identified and which are becoming increasingly accepted are low birth weight, which is evidence of prenatal growth deficiency, defective growth in infancy, small head size (microcephaly), mental deficiency, a very high incidence of cardiac septal defects, hemangiomas, and minor genital abnormalities.

The special features focus on craniofacial abnormalities of which the most common are short palpebral fissures, maxillofacial hypoplasia and epicanthic folds (Figure 17-2).

Of the 100 offspring of alcoholic mothers studied, approximately one quarter have one or more major malformations. The prevalence of severe chronic

FIGURE 17-2
Characteristic anatomic defects that are signs of fetal alcohol syndrome.

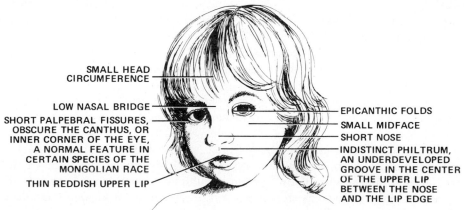

alcoholism during pregnancy in the western United States is thought to be at least 0.42 to 1.25 cases per 1000 pregnancies [25] and could possibly be higher in other parts of the nation. Maternal alcoholism thus becomes an important cause of persisting mental deficiency, and other evidence suggests that it may result in permanent alterations in brain development and function.

The possibility that nutrient deficiencies rather than the direct effect of ethanol are responsible for some or all of the abnormalities noted cannot be completely discounted, but nutrient deficiencies have not occurred consistently in the mothers of infants with the syndrome, the defects that occur have not been observed in relation to nutrient deficiencies in the absence of alcoholism (typically the fetal alcohol child is short for his or her weight), and the incidence of major defects in experimental animals correlates better with circulating ethanol levels than with the total amount consumed. However, a recent report has emphasized a possible association of fetal abnormalities and zinc deficiency in alcoholic mothers [26].

The maximal amount of alcohol which can safely be consumed in pregnancy is not known. In view of this, women should be strongly encouraged to stop drinking alcohol (and to stop smoking) as soon as they know they have conceived. Even better would be for those who are planning pregnancies to abstain from alcohol before embarking upon pregnancy. There have been strong recommendations made by many for early abortion in chronic alcoholics who cannot break the habit or who conceive accidentally.

ALCOHOL AND FASTING HYPOGLYCEMIA

Hypoglycemia may occur after ingesting alcohol in subjects in whom there is either minimal or no evidence of liver damage. These subjects are not necessarily alcoholics, but the phenomenon is more likely to be seen in chronic alcoholics and especially in those who are malnourished [27].

The patient usually is found stuporous or comatose, with the smell of alcohol on the breath. Hypothermia is frequently present.

A large amount of alcohol will have been ingested 10 to 24 hours beforehand, but this information may not be forthcoming for obvious reasons. Blood alcohol concentrations below 10 mg/dl suggest the diagnosis, which is strongly corroborated if the blood glucose concentration is less than 30 mg/dl. There may be a significant anion gap due to lactic acidosis, which occurs frequently but not invariably in this situation.

The most important and potentially lifesaving measure is to set up an intravenous infusion of 10% glucose, since the mortality rate may be 20 percent or higher.

The causes of the condition are multiple. Ethanol has an inhibitory effect on gluconeogenesis from arginine and other precursors. It has been shown that circulating insulin levels are low in ethanol-induced hypoglycemia but not to the degree which would be expected in relation to the degree of hypoglycemia were ethanol not present. The glucagon-secreting response is not abolished, and elevated circulating levels of glucagon are found. There is some evidence of disturbance of the normal adrenocortical-pituitary interaction, and circulating plasma cortisol and growth hormone levels, though elevated, are also not as high as would be found in hypoglycemia in the ethanol-free state.

ALCOHOL AND CIRCULATING LIPIDS

Chronic alcohol ingestion is one of the causes of hyperlipoproteinemia type IV, the hyperlipoproteinemia characterized by hypertriglyceridemia and elevated concentrations of very low density lipoprotein (VLDL). Type IV is associated with obesity, diabetes mellitus, and carbohydrate intolerance and with oral contraceptive use. When moderate alcohol consumers are compared with abstainers, the former tend also to have higher circulating concentrations of high density lipoprotein (HDL) [28]. The significance of these two disturbances in the prognosis of coronary heart disease or atherosclerosis is not yet clear.

INTERACTIONS OF ALCOHOL WITH DRUGS

Alcohol abuse significantly perturbs the use of therapeutic agents in two ways. First, alcoholics tend to be erratic in their compliance with therapeutic regimens. This behavioral problem can create serious and even life-threatening situations in such cases as insulin-dependent diabetics, in patients maintained on long-term anticoagulant therapy, and in sedative users. Frustrating relapses of ascites, hypertension, or heart failure may also occur in patients who disregard their low-salt regimen.

Second, alcohol, like many drugs, induces changes in smooth endoplasmic reticulum of liver parenchymal cells and increases the content of the microsomal drug-metabolizing enzyme, cytochrome P-450. The clearance of drugs such as barbiturates and tolbutamide is increased in consequence. Enzyme induction, however, shows marked individual variation. When this variability in enzyme induction is combined with the presence of a variable degree of liver damage, the result can be unpredictable responses to many drugs. There may be an enhancement of the drug-detoxifying pathway in the liver but hepatic damage may inhibit elimination. Further, the effects of enzyme enhancement may be evident in the chronic alcoholic when his or her circulating alcohol level is low, whereas when the circulating alcohol level is high, there may be a competitive effect between alcohol and the drug in the liver and a synergistic effect on the central nervous system. A range of possible interactions is shown in Table 17-3.

Some drugs inhibit the metabolism of alcohol. This effect is utilized in the disulfiram treatment of alcoholism. Disulfiram (Antabuse) blocks the metabolism of acetaldehyde in the alcohol oxidative pathway and accumulation of this matabolite results in nausea, vomiting, severe headache, and prostration.

A similar metabolic blocking action may occur when metronidazole (Flagyl), procarbazine, and some other similar drugs are taken. Thus while the patient is

TABLE 17-3
IMPORTANT INTERACTIONS OF ALCOHOL AND THERAPEUTIC DRUGS

Drug	Metabolic effects
Anticonvulsant Phenytoin (Dilantin)	Metabolism of drug enhanced. Larger doses than normal required
Sedatives Barbiturates Benzodiazepines	CNS depression enhanced or performance impaired due to synergism
Vasodilator Nitroglycerin	Vasodilation and risk of hypotensive collapse increased
Anticoagulants Warfarin (Coumadin)	Metabolism of drug blocked (acute ethanol intoxication) or rate of detoxification of drug increased (chronic alcoholism) or anticoagulant effect enhanced if liver damaged (cirrhosis)
Antibiotics and chemotherapeutic agents Metronidazole Quinacrine Chloramphenicol Griseofulvin	Alcohol metabolism inhibited by drug (Antabuse effect)
Hypoglycemic drugs Chlorpropamide Tolbutamide	Alcohol metabolism inhibited by drug (Antabuse effect)
Phenformin	Lactic acidosis produced
Hypotensives Methyldopa Hydralazine Rauwolfia	Alcohol potentiates drug's effect

using these drugs, alcohol is contraindicated because accumulation of acetaldehyde can occur.

If alcohol is taken simultaneously with some oral hypoglycemic agents, hypoglycemia, coma, and even death may occur. One such agent, phenformin, when given together with alcohol, has been reported frequently to produce marked lactic acidosis.

Alcohol may potentiate the action of a drug in other ways. It may, for instance, act synergistically with some antihypertensive drugs to produce marked vasodilation and a severe fall in blood pressure. Alcohol and aspirin taken together increase the chance of gastrointestinal bleeding as compared with aspirin taken alone. Alcoholics should always be warned about this. A popular remedy for a hangover, Alka-Seltzer, is now available in an aspirin-free form.

Alcohol may influence the effectiveness of coumadin anticoagulants in three ways. Acute intoxication inhibits their metabolism, so that an increased anticoagulant effect may lead to hemorrhage. Chronic alcohol abuse enhances coumadin detoxification, and thus effective coumadin levels may fall more rapidly than normal. Finally, in end-stage alcoholic cirrhosis the synthesis of prothrombin and factors VII, IX, and X may be impaired and synergism with coumadins may increase the danger of hemorrhage. These factors coupled with the problem of possible noncompliance may render the anticoagulant treatment of the alcoholic hazardous or impossible.

The timely recommendation of the surgeon general of the United States in the case of alcoholics is to "be alert to the possible interaction of prescribed, over-the-counter, or illicit drugs, singly or in combination, with alcohol."

TREATMENT OF ALCOHOLISM

Acute

The important principles are to protect both the acute alcoholic and innocent bystanders from the consequences of intoxication; to withhold alcohol but to observe the patient carefully for signs of incipient withdrawal symptoms; to attempt by any appropriate means to exclude causes other than alcohol of disturbed consciousness or behavior; to check serum electrolytes, looking particularly for deficiencies of potassium, magnesium, and phosphate; to give intravenous glucose; and when necessary, to maintain a good airway. Inhalation of vomitus is a life-threatening hazard. The main features are listed in Table 17-4.

Chronic

The main problems which have been discussed in various sections of this chapter have been tabulated (Table 17-4), and their treatment has been outlined.

From the foregoing a single unifying theme emerges. The most important component in the treatment of any alcohol-related disease is abstention from alcohol. Depending on the degree of organ damage which has occurred at the time alcohol is excluded from the diet, reversal or, at worst, some slowing of the progression of the pathological process results. The array of different regimens which have been devised and which are still used to achieve permanent abstention from or significantly curtailed consumption of alcohol is a clear expression of our relative ineffectiveness in treating this problem. Some successes have been and continue to be achieved, apparently by the application of a number of different techniques.

A basic requirement for successful treatment must be the patient's own motivation; without this no treatment is possible. Many workers in this field of therapy emphasize that abstention must be permanent and lifelong. Others

TABLE 17-4
TREATMENT OF EXCESSIVE ETHANOL INGESTION

Condition	Treatment
Acute disease	
Conscious	Withhold alcohol, observe patient, give careful sedation if necessary
Unconscious	Measure blood glucose and electrolytes including magnesium and anion gap
	Give intravenous glucose and electrolytes as indicated
Alcoholic hepatitis	Restore nutrition by using high-calorie low-sodium diet, observe patient
Wernicke's encephalopathy or Korsakoff's psychosis	Give IV thiamine
Polyneuropathy	Give thiamine
Chronic disease	
Anemia; thrombocytopenia	Withhold ethanol, give hematinics if deficient
Coagulopathies	Give vitamin K and fresh plasma
Cirrhosis	
Ascites	Restrict water and sodium, give diuretics
Encephalopathy	Restrict protein but aim for nitrogen balance, give lactulose, correct hypokalemia
Varices	Sclerosis
	Portal shunt

believe that the adoption of a moderate alcohol intake by the former alcoholic is possible and may be more successful than total abstention. Alcohol is a habituating drug and induces dependency. It possesses the property of eroding the will, so that many subjects lose control of their intake after a first drink and proceed to drink heavily.

The types of treatment which have been devised are behavioral therapy, individual or group psychotherapy, monitoring by peer group as practiced by Alcoholics Anonymous, pharmacotherapy, and various aversion therapies, some of which utilize pharmacological agents such as disulfiram. To date none seems to possess a clear advantage. There is even some controversy whether for some alcohol-dependent individuals total abstinence or reduced intake of alcohol is the better recommendation.

REFERENCES

1 Selzer, M. L.: The Michigan Alcoholism Screening Test: the quest for a new diagnostic instrument, Am. J. Psychiatry, 127:1653, 1971.

2 McGuiness, T.: An econometric analysis of total demand for alcoholic beverages in the U.K. 1956–75; J. Indust. Econom., 29:85, 1980.

3 Davies, P.: The U.K. and Europe: some comparative observations on alcohol consumption, alcohol related-problems and alcohol control policies in the United Kingdom and other countries of Europe, Br. J. Alcohol Alcoholism, 14:208, 1979.

4 *Alcohol and Health: First Special Report to the United States Congress from the Secretary of Health, Education and Welfare,* U.S. Department of Health, Education, and Welfare, U.S. Government Printing Office, Washington, 1971.

5 Jarman, C. M. B., and J. M. Kellett: Alcoholism in the general hospital, Br. Med. J., 2:469, 1979.

6 Kuller, L., K. Kramer, and R. Fisher: Changing trends in cirrhosis and fatty liver mortality, Am. J. Public Health and the Nation's Health, 59:1124, 1969.

7 Saunders, J. B., M. Davis, and R. Williams: Do women develop alcoholic liver disease more readily than men? Br. Med. J., 232:1140, 1981.

8 Morgan, M. Y., and S. Sherlock: Sex-related differences among 100 patients with alcoholic liver disease, Br. Med. J., 1:939, 1977.

9 Péquignot, G., C. Chabert, H. Eydoux, and M. A. Corcowl: Increased risk of liver cirrhosis with intake of alcohol, Revue in Alcoholism, 20:191, 1974.

10 Rubin, E., and C. S. Lieber: Alcohol-induced hepatic injury in nonalcoholic volunteers, N. Engl. J. Med., 278:869, 1968.

11 Palmer, E. D.: Gastritis: a re-evaluation, Medicine, 33:199, 1954.

12 Dinoso, V. P., W. Y. Chey, S. P. Braverman, A. P. Rosen, D. Ottenberg, and S. H. Lorber: Gastric secretion and gastric mucosal morphology in chronic alcoholics, Arch. Intern. Med., 130:715, 1972.

13 Halsted, C. H.: The small intestine in vitamin B-12 and folate deficiency, Nutr. Rev., 33:33, 1975.

14 Galambos, J. J.: Alcoholic hepatitis, in *The Liver and Its Diseases,* F. Schaffner, S. Sherlock, and C. M. Leevy (eds.), Intercontinental Medical Books, New York, 1974.

15 Garagliano, C. F., A. M. Lilienfeld, and A. I. Mendeloff: Incidence rates of liver cirrhosis and related diseases in Baltimore and selected areas of the United States, J. Chronic Dis., 32:543, 1979.

16 Anderson, B. B., H. O'Brien, G. E. Griffin, and D. L. Mollin: Hydrolysis of pyridoxal-5-phosphate in plasma in conditions with raised alkaline phosphatase, Gut, 21:192, 1980.

17 Alexander, C. S.: Electron microscopic observations in alcoholic heart disease, Br. Heart J., 29:200, 1967.

18 Burch, G. E., J. M. Harb, H. L. Colcolough, and C. Y. Tsui: The effect of prolonged consumption of beer, wine and ethanol on the myocardium of the mouse, Johns Hopkins Med. J., 129:130, 1971.

19 Wilkinson, P. K., A. J. Sedman, E. Sakmar, Y. J. Lin, and J. G. Wagner: Fasting and nonfasting blood alcohol concentrations following oral administration of ethanol to one adult male subject, J. Pharmacokinet. Biopharm., 5:41, 1977.

20 Victor, M.: Deficiency diseases of the nervous system secondary to alcoholism, Postgrad. Med. J., 50:75, 1971.

21 Blass, J. P., and G. E. Gibson: Abnormality of a thiamine-requiring enzyme in patients with Wernicke-Korsakoff syndrome, N. Engl. J. Med., 297:1367, 1977.

22 Eichner, E. R., B. Buchanan, J. W. Smith, and R. S. Hillman: Variations in the hematologic and medical states of alcoholics, Am. J. Med., 263:35, 1972.
23 Sullivan, L. W., and V. Herbert: Suppression of hematopoiesis by ethanol, J. Clin. Invest., 43:2048, 1964.
24 Jones, K. L., and D. W. Smith: Recognition of the fetal alcohol syndrome in early infancy, Lancet, 2:999, 1973.
25 Hanson, J. W., K. L. Jones, and D. W. Smith: Fetal alcohol syndrome—experience with 41 patients, J. Am. Med. Assoc., 235:1458, 1976.
26 Flynn, A., S. I. Miller, S. S. Martier, N. L. Golden, R. J. Sokol, and B. C. Del Villano: Zinc status of pregnant alcoholic women: a determinant of fetal outcome, Lancet, 1:572, 1981.
27 Madison, L. L.: Ethanol induced hypoglycemia, in *Advances in Metabolic Disorders*, vol. 3, R. Levine and R. Luft (eds.), Academic, New York, 1968.
28 Castelli, W. P., J. T. Doyle, T. Gordon, C. Hamnes, M. C. Hjortland, S. B. Hulley, A. Kagan, and W. J. Zukel: Alcohol and blood lipids. The cooperative phenotyping study, Lancet, 2:153, 1977.

CHAPTER 18

NUTRITIONAL ASPECTS OF MINERALS

CONTENTS

INTRODUCTION

The class of nutrients known as minerals are chemical elements known to be essential for nutritional health in humans and are required in milligram quantities in the daily diet. The *macrominerals,* or *major minerals,* are required in amounts of 100 mg or more per day; *microminerals,* or *trace minerals,* are required in amounts no greater than a few milligrams per day. The seven major minerals are calcium, phosphorus, magnesium, sodium, potassium, chlorine, and sulfur.

Unlike the macrominerals, which are more abundant in the body and often serve in a structural capacity, the microminerals generally perform a regulatory role, which is accomplished through a wide diversity of biochemical mechanisms. In fact, apart from their essentiality and scarcity the trace minerals share little in common to recommend their being grouped together. The list of trace minerals known to be essential in humans includes chromium, cobalt, copper, fluoride, iodine, iron, manganese, molybdenum, selenium, and zinc. Only deficiencies of iron, iodine, cobalt, copper, and zinc are known to cause disease in humans. As shown in Table 18-1 nutritional deficiencies arise from a variety of causes, which operate individually or in combination.

One of the major problems facing researchers who study minerals is the accurate determination of nutritional requirements. This problem is important because many trace elements, while essential in small amounts, can be toxic in larger quantities. Determining requirements is difficult, since the amounts needed in the body are small and because absorption of minerals is affected substantially by the composition of the diet (other nutrients, fiber, phytic acid,

TABLE 18-1
ETIOLOGICAL FACTORS CONTRIBUTING TO TRACE
ELEMENT DEFICIENCIES

Factor	Examples
Inadequate dietary intake	Protein-calorie malnutrition Low-income diets Old age Low environmental levels (e.g., fluorine, selenium)
Decreased availability	High-fiber–high-phytate diets Infant formulas
Decreased absorption	Malabsorption syndromes Steatorrhea Chemical interferences (calcium, phosphorus, other trace elements)
Excessive losses	Loss in urine Surgery Burns Increased sweating
Increased requirement	Rapid growth Pregnancy Lactation Tissue anabolism
Reduced stores	Prematurity
Iatrogenic factors	Chelating drugs Total parenteral nutrition, synthetic diets Dialysis
Genetic defects	Acrodermatitis enteropathica Menkes' kinky hair disease

Source: C. E. Casey and K. M. Hambridge, Trace element deficiencies in man, in Advances in Nutritional Research, vol. 3, H. H. Draper (ed.), Plenum, New York, 1980, p. 23.

and oxalates). In addition, only in recent years have techniques for accurate measurement of these elements in tissue and body fluids become available. Furthermore, the widespread use of processed foods from which trace elements have been removed is of concern because adequate intakes may be more difficult to achieve.

Each mineral required by human beings has been classified into one of three groups in the newest Recommended Dietary Allowances (RDAs) [1]: (1) those for which a well-defined allowance has been estabished (calcium, phosphorus, magnesium, iron, zinc, and iodine) (Table 18-2), (2) those for which "estimated adequate and safe intakes" have been established (sodium, potassium, chloride, copper, manganese, molybdenum, chromium, selenium, and fluoride) (Table 18-3), and (3) the "newer" trace elements which have been shown to be required by animal species but for which no requirement in humans has been established (silicon, vanadium, nickel, arsenic, tin, and cadmium).

Calcium and phosphorus are discussed in Chapter 13 of this text, while sodium and potassium are covered in Chapter 9. Iodine and cobalt function solely as

TABLE 18-2
UNITED STATES RECOMMENDED DIETARY ALLOWANCES FOR MINERALS

Age and sex group	Calcium, mg	Phos- phorus, mg	Mag- nesium, mg	Iron, mg	Zinc, mg	Iodine, μg
Infants						
0.0–0.5 yr	360	240	50	10	3	40
0.5–1.0 yr	540	360	70	15	5	50
Children						
1–3 yr	800	800	150	15	10	70
4–6 yr	800	800	200	10	10	90
7–10 yr	800	800	250	10	10	120
Males						
11–14 yr	1,200	1,200	350	18	15	150
15–18 yr	1,200	1,200	400	18	15	150
19–22 yr	800	800	350	10	15	150
23–50 yr	800	800	350	10	15	150˙
51+ yr	800	800	350	10	15	150
Females						
11–14 yr	1,200	1,200	300	18	15	150
15–18 yr	1,200	1,200	300	18	15	150
19–22 yr	800	800	300	18	15	150
23–50 yr	800	800	300	18	15	150
51+ yr	800	800	300	10	15	150
Pregnancy	+400	+400	+150	*	+5	+25
Lactation	+400	+400	+150	*	+10	+50

*The increased requirement during pregnancy cannot be met by the iron content of habitual American diets or by the existing iron stores of many women; therefore, the use of a 30- to 60-mg supplement is advisable in order to replenish stores depleted by pregnancy.

TABLE 18-3
ESTIMATED SAFE AND ADEQUATE DAILY DIETARY INTAKES OF ADDITIONAL SELECTED MINERALS*
(In Milligrams)

Age group	Trace elements						Electrolytes		
	Copper	Manganese	Fluoride	Chromium	Selenium	Molybdenum	Sodium	Potassium	Chloride
Infants									
0.0–0.5 yr	0.5–0.7	0.5–0.7	0.1–0.5	0.01–0.04	0.01–0.04	0.03–0.06	115–350	350–925	275–700
0.5–1.0 yr	0.7–1.0	0.7–1.0	0.2–1.0	0.02–0.06	0.02–0.06	0.04–0.08	250–750	425–1,275	400–1,200
Children and Adolescents									
1–3 yr	1.0–1.5	1.0–1.5	0.5–1.5	0.02–0.08	0.02–0.08	0.05–0.1	325–975	550–1,650	500–1,500
4–6 yr	1.5–2.0	1.5–2.0	1.0–2.5	0.03–0.12	0.03–0.12	0.06–0.15	450–1,350	775–2,325	700–2,100
7–10 yr	2.0–2.5	2.0–3.0	1.5–2.5	0.05–0.2	0.05–0.2	0.1 –0.3	600–1,800	1,000–3,000	925–2,775
11+ yr	2.0–3.0	2.5–5.0	1.5–2.5	0.05–0.2	0.05–0.2	0.15–0.5	900–2,700	1,525–4,575	1,400–4,200
Adults	2.0–3.0	2.5–5.0	1.5–4.0	0.05–0.2	0.05–0.2	0.15–0.5	1,100–3,300	1,875–5,625	1,700–5,100

*Because there is less information on which to base allowances, these figures are not given in the main table of the RDAs and are provided here in the form of ranges of recommended intakes.

†Since the toxic levels for many trace elements may be only several times usual intakes, the upper levels for the trace elements given in this table should not be habitually exceeded.

Source: From Recommended Dietary Allowances, Revised 1980, 9th ed., National Academy of Sciences, National Research Council, Food and Nutrition Board, Washington, 1980.

components of a hormone (thyroxine) and cobalamin, respectively; they have no other known function. Inadequate intake leads to specific abnormalities that are easily recognized and differentiated from other conditions. In Chapter 10 the role of iron and cobalamin in hematopoiesis are described. Further basic information regarding minerals can be found in Appendix 7. In this chapter, the clinically significant essential minerals (zinc, copper, chromium, selenium, magnesium, manganese, fluoride, and iodine) are discussed.

ZINC

Dietary Sources, Availability, and Requirements

The best sources of zinc are meats, shellfish, fish, whole-grain cereals, and legumes. As shown in Table 18-4 Atlantic oysters are the richest known source. Dairy products, fruits, and vegetables are generally poor sources. Refining of cereals decreases their zinc content, and the zinc found in whole-grain products may be largely unavailable because of the presence of phytic acid and fiber. Fermentation with yeast, as in leavened bread, markedly increases the physiological availability of zinc in whole wheat bread. This increase is attributed to the action of yeast in destroying phytate. Copper and iron, which are chemically similar divalent cations, appear to share common absorptive pathways and therefore compete with zinc in the intestine for absorption. Both calcium and

TABLE 18-4
ZINC CONTENT OF SELECTED FOODS

	Amount	Zinc content, mg
Oysters, fresh	6 medium	124.9
Turkey, dark meat	3 oz	3.7
Beef liver	3 oz	3.3
Lima beans, cooked	$\frac{1}{2}$ cup	2.7
Beef, ground, cooked	3 oz	2.1
Yogurt, plain	8 oz	1.3
Almonds	$\frac{1}{4}$ cup	1.2
Egg, whole	1 large	0.7
Spinach, cooked	$\frac{1}{2}$ cup	0.2
Orange juice	6 oz	0.1

Sources: L. P. Posati and M. L. Orr, Composition of Foods—Raw, Processed, Prepared—Dairy and Egg Products, U.S. Department of Agriculture Handbook no. 8-1, U.S. Government Printing Office, Washington, 1976; H. H. Sandstead, Zinc nutrition in the United States, Am. J. Clin. Nutr., 26:1257, 1973.

phosphate reduce the utilization of dietary zinc. The zinc in human milk has greater bioavailability than that in cow's milk, and this has been attributed to a low-molecular-weight zinc-binding ligand which probably facilitates absorption [2].

Precise minimum requirements for zinc for optimal health and growth are not known. Dietary requirements depend, in part, on the composition of the diet. The World Health Organization [3] has published provisional requirements for zinc that were estimated on a factorial basis and are adjusted for different levels (10 percent, 20 percent, and 30 percent) of available zinc in the diet. The RDAs (Table 18-2) are based on balance studies which indicated that 8 to 10 mg of zinc would maintain zinc equilibrium in healthy adults. On the assumption that 40 percent of the dietary zinc is available, a recommendation of 15 mg of zinc per day was made. No allowances are made for variations in availability, but the recommendation is "predicated on the consumption of a mixed diet containing animal products."

Absorption and Excretion

The exact site of zinc absorption in the small intestine is unknown; absorption ranges from 10 to 40 percent. In experiments with animals each portion of the small bowel has been proposed as the site of preferential zinc absorption. Low-molecular-weight (8000 to 10,000) zinc-binding ligands have been reported in experimental animals and in human milk [4,5], and it is thought that they facilitate zinc absorption from the intestinal lumen. The absorption of zinc, like that of iron, seems to be controlled by the nutritional state of the individual with respect to the mineral. The mechanism of control is not precisely understood, but metallothioneins, low-molecular-weight soluble proteins, may play a role. Metallothioneins are cytoplasmic proteins that have a rapid rate of turnover and a high affinity for binding zinc (and copper, cadmium, and mercury); their synthesis can be induced by parenteral or oral zinc administration [6]. Hence, a metallothionein may participate in the homeostatic regulation of zinc metabolism and absorption and may provide a source of zinc at times of deprivation.

Zinc is primarily excreted in the feces [7], and various gastrointestinal diseases can markedly increase zinc loss. Urine is generally a minor excretory pathway for zinc, but in certain conditions, such as following burns, surgery, or trauma or in hepatic disease, urinary excretion rises markedly [8].

Biological Functions

The biochemical functions of zinc are wide in scope. Zinc is an essential component in over 80 zinc metalloenzymes which participate in all major metabolic pathways. Mammalian metalloenzymes include carbonic anhydrase, carboxypeptidases, aminopeptidases, alkaline phosphatase, thymidine kinase, and alcohol, retinol, malate, lactate, glutamate, and glyceraldehyde-3-phosphate dehydrogenases. Zinc plays an essential role in the synthesis of deoxyribonucleic acid (DNA), ribonucleic acid (RNA), and protein. It also stabilizes cellular membranes and polyribosomes during protein synthesis. Zinc may play a physiological role in taste; gustin and nerve growth factor, two zinc metalloproteins, have been isolated from human and murine saliva, respectively [9]. Mobilization of vitamin A from the liver requires zinc, and the mineral also plays a part in wound healing, perhaps in the synthesis of collagen. Zinc is also required for the proper activity of DNA and RNA polymerases. It is essential for spermatogenesis and ova formation. Insulin is stored in the beta cells of the pancreas as a hexamer with two atoms of zinc [10]. Impaired glucose tolerance and insulin response have been associated with zinc deficiency in some studies [11]. Cell-mediated immunity is decreased in experimental zinc deficiency [12], and a study in Jamaica suggested that zinc deficiency is the cause of the impaired immunocompetence seen in protein-calorie malnutrition [13].

Human Zinc Deficiency

Etiologic Factors Responsible for Zinc Deficiency in Humans   Zinc deficiency can result from an inadequate dietary intake, malabsorption, increased body losses, intravenous feeding, or a combination of several of these predisposing factors.

Prasad and his colleagues [14] were the first to document human zinc deficiency in male adolescent Iranian and Egyptian villagers who subsisted on a high-phytate diet of unleavened bread and virtually no meat. The syndrome consisted of short stature, hepatosplenomegaly, and delay in sexual maturation. The first evidence that zinc deficiency might occur in otherwise well-nourished children was provided by Hambidge et al. [15]. They described ten children aged 4 to 13 years in Denver who had hair zinc concentrations more than three standard deviations below the adult mean. Seven of ten were at or below the 10th percentile for height, seven suffered from poor appetite, and of the six who were tested, five had objective evidence of impaired taste (hypogeusia). Therapy with zinc sulfate was followed by an objective improvement in taste sensation and by an increase in hair zinc concentration. However, no effect on growth was reported. Hambidge et al. [16] have also shown that children from low-income families in the Denver Headstart program have significantly lower hair and plasma zinc concentrations than do controls. Walravens and Hambidge [17] have reported the results of supplementing infant formula (Similac) with 4 mg of zinc per liter during the first 6 months of life. In the supplemented group, both boys and girls showed a significantly higher plasma zinc concentration than did controls but only the boys showed significant increases in length and weight. These data suggest that the provision of zinc in the diet of some children may be suboptimal.

The full consequences of profound zinc deficiency became evident when Moynahan, in 1973, recognized the similarity between the clinical findings in acrodermatitis enteropathica (AE) and those of experimental zinc deficiency in animals [18]. Acrodermatitis enteropathica (Color Figure 3) is a rare autosomal recessive trait that develops in the early months of life, soon after weaning from breast-feeding. If the disease is left untreated, the child dies within 3 years. The features of the disease include alopecia, vesicopustular lesions of the face, perineum, and extremities, esophagitis, diarrhea, a pronounced thymic atrophy, and a high incidence of *Candida albicans* infection. It can be cured by giving pharmacological doses of zinc. It is now appreciated that the principal defect consists of insufficient zinc absorption and that the earlier therapeutic success with diiodohydroxyquin depended on its capacity to complex zinc and to augment its absorption.

Protein-calorie malnutrition in the developing parts of the world is probably the most common cause of zinc deficiency, but western populations may be at risk as a consequence of marginal intake. This may be the case in some vegetarians, low socioeconomic groups subsisting on low-meat diets [15,16], and patients with chronic renal disease on low-protein diets [19].

Any individual with gastrointestinal disease is potentially at risk for developing zinc deficiency. Steatorrhea, protein-losing enteropathy, or any condition causing massive loss of intestinal secretions may result in increased zinc losses. Increased body losses may occur in a wide variety of conditions including burns, proteinuria, dialysis, chronic blood loss, or excessive sweating. Intravenous feeding, particularly if prolonged, carries a risk of zinc deficiency. This is in part due to the variable low content of zinc in the administered solutions [20]. It is particularly likely to occur during an anabolic phase in which there is an abrupt increase in the body requirement.

Since the zinc requirement increases with pregnancy, the suggestion has been made that pregnant women may be particularly susceptible to zinc deficiency [21]. Low hair zinc levels were found in a group of healthy pregnant women [22], but the physiological significance of these low levels during pregnancy is not clear. Except in several patients with acrodermatitis enteropathica [23] poor reproductive performance due to zinc deficiency has not been clearly shown in humans.

Clinical Manifestations of Zinc Deficiency   The variable clinical manifestations of zinc deficiency are listed in Table 18-5. Anorexia, growth retardation, and impaired taste and olfactory sensation are early features. Skin lesions are quite common. These may consist of parakeratosis or moist eczematoid dermatitis, most severe in the perioral, perianal, and periorbital areas, and alopecia.

Diagnosis   The parameters most commonly used to describe zinc status are the concentration of zinc in plasma (or serum) and in hair. Levels in whole blood, red cells, parotid saliva, and urine and activities of the zinc-dependent enzymes alkaline phosphatase and erythrocyte carbonic anhydrase have also been used. Laboratory measurements provide support for a diagnosis of zinc

TABLE 18-5
CLINICAL MANIFESTATIONS OF ZINC DEFICIENCY

Anorexia	Dysarthria
Impaired taste and smell	Jitteriness
Pica	Photophobia, night blindness, blepharitis
Growth retardation	Skin lesions (digits, perineum, parietal
Hypogonadism	areas, nasolabial folds)
Impotence in renal dialysis patients	Paronychia with monilial superinfection
Depression, mood lability, impaired	Nails (growth arrest, loss, Beau's lines)
concentration	Hair growth arrest or alopecia
Intention tremor	Delayed wound healing
Nystagmus	Diarrhea

Source: P. J. Aggett and J. T. Harries, Current status of zinc in health and disease states, Arch. Dis. Child., 54:909, 1979.

deficiency suggested by the presence of the clinical features described and the nutritional history. A response to therapy is probably the most reliable index for making a diagnosis of zinc deficiency in humans.

Treatment   Oral administration of 1 mg of zinc per kilogram of body weight per day is adequate to treat zinc deficiency under most circumstances [24]. Sulfate and acetate salts appear to be equally well absorbed, but the sulfate can be an irritant to the gastrointestinal tract. In these circumstances the zinc salt can be taken with a meal or in capsulated preparations, which may be better tolerated; but zinc is less efficiently absorbed in the presence of food or from capsules. Intravenous requirements appear to be about 20 to 40 μg of zinc per kilogram of body weight per day for children and adults and may be higher in infants [25].

Prevention   Prevention of nutritional zinc deficiency is best achieved by adequate nutritional advice. There are data to suggest that the average zinc intake on self-selected diets ranges from 8.5 to 13 mg per day [26]. It has been found that suboptimal levels of calories and low to marginal intakes of protein tend to be related to low zinc intakes. Also, high levels of energy and protein provided more than recommended levels of zinc. Statistical analysis of nutrient intakes showed that zinc was more closely correlated with the amount of protein in the diet than with the dietary energy level [27]. For a mixed diet, there was a ratio of 1.5 mg of zinc per 10 g of protein; thus, approximately 100 g of protein must be consumed to provide the recommended zinc intake. This level of protein represents the upper limit of normal protein intake and is almost 80 percent above the RDA for protein for the "reference man." However, the RDA for zinc is a *recommendation* not a requirement, and most individual needs are lower. In early postnatal life, breast-feeding provides the best means of protection from zinc deficiency.

Toxicity

Zinc salts are usually well tolerated. Ingestion of excess zinc has usually resulted from storage of food or beverages in galvanized containers and results in fever, nausea, vomiting, and diarrhea. If a corrosive form of zinc is ingested (zinc chloride), severe necrosis and ulceration of the gastrointestinal tract may occur.

COPPER

Dietary Sources, Availability, and Requirements

The estimate for the copper requirement of humans is based on balance studies. From these studies in adults, it has been determined that the body needs 1.5 to 2.0 mg per day. On the basis of these data and in order to allow for a margin of safety, the Food and Nutrition Board has recommended a dietary intake for adults of 2 to 3 mg per day. The World Health Organization [3] suggests that 40 μg per kilogram of body weight per day is adequate for older children and approximately 30 μg/kg daily is adequate for an adult male. This is about 2 mg per day. Slightly higher recommendations have been made for infants and young children; both agencies suggest an intake of 80 μg/kg per day. Addition of 20 to 30 μg/kg per day, up to about 1 mg of copper in the adult, to intravenous fluids is generally recommended for patients on long-term parenteral feeding [28].

The most abundant dietary sources of copper include liver, crustaceans, and shellfish, especially oysters (Table 18-6). Lesser concentrations are provided by nuts, wheat-based cereals, dried fruit, poultry, fish, meats, legumes, root and leafy vegetables, and fresh fruits. Cow's milk is one of the poorest sources of copper (less than 20 μg per 100 kcal) [29]. Adult human milk contains approximately 24 μg/dl or 36 μg per 100 kcal [30]. Tap water may provide a significant amount in the diet [31].

A number of factors influence the copper content of foods. Environmental factors include the copper content of soil, geographical location (such as nearness to industrial complexes that may release copper-containing wastes), use of copper containing fungicides and insecticides, use of fertilizers, and the origin of the water supply. Phytates found in whole-grain cereals form very stable complexes with copper and reduce the assimilation of this element.

Analysis of total daily intake indicates that many adults on self-chosen western-style diets obtain less than 2 mg of copper per day [32,33]. The median daily amount of copper in 20 American diets made from conventional foods was 0.8 mg [34]. Thus the daily intake of copper by U.S. adults apparently is well below recommended levels.

Absorption and Excretion

Dietary copper is absorbed from the lumen of the duodenum and stomach complexed to *l*-amino acids or other ligands. Other elements such as cadmium, mercury, silver, and zinc compete for absorption. Copper is transported from

TABLE 18-6
COPPER CONTENT OF SELECTED FOODS

	Amount	Copper content, mg
Oysters, fresh	6 medium	14.2
Beef liver	3 oz	2.4
Bran flakes, 40%	1 cup	0.5
Avocado	1 half	0.5
Potato	1 medium	0.4
Soybeans, cooked	½ cup	0.3
Pecans	1 oz	0.3
Green peas	½ cup	0.1
Raisins	1½ oz	0.1
Milk, whole	1 cup	0.1
Bread, whole wheat	1 slice	0.06
Beef, ground	3 oz	0.05
Cheddar cheese	1 oz	0.03

Source: J. T. Pennington and D. H. Calloway, Copper content of foods, J. Am. Diet. Assoc., 63:143, 1973.

the intestinal mucosa as a copper-albumin complex in the portal venous plasma to the liver. In the hepatic cells, copper is stored bound to a metallothionein, incorporated into ceruloplasmin (a copper-containing protein synthesized in the liver) or other copper enzymes, or excreted via the bile. Ceruloplasmin accounts for 95 percent of the copper found in serum and serves to transport copper to peripheral tissues, while albumin binds the remaining 5 percent. Copper is excreted in the bile complexed to amino acids and macromolecules, which prohibits any significant enterohepatic circulation.

Biological Functions

Copper is a component of a number of copper metalloenzymes. These enzymes generally bind between 1 and 8 gram-atoms of copper per mole. The function of the copper seems to be related to its ability to engage in oxidation-reduction reactions.

As a component of cytochrome oxidase, copper is important in mitochondrial oxidative phosphorylation. Cytochrome oxidase is the only enzyme that reduces molecular oxygen to water and is also an enzyme which produces adenosine triphosphate (ATP). Copper is essential for the function of lysyl oxidase, an enzyme required in the cross-linking that occurs in collagen and elastin. Tyrosinase is a copper-dependent enzyme required for the formation of melanin. As a component of the enzyme superoxide dismutase, copper may be very important in protecting cells from damage by superoxide radicals. Ceruloplasmin has as its main function the oxidation of ferrous iron to the ferric form, so that ferric iron can be incorporated into apotransferrin and transported to the bone marrow. Ceruloplasmin also serves as a transport protein for copper. Because of its enzymatic role in iron metabolism, ceruloplasmin is also called ferroxidase I.

Metallothioneins, low-molecular-weight proteins, are currently the subject of controversy. They are present in liver, intestinal mucosal epithelium, and kidney. Metallothioneins bind zinc, cadmium, mercury, and copper; their role in zinc homeostasis is better established than their suggested role in copper metabolism.

Human Copper Deficiency

Copper deficiency in humans is unusual; however, both genetic and acquired forms are now recognized. Each has features that resemble manifestations of spontaneous or experimental copper deficiency in animals.

Etiologic Factors Responsible for Copper Deficiency in Humans Clinically apparent copper deficiency in humans was first described in 1964 by Cordano and coworkers in severely malnourished infants in Peru with chronic diarrhea who were rehabilitated with low-copper, iron-fortified milk formula [35]. Copper depletion in infants with chronic diarrhea has also been reported in the United States [36]. One factor involved in development of copper deficiency is the prolonged administration of a diet based solely on cow's milk, which is one of the poorest sources of copper.

Another risk factor for copper deficiency is prematurity. The liver stores of the full-term neonate are generally adequate to supply the infant's copper needs for 4 to 6 months, by which age foods other than milk are generally introduced. However, since copper is mainly accumulated in the last 3 months of gestation, the premature infant is born with meager stores. Other factors involved in the development of copper deficiency include (1) generalized malnutrition, (2) prolonged diarrhea, (3) intestinal malabsorption, (4) long-term total parenteral nutrition (TPN) with copper-poor solutions, and (5) long-term use of chelating agents (e.g., D-penicillamine).

Severe deranged copper metabolism occurs in the fatal neurodegenerative disorder of infancy described in 1962 by Menkes et al. [37], known as the *kinky hair syndrome*. The extraordinary correspondence between the physiological defects and the reduced activity of copper metalloenzymes is striking. The pathognomonic feature—kinky hair or pili torti—can be ascribed to a defect in the formation of disulfide bonds as a consequence of deficiency of amine oxidase activity. The pale skin and depigmented hair are attributed to a defect in tyrosinase. Vascular tortuosity and diffuse aneurysms are due to defective elastin formation. The copper-containing enzyme lysyl oxidase is required to cross-link the precursors of elastin and collagen. The hypothermia has been related to deficient cytochrome c oxidase activity in mitochondrial oxidative metabolism. The neurological disorders—mental retardation, seizures, and hypotonia—are due, in part, to cytochrome c oxidase deficiency and perhaps to dopamine β-hydroxylase deficiency. Skeletal demineralization, resembling scorbutic bone disease, has been attributed to a deficient ascorbate oxidase activity, suspected of being copper-dependent in mammals as well as plants. This disease is transmitted in an X-linked manner, i.e., affects only males, and occurs in about 1 of 35,000 live births. Danks et al. [38] discovered that such patients have copper accumulated in the intestinal mucosal epithelium but very low serum copper and ceruloplasmin levels. Initially it was thought that Menkes' disease was a disorder simply of copper transport from the mucosa to the blood stream, but the failure of therapeutic trials with oral and parenteral copper has shown that the disease is more complex [39].

Clinical Manifestations   The earliest features of human copper deficiency are neutropenia and anemia that do not respond to oral iron. The anemia is initially hypochromic, and later, iron metabolism in the normoblast is disturbed and erythrocyte production becomes defective [40]. Later bone changes reminiscent of scurvy develop, with occasional fractures.

Other findings in copper deficiency include anorexia and failure to thrive in infants, diarrhea, depigmentation of hair and skin, skin lesions, and prominant dilated superficial veins. Neurological abnormalities that have been described in copper-deficient premature infants include hypotonia, lack of interest in outside surroundings, psychomotor retardation, and apparent lack of visual response.

With the exception of anemia, all the pathological abnormalities associated with copper deficiency have been observed in patients with Menkes' syndrome. In kinky hair disease, early symptoms include hypothermia, feeding difficulties, and occasionally, prolonged jaundice during the neonatal period. This disease is usually recognized when seizure activity starts at 2 to 3 months of age. The hair, which seems normal at birth, is progressively replaced by short, stubby, twisted growth of lighter pigmentation that feels like steel wool. Pallor and drowsiness are often present. As the disease progresses, seizure activity increases and rashes of the seborrheic dermatitis type appear. Death ensues during the early years of infancy, after increasing mental deterioration, infections, feeding difficulties, and failure to thrive.

Diagnosis   The diagnosis of copper deficiency should be considered in a patient when any of the predisposing factors are present and if anemia, leukopenia, and particularly neutropenia are found. Low levels of plasma copper and ceruloplasmin may help confirm the diagnosis. However, these plasma parameters may be affected by a number of conditions other than poor copper nutritional status. For example, hypocupremia occurs in Wilson's disease (a genetic defect of hepatic copper metabolism causing excessive copper storage) and in hypoproteinemia. Hair copper content may also be low, but it has not been generally accepted as a practical assay.

The discovery of an unexplained rib fracture in growing premature infants may also help to diagnose copper deficiency [41]. Other radiological changes include flaring of the anterior portion of the ribs, periosteal reactions, and the formation of spurs at the metaphysis of long bones. The bone changes are similar to those seen in the "battered-child syndrome" and also resemble the changes seen in scurvy.

Treatment   Nutritional copper deficiency in infants responds promptly to oral copper therapy. A 1% solution of anhydrous cupric sulfate given 1 to 3 mg per day (0.4 to 1.19 mg of Cu per day) has been efficacious orally [42]. Most infant formulas now contain 60 μg of Cu per 100 kcal. It has been suggested that formulas fed to preterm infants should contain copper at not less than 90 μg per 100 kcal (0.6 mg per liter) to provide approximately 100 μg of Cu per kilogram per day to prevent copper deficiency in preterm infants [43]. For patients on total parenteral nutrition (TPN), Green and colleagues [44] recommend inclusion in the fluid of 20 to 30 μg of Cu per kilogram per day for full-term infants, and for adults up to 0.5 to 1.0 mg of Cu per day appears to be adequate. This amount is probably also sufficient to treat existing copper deficiency.

In patients with Menkes' syndrome, some response has been obtained with parenteral copper but not with an oral form. Copper therapy restores ceruloplasmin and hepatic copper levels to normal, but the symptoms of the disease usually do not improve. This may be because in most of the cases reported to date the patients were at least 3 months old before they were identified and treatment was begun [45].

Prevention   Copper is widely distributed in foods, but the older analytical data reporting a daily intake between 2 and 5 mg are being reexamined and questioned. Recent surveys of a variety of diets have indicated much lower intakes, often substantially below 1 mg per day [46]. It is not known whether the discrepancy between the older and the more recent data is a true indication of a declining copper intake or whether it can be attributed to differences in analytical methodology. The prevention of nutritional copper deficiency is best achieved by consuming a *varied* diet.

Toxicity

Copper toxicity is not common in humans. Diets in the United States will rarely supply more than 5 mg daily. Toxicity occurs when a deliberate attempt has been made to ingest excessive amounts of some substances such as copper sulfate. The ingestion of more than 15 mg of elemental copper usually produces nausea, vomiting, diarrhea, and intestinal cramps. This phenomenon has been seen in renal dialysis units in which an excess of copper was transferred from the dialysis bath to the patient. Ingestion of gram quantities of copper causes serious gastrointestinal and systemic injuries and occasionally hepatic necrosis.

Wilson's disease (hepatolenticular degeneration) is an autosomal recessive disorder in which excessive copper accumulates in the liver, brain, kidney, and cornea and in which the concentrations of serum copper and ceruloplasmin decrease. It has an incidence of about 1 in 200,000. In affected patients copper slowly accumulates from birth. Almost half of the patients present with symptoms due to liver damage and may die before any neurological features become apparent. Even in presymptomatic subjects tests of liver function may already be abnormal. The accumulation of copper in the brain results in progressive mental deterioration with tremor, choreoarthritis, and loss of coordination. Deposits of metal about the cornea (Kayser-Fleischer rings) are uniformly present by the time neurological signs appear. These may be best detected using a slit-lamp microscope.

The basic defect is unknown. Serum ceruloplasmin levels are nearly always low, which renders the measurement of this protein a valuable diagnostic method; however, there are sufficient reports of patients with normal ceruloplasmin levels to demonstrate that the basic fault does not lie in this molecule. Absorption of copper from the gut and uptake into the liver are normal, but incorporation into ceruloplasmin and excretion in the bile are greatly reduced. D-Penicillamine (β,β-dimethylcysteine), which removes excessive copper through chelation and increased urinary excretion, appears to arrest the progress of the disease if instituted before damage is extensive. A low-copper diet is also desirable. Wilson's disease is further discussed in Chapter 16.

CHROMIUM

Chromium became of nutritional interest in 1959 when it was found that trace quantities of trivalent chromium are necessary for normal glucose tolerance in rats [47]. Subsequently, evidence developed that deficiency of chromium occurs in some human populations, presumably due to an inadequate intake and/or poor availability. Moreover, it is thought by some that suboptimal chromium nutrition could be contributing to the higher incidence in western populations of impaired glucose tolerance, hyperlipidemia, and associated cardiovascular disease. Presently, these concepts remain little more than tantalizing possibilities, neither confirmed nor disproven. Difficulties with analytical technique also hamper elucidation of the role of chromium in nutrition and metabolism.

Dietary Sources, Availability, and Requirements

Chromium is found in foods in two forms: as trivalent chromium (Cr^{3+}) or as an organic complex known as glucose tolerance factor (GTF). GTF is absorbed better from the gastrointestinal tract than Cr^{3+} (less than 1 percent of Cr^{3+} is absorbed), and the best dietary sources are brewer's yeast, liver, beef, cheese, whole grains, and black pepper. Refined foods contain little chromium; for example, sugar, polished rice, white flour, breakfast cereal, and spaghetti are poor sources.

Chromium requirements are usually estimated from urinary losses. The wide variation in reported values for urinary excretion, however, has made a precise definition of these requirements uncertain. The amount of chromium required in the diet also depends on the proportion present as the biologically active form (GTF). Within these limitations, the Committee on Recommended Allowances [1] has proposed that a daily intake of 50 to 200 μg of chromium should be adequate to meet the needs of most healthy adults. This range is based on the absence of signs of chromium deficiency in the major part of the U.S. population consuming on the average 60 μg of chromium per day. The safety of an intake of 200 μg has been established in long-term supplementation trials in human subjects receiving 150 μg per day in addition to the dietary intake [48]. The suggested range of intake is predicated on the assumption that a varied diet providing an adequate intake of other essential micronutrients will furnish chromium with an average availability of 1 to 2 percent. Recommendations for maintenance on total parenteral nutrition include 0.14 to 0.2 μg of Cr per kilogram of body weight per day for children and up to 10 to 15 μg per day for adults [28].

Absorption and Excretion

Little work has been done on the intestinal absorption of chromium in humans. Animal studies suggest that chromium is absorbed in the upper small intestine. Chromium (Cr^{3+}) is poorly absorbed and exhibits little biological activity in comparison to GTF chromium [49]. Chromium (Cr^{6+}) is absorbed more readily but does not occur in food. Absorption of chromium in GTF is 10 to 25 percent efficient in rats. Two forms of chromium circulate in the plasma compartments; some chromium is bound to transferrin and the other form is GTF-bound chromium [50]. Orally absorbed chromium is excreted mainly by the kidney.

Biological Functions

Chromium is essential as a component of nucleic acids and as a component of glucose tolerance factor. Neither the exact structure of glucose tolerance factor nor its mechanism of action is known. Toepfer et al. [51] recently described GTF as an organic chromium complex of low molecular weight containing Cr^{3+} liganded to nicotinic acid, glycine, glutamic acid, and cysteine. The current hypothesis is that GTF facilitates the interaction of glucose and its receptors [49] and thus helps dispose of ingested carbohydrate.

Chromium may also have a role in lipid metabolism. Rats maintained on a chromium-deficient diet had higher cholesterol levels, which were lowered by feeding chromium, and a higher incidence of aortic plaques than chromium-replete controls [52]. Furthermore, some subjects with impaired glucose tolerance tests showed a significant reduction in fasting serum cholesterol levels while on a GTF supplement [50].

Human Chromium Deficiency

Currently, there are no adequately established biochemical indexes of chromium nutriture, and confirmation of human chromium deficiency has been obtained largely by the observation of beneficial effects of dietary chromium supplementation. GTF chromium is not available for such studies; however, beneficial effects from Cr^{3+} administration have been reported.

Etiologic Factors Responsible for Chromium Deficiency in Humans   Infants suffering from marasmic protein-calorie malnutrition exhibit both hypoglycemia and impaired glucose tolerance. In three countries—Jordan, Nigeria, and Turkey—administration of chromium to infants improved the rate of removal of glucose given intravenously [53,54]. Oral inorganic Cr^{3+} supplementation improved the impaired glucose tolerance of middle-aged [55] and elderly people [56] in the United States and some patients with diabetes [57,58]. More recently, Jeejeebhoy et al. [59] have described an adult patient receiving total parenteral nutrition for more than 5 years in whom there developed an impairment of glucose tolerance and peripheral neuropathy that was reversed by chromium administration.

Certain population groups may be at risk for chromium depletion. Hair chromium is reduced in pregnancy, the decrease being most marked in multiparas [60]. Low hair levels, which suggest poor chromium nutrition, have also been observed in gestational diabetics and low-birth-weight infants [61]. In the United States, analysis of autopsy tissues revealed a decline in tissue chromium levels with increasing age [62,63], and adult levels were in general lower than those found in subjects in other countries (India, Japan, and Switzerland) [58]. These findings have been, in part, responsible for the unproven concept that suboptimal chromium nutrition may be common in the United States.

Clinical Manifestations   The principal effects of chromium deficiency in humans are impaired glucose tolerance, decreased nitrogen retention, ataxia, and defective peripheral nerve conduction [53,54,59].

Diagnosis   At present, diagnosis of chromium deficiency depends on demonstration of a chromium-responsive impairment of glucose tolerance. Precise measurement of chromium in body fluids and tissues is hampered by analytical difficulties and by the low levels present in tissues, which can best be expressed in parts per billion. Urinary chromium excretion has been suggested as a parameter for measuring nutritional status. Normal levels vary with age, with the highest levels being in preschool children. In recent studies a mean 24-hour chromium excretion of 0.8 ± 0.4 µg was found, with a range of 0.4 to 1.8 µg [64]. Although this value is lower by an order of magnitude than older published figures, it has been confirmed by independent methodology [65].

Levels of chromium in hair have also been used, but wide individual variations in hair chromium levels make these measurements more suitable for comparing the status of groups rather than for detecting deficiency in individuals. One study found levels of 240 ± 123 ng/g in the healthy adult and indicated that values below 200 ng/g may be suggestive of chromium depletion [66]. Values for newborns are considerably higher (400 ng/g), falling gradually throughout childhood [67].

Treatment   GTF chromium is the therapy of choice for chromium deficiency but is not available in a purified form. Food with a high concentration of GTF, e.g., brewer's yeast, probably is the best source. Inorganic trivalent chromium salts (chromium chloride), 50 µg three times daily, have been administered safely for many months.

Prevention   Prevention of dietary chromium deficiency is best assured by an adequate intake. Regrettably, reliable food composition data for chromium are not available. However, Mertz has produced a helpful qualitative estimate, by grouping foods that supply low, intermediate and high chromium density (Table 18-7). The relative chromium-energy ratios in Table 18-7 are based on the amount of chromium in 1000 kcal of the food lowest in chromium—refined sugar. The amount of chromium in 1000 kcal of refined sugar is arbitrarily set at 1, and the chromium content per 1000 kcal of all other foods is expressed on this basis. For example, skim milk and oysters furnish 6 and 65 times more chromium per 1000 kcal, respectively, than sugar.

Toxicity

Ingestion of chromium produces little toxicity.

TABLE 18-7
RELATIVE CHROMIUM-ENERGY RATIO OF
FOODS

	Relative index*
Low chromium density	
Sugar	1
Grits	3
Butter	4
Margarine	5
Skim milk	6
Corn meal	6
Corn flakes	7
Spaghetti	8
Intermediate chromium density	
Fish, shrimp, lobster	12
Flour	14

TABLE 18-7 (Continued)

	Relative index*
Grain, whole	17
Chicken breast	17
Bread	20
Fruit, fresh	20
Chicken legs	28
Cheese	32
Bread, whole-grain	32
Wheat bran	32
Vegetables, fresh	35
Beef	38
High chromium density	
Oysters	65
Potatoes with skin	72
Liver	78
Yeast, dried	80
Egg yolk	104

*Based on the amount of chromium in 1000 kcal of sugar, which equals an index of 1.
Source: W. Mertz, Mineral elements: new perspectives, J. Am. Diet. Assoc., 77:258, 1980.

SELENIUM

Selenium was known for its toxic effects long before it was recognized as an essential nutrient. Only recently was selenium designated an essential nutrient for humans. This fact was not established by demonstrating a deficiency condition but was established by proving that the element is part of human erythrocyte glutathione peroxidase.

Dietary Sources, Availability, and Requirements

There are few data on which to base an estimate of human selenium requirements. One study of selenium metabolism in women indicated a minimum daily requirement of 20 μg [68]. Long-term daily intakes of 28 to 32 μg have not been associated with any adverse human health effects in New Zealand [69]. The Food and Nutrition Board has set a safe and adequate range of selenium intake of 50 to 200 μg per day for adults [1]. These figures were derived by extrapolation from animal studies indicating that 0.1 ppm in the diet is a nutritionally adequate level. Most studies of North American diets have reported selenium levels in this range. Although the precise level of selenium intake causing toxicity in humans is not clear, the upper limit of the safe and adequate range was set in order to guard against possible selenium overdosing through nutritional supplements.

The two richest sources of selenium are seafoods and organ meats. Food selenium content is related to protein content and geographical origin. In most biological material, selenium is found largely in the protein fraction; foods low in protein, such as fruits, contain very little of the element. Geographical areas vary in the soil content of selenium. Once selenium is taken up by plants, it is passed up the food chain to animals and humans. Since crop plants are not known to require selenium, they are passive indicators of the selenium available in the soils of different regions. Thus, the selenium content of wheat, for example, has been shown to vary three orders of magnitude depending on where the grain was grown. Cooking has been shown not to cause major losses of selenium from most foods.

Absorption and Excretion

The absorption of selenium depends, to some extent, on the chemical form; selenomethionine is better absorbed than inorganic forms. Intestinal absorption of food selenium is about 80 percent [68] and does not appear to be homeostatically controlled. In humans homeostasis is achieved by the kidneys, the urine being the principal route of excretion. Fecal losses are not governed by selenium intake. In the rat very high intakes of selenium which can lead to toxicity are associated with a significant excretion of the element in the breath as dimethyl selenide [70].

Biological Functions

To date, the only established function of selenium in humans is as a component of the enzyme glutathione peroxidase. This enzyme is distributed widely in the cells of the body and in particular is present in high concentrations in red blood cells and in the liver. It catalyzes the reduction of hydrogen peroxide to water and of fatty acid hydroperoxides to hydroxy acids in the tissues and thus protects the lipids in cell membranes from peroxidation. This property is its principal function in the cell and accounts for its evident overlap in function with vitamin E, another important antioxidant. Selenium is essential for growth and reproduction in the rat and has an effect on growth in humans.

Human Selenium Deficiency

A number of selenium-responsive disorders have been observed in animals under both laboratory and free-living conditions. These include liver necrosis in rats and other species and muscular dystropy (white-muscle disease) in lambs, calves, and other young animals. Selenium deficiency has not been demonstrated unequivocally in humans, but several suggestive situations have been described.

Etiologic Factors and Clinical Manifestations   The uneven distribution of selenium in the soils of the United States could conceivably cause persons living in low-selenium areas and consuming only locally produced foods to develop a low-selenium state. Some epidemiologists have postulated that an increased incidence of certain diseases observed in human populations in certain regions may be associated with low levels of selenium in the soil. These epidemiological associations have led to the promotion of selenium as a cure-all for a variety of illnesses such as cancer, heart disease, sexual dysfunction, arthritis, skin and hair problems, and aging. But most nutrition authorities agree that there is currently no evidence of selenium deficiency in the United States, probably because of interregional food shipments. Furthermore, the addition of selenium to the feed of swine and poultry should help to maintain an adequate amount of selenium in our food supply [71].

Since selenium is usually associated with protein in foods, a low-protein diet may also be low in selenium. Low blood selenium levels have been reported in children with protein-calorie malnutrition [72] and in children on synthetic diets for phenylketonuria and maple syrup urine disease [73]. However, these children all had mean levels higher than the normal adult levels in New Zealand, and no condition has been discovered that could be attributed to these decreased concentrations.

A case of possible selenium deficiency has been reported in a woman from a low-selenium area in New Zealand who had received long-term total parenteral nutrition [74]. The patient developed severe muscular discomfort accompanied by loss of mobility that disappeared after supplemental selenium was added to the intravenous feeding solutions. Similar groups that might be vulnerable to selenium deficiency are children with metabolic disorders consuming synthetic protein diets, premature babies and infants during the first few months of life, and patients with cancer whose lowered dietary intake is a consequence of their disease.

In China, a cardiomyopathy called *Keshan disease* has been reported. This affects children primarily and is characterized by gallop rhythm, heart failure, cardiogenic shock, abnormal electrocardiograms, and heart enlargement [75]. It is associated with low levels of selenium in the blood and hair and is distributed in a region running from northeastern China to the southwest. Encouraging results were obtained in trials using sodium selenite to prevent the disease.

Diagnosis and Treatment   Blood levels of selenium have been used as an index of selenium status since the development of sensitive fluorometric assays. Studies in humans suggest that blood selenium is under homeostatic control. Normal adult levels of 0.1 to 0.34 μg/ml of blood have been reported for the United States [76], but lower values of 0.068 $\pm$ 0.013 μg/ml are found in New Zealand, where soil levels are generally low [77].

Measurement of the activity of the selenium-containing enzyme glutathione peroxidase may prove to be the best determinant of selenium status. In animals, glutathione peroxidase levels depend on dietary selenium intakes. They may also provide an indication of selenium status in humans; there is a strong correlation between blood enzyme levels and selenium levels [78].

Should a deficiency be discovered, it would be necessary to administer microgram quantities of a biologically active form such as sodium selenite.

Toxicity

The toxic effects of selenium have been recognized much longer than the nutritional ones. The discovery in the 1930s that certain geographical areas are seleniferous and produce plants with a high selenium content explained observations dating back centuries that foods grown in these areas cause sickness in human beings and beasts consuming it. Manifestations of chronic toxicity are often species-dependent and related to the form and amount of selenium ingested. Cattle that graze on selenium-rich land develop a condition with the descriptive name "blind staggers." In almost all species the liver is affected and cirrhosis develops. Frequently a cardiomyopathy is found. Loss of hair and sloughing of hoofs occurs. Very few cases of selenium toxicity in human beings have been reported. Increased dental caries among children have been attributed to high selenium intake. An isolated incidence of selenium poisoning by well water containing 9 ppm of selenium [79] caused alopecia, abnormal nails, and lassitude in an Indian family.

MAGNESIUM

Dietary Sources, Availability, and Requirements

Magnesium is one of the minerals needed by humans in relatively large amounts. Ordinarily not much attention is paid to it because it occurs widely in foods, especially those of vegetable origin. Of the commonly eaten foods and in the portions usually consumed, dairy products are the best sources of magnesium, followed by breads and cereals, vegetables, meats and poultry, and fruits. Of the vegetables, green leafy types are best, owing to their chlorophyll (a magnesium chelate of porphyrin) content. Highly purified foods such as sugars and starches and beverages such as soft drinks and alcohol have no magnesium. Table 18-8 gives the magnesium content of selected foods.

The magnesium content of the average American diet has been estimated at about 120 mg per 1000 kcal, and estimates of requirements for an adult man based on balance studies range from 200 mg per day (3.0 mg/kg per day) or 300 mg per day (4.3 mg/kg per day) up to as high as 700 mg per day [1]. Based on these studies and on usual dietary intakes, the allowance recommended for adult males is 350 mg per day and for adult females is 300 mg per day. The requirements for magnesium during pregnancy and lactation have received little attention. On the basis of limited information, an additional allowance of 150 mg per day is recommended for pregnant and lactating women.

TABLE 18-8
MAGNESIUM CONTENT OF SELECTED FOODS

	Amount	Magnesium content, mg
Peanuts, roasted	¼ cup	63
Banana	1 medium	58
Beet greens, raw	1 cup	58
Milk, whole	1 cup	33
Peanut butter	1 tbsp	28
Oysters, raw	6 medium	27
Pork, fresh, roasted	3 oz	25
Hamburger, lean, cooked	3 oz	20
Bread, whole wheat	1 slice	19
Orange	1 medium	15
Cheddar cheese	1 oz	8
Egg, whole	1 large	6

Sources: C. F. Adams, Nutritive Value of American Foods in Common Units, U.S. Department of Agriculture Handbook no. 456, U.S. Government Printing Office, Washington, 1975; L. P. Posati and M. L. Orr, Composition of Foods—Dairy and Egg Products—Raw, Processed, Prepared, U.S. Department of Agriculture Handbook no. 8-1, U.S. Government Printing Office, Washington, 1976; Consumer and Food Economics Institute, Composition of Foods, Raw, Processed, Prepared, U.S. Department of Agriculture Handbook no. 8, rev. ed., U.S. Government Printing Office, 1963.

Absorption and Excretion

Magnesium shares some of the attributes of calcium in its characteristics of absorption and storage in bone. The body absorbs about 35 to 40 percent of dietary magnesium by active transport from the intestine, mainly the ileum. The percentage absorbed varies inversely with dietary intake. Most of that portion of the magnesium that is absorbed in the body is excreted by the kidney; fecal magnesium represents largely the unabsorbed fraction. There is considerable secretion of magnesium into the gastrointestinal tract from bile and from pancreatic and intestinal juices. This secretion is followed by almost complete reabsorption.

Biological Functions

Magnesium plays a key role as a prosthetic group in many essential enzymatic reactions. The enzymes include those that hydrolyze and transfer phosphate groups (phosphokinases). Magnesium is involved in adenosine triphosphate (ATP) dependent reactions. Important ATP-dependent reactions include the anaerobic phosphorylation of glucose and the oxidative decarboxylation of glucose in the citric acid cycle. Magnesium is involved in protein synthesis through its role in the activation of amino acids, its action on ribosomal aggregation, its role in binding messenger RNA to 70 S ribosomes, and its role in the synthesis and degradation of DNA. Magnesium is required for the conversion of ATP to cyclic adenosine monophosphate (cAMP) by the enzyme adenylate cyclase. Magnesium also plays an important role in neuromuscular transmission and activity.

Human Magnesium Deficiency

Since magnesium is widely available in foodstuffs and efficient renal and gastrointestinal mechanisms control magnesium conservation, isolated magnesium deficiency is an uncommon entity. When it occurs, it is usually associated with disease states whose symptoms may obscure the presence of magnesium deficiency. Hence it is often missed or ignored.

Etiologic Factors Responsible for Deficiency in Humans Magnesium deficiency almost always is secondary to excessive losses of magnesium from the body. This loss most commonly occurs from the kidney or gastrointestinal tract. Nutritional magnesium deficiency is rarely seen, but reducing dietary magnesium intake during chronic illness will hasten the onset of symptomatic magnesium deficiency. Clinical conditions associated with depletion of magnesium include severe malabsorption of various etiologies, chronic alcoholism with malnutrition, prolonged magnesium-free parenteral feeding (usually in association with prolonged losses of gastrointestinal secretions), burns, renal disease involving tubular dysfunction, protein-calorie malnutrition, diabetic acidosis, and parathyroid disorders. A number of drugs may produce renal wasting of magnesium. Diuretics, particularly the loop diuretics furosemide and ethacrynic acid, may cause significant magnesium diuresis. Cardiac glycosides also cause an increase in urinary magnesium excretion.

Clinical Manifestations There has been considerable controversy about characteristic manifestations of magnesium deficiency. This situation is in part attributable to the fact that symptomatic human deficiency has always been reported in a setting of predisposing and complicating disease states. Furthermore, even severe hypomagnesemia may be totally asymptomatic and remain undetected clinically [80].

In the best study of experimental magnesium deficiency in humans to date, the six male subjects developed hypocalcemia; the one female subject did not [81]. Marked and persistent symptoms developed only in the presence of hypocalcemia. The serum potassium concentration decreased, but serum sodium was not altered significantly. Three of the four subjects with the severest symptoms also had metabolic alkalosis. A positive Trousseau's sign, which occurred in five of the seven subjects, was the most common neurological sign observed. Anorexia, nausea, and vomiting were frequently experienced.

The following manifestations have been reported.

1 Muscular twitching and tremor of any or all muscles
2 Muscle weakness
3 Convulsions
4 Sweating and tachycardia
5 Apathy, depression, and poor memory
6 Mild to severe delirium
7 Premature ventricular beats, ventricular tachycardia, and ventricular fibrillation
8 Positive Chvostek's sign
9 Positive Trousseau's sign

Diagnosis   In many patients the clinical symptoms and signs are nonspecific, but a low serum magnesium concentration confirms the diagnosis. Although about 30 percent of the magnesium in the circulation is bound to albumin, corrections of the total plasma magnesium concentration in hypoalbuminemic patients are not generally made. There is no routine method for measuring ionized magnesium concentration. Hypocalcemia and hypokalemia are also frequent findings in magnesium deficiency.

Treatment   Symptomatic magnesium deficiency should be treated with magnesium salts. Patients with mild deficiencies may receive sufficient magnesium from the diet if they are able to eat. Correction of hypocalcemia and hypokalemia also requires therapy with magnesium; treatment with vitamin D, calcium, or potassium will not correct the mineral imbalance. Prior to the administration of magnesium salts, renal function should be assessed. If the patient has a lowered glomerular filtration rate, the replacement dose of magnesium must be reduced or intoxication may result. Serum magnesium concentrations must be determined daily if renal function is impaired.

A suggested oral regimen of magnesium replacement is 1.0 g of $MgSO_4 \cdot 7H_2O$ (8.13 meq Mg) every 4 to six hours for 5 days [82]. If the intramuscular route is to be used, a 50% solution is available. If the patient requires intravenous infusions, up to 100 meq per day for 5 days can be safely administered to patients with normal renal function.

Toxicity

Magnesium intoxication and hypermagnesemia occur primarily in patients with serious renal insufficiency and in patients with eclampsia when magnesium salts are administered in large doses. An important cause of magnesium intoxication is the use of magnesium-containing antacids such as Gelusil and Maalox or cathartics (milk of magnesia) in patients with renal failure. The plasma magnesium concentration usually exceeds 4 meq per liter before any signs or symptoms of magnesium excess appear. Clinically, one of the earliest effects of intoxication is a decrease or disappearance of the deep tendon reflexes. Somnolence is seen at levels of 4 to 7 meq per liter, and paralysis of voluntary muscles at 10 meq per liter or greater. The latter may impair respiratory function. Although usually no treatment other than stopping exogenous magnesium is necessary, calcium gluconate or chloride can be used as a physiological antagonist in treating respiratory depression.

MANGANESE

Dietary Sources, Availability, and Requirements

Minimum requirements for manganese are not well-defined. Results of balance studies suggest 2.0 to 3.0 mg per day is adequate for adults; subjects receiving only 0.71 mg per day were in negative balance [3]. The Committee on Recommended Allowances [1] has recommended that the manganese intake of adults be in the range of 2.5 to 5 mg per day (Table 18-3). The daily intake for different groups of people in the United States varies from 2 to 9 mg per day in adults, depending on the composition of the diet [83].

Nuts and unrefined grains are rich sources of manganese; vegetables and fruit contain moderate amounts, whereas dairy products, meats, and seafoods contain only small concentrations. One cup of tea (1 tsp tea leaves) provides 1.3 mg of manganese. To date there are no official food tables for this element.

Absorption and Excretion

Manganese absorption tends to be inefficient (less than 20 percent) and varies inversely with the amount of dietary iron, calcium, and phosphorus. Absorbed manganese is excreted mainly in the bile; urinary losses are negligible.

Biological Functions

Manganese is known to be an activator of many enzymes; this effect is not specific, since many other metals, in particular magnesium, may substitute for manganese in most cases. Manganese is required for the synthesis of mucopolysaccharides in cartilage; it activates the galactotransferase that transfers the trisaccharide that links polysaccharide to the protein moiety and it activates the polymerase responsible for conversion of UDP-N-acetylgalactosamine to the polysaccharide. Manganese is also a component of two metalloenzymes, pyruvate carboxylase and mitochondrial superoxide dismutase.

Human Manganese Deficiency

In both mammals and birds, manganese deficiency is characterized by defective growth, bone abnormalities, sterility, stillbirths, and various congenital malformations. Abnormalities of glucose tolerance, lipid metabolism, growth, and brain function have also been reported. There was doubt that a deficiency could occur in humans until Doisy [84] recognized the first case in a volunteer undergoing a study of vitamin K deficiency in a metabolic ward. Failure to add manganese to a purified diet mixture resulted in weight loss, transient dermatitis, nausea, and slow growth of hair and beard with changes in hair color, and biochemically there was a striking hypocholesterolemia. The patient's depressed vitamin K-dependent clotting factors did not respond to therapy with vitamin K until manganese was given as well.

Low serum manganese levels have been reported in diabetes and in patients with pancreatic insufficiency, and liver manganese levels may be decreased in patients with kwashiorkor, suggesting that these groups may have a lowered nutritional status. The young infant receives a relatively low intake from breast milk [85].

Toxicity

Toxicity from dietary intake appears to be highly unlikely. However, toxicity does occur after long, continuous inhalation of large quantities of the element. For example, miners of manganese ores may develop a syndrome from inhaling ore dust. The clinical manifestations of the disease are both psychiatric and neurological. Clinical changes begin with asthenia, anorexia, apathy, headache, impotence, leg cramps, and speech disturbances. The disease progresses to a permanently crippling neurological disorder and is, in some ways, clinically similar to Parkinson's or Wilson's disease. In mild cases, symptoms are reversed by withdrawal from exposure or treatment with disodium dicalcium ethyl-enediaminetetraacetate (EDTA).

FLUORIDE

Fluoride is present in small but varying concentrations in practically all soils, water supplies, plants, and animals. It is therefore a constituent of all normal diets. Because of the ubiquity of this element, a fluoride deficiency severe enough to result in growth depression is difficult to produce. Fluoride is considered an essential element for humans on the basis of its proven beneficial effects on dental health.

Dietary Sources, Availability, and Requirements

The chief source of fluoride is usually drinking water, as a consequence of the water drunk and of the fluoride enrichment the cooking water gives the food. The concentration of fluoride in natural waters ranges from almost undetectable amounts to a reported value as high as 2800 ppm [86]. The optimal fluoride level for reduction of dental caries without undesirable mottling (see discussion under "Toxicity," below) is 1 ppm of fluoride for temperate climates, which provides a total daily intake of 0.5 to 1 mg of fluoride for children and 1.5 to 2 mg of fluoride for adults.

As compared with this source, the fluoride in foodstuffs is of minor importance. Very few foods contain more than 1 ppm. The exception is fish products, which can contain 5 to 15 ppm. Another significant source is tea; a cup of tea will supply 0.1 mg of fluoride.

Intake of fluoride by adults from foodstuffs (exclusive of drinking water) averages approximately 1 mg per day in nonfluoridated communities and 2 to 3 mg per day in fluoridated communities (1 ppm of fluoride) in the United States [86]. On the basis of consumption of 1500 ml of drinking water per day, the total fluoride intake for these two groups would average 1.2 mg of fluoride per day and 3.5 to 4.5 mg of fluoride per day, respectively. Intake by children is proportionally less, depending on their age and body weight.

Although RDAs for fluoride have not been established, the Food and Nutrition Board provisionally recommends that water supplies be fluoridated at the level of 1 ppm (1 mg per liter) to provide 1.5 to 4 mg per day for adults (Table 18-3). For younger age groups, the range is reduced to a maximal level of 2.5 mg in order to avoid the danger of mottling of the teeth. Infants may consume less than 0.1 mg from breast milk or cow's milk and as much as 1.2 mg from certain infant formulas [87].

Absorption and Secretion

Passive absorption of fluoride is rapid and takes place mainly in the stomach, but some may be absorbed from the intestine as well. Efficiency of absorption ranges from 75 to 90 percent of the amount ingested, with approximately half retained in the teeth and bones. The body excretes fluoride primarily in the urine, although small amounts are lost in sweat and feces.

Biological Functions

The function of fluoride appears to be the protection of dental tissue, an influence that it exercises primarily during prenatal life, infancy, and childhood. Fluoridated water also is of some benefit to adults as well as to children. The fluoride ion is incorporated into the crystalline structure of hydroxyapatite, resulting in increased resistance of the teeth to dental caries [88]. Some studies have suggested a possible function of fluoride in the maintenance of bone structure, but further investigation on this point is required.

Human Fluoride Deficiency

Fluoride augmentation of the diet has been reported to increase growth rates of rats [89] and mice [90]. No similar evidence is available for humans. However, a deficiency of fluoride during infancy and childhood leaves the teeth more vulnerable to dental caries. The reduction in dental caries by 50 to 70 percent as a result of water fluoridation is thoroughly documented [91]. Standardization of water supplies by addition of fluoride to bring the concentration to 1 ppm has proved to be a safe, economical, and efficient way to reduce the incidence of tooth decay—fluoridation is an important public health measure in areas where natural water supplies contain less than this amount.

Toxicity

Because fluoride occurs in such small amounts in food and is so rapidly excreted, fluoride toxicity from dietary ingestion is rare. In areas where fluoride is naturally present in the water supply at levels approximating 2 to 4 ppm, tooth enamel may have opaque, "paper-white" areas (so-called mottled enamel). With greater exposure brown stains will appear on the teeth, but no adverse health effects have been documented. When animals or humans are exposed to amounts of fluoride higher than 8 ppm over long periods of time, toxicity (fluorosis) manifested by deformed teeth and bones, erosion of tooth enamel, and other toxic symptoms can occur [92]. Mottling or staining of teeth results only from high flouride consumption by children (see Color Figure 20).

IODINE

Iodine is an essential nutrient for humans because it is an integral component of the thyroid hormones thyroxine (T_4) and triiodothyronine (T_3). Lack of dietary iodine (goiter) was a major public health problem in the United States 75 years ago, which was alleviated by the iodization of table salt. A disturbing recent finding is that the average intake in the American diet is now five to ten times more than the RDA. This finding has stimulated new debate concerning the use of iodized salt.

Dietary Sources, Availability, and Requirements

The ultimate source of iodine is the ocean. Seafood is rich in iodine, as are vegetables grown in an iodine-rich soil. The effects of glaciers and the weathering of the soil have removed much of the iodine from the soil over large portions of the earth's surface (Figure 18-1). Hence iodization of table salt was done in the state of Michigan in 1924 to prevent goiter in that region, and such salt eventually became available throughout the United States. Iodized salt must be labeled and contains up to the equivalent of 75 μg of iodine per gram of table salt. Thus, 2 g of iodized salt assures an adequate intake (adult RDA = 150 μg).

Since the turn of the century, changes have occurred in agricultural practices, food technology, medications, interstate commerce, and pollution which have increased tremendously the potential intake of iodine. The key food items responsible for the increase in available iodine are milk products and bread. Dairy cattle may be given iodine-supplemented feed or iodized-salt blocks. Also, iodine-containing veterinary medications, disinfectants, and sanitizers are used in the dairy industry. Milk iodine from these sources may reach levels as

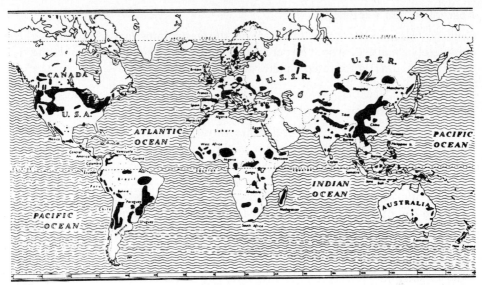

FIGURE 18-1
Goitrous areas of the world are shown in black. (*From World Goiter Survey: Iodine Facts, Iodine Educational Bureau, London, 1946, facts 271-380.*)

high as 450 µg per liter [93], and dairy products contribute as much as 38 percent of the daily iodine intake [94]. Concentrations of over 250 µg of iodine per slice of bread have been measured in products from bakeries using iodates, usually not specified on labels, as dough conditioners. Erythrosine (FD&C Red No. 3), a red food dye, is more than 50 percent iodine. The use of FD&C Red No. 3 has almost doubled since two other red dyes were taken off the market by the Food and Drug Administration in 1976.

The result of increased availability of iodine is that the average iodine intake of individuals is far greater than the nutritional requirement. For example, a study by the Food and Drug Administration in 1974 indicated that a teenage boy consuming 2850 kcal per day received an average of 830 µg of iodine. That is about 5½ times the current RDA [94]. Concern has been expressed that certain population groups (infants, toddlers, and teenagers) may be exposed to excessive levels of iodine which may lead to the development of goiter.

The daily iodine requirement for prevention of goiter in adults is 50 to 75 µg, or approximately 1 µg per kilogram of body weight [95]. In order to provide an extra margin of safety and to meet the increased demands that may be imposed by natural substances with antithyroid activity found in food (goitrogens are found in rutabagas, turnips, cabbage, and other members of the genus *Brassica*) under some conditions, an RDA of 150 µg is recommended for adolescents and adults (Table 18-2). Additional allowances of 25 to 50 µg for pregnant and lactating women, respectively, are suggested to cover the demands of the fetus and to provide the extra iodine excreted in milk.

Absorption and Excretion

Dietary iodine is converted to iodide in the gastrointestinal tract and is then completely absorbed. About 30 percent is removed by the thyroid gland, and the remaining iodine is excreted in the urine.

Biological Functions

The only known functions of iodine are those associated with its presence in thyroid hormones. Iodine is taken up by the thyroid gland as the iodide ion, is oxidized to elemental iodine, and is incorporated into the tyrosine residues of thyroglobulin, a large protein synthesized only in the thyroid gland. The monoiodotyrosine or diiodotyrosine residues are combined to form the active hormone thyroxine (tetraiodothyronine), or T_4, and triiodothyronine (T_3). All these reactions occur within the thyroglobulin molecule. For the active hormones to be released from the thyroid into the blood, thyroglobulin is broken down by proteolytic enzymes and the free hormones T_4 and T_3 and free iodotyrosines are released.

T_4 and T_3 regulate a large number of biological activities including (1) energy transformation through an effect on oxygen consumption and heat production, (2) growth (cretinism, a chronic condition due to congenital lack of thyroid secretion, is marked by arrested physical and mental development), (3) reproduction (cretins usually are sterile and thyroidectomized young animals remain infertile), (4) skin and hair growth, and (5) cellular metabolism, e.g., more than 100 enzyme systems respond to the administration of thyroid hormones by an alteration in activity.

Human Iodine Deficiency

With iodine deficiency the thyroid gland enlarges because the pituitary gland continues to form thyroid-stimulating hormone (TSH), which is responsible for stimulating the gland to synthesize and release thyroid hormones. Because of inadequate feedback inhibition in the absence of sufficient thyroid hormone, the gland hypertrophies. This condition is known as simple or endemic goiter (Color Figure 12). Simple goiter is a useful compensatory mechanism and generally does not pose any serious medical problem.

However, iodine deficiency is a very important global health problem, with an estimated 200 million persons affected [96]. A high incidence has been found in the Alps, the Pyrenees, the Himalaya mountains, the Thames Valley in England, Central America, the Great Lakes basin and northwestern sections of the United States. Of concern is not deficiency goiter and its attendant mild hypothyroidism but the concomitant cretinism of goitrous populations. This condition is present at birth in infants who are deprived of iodine during fetal development because their mothers are profoundly iodine-deficient. Since there is no significant transplacental transfer of thyroid hormones from maternal to fetal circulations the fetal thyroid must elaborate its own hormones. One form of cretinism is the "neurological" type which is characterized by mental retardation, deaf-mutism, spastic diplegia, and strabismus; clinical hypothyroidism is usually absent. The "myxedematous" type has the signs of congenital hypothyroidism and dwarfism but no goiter. The physical retardation may be corrected by the administration of thyroid hormone but the mental retardation is irreversible.

Simple goiters often regress somewhat in size under treatment with iodides. The response of large, long-standing goiters to iodides is often disappointing. The preferred treatment in such cases is thyroid hormone (0.1 to 0.3 mg daily).

Prevention Endemic goiter and cretinism are an enormous burden in some developing countries. Yet they are almost wholly preventable, since the major single factor is dietary iodine deficiency; goitrogens in the diet occasionally play a supplementary role. Iodization of table salt has greatly reduced the prevalence of goiter in many countries. Other supplementation measures including iodized bread, drinking water, milk, and chocolate [97] have been used. On the basis of the work of McCullagh [98] an alternative method of prophylaxis is intramuscular administration of up to 5 ml of iodized oil containing 400 mg of iodine per milliliter.

Toxicity

Normally excess iodine ingestion is regulated, within limits, by decreased iodine uptake by the thyroid and increased excretion of iodide in the urine. However, even normal individuals cannot cope adequately with grossly excessive intake. For example, thyrotoxicosis, an enlarged and hyperactive thyroid, has been noted among some inhabitants of Japan who consume as much as 25,000 μg of iodide per day in the form of iodide-rich seaweed. Iodine consumption in the United States does not approach this level unless an iodide-containing medication or large quantities of a very rich iodine source are consumed.

REFERENCES

1 Food and Nutrition Board: *Recommended Dietary Allowances,* 9th ed., National Academy of Sciences, Washington, 1980.
2 Eckhert, C. D., M. V. Sloan, J. R. Duncan, and L. S. Hurley: Zinc binding: a difference between human and bovine milk, Science, 195:789, 1977.
3 World Health Organization: *Trace Elements in Human Nutrition,* WHO Tech Rep. Ser. no. 532, 1973.
4 Evans, G. W.: Zinc absorption and transport, in *Trace Elements in Human Health and Disease,* vol. 1, A. S. Prasad and D. Oberleas (eds.), Academic, New York, 1976.
5 Hurley, L. S., J. R. Duncan, C. D. Eckhert, and M. V. Sloan: Zinc-binding ligands in

milk and their relationship to neonatal nutrition, in *Trace Element Metabolism in Man and Animals,* vol. 3, M. Kirchgessner (ed.), Technische Universitat Munchen, Freising-Weihenstephan, 1978.

6 Richards, M. P., and R. J. Cousins: Metallothionen and its relationship to the metabolism of dietary zinc in rats, J. Nutr., 106:1591, 1976.

7 Underwood, E. J.: *Trace Elements in Human and Animal Nutrition,* 4th ed., Academic, New York, 1977, p. 196.

8 Solomans, N. W.: Zinc and the gastroenterologist, Practical Gastroenterol., 4:15, 1980.

9 Henkin, R. I.: Zinc dependent control of food intake, taste and smell functions, in *Trace Element Metabolism in Man and Animals,* vol. 3, M. Kirchgessner (ed.), Technische Universitat Munchen, Freising-Weihenstephan, 1978.

10 Adams, M. J., T. L. Blundell, E. J. Dodson, G. G. Dodson, M. Vijayan, E. W. Baker, M. M. Harding, D. C. Hodgkin, B. Rimmer, and S. Sheat: Structure of rhombohedral 2 zinc insulin crystals, Nature, 224:491, 1969.

11 Kirchgessner, M., H. P. Roth, and E. Weigand: Biochemical changes in zinc deficiency, in *Trace Elements in Human Health and Disease,* vol. 1, A. S. Prasad and D. Oberleas (eds.), Academic, New York, 1976.

12 Gross, R. L., N. Osdin, L. Fong, and P. M. Newberne: 1. Depressed immunological function in zinc-deprived rats as measured by mitogen response of spleen, thymus and peripheral blood, Am. J. Clin. Nutr., 32:1260, 1979.

13 Golden, M. H. N., B. Golden, P. S. E. G. Harland, and A. A. Jackson: Zinc and immunocompetence in protein-energy malnutrition, Lancet, 1:1226, 1978.

14 Prasad, A. S.: Deficiency of zinc in man and its toxicity, in *Trace Elements in Human Health and Disease,* vol. 1, A. S. Prasad and D. Oberleas (eds.), Academic, New York, 1976.

15 Hambidge, K. M., C. Hambidge, M. Jacobs, and J. D. Baum: Low levels of zinc in hair, anorexia, poor growth and hypogeusia in children, Pediatr. Res., 6:868, 1972.

16 Hambidge, K. M., P. A. Walravens, R. M. Brown, J. Webster, S. White, M. Anthony, and M. L. Ross: Zinc nutrition of preschool children in Denver Headstart Program, Am. J. Clin. Nutr., 29:734, 1976.

17 Walravens, P. A., and K. M. Hambidge: Growth of infants fed a zinc supplemented formula, Am. J. Clin. Nutr., 29:1114, 1976.

18 Moynahan, H. E.: Acrodermatitis enteropathica. A lethal inherited human zinc deficiency disorder, Lancet, 2:399, 1974.

19 Rose, G. A. and E. G. Willden: Whole blood, red cell and plasma total and ultrafiltrable zinc levels in normal subjects and in patients with chronic renal failure with and without hemodialysis, Br. J. Urol., 44:281, 1972.

20 Van Callie, M., H. Deganhurt, I. Luijendijk, and J. Fernandes: Zinc content of intravenous solutions, Lancet, 2:200, 1978.

21 Sandstead, H. H.: Zinc nutrition in the United States, Am. J. Clin. Nutr., 26:1251, 1973.

22 Hambidge, K. M., and W. Droegemuller: Changes in plasma and hair concentrations of zinc, copper, chromium and manganese during pregnancy, Obstet. Gynecol., 44:666, 1974.

23 Nelder, K. H., and K. M. Hambidge: Zinc therapy of acrodermatitis enteropathica, N. Engl. J. Med., 292:879, 1975.

24 Hambidge, K. M., and P. A. Walravens: Trace elements in nutrition, Practical Pediatr., 1:1, 1975.

25 James, B. E., and R. A. MacMahon: Balance studies of nine elements during complete intravenous feeding of small premature infants, Aust. Paediatr., 12:154, 1976.

26 Holden, J. M., W. R. Wolf, and W. Mertz: Zinc and copper in self-selected diets, J. Am. Diet. Assoc., 75:23, 1979.

27 Swanson, C. A., and J. C. King: Human zinc nutrition, J. Nutr. Educ., 11:181, 1979.

28 Casey, C. E., and K. M. Hambidge: Trace element deficiencies in man, in *Advances in Nutritional Research,* vol. 3, H. H. Draper (ed.), Plenum, New York, 1980.

29 Morriss, F. H.: Trace minerals, Semin. Perinatol., 3:369, 1979.

30 Picciano, M. F., and H. A. Guthrie: Copper, iron and zinc contents of mature milk, Am. J. Clin. Nutr., 29:242, 1976.

31 Pennington, J. T., and D. H. Calloway: Copper content of foods, J. Am. Diet. Assoc., 63:143, 1973.

32 Guthrie, B. E., J. M. McKenzie, and C. E. Casey: Copper status of New Zealanders, in *Trace Element Metabolism in Man and Animals,* vol. 3, M. Kirchgessner (ed.), Technische Universitat Munchen, Freising-Weihenstephan, 1978.

33 Klevay, L. M.: Dietary copper and the copper requirement of man, in *Trace Element Metabolism in Man and Animals,* vol. 3, M. Kirchgessner (ed.), Technische Universitat Munchen, Freising-Weihenstephan, 1978.

34 Klevay, L. M., S. J. Reck, and D. F. Barcome: Evidence of dietary copper and zinc deficiencies, J. Am. Med. Assoc., 241:1916, 1979.

35 Cordano, A., J. M. Baertl, and G. G. Graham: Copper deficiency in infancy, Pediatrics, 34:324, 1964.

36 Holtzman, N. A., G. G. Graham, P. Charache, and R. Haslam: Effect of copper on serum ceruloplasmin concentrations (abstr.), Pediatr. Res., 1:219, 1967.

37 Menkes, J. H., M. Alter, G. K. Steigleder, D. R. Weakley, and J. H. Sung: A sex-linked, recessive disorder with retardation of growth, peculiar hair and focal cerebral and cerebellar degeneration, Pediatrics, 29:764, 1962.

38 Danks, D. M., P. E. Campbell, B. J. Stevens, V. Mayne, and E. Cartwright: Menkes' kinky hair syndrome. An inherited defect in copper absorption with widespread effects, Pediatrics, 50:188, 1972.

39 Bucknall, W. E., R. H. A. Haslam, and N. A. Holtzman: Kinky hair syndrome: Response to copper therapy, Pediatrics, 52:653, 1973.

40 Graham, G. G., and A. Cordano: Copper deficiency in human subjects, in *Trace Elements in Human Health and Disease,* vol. 1, A. S. Prasad and D. Oberleas (eds.), Academic, New York, 1976.

41 Walravens, P. A.: Nutritional importance of copper and zinc in neonates and infants, Clin. Chem., 26:185, 1980.

42 Ashkenazi, A., S. Levin, M. Djaldetti, E. Fishel, and D. Benvenisti: The syndrome of neonatal copper deficiency, Pediatrics, 52:525, 1973.

43 AAP Committee on Nutrition: Nutritional needs of low-birth-weight infants, Pediatrics, 60:519, 1977.

44 Heller, R. M., S. G. Kirchner, J. A. O'Neill, A. J. Hough, L. Howard, S. S. Kramer, and H. L. Green: Skeletal changes of copper deficiency in infants receiving prolonged total parenteral nutrition, J. Pediatr., 80:32, 1972.

45 Evans, G. W.: Metabolic disorders of copper metabolism, in *Advances in Nutritional Research,* vol. 1, H. H. Draper (ed.), Plenum, New York, 1977.

46 Klevay, L. M.: The ratio of zinc to copper of diets in the United States, Nutr. Rep. Int., 11:237, 1975.

47 Schwarz, K., and W. Mertz: Chromium (III) and the glucose tolerance factor, Arch. Biochem. Biophys., 85:292, 1959.

48 Glinsmann, W. H., and W. Mertz: Effect of trivalent chromium on glucose tolerance, Metabolism, 15:510, 1966.

49 Mertz, W., E. W. Toepfer, E. E. Roginski, and M. M. Polansky: Present knowledge of the role of chromium, Fed. Proc., 33:2275, 1974.

50 Doisy, R. J., D. H. P. Streeten, J. M. Freiberg, and A. J. Schneider: Chromium metabolism in man and biochemical effects, in *Trace Elements in Human Nutrition and Disease,* vol. 2, A. S. Prasad and D. Oberleas (eds.), Academic, New York, 1976.

51 Toepfer, E. W., W. Mertz, M. M. Polansky, E. E. Roginski, and W. R. Wolf: Preparation of chromium-containing material of glucose tolerance factor activity from brewer's yeast extracts and by synthesis, J. Agric. Food Chem., 25:162, 1977.

52 Schroeder, H. A., and J. J. Balassa: Influence of chromium, cadmium, and lead on rat aortic lipids and circulating cholesterol, Am. J. Physiol., 209:433, 1965.

53 Hopkins, L. L., O. Ransome-Kuti, and A. S. Majaj: Improvement of impaired carbohydrate metabolism by chromium III in malnourished infants, Am. J. Clin. Nutr., 21:195, 1968.

54 Gurson, C. T., and G. Saner: Effect of chromium supplementation on growth in marasmic protein-calorie malnutrition, Am. J. Clin. Nutr., 26:1313, 1973.

55 Hopkins, L. L., Jr., and M. G. Price: Effectiveness of chromium (III) in improving the impaired glucose tolerance of middle-aged Americans (abstr.), Proc. West. Hemisphere Nutr. Cong., 2:40, 1968.

56 Levine, R. A., D. H. P. Streeten, and R. J. Doisy: Effect of oral chromium supplementation on the glucose tolerance of elderly human subjects, Metab. Clin. Exp., 17:114, 1968.

57 Glinsmann, W. H., and W. Mertz: Effect of trivalent chromium on glucose tolerance, Metab. Clin. Exp., 15:510, 1966.

58 Schroeder, H. A.: The role of chromium in mammalian nutrition, Am. J. Clin. Nutr., 21:230, 1968.

59 Jeejeebhoy, K. N., R. C. Chu, E. B. Marliss, G. R. Greenberg, and A. Bruce-Robertson: Chromium deficiency, glucose intolerance and neuropathy reversed by chromium supplementation in a patient receiving long-term total parenteral nutrition, Am. J. Clin. Nutr., 30:531, 1977.

60 Hambidge, K. M., and D. O. Rogerson: Comparison of hair chromium levels of multiparous and parous women, Am. J. Obstet. Gynecol., 103:320, 1969.

61 Hambidge, K. M.: Chromium nutrition in man, Am. J. Clin. Nutr., 27:505, 1974.

62 Schroeder, H. A., J. J. Balassa, and I. H. Tipton: Abnormal trace metals in man, J. Chronic Dis., 15:941, 1962.

63 Tipton, I. H., and M. J. Cook: Trace elements in human tissue. II. Adult subjects from the United States, Health Physics, 9:103, 1963.

64 Guthrie, B. E., W. R. Wolf, C. Veillon, and W. Mertz: Chromium in urine, in *Trace Elements in Environmental Health,* D. D. Hemphill (ed.), University of Missouri, Columbia, 1978.

65 Veillon, C., W. R. Wolf, and B. E. Guthrie: Determination of chromium in biological materials by stable isotope dilution, Anal. Chem., 51:1022, 1979.

66 Gurson, C. T.: The metabolic significance of dietary chromium, in *Advances in Nutritional Research,* vol. 1, H. H. Draper (ed.), Plenum, New York, 1977.

67 Hambidge, K. W., and J. D. Baum: Hair chromium concentrations in human newborn and changes during infancy, Am. J. Clin. Nutr., 25:376, 1972.

68 Stewart, R. D. A., N. M. Griffiths, C. D. Thomson, and M. F. Robinson: Quantitative selenium metabolism in normal New Zealand women, Br. J. Nutr., 40:45, 1978.

69 Thomson, C. D., and M. F. Robinson: Selenium in human health and disease with emphasis on those aspects peculiar to New Zealand, Am. J. Clin. Nutr., 33:303, 1980.

70 McConnell, K. P., and O. W. Portman: Excretion of dimethyl selenide by the rat, J. Biol. Chem., 195:277, 1952.

71 Food and Nutrition Board: Selenium and human health, Nutr. Rev., 34:347, 1976.

72 Burk, R. F., W. N. Pearson, R. F. Wood, and F. Viteri: Blood-selenium levels and in vitro red blood cell uptake of ^{75}Se in kwashiorkor, Am. J. Clin. Nutr., 20:723, 1967.

73 Lombeck, I., K. Kasperek, H. D. Harbisch, K. Becker, E. Schumann, W. Schröter, L. E. Feinendegen, and H. J. Bremer: The selenium state of children II, Eur. J. Pediatr., 128:213, 1978.

74 Van Rij, A. M., C. D. Thomson, J. M. McKenzie, and M. F. Robinson: Selenium deficiency in total parenteral nutrition, Am. J. Clin. Nutr., 32:2076, 1979.

75 Keshan Disease Research Group: Observations on effect of sodium selenite in prevention of Keshan disease, Chinese Med. J. 92:471, 1979.

76 Allaway, W. H., J. Kubota, F. Losee, and M. Roth: Selenium, molybdenum and vanadium in human blood, Arch. Environ. Health, 16:342, 1968.

77 Robinson, M. F., C. D. Thomson, R. D. H. Stewart, H. M. Rea, and R. L. McKenzie: Selenium in human nutrition in New Zealand residents, in *Trace Element Metabolism in Man and Animals,* vol. 3, Kirchgessner (ed.), Technische Universitat Munchen, Freising-Weihenstephan, 1978.

78 Lombeck, I., K. Kasparek, H. D. Harbisch, L. E. Feinendegan, and H. J. Bremer: The selenium state of healthy children I., Eur. J. Pediatr., 125:81, 1977.

79 Rosenfeld, I., and O. A. Bealth: *Selenium: Geobotany, Biochemistry, Toxicity and Nutrition,* Academic, New York, 1964.

80 Flink, E. B.: Magnesium deficiency and magnesium toxicity in man, in *Trace Elements in Human Health and Disease,* vol. 2, A. S. Prasad and D. Oberleas (eds.), Academic, New York, 1976.

81 Shils, M. E.: Experimental human magnesium depletion. I Clinical observation and blood chemistry alterations, Am. J. Clin. Nutr., 15:133, 1964.

82 Rude, R. K., and F. R. Singer: Magnesium deficiency and excess, Ann. Rev. Med., 32:245, 1981.

83 Underwood, E. J.: *Trace Elements in Human and Animal Nutrition,* 4th ed., Academic, New York, 1977, p. 545.

84 Doisy, E. A.: Effects of deficiency in manganese upon plasma levels of clotting proteins and cholesterol in man and chicks, in *Trace Element Metabolism in Animals,* 2d ed., W. G. Hoekstra, J. W. Suttie, and H. E. Ganther (eds.), University Park Press, Baltimore, 1974.

85 McLeod, B. E., and M. F. Robinson: Dietary intake of manganese by New Zealand infants during the first six months of life, Br. J. Nutr., 27:221, 1972.

86 Messer, H. H., and L. Singer: Fluoride, in *Present Knowledge in Nutrition,* D. M. Hegsted (ed.), The Nutrition Foundation, New York, 1976.

87 Wiatrowski, E., D. Kramer, D. Osis, and H. Spencer: Dietary fluoride intake of infants, Pediatrics, 55:517, 1975.

88 Sognnaes, R. F.: Fluoride protection of bones and teeth, Science, 150:989, 1965.

89 Schwarz, K.: Recent dietary trace element research exemplified by tin, fluorine and silicon, Fed. Proc., 33:1748, 1974.

90 Schroeder, H. A., M. Mitchener, J. J. Balassa, M. Kanisaiva, and A. P. Nelson: Zirconium, niobium, antimony, and fluorine in mice: effect on growth, survival and tissue levels, J. Nutr., 95:95, 1968.

91 Horowitz, H. S.: A review of systemic and topical fluorides for the prevention of caries, Community Dent. Oral Epidemiol., 1:104, 1973.

92 Underwood, E. J.: *Trace Elements in Human and Animal Nutrition*, 4th ed., Academic, New York, 1977, p. 368.

93 Cullen, R. W., and S. M. Oace: Iodine: current status, J. Nutr. Educ., 8:101, 1976.

94 Taylor, F.: Iodine going from hypo to hyper, FDA Consumer, 15:15, 1981.

95 Food and Nutrition Board, National Research Council: *Iodine Nutriture in the United States,* National Academy of Sciences, Washington, 1970.

96 Moynahan, E. J.: Trace elements in man, Philos. Trans. R. Soc. London, Ser. B, 288:65, 1979.

97 Holman, J. C. M., and W. McCartey: Iodized Salt, WHO Monogr. Ser., 44:411, 1960.

98 McCullagh, S. F.: The effectiveness of an intramuscular depot of iodized oil in the control of endemic goitre, Med. J. Aust., 1:769, 1963.

SUGGESTED FURTHER READING

The aim of this text is to provide nutritional information which is applicable to the practice of clinical medicine. Consequently, many aspects of nutrition have been given only brief mention or have not been mentioned at all, not because they lack interest, but because they are not immediately relevant to clinical practice.

There is some merit in putting the necessarily restricted content of this book into the context of the whole field of human nutrition, which is a diverse and, for many, endlessly fascinating one. For those who wish to explore the area further this list of recommended reading is provided. This is necessarily selective, but it may provide a stimulus to exploration of new areas of knowledge.

British Medical Bulletin, vol. 37, no. 1, 1981 Special Issue on nutrition.

Darby, W J, H P Broquist and R E Olson (eds.): *Annual Review of Nutrition,* Palo Alto, CA, Annual Review Inc. 1981.

Davidson, S, R Passmore, J F Brock, and A S Truswell: *Human Nutrition and Dietetics,* 7th ed., Churchill Livingstone, New York, 1979.

Goodhart, R S, and M E Shils (eds.): *Modern Nutrition in Health and Disease,* 6th ed., Lea & Febiger, Philadelphia, 1980.

Human Nutrition Research, Beltsville Symposia in Agricultural Research No. 4, London, Allanheld, Osmun. Granada, 1981.

Lowenstein, F W: Major nutritional findings from the first health and nutrition examination survey in the United States of America, 1971–1974, Bibl. Nutr. Dieta., 30:1, 1981.

Lowenstein, F W: Review of the nutritional status of Spanish Americans based on published and unpublished reports between 1968 and 1978, Wld. Rev. Nutr. Diet., 37:1, 1981.

Nutrition & the M.D., PM, Inc., 6931 Van Nuys Boulevard, Van Nuys, CA 91405.

Nutrition Reviews, The Nutrition Foundation, 888 17th Street, NW, Washington, D.C. 20006.

GLOSSARY
OF TERMS

achlorhydria Inability of glands of stomach to produce hydrochloric acid, even when presented with a powerful stimulus.

analeptic A central nervous stimulant, revivifier, or tonic.

anemia Reduction in number of circulating red blood cells or of hemoglobin concentration. Aregenerative. Due to failure of bone marrow to make red blood cells.

anephric Lacking kidneys or, sometimes, kidney function.

angular stomatitis (perlèche) Inflammation at angles of mouth with resultant fissuring.

anisocytosis Inequality in size of red blood cells.

anuria Failure of kidneys to make urine.

aphthous ulcer (canker sore) Painful ulcers of mouth with white centers and red surrounding zones.

bulimia Excessive appetite, usually due to psychiatric disturbance or injury to the central nervous system.

cachexia Severe wasting associated with loss of subcutaneous fat and muscle mass.

cheilosis Fissuring of lips.

colostrum First milk from lactating breast following birth of child.

comatose Profoundly unconscious; not able to be aroused.

confabulation Fabrication of information, usually glib, to cover up gaps in memory or thought processes.

dyspepsia Discomfort which is usually felt in the chest or upper part of the front of the abdomen and which usually shows some relationship with eating or drinking.

dysphagia Difficulty with swallowing or inability to swallow food or drink; usually associated with discomfort or pain in the throat or front of the chest.

dyspnea Difficulty in breathing or "getting breath." Not necessarily painful. Frequently associated with a feeling of fear or apprehension. Difficult or labored breathing.

enteric Pertaining to the intestine.

epicanthus   Medial and downward fold of skin from upper eyelid.

epistaxis   Nosebleed; hemorrhage from the nose.

erythema   Redness of skin, usually patchy, due to dilatation of vascular capillaries.

escutcheon (pubic)   Distribution of hair in the pubic region, which displays secondary sexual differences.

fistula   An abnormal passage which is usually between two internal organs or which leads from an internal organ to the surface of the body.

friable   Abnormally susceptible to damage.

glossitis   Properly, inflammation of the surface of the tongue, the tongue appearing reddened and often raw, the surface structure (papillae) being reduced or absent.

hemangioma   A tumor, varying in size from a pin's head to a large mass, made up of blood vessels.

hematemesis   The vomiting of blood.

hypertension   Abnormally high blood pressure. Hence a hypertensive state.

hyponatremia   Abnormally low concentration of sodium ions in the blood.

hyposthenuria   Inability of kidneys to produce a urine of greater solute concentration than that of the blood plasma; therefore, the urine is of low specific gravity.

hypotension   Abnormally low blood pressure. Usually acute or short-term. Hence a hypotensive state.

icterus   Jaundice.

ileus   Obstruction of the intestines.

leukopenia   Reduced number of white cells in peripheral blood.

menorrhagia   Abnormally heavy menstrual loss of blood. Not easily quantified.

myelomatosis   A malignant disease of the bone marrow in which the main cell types involved are of the lymphocyte-plasma cell series; multiple myeloma.

normochromic   Having red cells with a normal hemoglobin content.

normocytic   Having red cells of a normal size, shape, and color.

nystagmus   Oscillatory movements, horizontal or vertical, of the eyes due to disturbed neurological control of the eye muscles responsible for fixing the gaze on an unmoving object. Produced by some drugs or nervous disease but may be congenital.

obtundation   Blunting or reduction of level of consciousness.

oliguria   Production of abnormally small quantities of urine.

palpebral fissure   Space between the eyelids extending from the outer to the inner canthus.

pancytopenia   Reduction in numbers of all three formed elements in the blood: red cells, white cells, and platelets.

paresthesia   Abnormal sensation, usually unpleasant.

pinguecula   Small, slightly elevated yellowish-white patch on the conjunctiva between the cornea and canthus of the eye. Due to degeneration of elastic collagen.

poikilocytosis   Abnormal variation in the shape of circulating red blood cells.

polydipsia   Increased thirst associated usually with polyuria (see next entry). Typical in diabetes insipidus or diabetes mellitus.

polyuria   Increased volume of urine.

porta hepatis   Transverse fissure of the liver in lower medial surface through which the portal vein and hepatic artery enter the liver and the ducts leave.

purpura   Hemorrhage into the skin or mucous membrane.

pyelonephritis   Disease associated with infection of the kidney.

ring sideroblasts   Precursors of red blood cells containing abnormal amounts of stainable iron in the form of rings.

sebum   The secretion of the sebaceous glands of the skin.

seborrheic dermatitis   Inflammation of the sebaceous glands.

spider angioma or nevus   Central, elevated, pinhead sized, red dot on the skin from which fine blood vessels radiate like a spider's web.

target cells   Circulating red blood cells which, in stained films, have the appearance of targets, exhibiting concentric rings of pigment and lack of pigment between the rings. Found after splenectomy and some forms of anemia.

telangiectasia   Dilatation of groups of blood capillaries in the skin or mucous membranes.

teratogenesis   The production of physical defects in offspring in utero.

thrombocytopenia   Decrease in the number of blood platelets.

tinnitus   A noise in the ears, as ringing, buzzing, roaring, or clicking, without external cause.

Trendelenburg's position   The position in which the patient is supine on a table or bed the head of which is tilted downward 30 to 40° and the foot of which is angled downward beneath the patient's knees.

Valsalva maneuver   Increase of intrathoracic pressure by forcible exhalation effort against the closed glottis.

vitiligo   Depigmentation of skin that is best seen in skin areas which are exposed to the sun and therefore tend to be otherwise pigmented.

ENERGY VALUE OF FOOD

The energy value of food is expressed in terms of a unit of heat, the kilocalorie (kcal). It represents the amount of heat required to raise the temperature of 1 kilogram (kg) of water 1 degree Celsius (1°C) at the temperature range 15 to 16°C. Much of the information on the energy value of food is obtained by combustion methods or direct calorimetry using an oxygen bomb calorimeter. When a dried sample of food is completely burned in the oxygen-rich environment of the combustion chamber, the heat produced is absorbed by a weighed amount of water surrounding the chamber. The change in temperature of the water is accurately measured, and the amount of heat resulting from the complete burning of the measured sample is calculated in kilocalories per gram.

The first column in Table 1 presents the heat of combustion obtained from the oxidation of 1 gram (g) of carbohydrate, fat, protein, and alcohol, respectively. The heat of combustion of food represents the total energy produced by the oxidation of the carbon to carbon dioxide, the hydrogen to water, and the nitrogen of the protein to nitrous oxide. In humans the cells oxidize digested food products. Unlike the bomb calorimeter, however, the animal cell cannot completely oxidize protein, and the nitrogen-containing product of protein, urea, is excreted in the urine. The latent heat of the excreted nitrogen must be subtracted from the heat of combustion of the protein (see column 2 in Table 1).

Since the human body is not 100 percent efficient in digesting and absorbing the major nutrients, it is necessary to determine the percentage of the nutrient ultimately available to the body as fuel. As shown in column 3 in Table 1, the availability or coefficient of digestibility is used to correct for the inefficiency of human digestion and absorption. Ethanol, although not usually considered a nutrient, contributes significantly to the total energy intake of many individuals. Ethanol does not require digestion and is absorbed very efficiently from the stomach and the rest of the gastrointestinal tract. This fact is

TABLE 1
HEATS OF COMBUSTION AND AVAILABILITY OF ENERGY IN
PRINCIPAL TYPES OF FOOD

	Heat of combustion, kcal/g	Loss in urine, kcal/g	Coefficient of digestibility	Atwater factor, kcal/g
Protein				
Meat	5.35	1.25	92	4
Egg	5.58			
Fat				
Butter	9.12	—	95	9
Animal fat	9.37			
Olive oil	9.38			
Carbohydrate				
Starch	4.12			
Sucrose	3.96	—	99	4
Glucose	3.81			
Ethanol	7.10	Trace*	100	7

*Traces are also lost in expired air.

reflected in the 100 percent coefficient of digestibility of ethanol listed in column 3 in Table 1. The actual physiological food values (Atwater factors) for the major energy-yielding groups are 4 kilocalories per gram (kcal/g) for carbohydrate and protein, 9 kcal/g for fat, and 7 kcal/g for ethanol.

To calculate the approximate energy value of the foods we eat, nutritionists determine its percentage composition of carbohydrate, protein, fat, and ethanol and then multiply by the appropriate Atwater factors. The exact proportions of nutrients may vary slightly among different samples of the same food, and since the efficiency of digestion differs among individuals, the energy provided by a serving of a particular food is only approximated and is not precisely known.

REFERENCE

1 Passmore, R. and J. S. Robson, *A Companion to Medical Studies,* Vol. 1, 3d printing, Blackwell, Oxford, 1971, pp. 4.1–4.5.

ESTIMATION OF HUMAN ENERGY REQUIREMENTS

Several factors contribute to the amount of energy required by an individual at a given time: basal metabolic rate, physical activity, and to a lesser extent, the specific dynamic action of food.

The energy expended to maintain the basal activities of the body such as respiration, circulation, maintenance of body temperature, and other cellular activities is termed *basal metabolic rate* (BMR). The basal metabolic rate is the number of kilocalories per unit time used by an individual to maintain life at rest. A quick, approximate figure for BMR is 1 kcal/kg of body weight per hour. Basal metabolic rates vary with age, sex, and the total body surface area of the subject. More accurate estimates can be determined when these three variables are accounted for. The Harris-Benedict equations for men and women calculate BMR, taking into account these variables;

$$\text{Men} \quad \text{BMR} = 66 + (13.7 \times W) + (5 \times H) - (6.8 \times A)$$
$$\text{Women} \quad \text{BMR} = 655 + (9.6 \times W) + (1.7 \times H) - (4.7 \times A)$$

where
$$W = \text{weight in kilograms}$$
$$H = \text{height in centimeters}$$
$$A = \text{age in years}$$

Another means of calculating BMR from height and weight data is as follows:

1 Determine body surface area from the accompanying nomogram (Figure 1).

2 Determine metabolic rate from predicted standards for age and sex of the subject (Table 1). These predicted standard metabolic rates are measured in kilocalories per square meter of body surface area per hour.

3 Multiply body surface areas by metabolic rate, or use the nomogram (Figure 2).

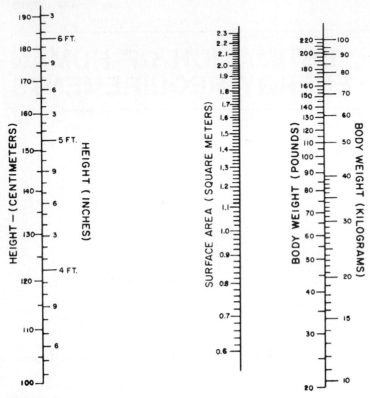

FIGURE 1
Surface area from height and weight. To determine body surface area
from the height on the left-hand scale and weight on the right-hand scale,
connect these points with a straightedge and read surface area from the
middle scale.

Total energy expenditure increases with physical activity. In fact, muscular work is the single most important factor that raises energy requirements above the basal metabolic rate in the healthy adult. The dominant factor leading to variability in energy needs is the proportion of time an individual devotes to moderate and heavy activities. The physical activity of people in the United States is generally considered to be light or sedentary, following typical patterns given in Table 2. For accurate estimates, the entire waking period should be considered in making adjustments and substituting different time spans for the activity categories given in Table 2.

In practice, a quick approximation of energy expenditure can be calculated by using the following guidelines:

Sedentary	BMR + 30%
Light to moderate activity	BMR + 40%
Strenuous activity	BMR + 50%

TABLE 1
DETERMINATION OF STANDARD METABOLIC RATES

Age in years	kcal/m^2 per hour		kJ*/m^2 per hour	
	Men	Women	Men	Women
1	53.0	53.0	222	222
2	52.4	52.4	219	219
3	51.3	51.2	215	214
4	50.3	49.8	211	208
5	49.3	48.4	206	203
6	48.3	47.0	202	197
7	47.3	45.4	198	190
8	46.3	43.8	194	183
9	45.2	42.8	189	179
10	44.0	42.5	184	178
11	43.0	42.0	180	176
12	42.5	41.3	178	173
13	42.3	40.3	177	169
14	42.1	39.2	176	164
15	41.8	37.9	175	159
16	41.4	36.9	173	154
17	40.8	36.3	171	152
18	40.0	35.9	167	150
19	39.2	35.5	164	149
20	38.6	35.3	162	148
25	37.5	35.2	157	147
30	36.8	35.1	154	147
35	36.5	35.0	153	146
40	36.3	34.9	152	146
45	36.2	34.5	152	144
50	35.8	33.9	150	142
55	35.4	33.3	148	139
60	34.9	32.7	146	137
65	34.4	32.2	144	135
70	33.8	31.7	141	133
75+	33.2	31.3	139	131

*Kilojoules.
Source: A. Fleisch, Le metabolisme basal standard et sa determination au moyen du "Metabocalculator," Helv. Med. Acta, 18:23, 1951.

Metabolic rate rises as a consequence of eating. The thermogenic effect of ingested food is termed *specific dynamic action* (SDA). The causes of SDA remain uncertain. Protein exerts the greatest increase in heat production; approximately 12 percent of ingested protein is dissipated as heat. The specific dynamic action for carbohydrates is 6 percent of ingested food, while that of fat is 2 percent. In the mixed diet approximately 6 percent of the potential fuel value is dissipated as heat. When calculating total energy expenditure, a value of 10 percent of the consumed calories is assigned to account for the SDA of food.

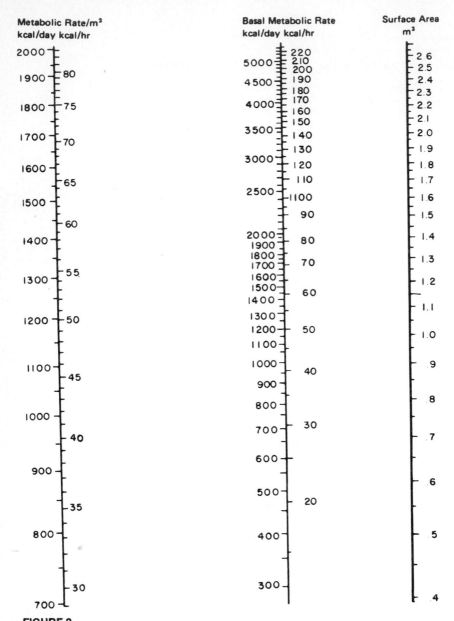

Metabolic Rate/m² kcal/day kcal/hr	Basal Metabolic Rate kcal/day kcal/hr	Surface Area m²

FIGURE 2

To predict daily metabolic requirements, determine surface area (right-hand scale) and metabolic requirements per square meter of body surface for age and sex (left-hand scale) (see Table 1). By connecting these points with a straightedge, the predicted daily or hourly requirements may be determined from the middle scale. (*From W. M. Boothby, J. Berkson, and H. L. Dunn, Am. J. Physiol., 116:468, 1936.*)

TABLE 2
EXAMPLES OF DAILY ENERGY EXPENDITURES OF ADULTS IN LIGHT OCCUPATIONS

Activity category*	Time, hours	Man, 70 kg		Woman, 58 kg	
		Rate, kcal/minute	Total, kcal	Rate, kcal/minute	Total, kcal
Sleeping, reclining	8	1.0–1.2	540	0.9–1.1	440
Very light Seated and standing activities, painting trades, auto and truck driving, laboratory work, typing, playing musical instruments, sewing, ironing	12	≤ 2.5	1300	≤ 2.0	900
Light Walking on level 2.5–3 mph, tailoring, pressing, garage work, electrical trades, carpentry, restaurant trades, cannery work, washing clothes, shopping with light load, golf, sailing, table tennis, volleyball	3	2.5–4.9	600	2.0–3.9	450
Moderate Walking 3.5–4 mph, plastering, weeding and hoeing, loading and stacking bales, scrubbing floors, shopping with heavy load, cycling, skiing, tennis, dancing	1	5.0–7.4	300	4.0–5.9	240
Heavy Walking with load uphill, tree felling, work with pick and shovel, basketball, swimming, climbing, football	0	7.5–12.0		6.0–10.0	
Total	24		2740		2030

*Data from J.V.G.A. Durnin and R. Passmore, Energy, Work and Leisure, Heinemann, London, 1967.
Source: Recommended Dietary Allowances, 9th ed., Food and Nutrition Board, National Academy of Sciences–National Research Council, Washington, D.C., 1980.

TABLE 3
RECOMMENDED ENERGY INTAKE

Category	Age, years	Weight, kg	Height, cm	Energy needs kcal	range
Infants	0.0–0.5	6	60	kg × 115	(95–145)
	0.5–1.0	9	71	kg × 105	(80–135)
Children	1–3	13	90	1300	(900–1800)
	4–6	20	112	1700	(1300–2300)
	7–10	28	132	2400	(1650–3300)
Male adults	11–14	45	157	2700	(2000–3700)
	15–18	66	176	2800	(2100–3900)
	19–22	70	177	2900	(2500–3300)
	23–50	70	178	2700	(2300–3100)
	51–75	70	178	2400	(2000–2800)
	76+	70	178	2050	(1650–2450)
Female adults	11–14	46	157	2200	(1500–3000)
	15–18	55	163	2100	(1200–3000)
	19–22	55	163	2100	(1700–2500)
	23–50	55	163	2000	(1600–2400)
	51–75	55	163	1800	(1400–2200)
	76+	55	163	1600	(1200–2000)
Pregnant women				+300	
Lactating women				+500	

Source: Recommended Dietary Allowances, 9th ed., Food and Nutrition Board, National Academy of Sciences–National Research Council, Washington, D.C., 1980.

Another resource for estimation of caloric requirement in the Recommended Dietary Allowances (RDA) established by the Food and Nutrition Board of the National Academy of Sciences. These energy allowances (Table 3) are approximations intended for general use. They represent proposals for healthy subjects whose weight is desirable and suitable for their height and whose physical activity is considered to be light to sedentary. For subjects who vary from this norm in activity, adjustments should be made accordingly. Caloric requirements may be estimated on the basis of desirable weight for age and height (Table 4) rather than actual weight for the obese or extremely thin person.

An alternate procedure for estimating caloric need is the use of the following figures, which include estimates for basal metabolism:

Activity level	kcal/kg ideal weight
Sedentary	30
Light	35
Moderate	40
Heavy	45

Special guidelines should be considered when calculating energy allowances for infants, children, and pregnant and lactating women. For the thriving infant during the

TABLE 4
DESIRABLE WEIGHT FOR HEIGHT*

Height, cm	Weight, kg	
	Men	Women
147	—	46 (42–54)
152	—	49 (44–57)
158	56 (51–64)	51 (46–59)
163	59 (54–67)	55 (49–63)
168	62 (56–71)	58 (52–66)
173	66 (60–75)	62 (55–70)
178	70 (64–79)	65 (59–74)
183	74 (67–84)	69 (63–79)
188	78 (71–88)	—
193	82 (74–93)	—

*Height without shoes, weight without shoes and clothing. Average weight ranges are given in parentheses.
Source: Recommended Dietary Allowances, 9th ed., Food and Nutrition Board, National Academy of Sciences–National Research Council, Washington, D.C., 1980.

first year of life, energy allowances are reduced in suitable steps from an initial level of 115 kcal per kilogram of body weight to 105 kcal/kg by the end of the infant's first year. Energy allowances for children of both sexes decline gradually to about 80 kcal/kg over the first 10 years of age. During the teenage years, energy allowances decline further to 45 kcal/kg for males in their late teens and to 38 kcal/kg for females in their late teens. Conditions such as pregnancy and lactation require additional energy intake. The RDAs suggest an additional 300 kilocalories per day during pregnancy and an additional 500 kcal per day for lactation. These figures may need adjustment to account for changes in activity or body stores.

REFERENCES

1 *Recommended Dietary Allowances,* 9th ed. Food and Nutrition Board, National Academy of Sciences–National Research Council. Washington, D.C., 1980, pp. 16–30.
2 Wilmore, D. W. Energy and energy balance, in *The Metabolic Management of the Critically Ill,* T. King and K. Reemtsma (eds.), Plenum, New York, 1977, pp. 1–50.

HUMAN PROTEIN REQUIREMENTS AND RECOMMENDATIONS

The body's requirement for dietary protein can best be explained in terms of its requirements for (1) essential amino acids and (2) nitrogen. Dietary protein supplies the 20 amino acids that are needed for the synthesis of body protein (Table 1). The amino acids are designated either as essential (those which must be supplied in the diet since they cannot be synthesized in the body in adequate amounts) or nonessential (those which can be synthesized in the body in adequate amounts). For adults there are eight essential amino acids; however, infants require a ninth, histidine. Protein nitrogen is lost continuously through the urine, feces, skin, hair, and nails. The daily protein supply for tissue protein synthesis must, therefore, be continuously replenished.

The requirement for protein in the diet can be estimated by either the factorial method or the nitrogen balance technique. The *factorial method* is based on adding up the series of factors that represent obligatory nitrogen losses from the body when the diet is devoid of protein but contains adequate energy and then assuming that sufficient nitrogen from high-quality dietary protein to replace these obligatory losses will provide the subject with the body's requirements. This calculation is summarized in the following equation:

$$R_N = U + F + S + G$$

where R_N is the requirement of nitrogen (grams per kilogram of body weight per day); U, F, and S are the urinary, fecal, and skin nitrogen losses, respectively; and G is the nitrogen increment during growth. Since about 16 percent of protein is nitrogen, protein loss can be estimated by multiplying the grams of nitrogen lost by the body by 100/16 or 6.25.

When a protein-free diet is administered to a human subject there is an initial, rapid decrease in urinary nitrogen output over the first 4 or 5 days (Figure 1). Following adaptation to the protein-free diet, daily urinary nitrogen loss reaches a plateau between

TABLE 1
AMINO ACIDS

Essential	Nonessential
Isoleucine	Glycine
Leucine	Alanine
Threonine	Serine
Lysine	Tyrosine
Methionine	Cysteine
Phenylalanine	Cystine
Tryptophan	Aspartic acid
Valine	Glutamic acid
Histidine*	Arginine
	Proline
	Hydroxyproline

*Histidine is essential for infants only.

FIGURE 1
Obligatory daily urinary nitrogen loss of 83 young men given minimal protein diet for 14 days. (*From N. S. Scrimshaw, M. A. Hussein, E. Murray and V. R. Young, J. Nutr., 102:1595, 1972.*)

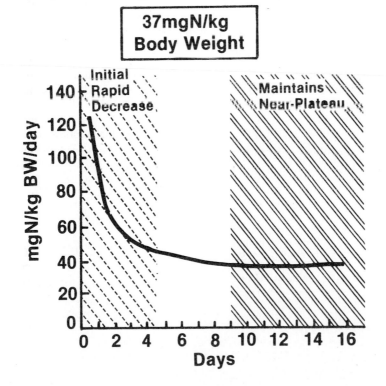

37mgN/kg Body Weight

the ninth and sixteenth days. At that point urinary nitrogen loss averages 37 mg of nitrogen per kilogram of body weight per day. Even on a diet without protein, there is an obligatory loss of nitrogen in the feces, representing enzymes, bacterial flora, and shed intestinal cells. This obligatory fecal nitrogen output of adults is about 12 mg of nitrogen per kilogram of weight per day (Table 2). Nitrogen is also lost from the skin in the form of sweat, hair, and nail clippings and shed skin cells. Recent studies indicate that daily skin nitrogen losses by adult men on a protein-free diet in a temperate environment is about 3 mg of nitrogen per kilogram of body weight. In addition to the major channels of nitrogen loss, there are a series of minor routes of nitrogen excretion. These minor channels include ammonia excreted in the breath, menstrual losses by the female, seminal ejaculations by the male, and nasal secretions and sputum. For all these minor channels, a daily estimate of 2 mg of nitrogen per kilogram of body weight for men and 3 mg of nitrogen per kilogram of body weight for women is used. As shown in Table 2, the sum of urinary, fecal, skin, and minor channels of nitrogen loss is 54 mg of nitrogen per kilogram of body weight. These estimates of nitrogen loss can be expressed as amounts of body protein, that is, 0.34 g of protein per kilogram of body weight. This mimimum daily requirement is in terms of protein that is fully utilized by the body.

Alternatively, use of the *nitrogen balance* technique makes it possible to determine the minimum amount of protein that must be ingested to maintain nitrogen equilibrium, in other words, nitrogen intake is balanced by nitrogen output. The determination of nitrogen balance requires a careful estimate of intake I and nitrogen loss through feces F and urine U:

$$\text{Nitrogen balance} = I - (U + F)$$

Skin losses are seldom measured. Most investigators rely on previously published observations to make an estimated correction for skin losses.

In a nitrogen balance study, Scrimshaw and colleagues (J. Nutr. 103:1164, 1973) fed young men egg protein at seven different levels ranging from 7 to 85 mg of nitrogen per kilogram of body weight for 14-day periods. Regression analysis of the data (Figure 2) showed that the mean requirement for egg protein was 73 mg of nitrogen per kilogram of body weight or 0.456 g of protein per kilogram of body weight.

The National Academy of Sciences RDA is based on an estimated mean daily requirement of 0.47 g of protein per kilogram of body weight. This value has been

TABLE 2
FACTORIAL METHOD

	Channels for nitrogen loss, milligrams of nitrogen per kilogram of body weight
Urine	37
Fecal	12
Skin	3
Minor channels	2
Total nitrogen loss	54

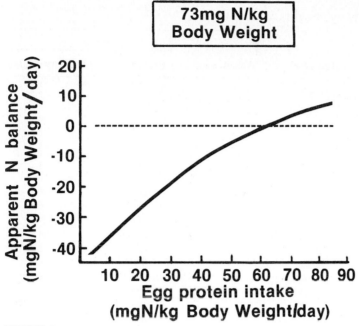

FIGURE 2
Relationship between apparent nitrogen balance and egg protein intake within the submaintenance range of nitrogen intake in young men.
(*From V. R. Young, Y. S. Taylor, W. M. Rand and N. S. Scrimshaw, J. Nutr., 103:1164, 1973.*)

obtained by nitrogen balance studies and has been increased by 30 percent to account for individual variability, giving daily allowances of 0.6μ/kg of high-quality protein. This amount of protein covers the range of individual needs for 97.5 percent of the population (mean ± 2 Standard Deviations). This value has been further increased by allowing for a 75 percent efficiency of utilization for a diet of mixed proteins. The total recommended RDA is 0.8 g per kilogram of body weight.

For a man weighing 70 kg, the daily protein allowance is 56 g and for a 55-kg woman, 44 g. Most recent studies indicate that the average American consumption of protein is 102 g of protein per day. Two-thirds of this intake is from sources of high biological value such as meat, eggs, and dairy products. The remaining portion is derived mainly from grains and vegetables.

Protein allowances have also been issued to cover the special needs of pregnant and lactating women. An additional 30 g of protein per day is recommended for the pregnant woman from the second month until the end of gestation. Lactation requires an additional 20 g of protein per day above the maintenance allowance to cover the requirement for milk production and to allow for 70 percent efficiency of protein utilization.

The allowance for infants is based on the amount of milk consumed and the amount known to ensure a satisfactory rate of growth. For ages up to 6 months, the allowance is 2.2 g of protein per kilogram of body weight. This figure declines to 2.0 g of protein per

TABLE 3
RECOMMENDED DIETARY PROTEIN ALLOWANCES

			Allowances	
	Age, years	Weight, kg	Protein, g	Protein, g/kg
Infants	0.0–0.5	6	kg X 2.2	2.2
	0.5–1.0	9	kg X 2.0	2.0
Children	1–3	13	23	1.8
	4–6	20	30	1.5
	7–10	28	34	1.2
Males	11–14	45	45	1.0
	15–18	66	56	0.8
	19–22	70	56	0.8
	23–50	70	56	0.8
	51+	70	56	0.8
Females	11–14	46	46	1.0
	15–18	55	46	0.8
	19–22	55	44	0.8
	23–50	55	44	0.8
	51+	55	44	0.8
Pregnant women			+30	
Lactating women			+20	

Source: Recommended Dietary Allowances, 9th ed., Food and Nutrition Board, National Academy of Sciences–National Research Council, Washington, D.C., 1980.

kilogram of body weight from 6 months to 1 year. A complete listing of the protein RDAs throughout the life cycle is given in Table 3.

In the clinical setting, a reasonably good estimate of nitrogen balance can be obtained by measuring the urinary urea nitrogen (UUN) in an aliquot of a 24-hour urine collection. Approximately 90 percent of daily nitrogen loss is excreted via the urine. Seventy to 90 percent of this urinary nitrogen is in the form of urea. The remainder represents uric acid, ammonia, creatinine, amino acids, and other nitrogenous waste products. Rather than the clinically impracticable, time-consuming, expensive, standard Kjeldahl method for measuring total nitrogen, nitrogen balance can be determined by the formula:

$$\text{Nitrogen balance} = (\text{Nitrogen intake}) - (\text{nitrogen output})$$
$$= \frac{\text{protein intake (g)}}{6.25} - (\text{UNN} + 4)$$

where 4 represents a constant for skin, fecal, and urinary nonurea nitrogen losses. It is not reasonable to use this formula if a patient has additional nitrogen loss from wounds, burns, or hemorrhage.

Normally adults are in nitrogen balance. When protein anabolism exceeds protein catabolism (pregnancy, growth, recovery from illness, athletic training), nitrogen balance is positive. When nitrogen excretion exceeds intake (poor-quality diet, inadequate protein, inadequate energy intake, accelerated protein catabolism), nitrogen balance is negative.

REFERENCES

1 *Recommended Dietary Allowances,* 9th ed., Food and Nutrition Board, National Academy of Sciences–National Research Council, Washington, D.C., 1980, pp. 39–54.
2 Young, V. R., Y. S. Taylor, W. M. Rand, and N. S. Scrimshaw: Protein requirements of man: efficiency of egg protein utilization at maintenance and submaintenance levels in young men, J. Nutr. 103:1164, 1973.
3 N. S. Scrimshaw: An analysis of past and present recommended dietary allowances for protein in health and disease, New Engl. J. Med. 294:136, 198, 1976.

ESTIMATION OF DIETARY PROTEIN QUALITY

The "quality" of protein refers to the amount of essential amino acids (Table 1) that it contains in relation to the amount required for new tissue formation. Therefore, the quality of a specific protein is determined primarily by two factors: (1) the digestibility of that protein, or how well it is broken down and made available for absorption; and (2) the essential amino acid content of the protein. Methods of evaluation of protein quality are usually biological since it is the ability of a protein to support growth and maintenance that determines its ultimate value. Some methods, such as those using nitrogen balance or growth as criteria of nitrogen retention, can be applied to studies with human subjects. The majority of studies, however, are performed with experimental animals and sometimes use techniques such as carcass analysis that are not suitable for human studies.

PROTEIN EFFICIENCY RATIO

The protein efficiency ratio (PER) was introduced over 60 years ago as a method of expressing numerically the growth-promoting value of protein. It is defined as the weight gain of growing animals divided by the weight of protein they consume:

$$PER = \frac{\text{weight gain, g}}{\text{protein consumed, g}}$$

In the assay, young growing animals of the same age, usually rats, are fed the protein source at a standard level of 9.09 percent for 10 or more days, and weight gain and food intake are measured. For example, in one series of tests the usual standard protein,

TABLE 1
ESSENTIAL AMINO ACIDS

Isoleucine	Phenylalanine
Leucine	Tryptophan
Threonine	Valine
Lysine	Histidine*
Methionine	

*Histidine is essential for in-
fants only.

casein, a milk protein, had a PER of 2.8, soy protein 2.4, and wheat gluten 0.4. This means that young rats gained 2.4 g for every gram of soy eaten, but only 0.4 g for every gram of wheat gluten eaten. This method has several shortcomings: (1) dietary protein required for the maintenance of the animal is not credited in the measurement of PER; (2) variation in body composition may occur, in which case PER would not afford an adequate measure of *nitrogen* retention; and (3) PER also varies with the *amount* of food consumed.

BIOLOGICAL VALUE

The classic procedure for measuring protein quality which estimates changes in total body *protein* rather than body weight is the determination of biological value (BV). Biological value is an expression of nitrogen retained for growth or maintenance divided by nitrogen absorbed. It is determined by nitrogen balance and is applicable to humans as well as laboratory animals:

$$BV = \frac{\text{retained nitrogen}}{\text{absorbed nitrogen}} = \frac{I - (F - F_0) - (U - U_0)}{I - (F - F_0)}$$

where I is nitrogen intake, U is urinary nitrogen, F is fecal nitrogen, and U_0 and F_0 respectively are urinary and fecal nitrogen excreted when subjects are maintained on a nitrogen-free diet. Biological value calculated from this equation takes into account obligatory nitrogen losses when subjects are fed a nitrogen-free diet. If this correction is not made, that is, if U_0 and F_0 are not in the equation, the BV obtained is designated the *apparent biological value:*

$$BV = \frac{I - F - U}{I - F}$$

This method does not take into consideration (1) poor digestibility of a protein or (2) incomplete absorption. The biological value of various food items is given in Table 2.

TABLE 2
BIOLOGICAL VALUE OF FOOD

Food item	Biological value
Hen's eggs	100
Cow's milk	93
Rice	86
Fish	75
Beef	75
Corn	72
Peanut flour	56
Wheat gluten	44

TRUE VERSUS APPARENT DIGESTIBILITY

Digestion and absorption are not ordinarily major considerations unless the diet is rich in foods that are not easily digested. The percentage of food protein consumed which is actually digested and absorbed is termed *protein digestibility*. It is calculated as follows:

$$\text{Digestibility apparent} = \frac{\text{absorbed nitrogen}}{\text{nitrogen intake}} \times 100 = \frac{(I - F) \times 100}{I}$$

where I is nitrogen intake and F is fecal nitrogen.

If a correction for the obligatory nitrogen losses for a subject fed a protein-free diet is made, the value is termed the *true digestibility of nitrogen* rather than the *apparent digestibility*.

$$\text{Digestibility true} = \frac{I - (F - F_0) \times 100}{I}$$

Some estimates of protein digestibility are given in Table 3.

TABLE 3
DIGESTIBILITY OF FOOD

Food item	Digestibility
Hen's eggs	99
Cow's milk	97
Rice	97
Fish	98
Beef	99
Corn	90
Peanut flour	87
Wheat gluten	99
Beans	73

NET PROTEIN UTILIZATION

The net protein utilization (NPU) is the proportion of food nitrogen retained in the body. It is the product of biological value and digestibility:

$$\underset{\text{(BV)}}{\frac{\text{Retained N}}{\text{Absorbed N}}} \times \underset{\text{(Digestibility)}}{\frac{\text{Absorbed N}}{\text{N intake}}} = \underset{\text{(NPU)}}{\frac{\text{Retained N}}{\text{N intake}}}$$

where NPU represents the proportion of *food* nitrogen retained, whereas BV represents the proportion of *absorbed* nitrogen retained. Net protein utilization, therefore, is related directly to dietary intake of nitrogen. Nitrogen retention may be measured by nitrogen balance studies or by direct analysis of the animal body. The formula for calculating NPU by use of nitrogen balance studies is as follows:

$$\text{NPU} = \frac{I - (F - F_0) - (U - U_0)}{I}$$

where I is nitrogen intake, U is urinary nitrogen, F is fecal nitrogen, and U_0 and F_0 respectively are urinary and fecal nitrogen excreted when subjects are maintained on a nitrogen free diet.

COMPOSITION OF DIETARY PROTEIN

Definitions:

Complete protein—term for dietary protein that contains all the essential amino acids in amounts sufficient for growth and maintenance. Examples include eggs, milk, and meat.

Incomplete protein—dietary protein that contains less than the optimal amounts of essential amino acids.

Limiting amino acid—the essential amino acid of protein that shows the greatest percentage deficit in comparison with the amino acids contained in the same quantity of another protein selected as a standard.

REFERENCES

1 *Improvement of Protein Nutriture,* Food and Nutrition Board, National Academy of Sciences–National Research Council: Washington, D.C., 1974.
2 WHO/FAO Report: *Protein Requirements,* WHO Technical Report Series No. 301, WHO, Geneva, 1965.

FAT-SOLUBLE VITAMINS AND ESSENTIAL FATTY ACID

VITAMIN A

CHEMICAL FORMS	Retinol, retinal; retinoic acid. Precursor: carotenes.
STRUCTURE	

Retinol

FUNCTION	Visual cycle: formation of the visual pigments rhodopsin and iodopsin; growth, reproduction, and maintenance of epithelial cells.
ABSORPTION	Primarily jejunum; adversely affected by drugs that bind bile acids (e.g., cholestyramine).
CHARACTERISTICS OF DEFICIENCY STATE	Xerosis of eye and skin, xerophthalmia, Bitot's spot, follicular hyperkeratosis, and increased dark adaptation time.
DEFICIENCY MAY OCCUR IN	Children in developing countries where dietary staple is often rice or wheat; patients with intestinal malabsorption, liver disease,

	or protein-calorie malnutrition or using mineral oil or cholestyramine.
RDA	Adult male, 1000 RE or 1000 μg of retinol; adult female, 800 RE or 800 μg of retinol.
DIETARY SOURCES	Liver, green leafy vegetables, cantaloupes, sweet potato, and carrots.
STORAGE	Liver.
ESTIMATION OF STATUS	Direct: spectrophotometric ultraviolet (UV) absorption. Fasting serum; avoid hemolysis; plasma retinol (normal >30 μg/dl).
TOXICITY	Large doses of vitamin A during pregnancy produce severe skeletal malformations in newborns. Acute toxicity: headaches, vomiting, dizziness, and drowsiness. Chronic toxicity: anemia, pruritus, alopecia, and occasionally hepatomegaly.
THERAPY	9000 RE orally for a few days.

REFERENCES

1 Roels, O. A.: Vitamin A physiology, J. Am. Med. Assoc., 214:1047, 1970.
2 Bjelke, E.: Dietary vitamin A and human lung cancer, Internatl. J. Cancer., 15:561, 1975.
3 Wald, G.: Molecular basis of visual excitation, Science, 162:230, 1968.
4 Oomen, H. A. P. C.: Vitamin A deficiency, xerophthalmia and blindness, Nutr. Rev., 32:161, 1974.
5 McLaren, D. S., W. W. C. Read, Z. I. Awdeh, and M. Tchalian: Microdetermination of vitamin A and carotenoids in blood and tissue, in *Methods of Biochemical Analysis*, Vol. XV, D. Glick (ed.), Wiley, New York, 1967, p. 1.

VITAMIN D

CHEMICAL FORMS	Plant: ergocalciferol (Vitamin D_2). Animal: cholecalciferol (Vitamin D_3). Most active form: 1,25-dihydroxycholecalciferol.
STRUCTURE	

Vitamin D_3

FUNCTION	Intestinal absorption of calcium and phosphorus; calcium mobilization from bone.
ABSORPTION	Jejunum; adversely affected by ingestion of mineral oil and drugs that bind bile acids (e.g., cholestyramine).
CHARACTERISTICS OF DEFICIENCY STATE	Faulty mineralization of bones and teeth; rickets (children) and osteomalacia (adults).
DEFICIENCY MAY OCCUR IN	People with limited exposure to sun; breast-fed infants of vegan mothers; patients with intestinal malabsorption, liver disease, or kidney disease or using anticonvulsant drugs.
RDA	Birth to 18 years, 10 μg (400 IU); 19 to 22 years, 7.5 μg (300 IU); adults; 5 μg (200 IU).
DIETARY SOURCES	Vitamin D-fortified milk, egg yolk, butter, liver, and fish-liver oils.
STORAGE	Liver.
ESTIMATION OF STATUS	Indirect: serum alkaline phosphatase is elevated; serum calcium and phosphorus levels are low. Direct: methods for estimating plasma 25-OH vitamin D are becoming available.
TOXICITY	Occurs with excessive intake of cod-liver oil; symptoms due to hypercalcemia include nausea, weight loss, anorexia, and calcification of bone and soft tissues.
THERAPY	Vitamin D_2 or D_3 orally: 0.05 to 0.1 mg daily for 6 to 12 weeks.
ADDITIONAL COMMENTS	Vitamin D_3 synthesized from 7-dehydrocholesterol in skin by ultraviolet irradiation.

REFERENCES

1 Norman, A.: *Vitamin D. The Calcium Homeostatic Steroid Hormone,* Academic Press, New York, 1979.
2 Haussler, M. R. and T. A. McCain: Basic clinical concepts related to vitamin D metabolism and action, New Engl. J. Med., 297:974; 297:1041, 1977.
3 DeLuca, H. F.: The Vitamin D system in the regulation of calcium and phosphorus metabolism, Nutr. Revs., 37:161, 1979.

VITAMIN E

CHEMICAL FORMS	α-Tocopherol, β-tocopherol, γ-tocopherol, α-tocotrienol.

STRUCTURE

α-Tocopherol

FUNCTION	Antioxidant, heme synthesis.
ABSORPTION	Jejunum; 50 to 85 percent.
CHARACTERISTICS OF DEFICIENCY STATE	Not clearly defined in adults; increased fragility of red blood cells, hemolytic anemia, edema, irritability in premature infants.
DEFICIENCY MAY OCCUR IN	Premature infants and patients with intestinal fat malabsorption due to cystic fibrosis or abetalipoproteinemia.
RDA	Adult male, 10-mg α-tocopherol equivalents; adult female, 8 mg α-tocopherol equivalents.
DIETARY SOURCES	Vegetable oils and margarine.
STORAGE	Liver and adipose tissue.
ESTIMATION OF STATUS	Direct: plasma α-tocopherol (normal >0.5 mg/dl).
TOXICITY	None known.

REFERENCES

1 Graber, J. E., M. L. Williams, and F. A. Oski: The use of intramuscular vitamin E in the premature infant, J. Pediatr., 90:282, 1977.
2 Bieri, J. G.: Vitamin E, Nutr. Rev., 33:161, 1975.
3 Hashim, S. A. and G. R. Schuttringer: Rapid determination of tocopherol in macro- and microquantities of plasma. Results obtained in various nutrition and metabolic studies, Am. J. Clin. Nutr., 19:137, 1966.

VITAMIN K

CHEMICAL FORMS	Naphthoquinone derivatives. Plants: phylloquinone (vitamin K_1). Bacteria and animal: menaquinones (vitamin K_2). Synthetic: menadione.

STRUCTURE

Vitamin K_1

FUNCTION	Cofactor in synthesis of prothrombin(II), proconvertin(VII), Christmas factor(IX), Stuart factor(X), and osteocalcin.
ABSORPTION	Jejunum.
CHARACTERISTICS OF DEFICIENCY STATE	Bleeding diathesis with prolonged prothrombin time.
DEFICIENCY MAY OCCUR IN	Newborn infants; chronic alcoholics; patients with intestinal malabsorption, biliary obstruction, or severe liver disease or taking antibiotics, mineral oil, or cholestyramine.
RDA	Estimated safe and adequate daily intake for adults, 70 to 140 μg.
DIETARY SOURCES	Green leafy vegetables, broccoli, lettuce, spinach, and beef liver.
STORAGE	Liver.
ESTIMATION OF STATUS	Indirect: increased prothrombin time (no biochemical analysis available).
TOXICITY	Jaundice and hemolytic anemia in infants given excessive doses of menadione; the natural vitamins K_1 and K_2 are nontoxic in large doses.
THERAPY	Oil-soluble vitamin K_1 (oral and intravenous forms) or synthetic vitamin K.
ADDITIONAL COMMENTS	Bacterial synthesis of vitamin K_2 in the intestine is an important source of vitamin K in humans.

REFERENCES

1 Ansell, J. E., R. Kumar, and D. Deykin: The spectrum of vitamin K deficiency, J. Am. Med. Assoc., 238:40, 1977.
2 Gallopa, P. M., J. B. Lian, and P. V. Hauschka: Carboxylated calcium-binding proteins and vitamin K, New Engl. J. Med., 302:1460, 1980.
3 Quick, A. J.: *Bleeding Problems in Clinical Medicine,* Saunders, Philadelphia, 1970.

ESSENTIAL FATTY ACID (EFA)

CHEMICAL NAME	Linoleic acid (18:2, *cis*-9,12-octadecadienoic acid).
STRUCTURE	

$$CH_3(CH_2)_4\overset{\overset{H}{|}}{C}=\overset{\overset{H}{|}}{C}-CH_2-\overset{\overset{H}{|}}{C}=\overset{\overset{H}{|}}{C}(CH_2)_7COOH$$

FUNCTIONS	Essential precursor of longer-chain, polyunsatured fatty acids from which prostaglandins (PG), prostacyclin (PGI$_2$), and thromboxane A$_2$ (TXA$_2$) are derived. Also required to maintain normal phospholipid membrane function and normal coupling in oxidative phosphorylation.
ABSORPTION	Same mechanism as in other fatty acids.
CHARACTERISTICS OF DEFICIENCY STATE	Scaling of skin; possibly poor healing of wounds.
DEFICIENCY MAY OCCUR IN	Chronic inflammatory bowel disease, bowel resection, or long-term total parenteral feeding without fat preparations.
RDA	It has been suggested tentatively that 3 percent of total energy should be EFA at total fat intakes of 25 percent of total energy or less. At fat consumption of 35 to 40 percent of total energy, 8 to 10 percent of total energy as EFA is recommended. This is currently speculative.
DIETARY SOURCES	Vegetable oils, with some exceptions (coconut, palm).
STORAGE	Adipose tissue.
ESTIMATION OF STATUS	Currently not well defined; analyses of fatty acid content of subcutaneous fat, plasma, or erythrocytes by gas or thin-layer chromatography. From estimations of methylated 5,8,11-eicosatrienoic and arachidonic acids in plasma, a triene-tetraene ratio is derived; if >0.4, indicative of EFA deficiency.
THERAPY	Vegetable oils by mouth, intravenously, or inunction on skin surface.

REFERENCES

1 Collins, F. D., A. J. Sinclair, J. P. Royle, D. A. Coats, A. T. Maynard, and R. F. Leonard: Plasma lipids in human linoleic acid deficiency, Nutr. Metab. 13:150, 1971.
2 Fleming, C. R., L. M. Smith, and R. E. Hodges: Essential fatty acid deficiency in adults receiving total parenteral nutrition, Am. J. Clin. Nutr., 29:976, 1976.

WATER-SOLUBLE VITAMINS

VITAMIN B₁

CHEMICAL FORMS

Thiamine pyrophosphate [3-(2'-methyl-4'
-amino-5'-pyrimidylmethyl)-5-(2-hydroxyethyl)
-4-methyl thiazole].

STRUCTURE

Thiamine chloride

FUNCTIONS

Coenzyme: oxidative decarboxylation of pyruvate to acetyl CoA: transketolase.

ABSORPTION

Proximal small intestine.

CHARACTERISTICS OF
DEFICIENCY STATE

Disturbances of neural function: central, peripheral, and autonomic nervous system disorders (dry beriberi, Wernicke's encephalopathy), including confusion, weakness and paralysis, ophthalmoplegia, ataxia, muscle wasting, paresthesia, and peripheral vasodilatation. Disturbance of cardiovascular system: myocardial damage, heart enlargement, and failure with resulting edema (wet beriberi).

DEFICIENCY MAY OCCUR IN	Alcoholism, prolonged starvation, and chronic renal dialysis.
RDA	Related to energy expenditure. Adults and infants: 0.5 mg per 1000 kcal; minimal intake on restricted activity (older persons): 1 mg. Pregnancy, lactation: 0.6 mg per 1000 kcal.
DIETARY SOURCES	Animal: meat, especially pork. Plant: yeasts, pericarp of grains, rice, and nuts.
STORAGE	Muscle. Stores small, with short biological half-life.
ANALYSIS OF STATUS	Indirect: hemolyzed red cell transketolase activity, basic and following activation with added thiamine pyrophosphate.
THERAPY	Thiamine hydrochloride.

REFERENCE

1 Warnock, L. G., V. Frattali, and A. M. Preston: Transketolase activity of blood hemolysate, a useful index for diagnosing thiamine deficiency, Clin. Chem., 21:432, 1975.

VITAMIN B₂

CHEMICAL FORM	Riboflavin—a flavoprotein [6,7-dimethyl-9-(DL'-ribityl) isoalloxazine].

STRUCTURE

$$CH_2\text{---}C\text{---}C\text{---}C\text{---}CH_2OH$$

(with OH, OH, OH above and H, H, H below; attached to isoalloxazine ring system with CH_3, CH_3 substituents, N, N, C=O, C-NH, O)

FUNCTIONS	Reactive part of flavoprotein enzymes involved in biological oxidations (electron transfer).
ABSORPTION	Small intestine.
CHARACTERISTICS OF DEFICIENCY STATE	Angular stomatitis; cheilosis; seborrheic dermatitis.
DEFICIENCY MAY OCCUR IN	Severe undernourished states, particularly in chronic alcoholics omitting animal protein and dairy foods from diet and after trauma. Rare in the United States.

RDA	Controversy about relating stated requirements to carbohydrate or protein consumption: currently 0.6 mg per 1000 kcal but 1.2 mg minimum in elderly people. Pregnancy, add 0.3 mg; lactation, add 0.5 mg.
DIETARY SOURCES	Milk, meat, green vegetables, whole grains, fish, and eggs.
STORAGE	Small reserves—short biological half-life.
ANALYSIS OF STATUS	Erythrocyte glutathione reductase; basal and activation coefficient. Current uncertainty about interpretation of results and also of urinary riboflavin concentrations.
THERAPY	As part of anticipated or established B-complex deficiency. May be given orally or intramuscularly.

REFERENCE

1 Horwitt, M. K.: Nutritional requirements of man, with special reference to riboflavin, Am. J. Clin. Nutr., 18:458, 1966.

NIACIN

CHEMICAL FORMS	Niacin (β-pyridine carboxylic acid); niacinamide.
STRUCTURE	

$$\text{pyridine ring}-COOH \quad (N)$$

FUNCTIONS	As diphosphopyridine [nicotinamide adenine dinucleotide (NAD)] and triphosphopyridine [nicotinamide adenine dinucleotide phosphate (NADP)] nucleotides, function as prosthetic groups in dehydrogenase reactions in tricarboxylic acid cycle, ethanol oxidation, and many other reactions.
ABSORPTION	Small intestine.
CHARACTERISTICS OF DEFICIENCY STATE	Pellagra: weakness, lassitude, anorexia, diarrhea, dermatitis (especially in skin exposed to sun), glossitis, dementia, and death.
DEFICIENCY MAY OCCUR IN	Alcoholism associated with poor diet, especially corn-based. Rarely occurs in patients with carcinoid tumors secreting excessive amounts of serotonin and depleting tryptophan, a precursor of endogenous niacin.

	Intestinal disease, with malabsorption. Hartnup disease (defective absorption of tryptophan).
RDA	Adults and children: 6.6 niacin equivalents per 1000 kcal (1 niacin equivalent = 1 mg of niacin or 60 mg of tryptophan). Not less than 13 niacin equivalents. Infants: 8 niacin equivalents per 1000 kcal. Pregnancy: add 2 niacin equivalents. Lactation: add 5 niacin equivalents.
DIETARY SOURCES	Animal: meat, liver, fish, and eggs. Plants: some green leaves, peanuts.
STORAGE	Not documented because of interrelationship of tryptophan and niacin.
ANALYSIS OF STATUS	Measurement of urinary excretion of N'-methylnicotinamide and N'-methyl-2-pyridone-5-carboxylamide: interpretation not well established (normal >3 mg per 24 hours).
THERAPY	Niacinamide used in preference to niacin since it does not cause flushing. A daily dose of 50 to 250 mg can be administered until an adequate diet is restored.

REFERENCES

1 de Lange, D. J. and C. P. Joubert: Assessment of nicotinic acid status of population groups, Am. J. Clin. Nutr., 15:169, 1964.
2 Herman, R. H., F. B. Stifel, and H. L. Greene: Nicotinic acid and nicotinic acid deficiency (pellagra), in *The Science and Practice of Clinical Medicine*, vol. I, J. M. Dietschy (ed.), Grune and Stratton, New York, 1976.

VITAMIN B₆ (PYRIDOXIN)

CHEMICAL FORMS	Pyridoxol; pyridoxal; pyridoxamine.
STRUCTURE	

Pyridoxol

FUNCTIONS	As pyridoxal-5-phosphate, constitutes coenzyme of large number of enzyme-mediated reactions, chiefly transaminations and decarboxylations. Conversion of tryptophan to niacin is pyridoxal-5-phosphate-dependent.

ABSORPTION	Small intestine.
CHARACTERISTICS OF DEFICIENCY STATE	Convulsions described in infants. Peripheral neuritis in adults, possibly depression, and convulsions. Leucopenia. Rarely anemia. Seborrheic dermatitis.
RDA	Data on bioavailability are incomplete. Increased requirements when dietary protein intake is increased. Currently 2.2 mg daily for adult males and 2.0 mg daily for females are proposed. In pregnancy 2.6 mg is recommended and during lactation, 2.5 mg.
DEFICIENCY MAY OCCUR IN	Possibly subjects using oral steroid contraceptives; also in chronic alcoholism. Has been described in association with vitamin B_6-deficient infant formulas.
DIETARY SOURCES	Fish, poultry, and meats.
STORAGE	No published information.
ANALYSIS OF STATUS	Urinary excretion of kynurenine and kynurenic and xanthurenic acids is markedly increased following a test dose of tryptophan in vitamin B_6-deficient subjects. Red cell aminotransferase activity in vitro, using the principle of the activation coefficient (comparing activity without and with added pyridoxal 5-phosphate). There is currently difficulty in establishing normal range.
THERAPY	Pyridoxin hydrochloride, orally or by injection.

REFERENCE

1 Bauernfeind, J. C. and O. N. Miller: Vitamin B_6: nutritional and pharmaceutical usage, stability, bioavailability, antagonists, and safety, in *Human Vitamin B_6 Requirements*, National Academy of Sciences, Washington, D. C., 1978, pp. 78–110.

BIOTIN

CHEMICAL FORMS	Biotin.
STRUCTURE	

FUNCTIONS	Component of pyruvate carboxylase and acetyl coenzyme A carboxylase. Carboxyl transport; carbon dioxide fixation as tissue bicarbonate. Regulates carbohydrate–fatty acid metabolic interactions, especially lipid synthesis.
ABSORPTION	Small intestine, probably proximal.
CHARACTERISTICS OF DEFICIENCY STATE	Anorexia, nausea, depression, dermatitis, and glossitis. Seborrheic dermatitis in infants.
RDA	Not established, partly because evidence favors intestinal microflora making a significant contribution. Estimated safe and adequate daily dietary intake for an adult is 100 to 200 µg.
DEFICIENCY MAY OCCUR IN	Adults consuming excessive amounts of raw egg white, which contains a glycoprotein, avidin, which binds biotin. Infants fed formulas lacking biotin.
DIETARY SOURCES	Liver, kidney, egg yolk, and some vegetables.
STORAGE	Presumably liver. Total body stores have not been estimated.
ANALYSIS OF STATUS	Concentration of biotin in serum and urine are depressed in biotin-deficient infants.
THERAPY	In infants 5 mg daily intravenously (IV) or intramuscularly (IM) produces rapid disappearance of seborrheic dermatitis.

REFERENCES

1 Baugh, C. M., J. H. Malone, and C. E. Butterworth, Jr.: Human biotin deficiency. A case history of biotin deficiency induced by raw egg consumption in a cirrhotic patient, Am. J. Clin. Nutr., 21:173, 1968.
2 McCormick, D. B.: Biotin, Nutr. Rev., 33:97, 1975.

PANTOTHENIC ACID

CHEMICAL FORMS	Pantothenic acid.
STRUCTURE	

$$H-\underset{\underset{H}{|}}{\overset{\overset{OH}{|}}{C}}-\underset{\underset{CH_3}{|}}{\overset{\overset{CH_3}{|}}{C}}-\underset{\underset{H}{|}}{\overset{\overset{OH}{|}}{C}}-\overset{\overset{O}{\|}}{C}-\underset{\underset{H}{|}}{N}-\underset{\underset{H}{|}}{\overset{\overset{H}{|}}{C}}-\underset{\underset{H}{|}}{\overset{\overset{H}{|}}{C}}-COOH$$

FUNCTIONS	Component of coenzyme A; essential role in acyl transport, metabolic energy release, and fatty acid synthesis. Synthesis of steroid hormones, porphyrins, and acetylcholine.
ABSORPTION	Small intestine.
CHARACTERISTICS OF DEFICIENCY STATE	Rare. Hypotension. "Burning feet" syndrome. Paresthesia in hands and feet; muscle weakness.
RDA	Estimated safe and adequate daily dietary intake for infants is 2 mg to age 6 months and 3 mg to age 3 years and for adults, 4 to 7 mg.
DEFICIENCY MAY OCCUR IN	Prolonged partial starvation and deficiency of B vitamins has been associated with the burning feet syndrome. Otherwise almost unknown since pantothenate ubiquitous. Produced in humans experimentally by giving a metabolic antagonist.
DIETARY SOURCES	Widely distributed in animal tissues, whole-grain cereals, and legumes.
STORAGE	No published studies. Symptoms of deficiency have been produced by feeding a pantothenate-free, semisynthetic diet for 10 weeks.
ANALYSIS OF STATUS	—
THERAPY	Calcium pantothenate may be given orally or by IM or IV injection.

REFERENCE

1 Fry, P. C., H. M. Fox, and H. G. Tao: Metabolic response to a pantothenic acid deficient diet in humans, J. Nutr. Sci. Vitaminol., 22:339, 1976.

FOLIC ACID; FOLACINS

CHEMICAL FORMS	Pteroylglutamic acid (PGA). Tetrahydrofolates in tissues; polyglutamates in food.
STRUCTURE	

FUNCTIONS	PGA-containing coenzymes are responsible for intermolecular transfer of single carbon atom-containing groups. These transfers are essential for nucleic acid synthesis and metabolism of some amino acids.
ABSORPTION	Mainly proximal third of small intestine. Glutamates split off side chain by conjugases present on brush border. Monoglutamyl folate absorbed by active process.
CHARACTERISTICS OF DEFICIENCY STATE	Macrocytic and megaloblastic anemia; reduction in number of polymorphonuclear white blood cells and blood platelets. Hypersegmentation of nuclei of polymorphs. Irritability and depression.
RDA	Adults, 400 μg of total folacin activity in diet (assuming that 100 to 200 μg is absorbed); infants, 5 μg per kilogram of body weight; pregnant and lactating women, 800 and 500 μg of total folacin activity, respectively.
DEFICIENCY MAY OCCUR IN	Intestinal malabsorption such as gliadin-sensitive enteropathy and tropical sprue, pregnancy, and possibly lactation.
DIETARY SOURCES	Liver, meat, fresh green vegetables, yeast, and some fruits.
STORAGE	Total adult body pool may be as high as 50 mg (7.5 to 10 mg in liver).
ANALYSIS OF STATUS	Folate activity in serum and erythrocytes by microbiological assay or competitive binding techniques.
THERAPY	Folic acid: oral or IM. Exclude cobalamin deficiency before commencing therapy with folic acid.

REFERENCE

1 Herbert, V., N. Colman, and E. Jacob: Folic acid and vitamin B_{12}, in *Modern Nutrition in Health Disease,* R. S. Goodhart and M. E. Shils (eds.), Lea and Febiger, Philadelphia, 1980.

VITAMIN B_{12} (COBALAMINS)

CHEMICAL FORMS	Cobalt-containing corrinoids; methyl, -hydroxo-, -adenosyl-cobalamins.

STRUCTURE

FUNCTIONS	As coenzymes: 5'-deoxyadenosylcobalamin, methylcobalamin. Transmethylation reactions (e.g., methyl malonyl-CoA to succinyl-CoA). Regeneration of folacin from 5-methyl-tetrahydrofolate pool.
ABSORPTION	Distal small intestine (ileum). Mediated by specific transport glycoprotein of gastric origin, termed *intrinsic factor.*
CHARACTERISTICS OF DEFICIENCY STATE	Macrocytic-megaloblastic anemia. Damage to and impaired function of central and peripheral nervous systems.
DEFICIENCY MAY OCCUR IN	Chronic atrophic gastritis and gastric atrophy (pernicious anemia); following total or partial gastrectomy or inflammatory bowel disease; strict vegetarians.
RDA	Adults, 3 μg; infants, 0.15 μg per 100 kcal; pregnancy and lactating women, 4 μg.
DIETARY SOURCES	Animal: liver and other meat. Some fermented fish and vegetable seasonings and sauces.

STORAGE	Liver; biological half-life 1.5 to 3.0 years.
ANALYSIS OF STATUS	Serum activity. Estimated microbiologically (lactobacilli of various strains) or by competitive binding techniques using radio-cobalt labeled cyanocobalamin and intrinsic factor. Deficiency <100 pg/ml; normal range 150 to 1500 pg/ml.
THERAPY	In pernicious anemia, following gastrectomy, in disease, or following resection of ileum 100 to 1000 μg IM per month; in strict vegetarians 5 μg daily by mouth.

REFERENCE

1 Herbert, V., N. Colman, and E. Jacob: Folic acid and vitamin B_{12}, in *Modern Nutrition in Health and Disease*, R. S. Goodhart and M. E. Shils (eds.), Lea and Febiger, Philadelphia, 1980.

VITAMIN C

CHEMICAL FORMS	Ascorbic acid; dehydroascorbic acid.
STRUCTURE	

FUNCTION	Ascorbic acid is potent reducing agent: involved in collagen synthesis (proline → hydroxyproline); hydroxylation reactions in synthesis of adrenal corticosteroids.
ABSORPTION	Distal small intestine.
CHARACTERISTICS OF DEFICIENCY STATE	Scurvy; faulty collagen synthesis: weakness of walls of blood capillaries, resulting in hemorrhage at multiple sites; poor wound healing.
DEFICIENCY MAY OCCUR IN	Infants fed ascorbate-deficient diets (cow's milk without supplementation); elderly people on poor diets; alcoholics; faulty food preparation (prolonged heating, especially in iron or copperware, destroys ascorbic acid).
RDA	Adults, 60 mg (achieves saturation of leucocytes), pregnant and lactating women, 80 and 100 mg, respectively.
DIETARY SOURCES	Plants: green leaves, fruits, and skin of tubers. Animal: liver and all fresh meat.

STORAGE	Total body pool in adults 1500 mg.
ANALYSIS OF STATUS	Measurements of ascorbate in serum and blood leucocytes. Low serum levels (<0.3 mg/dl) indicate inadequate recent dietary intake of vitamin C. Leucocyte ascorbate concentrations are better indication of tissue stores—method requires large quantities of blood, however.
THERAPY	Ascorbic acid: oral or IM.

REFERENCES

1 *Recommended Dietary Allowances,* 9th ed., Food and Nutrition Board, National Academy of Sciences–National Research Council, Washington, D. C., 1980.
2 Hodges, R. E., J. Hood, J. E. Canham, H. E. Sauberlich, and E. M. Baker: Clinical manifestations of ascorbic acid deficiency in man, Am. J. Clin. Nutr., 24:432, 1971.

MINERALS AND TRACE ELEMENTS

CALCIUM

FUNCTION	Formation of bones and teeth, regulation of excitable tissues (striated, cardiac and smooth muscle, nerves), activation of some enzymes, blood clotting.
ABSORPTION	Twenty to thirty percent; vitamin D and lactose increase; dietary protein, oxalate, and phytic acid decrease.
MAJOR ROUTE OF EXCRETION	Urine and feces.
CHARACTERISTICS OF DEFICIENCY STATE	Rickets, osteomalacia, osteoporosis; tetany (in acute hypocalcemia).
DEFICIENCY MAY OCCUR IN	Postmenopausal women; children on vegan diet; patients with celiac-sprue and other intestinal malabsorption syndromes, vitamin D deficiency, or nephritis.

RDA

Males (1 to 10 years)	800 mg
Males (11 to 18 years)	1200 mg
Males (>19 years)	800 mg
Females (1 to 10 years)	800 mg
Females (11 to 18 years)	1200 mg
Females (>18 years)	800 mg
Pregnant women	+400 mg
Lactating women	+400 mg

DIETARY SOURCES	Milk, hard cheeses, green leafy vegetables.
STORAGE	Bone.

ANALYSIS OF STATUS	Serum levels (normal range 9 to 11 mg/dl).
TOXICITY	Intakes from 1 to 2.5 g/day well tolerated; larger amounts result in hypercalcemia and deterioration of renal function and levels of consciousness.
INBORN ERRORS	None known.
THERAPY	Oral calcium gluconate, carbonate, and lactate.

REFERENCES

1 Nordin, B. E. C., P. J. Heyburn, M. Peacock, A. Horsman, J. Aaron, D. Marshall, and R. G. Crilly: Osteoporosis and osteomalacia, Clin. Endocrinol. Metab. 9:177, 1980.
2 Avioli, L.: What to do with postmenopausal osteoporosis?, Am. J. Med. 65:881, 1978.

CHROMIUM

FUNCTION	Component of glucose tolerance factor (GTF).
ABSORPTION	GTF: 10 to 25 percent, competes with zinc; $Cr^{3+} < 1$ percent.
MAJOR ROUTE OF EXCRETION	Urine.
CHARACTERISTICS OF DEFICIENCY STATE	Impaired glucose tolerance.
DEFICIENCY MAY OCCUR IN	Reduced glucose tolerance observed in some patients receiving total parenteral nutrition, undernourished infants.
RDA	Estimated safe and adequate daily intake for adults 0.05 to 0.20 mg.
DIETARY SOURCES	GTF: brewer's yeast, cheese, bread, beef. Chromium: molasses, nuts, whole grains, and seafoods.
STORAGE	Spleen and heart.
ANALYSIS OF STATUS	Serum levels; normal range 1 to 5.5 µg/dl.
TOXICITY	Low.
INBORN ERRORS	None known.
THERAPY	Chromium chloride, 50 mg, three times daily, has been used in elderly diabetics with inconclusive results.

REFERENCES

1 Shaw, J. L.: Trace elements in the fetus and young infant. II. Copper, manganese, selenium, and chromium, Am. J. Dis. Childh. 134:74, 1980.

2 Mertz, W.: Effects and metabolism of glucose tolerance factor, in *Present Knowledge in Nutrition,* 4th ed., D. M. Hegstead (ed.), Nutrition Foundation, Inc., Washington, D. C., 1976.

COPPER

FUNCTION	Copper enzymes (cytochrome c oxidase, tyrosinase, dopamine β hydroxylase); ceruloplasmin; necessary for iron mobilization; cross-linking of elastin.
ABSORPTION	Thirty to sixty percent; decreased by calcium, zinc, and phytic acid.
MAJOR ROUTE OF EXCRETION	Bile.
CHARACTERISTICS OF DEFICIENCY STATE	Hypochromic, microcytic anemia; neutropenia.
DEFICIENCY MAY OCCUR IN	Preterm infants or infants with chronic diarrhea or malabsorption or on a diet consisting exclusively of cow's milk; patients with malnutrition, malabsorption states, prolonged diarrhea, and prolonged total parenteral nutrition.
RDA	Estimated safe and adequate intake for adults 2 to 3 mg/day.
DIETARY SOURCES	Liver, shellfish, dried beans, whole-grain cereals, and nuts.
STORAGE	Liver.
ANALYSIS OF STATUS	Serum levels (normal range 90 to 140 mg/dl).
TOXICITY	Not common—occurs only with deliberate attempt to ingest excessive copper sulfate.
INBORN ERRORS	Hepatolenticular degeneration (Wilson's disease)—excess copper deposited in tissues (autosomal recessive); Menkes's kinky hair syndrome—congenital copper deficiency (X-linked recessive).
THERAPY	A varied diet; in patients with Menkes's syndrome, some response can be obtained with parenteral copper, but not oral form.

REFERENCES

1 Shaw, J. L.: Trace elements in the fetus and young infant. II. Copper, manganese, selenium, and chromium, Am. J. Dis. Childh., 134:74, 1980.
2 Burch, R. E. and H. Hahn: Trace elements in human nutrition, Med. Clin. N. Am., 63:1057, 1979.

FLUORIDE

FUNCTION	Structural component in calcium hydroxyapatite of bones and teeth.
ABSORPTION	Seventy-five to ninety percent.
MAJOR ROUTE OF EXCRETION	Urine.
CHARACTERISTICS OF DEFICIENCY STATE	Reduced resistance to dental caries and osteoporosis.
DEFICIENCY MAY OCCUR IN	Individuals with insufficient intake from diet or water supplies.
RDA	Estimated safe and adequate daily intake for adults 1.5 to 4.0 mg.
DIETARY SOURCES	Seafood, meat, water, and tea.
STORAGE	Bone.
ANALYSIS OF STATUS	Blood concentration, normal range 10 to 20 $\mu g/dl$.
TOXICITY	Low; dental fluorosis (mottling of teeth in growing children).
INBORN ERRORS	None known.
PROPHYLAXIS	One part per million of fluoride in water supply.

REFERENCE

1 Messer, H. H. and L. Singer: Fluoride, in *Present Knowledge in Nutrition,* 4th ed., D. M. Hegsted (ed.), Nutrition Foundation, Inc., Washington, D. C., 1976.

IODINE

FUNCTION	Constituent of thyroxine and triiodothyronine.
ABSORPTION	Nearly 100 percent.
MAJOR ROUTE OF EXCRETION	Urine.
CHARACTERISTICS OF DEFICIENCY STATE	Goiter, cretinism, and myxedema.
DEFICIENCY MAY OCCUR IN	Individuals living in geographic areas remote from sea and where soil is iodine-poor and iodized salt is not used.
RDA	Adults 150 $\mu g/day$.
DIETARY SOURCES	Iodized salt and seafood.
STORAGE	Thyroid.

ANALYSIS OF STATUS	Protein-bound iodine (PBI), normal range 4.0 to 8.0 µg/dl.
TOXICITY	Ingestion of large amounts (25 to 50 × RDA) over long periods of time can suppress synthesis of thyroid hormones, resulting in hyperactive and enlarged thyroid gland (thyrotoxicosis).
INBORN ERRORS	—
THERAPY	Iodized salt.

REFERENCES

1 Cullen, R. W. and S. Oace: Iodine: Current status, J. Nutr. Educ., 8:100, 1976.
2 Taylor, F.: Iodine going from hypo to hyper, FDA Consumer, 5:15, 1981.

IRON

FUNCTION	Structural component of hemoglobin, myoglobin, cytochrome, and other enzymes.
ABSORPTION	Inorganic form 5 to 15 percent, increased by vitamin C, decreased by antacids, phytic acid; organic form 30 to 70 percent, increased in presence of animal protein.
MAJOR ROUTE OF EXCRETION	Cells shed from internal and external body surfaces; bile.
CHARACTERISTICS OF DEFICIENCY STATE	Hypochromic, microcytic anemia; listlessness.
DEFICIENCY MAY OCCUR IN	Children, teenagers, pregnant females, elderly; patients with an iron-poor diet, increased blood loss, malabsorption (postgastrectomy, small bowel disease).
RDA	Adult males 10 mg; adult females 18 mg.
DIETARY SOURCES	Meat, poultry, fish, beans, and raisins.
STORAGE	Bone marrow, liver, spleen.
ANALYSIS OF STATUS	Serum iron [normal (men), 90 to 180 mg/dl; normal (women), 70 to 150 mg/dl]. Percent saturation of transferrin (normal 20 to 50).
TOXICITY	Occurs accidentally in children who ingest medicinal tablets, resulting in convulsions, circulatory collapse and death; chronic toxicity occurs with use of iron cooking pots.
INBORN ERRORS	Hereditary hemochromatosis (excessive iron storage in liver and spleen).
THERAPY	Ferrous sulfate (oral), Imferon (50 mg of elemental iron per milliliter IM).

REFERENCES

1 *Recommended Dietary Allowances,* 9th ed., Food and Nutrition Board, National Academy of Sciences–National Research Council, Washington, D. C., 1980, pp. 137–144.
2 Crosby, W. H.: Current concepts in nutrition: who needs iron?, New Engl. J. Med., 297:543, 1977.

MAGNESIUM

FUNCTION	Part of enzyme systems—especially reactions involving ATP; maintaining electrical potential in nerves and muscle membranes.
ABSORPTION	Thirty-five to forty percent.
MAJOR ROUTE OF EXCRETION	Urine and feces.
CHARACTERISTICS OF DEFICIENCY STATE	Neurological manifestations, especially anxiety, hyperirritability, disorientation, confusion, hallucinations, and seizures.
DEFICIENCY MAY OCCUR IN	Chronic alcoholics; some patients with celiac-sprue or diarrhea; prolonged magnesium-free parenteral feeding.
RDA	Adult males, 350 mg/day; adult females, 300 mg/day.
DIETARY SOURCES	Universally present in most foods; nuts, fruits, vegetables, cereals are best sources.
STORAGE	Bone.
ANALYSIS OF STATUS	Serum magnesium levels (normal range 1.5 to 2.5 meq/liter).
TOXICITY	None in people with normal renal function; patients with renal failure treated with magnesium-containing antacids (Gelusil, Maalox) and cathartics (milk of magnesia).
INBORN ERRORS	None known.
THERAPY	Magnesium sulfate administered by IV, IM, or orally.

REFERENCES

1 Seelig, M. S.: *Magnesium Deficiency in the Pathogenesis of Disease,* Plenum, New York, 1980.
2 Aikawa, J. K.: Biochemistry and physiology of magnesium, Wld. Rev. Nutr. Diet., 28:112, 1978.
3 Rude, R. K. and F. R. Singer: Magnesium deficiency and excess, Ann. Rev. Med., 32:245, 1981.
4 Flink, E. B.: Magnesium deficiency and magnesium toxicity in man, in *Trace Elements in Human Health and Disease,* Vol. II, A. S. Prasad and D. Oberleas (eds.), Academic Press, New York, 1976.

MANGANESE

FUNCTION	Formation of mucopolysaccharides; activation of many enzymes.
ABSORPTION	Ten to forty percent.
MAJOR ROUTE OF EXCRETION	Bile.
CHARACTERISTICS OF DEFICIENCY STATE	A single patient placed on a manganese-deficient diet in a metabolic ward developed a striking hypocholesterolemia, weight loss, dermatitis, nausea, and vomiting.
DEFICIENCY MAY OCCUR IN	—
RDA	Estimated safe and adequate intake for adults 2.5 to 5 mg/day.
DIETARY SOURCES	Cereal grains, leafy green vegetables, wheat germ, coffee, and tea.
STORAGE	Liver and bone.
ANALYSIS OF STATUS	Ill-defined (serum levels, reversal of symptoms with treatment).
TOXICITY	Low; toxicity recognized in miners after prolonged inhalation of manganese; produces profound neurological disturbances similar to those due to Parkinson's disease.
INBORN ERRORS	None known.
THERAPY	—

REFERENCES

1 Hurley, L. S.: Manganese and other trace elements, in *Present Knowledge in Nutrition,* D. M. Hegsted (ed.), Nutrition Foundation, Inc., Washington, D. C., 1976.
2 Schroeder, H. A., J. J. Balassa, and I. H. Tipton: Essential trace metals in man: Manganese. J. Chron. Dis., 19:545, 1966.

MOLYBDENUM

FUNCTION	Xanthine oxidase; aldehyde oxidase.
ABSORPTION	Forty to one hundred percent.
MAJOR ROUTE OF EXCRETION	Urine.
CHARACTERISTICS OF DEFICIENCY STATE	No definite deficiency demonstrated
DEFICIENCY MAY OCCUR IN	—
RDA	Estimated adequate and safe intake for adults 0.15 to 0.5 mg/day.
DIETARY SOURCES	Legumes, whole grains, and wheat.
STORAGE	Liver.

ANALYSIS OF STATUS	—
TOXICITY	None documented in humans.
INBORN ERRORS	None known.
THERAPY	—

REFERENCE

1 *Recommended Dietary Allowances,* 9th ed., Food and Nutrition Board, National Academy of Sciences–National Research Council, Washington, D. C., 1980, pp. 164–165.

PHOSPHORUS

FUNCTION	Mineralization of bones and teeth; component of DNA and RNA; regulation of acid-base balance; component of phosphorylated vitamins (thiamin, niacin, riboflavin, pyridoxine) and ATP; component in phospholipids.
ABSORPTION	Decreased by magnesium, iron, and phytic acid.
MAJOR ROUTE OF EXCRETION	Urine.
CHARACTERISTICS OF DEFICIENCY STATE	Weakness, anorexia, malaise, skeletal pain, bone demineralization and increase in calcium excretion, and decreased tissue oxygenation.
DEFICIENCY MAY OCCUR IN	Patients with an excessive intake of nonabsorbable antacids containing aluminum hydroxide or kidney disorders or malabsorption.
RDA	About 800 mg.
DIETARY SOURCES	Milk, poultry, fish, meat, and carbonated beverages.
STORAGE	Bones.
ANALYSIS OF STATUS	Plasma phosphate; normal range for adults 2.5 to 4.4 mg/dl.
TOXICITY	Hyperphosphatemia can result from renal disease.
INBORN ERRORS	—
THERAPY	Oral sodium or potassium phosphate.

REFERENCES

1 Harrison, H. E.: Phosphorus, in *Present Knowledge in Nutrition,* 4th ed., D. M. Hegsted (ed.), Nutrition Foundation, Inc., Washington, D. C., 1976.
2 Harrison, H. E.: Dietary phosphorus, PTH, and bone resorption, Nutr. Rev., 31:124, 1973.

POTASSIUM

FUNCTION	Regulation of osmotic pressure and acid-base balance; activation of a number of intracellular enzymes; regulation of nerve and muscle excitability.
ABSORPTION	Nearly 100 percent.
MAJOR ROUTE OF EXCRETION	Urine.
CHARACTERISTICS OF DEFICIENCY STATE	Muscle weakness, anorexia, and tachycardia.
DEFICIENCY MAY OCCUR IN	Patients with deficient intake, diarrhea, diabetic acidosis, diuretic therapy, or nephropathy.
RDA	Estimated safe and adequate daily intake for adults 1875 to 5625 mg.
DIETARY SOURCES	Meat, fish, poultry, cereals, fruits, and vegetables.
STORAGE	Minimal.
ANALYSIS OF STATUS	Plasma levels (normal range 2.5 to 5.5 meq/liter).
TOXICITY	Can occur as a result of decreased renal excretion or severe dehydration, leading to cardiac arrhythmias, including fibrillation, and seizures.
INBORN ERRORS	None known.
THERAPY	Potassium chloride except for patient with renal tubular acidosis.

REFERENCES

1 *Recommended Dietary Allowances,* 9th ed., Food and Nutrition Board, National Academy of Sciences–National Research Council, Washington, D. C., 1980, pp. 166–178.
2 Meneely, G. R. and H. D. Battarbee: Sodium and potassium, in *Present Knowledge in Nutrition,* 4th ed., The Nutrition Foundation, New York, 1976.

SELENIUM

FUNCTION	Active part of glutathione peroxidase.
ABSORPTION	Thirty-five to eighty-five percent.
MAJOR ROUTE OF EXCRETION	Urine and feces.
CHARACTERISTICS OF DEFICIENCY STATE	One case: painful muscular symptoms. Keshan disease: cardiomyopathy in children in China.

DEFICIENCY MAY OCCUR IN	Patients taking long-term total parenteral nutrition with negligible selenium intake, low dietary intake.
RDA	Estimated safe and adequate intake for adults 0.05 to 0.20 mg/day.
DIETARY SOURCES	Seafood, organ meats, muscle meats, cereals, and milk.
STORAGE	Probably in kidney.
ANALYSIS OF STATUS	Blood selenium levels, normal range 10 to 30 mg/dl; blood glutathione peroxidase levels.
TOXICITY	Rarely reported in humans.
INBORN ERRORS	None known.
THERAPY	—

REFERENCES

1 Stadtman, T. C.: Biological function of selenium, Nutr. Rev., 35:161, 1977.
2 Food and Nutrition Board, Selenium and human health, Nutr. Rev., 34:347, 1976.
3 Shaw, J. L.: Trace elements in the fetus and young infant, Am. J. Dis. Childh., 134:74, 1980.
4 Thomson, C. D. and M. F. Robinson: Selenium in human health and disease with emphasis on those aspects peculiar to New Zealand, Am. J. Clin. Nutr., 33:303, 1980.

SODIUM

FUNCTION	Regulation of pH, osmotic pressure and water balance; conductivity or excitability of nerves and muscles; active transport of glucose and amino acids.
ABSORPTION	Nearly 100 percent.
MAJOR ROUTE OF EXCRETION	Urine and feces.
CHARACTERISTICS OF DEFICIENCY STATE	Nausea, anorexia, muscle weakness and cramps, and hypotension.
DEFICIENCY MAY OCCUR IN	Patients with diarrhea, vomiting, prolonged excessive sweating, or insufficient adrenocortical hormone production.
RDA	Estimated safe and adequate intake for adults 1100 to 3000 mg/day.
DIETARY SOURCES	Table salt (sodium chloride), soy sauce, seafoods, and dairy products.
STORAGE	Probably in bone.
ANALYSIS OF STATUS	Serum sodium concentration (normal range 135 to 145 meq/liter).

TOXICITY	Prolonged feeding of high-salt diets leads to development of hypertension in experimental animals, and in humans with predisposition to hypertension it can cause edema, seizures, coma, and possibly death.
INBORN ERRORS	None known.
THERAPY	Isotonic or hypertonic saline for deficiency.

REFERENCES

1 *Recommended Dietary Allowances,* 9th ed., Food and Nutrition Board, National Academy of Sciences–National Research Council, Washington, D. C., 1980, pp. 166–178.
2 Weinsier, R. L.: Overview: salt and the development of essential hypertension, Prevent. Med., 5:7, 1976.
3 Meneely, G. R. and H. D. Battarbee: Sodium and potassium, in *Present Knowledge in Nutrition,* 4th ed., The Nutrition Foundation, New York, 1976.

ZINC

FUNCTION	Component of over 80 metalloenzymes (carbonic anhydrase, carboxypeptidases A and B, alkaline phosphatase, alcohol dehydrogenase); activates many others. Wound healing. Metabolism of nucleic acids (thymidine kinase).
ABSORPTION	Ten to forty percent; fiber and phytate decrease.
MAJOR ROUTE OF EXCRETION	Feces.
CHARACTERISTICS OF DEFICIENCY STATE	Dwarfism, hypogonadism, hepatosplenomegaly, parakeratosis, alopecia (hair loss), hypogeusia (loss of taste and smell acuity), slow rate of wound healing.
DEFICIENCY MAY OCCUR IN	Children and teenagers, pregnant females, preterm infants, patients with alcoholic cirrhosis or intestinal malabsorption syndrome; patients on long-term TPN.
RDA	Adults 15 mg.
DIETARY SOURCES	Red meat; seafood, especially oysters; beans.
STORAGE	Very little of bone and muscle zinc available; constant dietary supply essential.
ANALYSIS OF STATUS	Deficiency: plasma, less than 90 µg/dl; hair, less than 140 µg/g; urine, less than 100 µg/day.

TOXICITY	Only with accidental or intentional (suicidal) ingestion; rare; causes vomiting.
INBORN ERRORS	Acrodermatitis enteropathica (zinc malabsorption).
THERAPY	Zinc sulfate up to 220 mg, three times daily (50 mg of elemental zinc per tablet) orally.

REFERENCES

1 Swanson, C. A. and J. C. King: Human zinc nutrition, J. Nutr. Educ., 11:181, 1979.
2 Shaw, J. C. L.: Trace elements in the fetus and young infant. I. Zinc, Am. J. Dis. Childh., 133:1260, 1979.
3 Prasad, A. S.: Zinc deficiency in man, in *Zinc and Copper in Clinical Medicine,* K. M. Hambidge and B. L. Nichols, Jr. (eds.), S. P. Medical Science Books, New York, 1978.

RECOMMENDED DAILY DIETARY ALLOWANCES, REVISED 1980 FOOD AND NUTRITION BOARD, NATIONAL ACADEMY OF SCIENCES– NATIONAL RESEARCH COUNCIL

	Age, Years	Weight		Height		Pro-tein, g	Fat-soluble vitamins			Water soluble vitamins	
		kg	lb	cm	in		Vita-min A, µg RE†	Vita-min D, µg‡	Vita-min E, mg α TE§	Vita-min C, mg	Thia-min, mg
Infants	0.0–0.5	6	13	60	24	kg × 2.2	420	10	3	35	0.3
	0.5–1.0	9	20	71	28	kg × 2.0	400	10	4	35	0.5
Children	1–3	13	29	90	35	23	400	10	5	45	0.7
	4–6	20	44	112	44	30	500	10	6	45	0.9
	7–10	28	62	132	52	34	700	10	7	45	1.2
Males	11–14	45	99	157	62	45	1000	10	8	50	1.4
	15–18	66	145	176	69	56	1000	10	10	60	1.4
	19–22	70	154	177	70	56	1000	7.5	10	60	1.5
	23–50	70	154	178	70	56	1000	5	10	60	1.4
	51+	70	154	178	70	56	1000	5	10	60	1.2
Females	11–14	46	101	157	62	46	800	10	8	50	1.1
	15–18	55	120	163	64	46	800	10	8	60	1.1
	19–22	55	120	163	64	44	800	7.5	8	60	1.1
	23–50	55	120	163	64	44	800	5	8	60	1.0
	51+	55	120	163	64	44	800	5	8	60	1.0
Pregnant						+30	+200	+5	+2	+20	+0.4
Lactating						+20	+400	+5	+3	+40	+0.5

*The allowances are intended to provide for individual variations among most normal persons as they live in the United States under usual environmental stresses. Diets should be based on a variety of common foods in order to provide other nutrients for which human requirements have been less well defined.

†Retinol equivalents. 1 Retinol equivalent = 1 µg of retinol or 6 µg of β-carotene.

‡As cholecalciferol; 10 µg of cholecalciferol = 400 IU of vitamin D.

§α-Tocopherol equivalents; 1 mg D-α-tocopherol = 1 α TE.

‖NE (niacin equivalent) is equal to 1 mg of niacin or 60 mg of dietary tryptophan.

¶The folacin allowances refer to dietary sources as determined by Lactobacillus casei assay after treatment with enzymes ("conjugases") to make polyglutamyl forms of the vitamin available to the test organism.

**The RDA for vitamin B_{12} in infants is based on average concentration of the vitamin in human milk. The allowances after weaning are based on energy intake (as recommended by the American Academy of Pediatrics) and consideration of other factors such as intestinal absorption.

††The increased requirement during pregnancy cannot be met by the iron content of habitual American diets nor by the existing iron stores of many women; therefore, the use of 30 to 60 mg of supplemental iron is recommended. Iron needs during lactation are not substantially different from those of nonpregnant women, but continued supplementation of the mother for 2 to 3 months after parturition is advisable in order to replenish stores depleted by pregnancy.

ESTIMATED SAFE AND ADEQUATE DAILY DIETARY INTAKES OF ADDITIONAL SELECTED VITAMINS AND MINERALS*

	Vitamins			Trace elements[†]		
Age, years	Vitamin K, μg	Biotin, μg	Pantothenic acid, mg	Copper, mg	Manganese, mg	Fluoride, mg
Infants						
0–0.5	12	35	2	0.5–0.7	0.5–0.7	0.1–0.5
0.5–1	10–20	50	3	0.7–1.0	0.7–1.0	0.2–1.0
Children and adolescents						
1–3	15–30	65	3	1.0–1.5	1.0–1.5	0.5–1.5
4–6	20–40	85	3–4	1.5–2.0	1.5–2.0	1.0–2.5
7–10	30–60	120	4–5	2.0–2.5	2.0–3.0	1.5–2.5
11+	50–100	100–200	4–7	2.0–3.0	2.5–5.0	1.5–2.5
Adults	70–140	100–200	4–7	2.0–3.0	2.5–5.0	1.5–4.0

	Electrolytes			Trace elements[†]		
Age, years	Sodium, mg	Potassium, mg	Chloride, mg	Chromium, mg	Selenium, mg	Molybdenum, mg
Infants						
0–0.5	115–350	350–925	275–700	0.01–0.04	0.01–0.04	0.03–0.06
0.5–1	250–750	425–1275	400–1200	0.02–0.06	0.02–0.06	0.04–0.08
Children and adolescents						
1–3	325–975	550–1650	500–1500	0.02–0.08	0.02–0.08	0.05–0.1
4–6	450–1350	775–2325	700–2100	0.03–0.12	0.03–0.12	0.06–0.15
7–10	600–1800	1000–3000	925–2775	0.05–0.2	0.05–0.2	0.1–0.3
11+	900–2700	1525–4575	1400–4200	0.05–0.2	0.05–0.2	0.15–0.5
Adults	1100–3300	1875–5625	1700–5100	0.05–0.2	0.05–0.2	0.15–0.5

*Because there is less information on which to base allowances, these figures are not given in the main table of the RDA and are provided here in the form of ranges of recommended intakes.

[†]Since the toxic levels for many trace elements may be only several times usual intakes, the upper levels for the trace elements given in this table should not be habitually exceeded.

MEAN HEIGHTS AND WEIGHTS AND RECOMMENDED ENERGY INTAKE*

Category	Age, years	Weight		Height		Energy needs (with range)		
		kg	lb	cm	in	kcal	kcal	Mj
Infants	0.0-0.5	6	13	60	24	kg × 115	(95-145)	kg × 0.48
	0.5-1.0	9	20	71	28	kg × 105	(80-135)	kg × 0.44
Children	1-3	13	29	90	35	1300	(900-1800)	5.5
	4-6	20	44	112	44	1700	(1300-2300)	7.1
	7-10	28	62	132	52	2400	(1650-3300)	10.1
Males	11-14	45	99	157	62	2700	(2000-3700)	11.3
	15-18	66	145	176	69	2800	(2100-3900)	11.8
	19-22	70	154	177	70	2900	(2500-3300)	12.2
	23-50	70	154	178	70	2700	(2300-3100)	11.3
	51-75	70	154	178	70	2400	(2000-2800)	10.1
	76+	70	154	178	70	2050	(1650-2450)	8.6
Females	11-14	46	101	157	62	2200	(1500-3000)	9.2
	15-18	55	120	163	64	2100	(1200-3000)	8.8
	19-22	55	120	163	64	2100	(1700-2500)	8.8
	23-50	55	120	163	64	2000	(1600-2400)	8.4
	51-75	55	120	163	64	1800	(1400-2200)	7.6
	76+	55	120	163	64	1600	(1200-2000)	6.7
Pregnancy						+300		
Lactation						+500		

Source: Recommended Dietary Allowances, 9th ed., Food and Nutrition Board, National Academy of Sciences-National Research Council, Washington, D.C., 1980.

*The energy allowances for the young adults are for men and women doing light work. The allowances for the two older age groups represent mean energy needs over these age spans, allowing for a 2 percent decrease in basal (resting) metabolic rate per decade and a reduction in activity of 200 kcal/day for men and women between 51 and 75 years, 500 kcal for men over 75 years, and 400 kcal for women over 75. The customary range of daily energy output is shown for adults in parentheses and is based on a variation in energy needs of ± 400 kcal at any one age—emphasizing the wide range of energy intakes appropriate for any group of people.

Energy allowances for children through age 18 are based on median energy intakes of children of these ages followed in longitudinal growth studies. The values in parentheses are 10th and 90th percentiles of energy intake, to indicate the range of energy consumption among children of these ages.

Water-soluble vitamins					Minerals					
Ribo-flavin, mg	Niacin, mg NE‖	Vita-min B_6, mg	Fola-cin, ¶ μg	Vita-min B_{12}, μg	Cal-cium, mg	Phos-phorus mg	Magne-sium, mg	Iron, mg	Zinc, mg	Io-dine, μg
0.4	6	0.3	30	0.5**	360	240	50	10	3	40
0.6	8	0.6	45	1.5	540	360	70	15	5	50
0.8	9	0.9	100	2.0	800	800	150	15	10	70
1.0	11	1.3	200	2.5	800	800	200	10	10	90
1.4	16	1.6	300	3.0	800	800	250	10	10	120
1.6	18	1.8	400	3.0	1200	1200	350	18	15	150
1.7	18	2.0	400	3.0	1200	1200	400	18	15	150
1.7	19	2.2	400	3.0	800	800	350	10	15	150
1.6	18	2.2	400	3.0	800	800	350	10	15	150
1.4	16	2.2	400	3.0	800	800	350	10	15	150
1.3	15	1.8	400	3.0	1200	1200	300	18	15	150
1.3	14	2.0	400	3.0	1200	1200	300	18	15	150
1.3	14	2.0	400	3.0	800	800	300	18	15	150
1.2	13	2.0	400	3.0	800	800	300	18	15	150
1.2	13	2.0	400	3.0	800	800	300	10	15	150
+0.3	+2	+0.6	+400	+1.0	+400	+400	+150	††	+5	+25
+0.5	+5	+0.5	+100	+1.0	+400	+400	+150	††	+10	+50

*The allowances are intended to provide for individual variations among most normal persons as they live in the United States under usual environmental stresses. Diets should be based on a variety of common foods in order to provide other nutrients for which human requirements have been less well defined.

†Retinol equivalents. 1 Retinol equivalent = 1 μg of retinol or 6 μg of β-carotene.

‡As cholecalciferol; 10 μg of cholecalciferol = 400 IU of vitamin D.

§α-Tocopherol equivalents; 1 mg D-α-tocopherol = 1 α TE.

‖NE (niacin equivalent) is equal to 1 mg of niacin or 60 mg of dietary tryptophan.

¶The folacin allowances refer to dietary sources as determined by Lactobacillus casei assay after treatment with enzymes ("conjugases") to make polyglutamyl forms of the vitamin available to the test organism.

**The RDA for vitamin B_{12} in infants is based on average concentration of the vitamin in human milk. The allowances after weaning are based on energy intake (as recommended by the American Academy of Pediatrics) and consideration of other factors such as intestinal absorption.

††The increased requirement during pregnancy cannot be met by the iron content of habitual American diets nor by the existing iron stores of many women; therefore, the use of 30 to 60 mg of supplemental iron is recommended. Iron needs during lactation are not substantially different from those of nonpregnant women, but continued supplementation of the mother for 2 to 3 months after parturition is advisable in order to replenish stores depleted by pregnancy.

NUTRITIVE VALUES OF THE EDIBLE PART OF FOODS

APPENDIX 9
NUTRITIVE VALUES OF THE EDIBLE PART OF FOODS

Food and approximate measure		Weight, g	Food energy kcal	Food energy kJ	Protein, g	Fat (total lipids), g	Saturated (total), g	Unsaturated Oleic, g	Unsaturated Lino-leic, g	Carbohydrate, g	Calcium, mg	Iron, mg	Vitamin A value, IU	Thiamine, mg	Riboflavin, mg	Niacin, mg	Ascorbic acid, mg
Milk, cream, cheese (related products)																	
Milk, cow's																	
Fluid, whole (3.5% fat)	1 cup	244	160	672	9	9	5	3	Trace	12	288	0.1	350	0.08	0.42	0.1	2
Fluid, nonfat (skim)	1 cup	246	90	378	9	Trace	—	—	—	13	298	0.1	10	0.10	0.44	0.2	2
Cheddar, process	1 oz	28	105	441	7	9	5	3	Trace	1	219	0.3	350	Trace	0.12	Trace	0
Cottage, creamed	1 cup	225	240	1008	31	9	5	3	Trace	7	212	0.7	380	0.07	0.56	0.2	0
Ice cream, plain, factory-packed container	8 fl oz	142	295	1239	6	18	10	6	1	29	175	0.1	740	0.06	0.27	0.1	1
Yogurt, from partially skimmed milk	1 cup	246	120	504	8	4	2	1	Trace	13	295	0.1	170	0.09	0.43	0.2	2
Eggs																	
Whole, without shell	1 egg	50	80	336	6	6	2	3	Trace	Trace	27	1.1	590	0.05	0.15	Trace	0
Meat, poultry, fish, shell-fish (related products)																	
Hamburger (ground beef), broiled, regular	3 oz	85	245	1029	21	17	8	8	Trace	0	9	2.7	30	0.07	0.18	4.6	—
Steak, broiled, lean and fat	3 oz	85	330	1386	20	27	13	12	1	0	9	2.5	50	0.05	0.16	4.0	—
Chicken, cooked																	
Flesh only, broiled	3 oz	85	115	483	20	3	1	1	1	0	8	1.4	80	0.05	0.16	7.4	—
With bone	3.3 oz	94	155	651	25	5	1	2	1	1	9	1.3	70	0.04	0.17	11.2	—
Lamb leg roasted, lean and fat	3 oz	85	235	987	22	16	9	6	Trace	0	9	1.4	—	0.13	0.23	4.7	—

APPENDIX 9 (Continued)

Food and approximate measure	Weight, g	Food energy		Protein, g	Fat (total lipids), g	Fatty acids			Carbohydrate, g	Calcium, mg	Iron, mg	Vitamin A value, IU	Thiamine, mg	Riboflavin, mg	Niacin, mg	Ascorbic acid, mg
						Saturated (total), g	Unsaturated									
		kcal	kJ				Oleic, g	Lino-leic, g								
Pork, fresh trimmed to retail basis, cooked																
Chop, thick, with bone	3.5 oz	98	260	1092	16	21	8	9	2	0	8	2.2	0	0.63	0.18	3.8	—
Bluefish, baked or broiled	3 oz	85	135	567	22	4	—	—	—	0	25	0.6	40	0.09	0.08	1.6	—
Haddock, fried	3 oz	85	140	588	17	5	1	—	—	5	34	1.0	—	0.03	0.06	2.7	2
Tuna, canned in oil	3 oz	85	170	714	24	7	—	3	—	0	7	1.6	70	0.04	0.10	10.1	—
Mature dry beans and peas, nuts, peanuts (related products)																
Red beans	1 cup	256	230	966	15	1	—	—	—	42	74	4.6	Trace	0.13	0.10	1.5	—
Lima beans, cooked	1 cup	192	260	1092	16	1	—	—	—	48	56	5.6	Trace	0.26	0.12	1.3	Trace
Cashew nuts, roasted	1 cup	135	760	3192	23	62	10	43	4	40	51	5.1	140	0.58	0.33	2.4	—
Peanut butter	1 tbsp	16	95	399	4	8	2	4	2	3	9	0.3	—	0.02	0.02	2.4	0
Peas, split, dry, cooked	1 cup	250	290	1218	20	1	—	—	—	52	28	4.2	100	0.37	0.22	2.2	—
Vegetables and vegetable products																
Asparagus, canned green	6 spears	96	20	84	2	Trace	—	—	—	3	18	1.8	770	0.06	0.10	0.8	14
Snap beans, green, cooked short time in small amount of water	1 cup	125	30	126	2	Trace	—	—	—	7	62	0.8	680	0.08	0.11	1.2	16
Broccoli spears, cooked	1 cup	150	40	168	5	Trace	—	—	—	7	132	1.2	3750	0.14	0.29	1.2	135
Carrots, cooked, diced	1 cup	145	45	189	1	Trace	—	—	—	10	48	0.9	15,220	0.08	0.07	0.7	9
Peas, green, cooked	1 cup	160	115	483	9	1	—	—	—	19	37	2.9	860	0.44	0.17	3.7	33

Food	Measure															
Potato, baked, peeled after baking	1	99	90	378	3	Trace	—	—	21	9	0.7	Trace	0.10	0.04	1.7	20
Spinach, cooked	1 cup	180	40	168	5	1	—	—	6	167	4.0	14,580	0.13	0.25	1.0	50
Squash, winter, baked, mashed	1 cup	205	130	546	4	1	—	—	32	57	1.6	8610	0.10	0.27	1.4	27
Sweet potatoes, boiled, peeled after boiling	1	147	170	714	2	1	—	—	39	47	1.0	11,610	0.13	0.09	0.9	25
Tomato juice, canned	1 cup	242	45	189	2	Trace	—	—	10	17	2.2	1940	0.13	0.07	1.8	39
Fruits and fruit products																
Apple, raw, 2½-in diameter	1	150	70	294	Trace	Trace	—	—	18	8	0.4	50	0.04	0.02	0.1	3
Fruit cocktail, canned in heavy syrup	1 cup	256	195	819	1	1	—	—	50	23	1.0	360	0.04	0.03	1.1	5
Grapefruit, white, raw, medium, 4½-in diameter	½	285	55	231	1	Trace	—	—	14	22	0.6	10	0.05	0.02	0.2	52
Orange, raw California, navel, 2⅘-in diameter	1	180	60	252	2	Trace	—	—	16	49	0.5	240	0.12	0.05	0.5	75
Orange juice, frozen concentrate, diluted with 3 parts water, by volume	1 cup	248	110	462	2	Trace	—	—	27	22	0.2	500	0.21	0.03	0.8	112
Raisins, dried	1 cup	160	460	1932	4	Trace	—	—	124	99	5.6	30	0.18	0.13	0.9	2
Strawberries, raw, capped	1 cup	149	55	231	1	1	—	—	13	31	1.5	90	0.04	0.10	1.0	88
Tangerine raw, medium	1	114	40	166	1	Trace	—	—	10	34	0.3	350	0.05	0.02	0.1	26
Bread (related products)																
White bread, enriched	1 slice	23	60	252	2	1	Trace	Trace	12	16	0.6	Trace	0.06	0.04	0.5	Trace
Whole-wheat bread, made with 2% nonfat dry milk	1 slice	23	55	231	2	1	Trace	Trace	11	23	0.5	Trace	0.06	0.03	0.7	Trace
Macaroni, enriched, cooked firm stage (8–10 min; undergoes additional cooking in a food mixture)	1 cup	130	190	798	6	1	—	—	39	14	1.4	0	0.23	0.14	1.9	0
Rice, white (fully milled or polished) cooked, common commercial	1 cup	168	185	777	3	Trace	—	—	41	17	1.5	0	0.19	0.01	1.6	0
Wheat flakes, with added nutrients	1 oz	28	100	420	3	Trace	—	—	23	12	1.2	0	0.18	0.04	1.4	0

APPENDIX 9 (Continued)

Food and approximate measure		Weight, g	Food energy		Protein, g	Fat (total lipids), g	Fatty acids			Carbohydrate, g	Calcium, mg	Iron, mg	Vitamin A value, IU	Thiamine, mg	Riboflavin, mg	Niacin, mg	Ascorbic acid, mg
								Unsaturated									
			kcal	kJ			Saturated (total), g	Oleic, g	Lino-leic, g								
Fats, oils																	
Butter, pat or square (64 per pound)	1 pat	7	50	210	Trace	6	3	2	1	Trace	1	0	230	—	—	—	0
Margarine, pat or square (64 per pound)	1 pat	7	50	210	Trace	6	1	3	1	Trace	1	0	230	—	—	—	0
Corn oil	1 tbsp	14	125	525	0	14	1	4	7	0	0	0	—	0	0	0	0
Mayonnaise	1 tbsp	15	110	462	Trace	12	2	3	6	Trace	3	0.1	40	Trace	0.01	Trace	—
Sugars, sweets																	
Candy, fudge plain	1 oz	28	115	483	1	3	2	1	Trace	21	22	0.3	Trace	0.01	0.03	0.1	Trace
Jellies	1 tbsp	20	55	231	Trace	Trace	—	—	—	14	4	0.3	Trace	Trace	0.01	Trace	1
Sugar, cane or beet, granulated	1 tbsp	12	45	189	0	0	—	—	—	12	0		0	0	0	0	0
Beverages																	
Carbonated																	
Cola type	1 cup	240	95	399	0	0	—	—	—	24	—	—	0	0	0	0	0
Ginger ale	1 cup	230	70	294	0	0	—	—	—	18	—	—	0	0	0	0	0
Coffee	1 cup	180	2	8	Trace	Trace				Trace	4	0.2	0	0	Trace	0.5	0

Source: U.S. Department of Agriculture, Nutritive Values of Food, Home and Garden Bulletin No. 72, 1971.

CHEMICAL DEFINITIONS
AND CONVERSIONS

1 Moles and Equivalents.
  A *Mole:* molecular weight in grams:

$$
\begin{array}{ll}
1 \text{ mol NaCl} = 58.5 \text{ g} & 1 \text{ mol NaHCO}_3 = 94 \text{ g} \\
\qquad\qquad \text{Na} = 23 & \qquad\qquad \text{Na} = 23 \\
\qquad\qquad \text{Cl} = \underline{35.5} & \qquad\qquad \text{H} = 1 \\
\qquad\qquad\quad\ \ 58.5 \text{ g} & \qquad\qquad \text{C} = 12 \\
& \qquad\qquad 3\text{O} = \underline{48} \\
\text{and } 1 \text{ mmol} = 58.5 \text{ mg} & \qquad\qquad\qquad 94 \text{ g}
\end{array}
$$

B *Equivalent:* molecular weight divided by valence (where valence is number of hydrogen atoms that a molecule can exchange):

$$
1 \text{ eq Na}^+ = \frac{23 \text{ g}}{1} = 23 \text{ g}
$$

$$
1 \text{ eq Ca}^{2+} = \frac{40 \text{ g}}{2} = 20 \text{ g}
$$

$$
1 \text{ eq H}_2\text{SO}_4 = \frac{98 \text{ g}}{2} = 49 \text{ g}
$$

To convert milligrams (mg) to milliequivalents (meq), the following formula is used:

$$\frac{\text{Milligrams}}{\text{Atomic weight}} \times \text{valence} = \text{milliequivalents}$$

Example: Convert 2000 mg of sodium to milliequivalents of sodium:

$$\frac{2000}{23} \times 1 = 87 \text{ meq sodium}$$

To change milliequivalents back to milligrams, multiply the milliequivalents by the atomic weight and divide by the valence.

Example: Convert 20 meq of sodium to milligrams of sodium:

$$\frac{20 \times 23}{1} = 460 \text{ mg sodium}$$

Minerals	Atomic weights	Valence
Calcium	40.00	2
Chlorine	35.40	1
Magnesium	24.30	2
Phosphorus	31.00	2
Potassium	39.00	1
Sodium	23.00	1
Sulfur	32.00	2
Zinc	65.37	2

2 Molarity and Normality: Measure of concentration of solutions.

A. A *molar* solution (1.0 *M*) contains 1 mol/liter of made-up solution:

$$1.0 \; M \; KH_2PO_4 = \frac{136 \text{ g}}{\text{liter}}$$

$$
\begin{aligned}
K &= 39 \\
2H &= 2 \\
P &= 31 \\
4O &= \frac{64}{136 \text{ g}} = 1 \text{ mol}
\end{aligned}
$$

B. A *normal* solution (1.0 N) contains 1 equivalent per liter of made-up solution:

$$1.0 \text{ } M \text{ sulfuric acid (H}_2 \text{ SO}_4) = \frac{96 \text{ g}}{\text{liter}}$$

$$
\begin{array}{r}
2H = 2 \\
S = 32 \\
4O = 64 \\
\hline
98
\end{array}
$$

$$1 \text{ eq of H}_2\text{SO}_4 = \frac{98 \text{ g}}{2} = 49 \text{ g}$$

3. Osmolality and osmolarity.

A. *Osmolality:* concentration of particles in solution per 1000 g of water (solvent).

B. *Osmolarity:* concentration of particles in solution per liter of made-up solution. For nonionized solutes such as urea and glucose, 1 mole of solid gives 1 mole of solute particles. For sodium chloride the molecule dissociates into two charged particles when dissolved so that 1 mole of NaCl behaves in osmosis as if there were two, Na^+ and Cl^-. The concentration of solute particles is therefore identified as the osmolarity of the solution. The following examples illustrate the relationship between molarity and osmolarity:

1 M solution of glucose	= 1 Osm
1 mM solution of urea	= 1 mOsm
1 meq Na^+ per liter	= 1 mOsm
1 mmol NaCl per liter	= 2 mOsm
1 mmol Na_2SO_4 per liter	= 3 mOsm
1 mmol $MgSO_4$ per liter	= 2 mOsm

In each case it is the number of particles produced in solution, not their charge, that governs the osmotic pressure and osmolarity.

INDEX